Cardiac Catheterization,
Angiography, and Intervention

Cardiac Catheterization, Angiography, and Intervention

Edited by WILLIAM GROSSMAN, M.D.

Dana Professor of Medicine, Harvard Medical School;
Chief, Cardiovascular Division,
Beth Israel Hospital, Boston, Massachusetts

and

DONALD S. BAIM, M.D.

Associate Professor of Medicine,
Harvard Medical School;
Director, Invasive Cardiology,
Beth Israel Hospital
Boston, Massachusetts

Fourth Edition

LEA & FEBIGER • PHILADELPHIA • LONDON • 1991

Lea & Febiger
200 Chester Field Parkway
Malvern, Pennsylvania   19355-9725
U.S.A.
(215) 251-2230

Library of Congress Cataloging-in-Publication Data

Cardiac catheterization, angiography, and intervention/edited by
   William Grossman and Donald S. Baim.—4th ed.
      p.   cm.
   Rev. ed. of: Cardiac catheterization and angiography. 3rd ed.
1986.
   Includes bibliographical references.
   ISBN 0-8121-1342-X
   1. Heart catheterization. 2. Angiography. I. Grossman, William,
1940–   . II. Baim, Donald S. III. Cardiac catheterization and
angiography.
   [DNLM: 1. Angiocardiography. 2. Heart Catheterization. WG
141.5.C2 C267]
RC683.5.C25C38   1990
616.1′207572—dc20
DNLM/DLC
for Library of Congress   90-5835
                                                                      CIP

First Edition, 1974
   Reprinted, 1976
Second Edition, 1980
   Reprinted, 1981, 1983, 1985
Third Edition, 1986
   Reprinted, 1987, 1988
Fourth Edition, 1991

PRINTED IN THE UNITED STATES OF AMERICA

Print number: 5   4   3

Reprints of chapters may be purchased from Lea & Febiger in quantities of 100 or more.

To my wife, Melanie,
and my children, Jennifer, Edward, and Jessica
W. Grossman

To my wife, Peggy,
and my son, Adam
D. Baim

Preface

This textbook, in both its conception and design, is aimed at the instruction of physicians training to become cardiologists. The intent was to compile a book that would be practical and bring together clear and concise descriptions of the major techniques currently used in cardiac catheterization angiography and the growing field of interventional cardiology. No effort was made to be exhaustive or to construct a compendium of every technique that has been reported; instead, we have concentrated on the detailed description of a few methods that are moderately successful and practical, and whose strengths and weaknesses are well known.

The book begins with a section on "General Principles of Cardiac Catheterization and Angiography." The second section deals with "Techniques of Catheter Placement," including discussions of arteriotomy, percutaneous catheterization, transseptal catheterization, balloon-tipped flow-directed catheters, and special considerations in the catheterization of infants and children. Subsequent sections on "Hemodynamic Principles" and "Angiographic Techniques" attempt to cover basic knowledge in these areas, with an emphasis on practical application and avoidance of commonly encountered mistakes and pitfalls.

A unique section on "Evaluation of Cardiac Function" offers pragmatic discussions of recent advances and the current state of the art in evaluation of systolic and diastolic ventricular function, atrial pacing, ventricular volume analysis, and dynamic and isometric exercise.

In this edition, the section on "Special Catheter Techniques" (Part VI) has been reorganized and now contains chapters on percutaneous placement of intraaortic balloon pump, endomyocardial biopsy, placement of temporary and permanent pacemakers, myocardial blood flow, and electrophysiologic techniques.

Coronary angioplasty and laser therapy, having grown greatly since the third edition, have been relocated to a new section on "Interventional Techniques" (Part VII), along with chapters on new angioplasty technologies (stents and atherectomy), balloon valvuloplasty, and pediatric interventions. The importance of this field has also been recognized in the new title of the book, *Cardiac Catheterization, Angiography, and Intervention*, and in the addition of Dr. Donald S. Baim as coeditor.

Discussion of the interpretation of hemodynamic and angiographic findings has been largely separated from the description of techniques. Interpretation is discussed and illustrated at the end of the book in the chapters on profiles of characteristic hemodynamic and angiographic abnormalities in specific disorders (Part VIII). This separation is purposeful, and serves to emphasize the importance of considering hemodynamic and angiographic data together when analyzing the physiologic and anatomic abnormalities presented by a given disorder.

This book could not have been written without the help of many individuals whose names do not appear in the list of contributors. In particular, we are grateful to Dr. Eugene Braunwald; our many colleagues in the Departments of Medicine at Harvard Medical

School and the Beth Israel Hospital, who gave us encouragement and advice; to our Cardiology Fellows whose thoughtful questions and comments stimulated us to undertake this task in the first instance; and to the technicians and staff of our laboratory whose hard work and dedication allow the precepts of this book to be transformed into action each day.

We hope that this book will be of value not only to those involved in the daily practice of cardiac catheterization and angiography but to all who are involved in the care of patients with serious heart disease. Most of all, we sincerely hope that the lessons of this book will benefit the patients themselves; without this final result, it will have been a sterile venture.

William Grossman, M.D.
Donald S. Baim, M.D.
Boston, Massachusetts

Contributors

Julian M. Aroesty, M.D.
Associate Clinical Professor of Medicine,
Harvard Medical School;
Cardiovascular Division,
Beth Israel Hospital,
Boston, MA

Donald S. Baim, M.D.
Associate Professor of Medicine,
Harvard Medical School;
Director, Invasive Cardiology,
Beth Israel Hospital,
Boston, MA

Joseph R. Benotti, M.D.
Associate Professor of Medicine,
University of Massachusetts Medical Center;
Director, Cardiac Catheterization Laboratory,
Saint Vincent Hospital,
Worcester, MA

Blase A. Carabello, M.D.
Professor of Medicine,
Medical University of South Carolina,
Charleston, SC

Stafford I. Cohen, M.D.
Associate Clinical Professor of Medicine,
Harvard Medical School;
Cardiovascular Division,
Beth Israel Hospital,
Boston, MA

John P. DiMarco, M.D., Ph.D.
Associate Professor of Medicine,
Director, Clinical Electrophysiology Laboratory,
Division of Cardiology,
University of Virginia Health Sciences Center,
Charlottesville, VA

Michael A. Fifer, M.D.
Assistant Professor of Medicine,
Harvard Medical School;
Cardiovascular Unit,
Massachusetts General Hospital,
Boston, MA

Peter Ganz, M.D.
Assistant Professor of Medicine,
Harvard Medical School;
Associate Director, Cardiac Catheterization Laboratory,
Brigham and Women's Hospital,
Boston, MA

William Ganz, M.D., C.Sc.
Professor of Medicine,
University of California at Los Angeles School of Medicine;
Senior Scientist,
Department of Cardiology,
Cedars-Sinai Medical Center,
Los Angeles, CA

William Grossman, M.D.
Dana Professor of Medicine,
Harvard Medical School;
Chief, Cardiovascular Division,
Beth Israel Hospital,
Boston, MA

L. David Hillis, M.D.
Professor of Internal Medicine,
University of Texas Southwestern Medical School;
Director, Cardiac Catheterization Laboratory,
Parkland Memorial Hospital,
Dallas, TX

John F. Keane, M.D.
Associate Professor of Pediatrics,
Harvard Medical School;
Senior Associate in Cardiology;
Co-Director, Cardiac Catheterization Laboratory,
The Children's Hospital,
Boston, MA

Arlene B. Levine, M.D.
Director, Interventional Cardiology,
William Beaumont Hospital,
Royal Oak, MI

Marc J. Levine, M.D.
Instructor in Medicine,
Harvard Medical School;
Cardiovascular Division,
Beth Israel Hospital,
Boston, MA

James E. Lock, M.D.
Associate Professor of Pediatrics,
Harvard Medical School;
Director, Cardiac Catheterization Laboratory,
The Children's Hospital,
Boston, MA

Beverly H. Lorell, M.D.
Associate Professor of Medicine,
Harvard Medical School;
Co-Director, Hemodynamic Research Laboratory,
Beth Israel Hospital,
Boston, MA

Raymond G. McKay, M.D.
Director, Cardiac Laboratory,
Hartford Hospital,
Hartford, CT

Richard C. Pasternak, M.D.
Assistant Professor of Medicine,
Harvard Medical School;
Director, Coronary Care Unit,
Beth Israel Hospital,
Boston, MA

Sven Paulin, M.D.
Stoneman Professor of Radiology,
Harvard Medical School;
Chairman, Department of Radiology,
Beth Israel Hospital,
Boston, MA

Stanton B. Perry, M.D.
Assistant Professor of Pediatrics,
Harvard Medical School;
Associate in Cardiology,
The Children's Hospital,
Boston, MA

Gregg J. Reis, M.D.
Instructor in Medicine,
Harvard Medical School;
Cardiovascular Division,
Beth Israel Hospital,
Boston, MA

Robert D. Safian, M.D.
Assistant Professor of Medicine,
Harvard Medical School;
Assistant Director, Cardiac Catheterization Laboratory,
Beth Israel Hospital,
Boston, MA

J. Richard Spears, M.D.
Associate Professor of Medicine,
Wayne State University;
Director, Cardiac Laser Laboratory,
Harper Hospital,
Detroit, MI

H.J.C. Swan, M.D., Ph.D., F.R.C.P.
Professor of Medicine Emeritus,
University of California at Los Angeles School of Medicine;
Department of Cardiology,
Cedars-Sinai Medical Center,
Los Angeles, CA

Contents

Part VII:
Interventional Techniques

Part VIII:
Profiles of Hemodynamic and Angiographic Abnormalities in Specific Disorders

Index

Part I

General Principles of Cardiac Catheterization and Angiography

1

Cardiac Catheterization: Historical Perspective and Present Practice

WILLIAM GROSSMAN

I t is difficult to imagine what our concepts of heart disease might be like today if we had to construct them without the enormous reservoir of physiologic and anatomic knowledge derived during the past 50 years in the cardiac catheterization laboratory. As Andre Cournand remarked in his Nobel Lecture of December 11, 1956: "the cardiac catheter was . . . the key in the lock."[1] By turning this key, Cournand and his colleagues led us into a new era in the understanding of normal and disordered cardiac function in man.

HISTORICAL REVIEW

According to Cournand,[2] cardiac catheterization was first performed (and so named) by Claude Bernard in 1844. The subject was a horse, and both the right and left ventricles were entered by a retrograde approach from the jugular vein and carotid artery. An era of investigation of cardiovascular physiology in animals then followed, resulting in the development of many important techniques and principles (pressure manometry, the Fick cardiac output method), which awaited direct application to the patient with heart disease.

Although others had passed catheters into the great veins previously, Werner Forssmann is generally credited with being the first person to pass a catheter into the heart of a living person—himself.[3] At age 25, while receiving clinical instruction in surgery at Eberswalde, near Berlin, he passed a catheter 65 cm through one of his left antecubital veins, guiding it by fluoroscopy (he looked through a mirror held by his nurse in front of the fluoroscope screen) until it entered his right atrium. He then walked to the Radiology Department (which was on a different level, requiring that he climb stairs), where the catheter position was documented by a chest roentgenogram (Fig. 1–1). During the next two years, Forssmann continued to perform catheterization studies, including six additional attempts to catheterize himself. Bitter criticism, based on an unsubstantiated belief in the danger of his experiments, caused Forssmann to turn his attention to other concerns, and he eventually pursued a career as a urologist.

It is of interest that Forssmann's primary goal in his catheterization studies was to develop a therapeutic technique for the direct delivery of drugs into the heart. He wrote: "If cardiac action ceases suddenly, as is seen in acute shock or in heart disease, or during an-

3

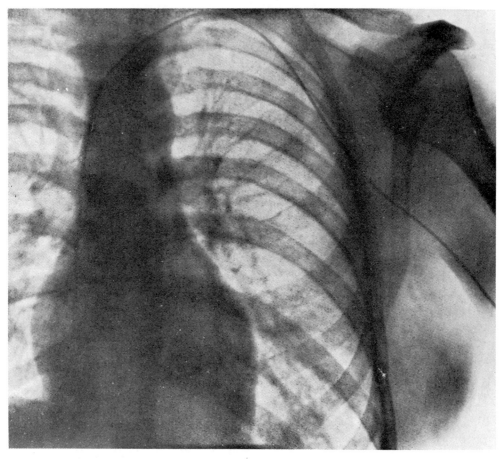

Fig. 1–1. The first documented cardiac catheterization. At age 25, while receiving clinical instruction in surgery at Eberswalde, Werner Forssmann passed a catheter 65 cm through one of his left antecubital veins until its tip entered the right atrium. He then walked to the Radiology Department, where this roentgenogram was taken.[2] (Klin Wochenschr 8:2085, 1929. © Springer-Verlag Berlin, Heidelberg, New York)

esthesia or poisoning, one is forced to deliver drugs locally. In such cases the intracardiac injection of drugs may be life saving. However, this may be a dangerous procedure because of many incidents of laceration of coronary arteries and their branches leading to cardiac tamponade, and death. . . . Because of such incidents, one often waits until the very last moment and valuable time is wasted. Therefore I started to look for a new way to approach the heart, and I catheterized the right side of the heart through the venous system.''[3]

The potentials of Forssmann's technique as a diagnostic tool were appreciated by others. In 1930, Klein reported 11 right heart catheterizations, including passage to the right ventricle and measurement of cardiac output using Fick's principle.[4] The cardiac outputs were 4.5 and 5.6 L/min in two patients without heart disease. In 1932 Padillo and co-workers reported right heart catheterization and measurement of cardiac output in two subjects.[2] Except for these few studies, application of cardiac catheterization to study of the circulation in normal and disease states was fragmentary until the work of Andre Cournand and Dickinson Richards, who separately and in collaboration produced a remarkable series of investigations of right heart physiology in man.[5–7] In 1947 Dexter reported his studies on congenital heart disease.[8] He went further than his predecessors by passing the catheter to the pulmonary artery, and in addition mentioned some observations on "the oxygen saturation and source of pulmonary capillary blood" obtained from the pulmonary artery "wedge" position.[8,9] Subsequent studies from Dexter's laboratory[10] and by Werko[11] elaborated on this pulmonary artery "wedge" position, and pressure measured at this position was reported to be a good estimate of pulmonary venous and left atrial pressure. During this exciting early period, catheterization was used to investigate problems in cardiovascular physiology by McMichael in England,[12] Lenègre in Paris,[13] and Warren, Stead, Bing, Dexter, Cournand, and others in this country.[14-23]

Further developments came rapidly. To touch briefly on some of the highlights: Retrograde left heart catheterization was first reported by Zimmerman[24] and Limon Lason[25] in 1950. The percutaneous technique developed by Seldinger in 1953 was soon applied to cardiac catheterization of both the left and right heart chambers.[26] Transseptal catheterization was first developed in 1959 by Ross[27] and Cope[28] and quickly became accepted as a standard technique. Selective coronary arteriography was developed by Sones in 1959 and perfected to a remarkable excellence over the ensuing years.[29,30] This technique was modified for a percutaneous approach by Ricketts and Abrams[31] in 1962 and Judkins[32] in 1967. In 1970 a practical balloon-tipped, flow-guided catheter technique was introduced by Swan and Ganz, making possible the applicability of catheterization outside the laboratory.[33]

In the more recent past, investigators have focused once again on the therapeutic potential of the cardiac catheter. In 1977, Grüntzig introduced the technique of coronary angioplasty.[34,35] In the ensuing years, the method was widely applied and with rapidly evolving technology has developed a firm position rivaling coronary bypass surgery as a therapeutic modality for coronary artery disease. Angioplasty itself is rapidly being modified by the addition of stents,[36] atherectomy,[37] and laser techniques[38,39] to the treatment of atherosclerotic vascular disease.

There are many other landmarks that could be mentioned, and many individuals whose contributions should be recognized. The interested reader is referred elsewhere for details.[40]

Indications for Cardiac Catheterization

As performed today, cardiac catheterization may be defined as a combined hemodynamic and angiographic procedure undertaken for diagnostic or therapeutic purposes.

As with any invasive procedure, the decision to perform cardiac catheterization must be based upon a careful balance of the risk of the procedure against the anticipated benefit to the patient. Cardiac catheterization is generally recommended when there is a need to confirm the presence of a clinically suspected condition, define its anatomic and physiologic severity, and determine the presence or absence of associated conditions. This need most commonly arises when the clinical assessment suggests that the patient is approaching the stage of rapid deterioration, incapacitation, and death when viewed in the context of the natural history of his or her specific disorder. Cardiac catheterization may yield information that will be crucial in defining the need for cardiac surgery, coronary angioplasty, or other therapeutic interventions as well as timing, risks, and anticipated benefit in a given patient.

Is Cardiac Catheterization Necessary in All Patients Being Considered for Cardiac Surgery? Although few would disagree that consideration of heart surgery is an adequate reason for the performance of catheterization, there are differences of opinion about whether *all* patients being considered for heart surgery should undergo preoperative cardiac catheterization. In this regard, at least one study[41] concluded that routine cardiac catheterization is unnecessary before valve replacement but can be reserved for specific indications in some patients. There has been sharp disagreement with this conclusion by at least two authorities,[42-43] who pointed out that information concerning concomitant coronary artery obstruction, pulmonary hypertension, and other associated conditions cannot be precisely obtained without cardiac catheterization. In a study of 108 consecutive patients referred for cardiac catheterization, noninvasive evaluation led to diagnostic predictions that were completely correct in 86% of patients.[44] A "management strategy" (choice of (1) no catheterization, no operation; (2) no catheterization, operation; (3) cardiac catheterization required before decision regarding operation) was decided upon, based on the clinical and noninvasive evaluation, and this management strategy was subsequently evaluated by comparison with the findings of the actual cardiac catheterization, which followed noninvasive evaluation in every patient.[44] The results are summarized in Table 1–1.

Thus, although clinical and noninvasive evaluation are usually adequate for clinical decision making, there was a 16% error rate in devising an appropriate management strategy in one category of strategy. In this regard I would emphasize that the risks of catheterization are small compared to those of cardiac surgery in a patient with an incorrect clinical diagnosis or in whom the presence of an unsuspected additional condition greatly prolongs and complicates the planned surgical approach. *The operating room is not a good place for surprises:* cardiac catheterization can provide the surgical team with a precise and complete roadmap of the course ahead and thereby permit a carefully reasoned and maximally efficient operative procedure. Furthermore, information obtained by cardiac catheterization may be invaluable in the assessment of crucial determinants of prognosis, such as left ventricular function and the patency of the coronary arteries. For these reasons, I recommend cardiac catheterization in the majority of patients in whom heart surgery is contemplated.

Other major therapeutic considerations besides heart surgery may depend upon the type of information afforded by cardiac catheterization. For example, pharmacologic intervention with heparin in suspected acute pulmonary embolism, or with high doses of propranolol and/or calcium antagonists in suspected hypertrophic subaortic stenosis might well be considered decisions of sufficient magnitude to warrant confirmation of the diagnoses by angiographic and hemodynamic investigation.

A second broad indication for performing cardiac catheterization is diagnosis of obscure or confusing problems in heart disease, even when a major therapeutic decision is not imminent. Currently, the most common instance of this indication in our laboratory is presented by the patient with chest pain of uncertain cause, about whom there is confusion regarding the presence of obstructive coronary artery disease. Both management and prognosis of this difficult problem are greatly simplified when it is known, for example, that the coronary arteries are widely patent. Another example within this category might be the symptomatic patient with a suspected diagnosis of cardiomyopathy. Although some may feel satisfied with a clinical diagnosis of this condition, the implications of such a diagnosis in terms of prognosis and therapy (such as long-term bed rest or chronic anticoagulant therapy) are so important that I feel it worthwhile to be aggressive in ruling out potentially correctable conditions with certainty (e.g., pericardial effusive-constrictive disease), even though the likelihood of their presence may appear remote on clinical grounds.

Research. On occasion, cardiac catheterization is performed primarily as a research procedure. Although research is conducted to some degree in many of the routine diagnostic studies performed in our laboratory, this is

Table 1–1. *Correctness of Suggested Management Strategies Based on Clinical and Full Noninvasive Studies in 108 Patients*

Suggested Strategy	Number of Patients	Errors
No catheterization; no operation	19/108 (18%)	3/19 (16%)
No catheterization; operation	30/108 (28%)	0/30 (0%)
Catheterization	59/108 (54%)	0/59 (0%)

quite different from catheterization for the sole purpose of a research investigation. Such studies should be carried out only under the direct supervision of an experienced investigator who is expert in cardiac catheterization, using a protocol that has been carefully scrutinized and approved by the Human Studies Committee at the investigator's institution, and after a thorough explanation has been made to the patient detailing the risks of the procedure and the fact that the purpose of the investigation is to gather research information.

CONTRAINDICATIONS

If it is important to carefully consider the indications for cardiac catheterization in each patient, it is equally important to determine whether there are any contraindications. Over the past several years, our concepts of contraindications have been modified because patients with acute myocardial infarction, cardiogenic shock, intractable ventricular tachycardia, and other extreme conditions have tolerated catheterization and coronary arteriography surprisingly well. At present the only absolute contraindication to cardiac catheterization in our laboratory is the refusal of a mentally competent patient to consent to the procedure.

A long list of *relative* contraindications must be kept in mind, however, and these include all intercurrent conditions that can be corrected and whose correction would improve the safety of the procedure. These relative contra-

indications are listed in Table 1–2. For example, ventricular irritability can increase the risk and difficulty of left heart catheterization and can greatly interfere with interpretation of ventriculography (see Chapter 14); it should be suppressed medically prior to catheterization. Hypertension increases predisposition to ischemia and/or pulmonary edema, and should be controlled before and during catheterization. Other conditions that should be controlled before elective catheterization include intercurrent febrile illness, decompensated left heart failure, correctable anemia, digitalis toxicity, and hypokalemia. *Allergy to radiographic contrast agent* is a relative contraindication to cardiac angiography, but with proper premedication the risks of a major adverse reaction can be substantially reduced, as discussed in Chapter 2.

Anticoagulant therapy is more controversial as a contraindication. As pointed out in Chapters 5 and 13, heparin may lower the incidence of thromboembolic complications during coronary angiography.[45] It is important to distinguish anticoagulation with oral anticoagulants (e.g., coumadin) from that with heparin. Heparin anticoagulation can be reversed rapidly during catheterization if necessary (e.g., perforation of the heart or great vessels, uncontrolled bleeding from femoral or brachial sites). Reversal of the prolonged prothrombin time of oral anticoagulation before or during cardiac catheterization represents a more complex problem. *I strongly oppose acute reversal of oral anticoagulation with parenteral vita-*

Table 1–2. *Relative Contraindications to Cardiac Catheterization and Angiography*

1. Uncontrolled ventricular irritability: the risk of ventricular tachycardia/fibrillation during catheterization is increased if ventricular irritability is uncontrolled.
2. Uncorrected hypokalemia or digitalis toxicity.
3. Uncorrected hypertension: predisposes to myocardial ischemia and/or heart failure during angiography.
4. Intercurrent febrile illness.
5. Decompensated heart failure: especially acute pulmonary edema, unless catheterization can be done with patient sitting up.
6. Anticoagulated state: prothrombin time >18 seconds.
7. Severe allergy to radiographic contrast agent.
8. Severe renal insufficiency and/or anuria: unless dialysis is planned to remove fluid and radiographic contrast load.

min K because of the occasional induction of a hypercoagulable state. This in turn may result in thrombosis of prosthetic valves or thrombus formation within cardiac chambers, arteries, or veins. If reversal of oral anticoagulation is required, I recommend administration of fresh frozen plasma. For patients chronically anticoagulated with an oral agent, I routinely recommend discontinuation of the oral anticoagulant 48 hours prior to cardiac catheterization, with heparin given during these 48 hours for the patients who have a strong indication for continuous anticoagulation (e.g., mechanical cardiac valve prosthesis). I prefer to have the prothrombin time less than 18 seconds and no heparin administration for 4 hours before the catheterization. If anticoagulant therapy cannot be interrupted at all, I prefer heparin for the reasons just mentioned.

FACTORS INFLUENCING CHOICE OF APPROACH

Of the various approaches to cardiac catheterization, certain ones have only historical interest (transbronchial approach, posterior transthoracic left atrial puncture, suprasternal puncture of the left atrium). In this book we will discuss in detail only (a) catheterization by direct exposure of artery and vein, and (b) catheterization by percutaneous approach (including transseptal catheterization and apical left ventricular puncture).

By either the direct or percutaneous approach (or a combination of both), the great vessels and all cardiac chambers can be entered in nearly all cases. Each method has its advantages and disadvantages, its adherents and detractors. In reality, the methods are not mutually exclusive but rather complementary, and the physician performing cardiac catheterization should be well versed in both methods.

Advantages of the Brachial Approach. The direct exposure approach usually utilizes cutdown on the brachial artery and basilic vein at the elbow, whereas the percutaneous approach of Seldinger traditionally involves entry of the femoral artery and vein at the groin.[26]

The direct brachial approach may have advantages in a patient with peripheral vascular disease involving the abdominal aorta, iliac, or femoral arteries, suspected femoral vein or inferior vena caval thrombosis, or coarctation of the aorta. The direct brachial approach may also have advantages in the very obese patient, in whom the percutaneous femoral technique may be technically difficult and bleeding hard to control after catheter removal. Some prefer the brachial approach in patients who have significant hypertension, aortic regurgitation, or wide pulse pressure from other causes, or who are receiving anticoagulants. In these three circumstances, an increased hazard of bleeding has been reported with the percutaneous femoral technique. Other advantages occasionally cited for the direct brachial approach include use of a single left heart catheter (Sones catheter) for left ventriculography and coronary angiography.

Advantages of the Femoral Approach. In contrast, the percutaneous femoral approach has its own broad set of advantages and indications. Arteriotomy and arterial repair are not required; it can be performed repeatedly in the same patient at intervals, whereas the brachial approach can rarely be repeated more than two or three times with safety; infection and thrombophlebitis at the catheterization site are rare; there is no need for surgical (suture) closure of the skin and it is readily adaptable to other entry vessels (internal jugular vein, axillary artery, etc.). Larger caliber devices (i.e., valvuloplasty balloons or intraaortic counterpulsation catheters) can be introduced into the femoral artery, but generally not into the smaller brachial artery. It is clearly the method of choice in a patient with absent or diminished radial and brachial pulsations, or when direct brachial approach has been unsuccessful. In the patient with tight aortic stenosis in whom retrograde catheterization may prove impossible, percutaneous transseptal catheterization of the left atrium and ventricle is helpful; in the rare instance when retrograde arterial and transseptal catheterization have not been successful in gaining entry into the left ventricle (or is contraindicated by the presence of a disc mitral prosthesis or left atrial thrombus), direct transthoracic puncture of the left ventricle may be considered (see Chapter 5).

DESIGN OF THE CATHETERIZATION PROTOCOL

Every cardiac catheterization should have a *protocol,* that is, a carefully reasoned sequential plan designed specifically for the individual patient being studied. Although this protocol may exist only in the mind of the operator, it is often helpful to prepare a written protocol and post it in the catheterization suite so that all personnel in the laboratory may be aware of exactly what is planned and thus may be reasonably expected to anticipate the needs of the operator.

Certain *general principles* should be considered in the design of a protocol. *First,* we prefer to have an arterial monitor line present in virtually all cases; when complications develop (and they do, no matter how skilled the operator), it is helpful to be able to monitor arterial pressure continuously. In our laboratory, an arterial monitor line (usually a percutaneously introduced radial artery cannula) is placed at the start of each brachial cardiac catheterization. For catheterizations done by the percutaneous femoral approach, we use introducer arterial sheaths (see Chapter 5), using the sidearm of the sheath to monitor arterial pressure. *Second,* hemodynamic measurements should precede angiographic studies, whenever possible, so that the physiologic values may be as basal as possible at the time of crucial pressure and flow measurements. *Third,* pressures and oxygen saturations should be measured and recorded in each chamber immediately after entry and before passing on to the next chamber. If problems should develop during the later stages of a catheterization procedure (atrial fibrillation or other arrhythmia, pyrogen reaction, hypotension, or reaction to contrast material), the investigator will wish that he had measured pressures and saturations "on the way in," rather than waiting until the time of catheter pullback. A *fourth principle* is that pressure and cardiac output

measurements should be made as simultaneously as possible. A simple routine for recording pressure during the cardiac output measurement can be learned by the laboratory personnel and performed efficiently in every case.

Beyond these general guidelines, the protocol will reflect individual differences from patient to patient. With regard to angiography, it is important to keep Sutton's Law* in mind, and order the contrast injections in relation to the most important diagnostic considerations in a given patient.

PREPARATION AND PREMEDICATION OF THE PATIENT

It goes without saying that the emotional as well as the "medical" preparation of the patient for cardiac catheterization is the responsibility of the operator. We believe it is our firm obligation to fully explain the proposed procedure in such terms that the patient will be in a position to give truly informed consent. We *always* tell the patient and his family that there is some risk involved, depending on the specific procedure and the patient's clinical situation. If appropriate, we generally reassure them that we do not anticipate any special problems in their case. Our consent form lists these specific risks and informs the patient that "there is a less than 1% risk of serious complications (stroke, heart attack, or death)." If the patient and his family want to know more about these risks, they will ask for details. We do not understate the discomfort or duration of the procedure and believe that to do so runs the risk of losing one's credibility. We have been satisfied with this overall approach and can heartily recommend it. A recent study of psychologic preparation for cardiac catheterization[46] found that patients who received careful psychologic preparation had lower levels of autonomic arousal both during and after

---

*When once asked why he robbed banks, Willie Sutton is reported to have replied: "because that's where the money is."

cardiac catheterization than did control subjects.

Once the question of indications and contraindications has been dealt with and the patient's consent obtained, attention can be directed toward the matter of medications. As mentioned earlier, we prefer to have the prothrombin time less than 18 sec and no heparin administered for 4 hours. One exception is the patient with unstable angina, in whom a therapeutic heparin infusion may be continued until arterial entry, and then supplemented by 3000 to 5000 additional units. For patients on chronic anticoagulation, we discontinue oral anticoagulants the day before hospitalization (or 48 hours before study for outpatient catheterizations) and on admission we begin intravenous heparin, which is stopped after midnight on the night preceding the catheterization. Heparin and oral anticoagulants are reinstituted following the catheterization, and heparin is stopped once adequate prothrombin time prolongation has been achieved.

The question of administering antibiotics prophylactically is frequently raised, and some laboratories routinely administer them before catheterization. We do not administer antibiotics prophylactically before cardiac catheterization, and we know of no controlled studies to support their use.

A wide variety of sedatives has been employed for premedication. We routinely use diazepam (Valium), 5 to 10 mg p.o., and diphenhydramine (Benadryl), 25 to 50 mg p.o., one-half hour before starting the procedure. For coronary angiography, atropine, 0.4 mg subcutaneously, is recommended by some.[45] In a patient in whom unusual anxiety or discomfort is anticipated, meperidine (Demerol) may be added in doses from 25 to 100 mg IM, depending on body size.

It is our practice to have the patient fasting (except for his oral medications) after midnight, but many laboratories allow a light tea and toast breakfast without ill effects. It is important to have complete vital signs recorded by the nurse before the patient leaves the ward (for inpatients), or shortly after arriving at the Ambulatory Center (for outpa-

tients), so that the procedure may be aborted if a change has occurred in the patient's condition since he or she was last seen. The patient should be sent to the catheterization laboratory with his or her eyeglasses and dentures (if any) when Fick cardiac output and Douglas bag collection of expired air are planned.

In a typical inpatient, our precatheterization orders might be:

1. To Cardiac Catheterization Laboratory at 7:30 AM tomorrow by stretcher; patient to be in hospital gown, and with eyeglasses and dentures, if any.
2. Fasting after midnight except for regularly scheduled oral medications.
3. Have patient void before leaving for catheterization laboratory.
4. Record complete vital signs before patient leaves for catheterization laboratory.
5. Premedication: Valium 10 mg p.o. and Benadryl 50 mg p.o. as the patient leaves the floor.

This list must be regarded as a general procedure guide and obviously will have to be modified as the details of specific situations require.

THE CARDIAC CATHETERIZATION FACILITY

A modern cardiac catheterization laboratory requires an area of 500 to 700 sq. feet, within which will be housed a conglomeration of highly sophisticated electronic and radiographic equipment. Reports of the Inter-Society Commission for Heart Disease Resources on optimal resources for cardiac catheterization facilities have appeared in 1971, 1976, and 1983. In the 1983 report,[47] a variety of issues are dealt with, some of which are listed:

1. Location of a catheterization laboratory: within a hospital vs. freestanding
2. Outpatient catheterization
3. Administration, staff organization, and criteria for professional privileges

4. Optimal annual caseload for physicians and for the laboratory
5. Radiation safety and radiologic techniques
6. Physiologic measurements, patient safety

The reader is referred to this report[47] for detailed discussion of these issues. Certain points, however, are worth repeating here.

Location Within a Hospital versus Free-Standing. The issue of whether cardiac catheterization laboratories should be hospital-based, free-standing, or mobile has been addressed by numerous groups, and much of the debate on this subject has been summarized succinctly in a recent editorial by Conti.[48] As he points out, there are many potential concerns about performance of cardiac catheterization in a free-standing facility, although the available data from such facilities are limited. Mobile cardiac catheterization laboratories may be either free-standing *or* hospital-based (as is the case for mobile MRI and other mobile diagnostic units), and it is important not to equate mobile and free-standing units automatically. Careful prospective studies of the safety and cost-effectiveness of these innovative approaches to diagnostic cardiac catheterization must be done before meaningful policies can be drafted.

Outpatient Cardiac Catheterization. This has been demonstrated by a variety of groups to be safe, practical, and highly cost-efficient. Some laboratories that have had extensive experience with outpatient catheterization[49] have utilized the brachial approach, which allows the patient to be ambulatory within minutes of the completion of the catheterization study. However, outpatient catheterization can be accomplished safely using percutaneous femoral technique.[50–52] In one study,[50] 2207 patients underwent elective outpatient cardiac catheterization at the Kaiser Permamente Regional Cardiac Catheterization Laboratory in Los Angeles, California. Ninety-seven percent of the procedures were done by percutaneous femoral approach, using 7 Fr catheters without sheaths. Heparin was given intra-arterially in a relatively low dose (2000 to 3000 units) and was not reversed with protamine at the end of the

procedure. Hemostasis was obtained by manual compression for 10 minutes over the femoral artery, followed by placement of a pressure dressing and sandbag for 4 hours. Patients were checked at 15-minute intervals during the 4-hour surveillance period and discharged after they had become ambulatory. Each patient was contacted at home by telephone on the following day by a nurse from the Outpatient Observation Area, and patients were seen in 1 to 2 weeks by their referring cardiologist for follow-up consultation and discussion of results. Complication rates were extremely low, and were in fact lower than rates generally reported for inpatient diagnostic catheterization (see Chapter 3). A report of 1000 cases of outpatient catheterization reported by Pink et al.[51] utilized a similar protocol, except that 8 Fr catheters were used and protamine was given at the time of catheter removal. Thirty-nine patients (3.9%) were admitted because of complications of the procedure, including 17 patients with local vascular complications; an additional 59 patients (5.9%) were admitted directly for revascularization procedures (e.g., left main disease).

A prospective randomized trial of outpatient (n = 192) versus inpatient (n = 189) cardiac catheterization was carried out in three university hospitals in Massachusetts, where cardiology trainees were involved in the procedures.[52] In the outpatient group, catheterization was performed by percutaneous femoral technique in 98% of cases, using 7 Fr or 8 Fr catheters. Patients recovered in an Ambulatory Center, lying supine for 4 to 5 hours and then walking to a lounge where they were observed for an additional hour before being sent home or to nearby lodging (7% stayed with relatives and 5% stayed in nearby hotels). All outpatients were interviewed by phone the next day, and answered a standardized list of questions. There was a slightly higher risk of hematoma (12% vs. 8.5%), cold or blue extremity (1.6% vs. 1.1%) and myocardial infarction (1.6% vs. 0.5%) in patients undergoing outpatient catheterization, but these differences were not statistically significant. In the outpatient group, 23 (12%) of 192 patients were admitted be-

Table 1–3. *Suggested Criteria for Exclusion from Outpatient Cardiac Catheterization*

1. Unstable angina
2. Suspected left main coronary disease
3. Known left ventricular dysfunction (LVEF < 40%) or symptomatic congestive heart failure
4. Significant ventricular arrhythmias
5. Uncontrolled systemic hypertension
6. Renal disease (creatinine > 2.0 mg% or BUN > 40 mg%)
7. Anticoagulant therapy or coagulation disorder
8. Age greater than 70 years
9. Patients living more than 45 minutes from the hospital, and patients with an inadequate home environment

Table 1–4. *Inter-Society Recommendations for Catheterization Laboratory and Physician Caseloads*[47]

1. Adult Catheterization Laboratories	≥300 cases/year
2. Pediatric Catheterization Laboratories	≥150 cases/year
3. Physician Caseload:	
Adult catheterizations	≥150 but ≤600
Pediatric catheterizations	≥50

Note: The report indicates that physicians with extensive experience (e.g., more than 1000 independently performed catheterizations) can perform fewer catheterizations to maintain their skill levels.

cause of bleeding or hematoma (7), chest pain (3), the need for coronary bypass surgery (3), syncope (1), allergy to contrast medium (1), nausea (1), the need for heparin for thrombus (1), and miscellaneous causes. Based on a variety of considerations, a proposed set of exclusions from outpatient catheterization is presented in Table 1–3. In the context of these guidelines, outpatient cardiac catheterization appears to be a safe and practical approach with much to recommend it.

Another issue addressed in the Inter-Society Report concerns the question of proximity and availability of *cardiac surgical facilities*. The report states that "Optimally, cardiovascular catheterization laboratories should be located only in institutions with well organized and closely related programs of cardiovascular surgery.[47] Experience in many community-based catheterization laboratories, however, has demonstrated that properly selected patients can undergo catheterization safely in hospitals *without* on-site heart surgery programs. Immediately available cardiac surgical back-up is particularly critical for laboratories perform-

ing coronary angioplasty, endomyocardial biopsy, or transseptal catheterization.

Utilization levels as well as optimal *physician caseload* represent a third issue of general interest addressed in the Inter-Society Report.[47] The report recommends certain levels of utilization for cost-effectiveness and maintenance of skills (Table 1–4). It is important to note that there is an upper limit as well as a lower limit to the optimal caseload. This is important because a cardiologist should not have such an excessive caseload that it interferes with proper precatheterization evaluation of the patient and adequate postcatheterization interpretation of the data, report preparation, patient follow-up, and continuing medical education.

Having carefully considered indications and contraindications, chosen a method of approach, designed the catheterization protocol and prepared the patient, the next step is to perform the cardiac catheterization itself and thereby gain the anatomic and physiologic information needed in the individual case. Chapters 4 to 6 offer detailed descriptions of how this may be done. These descriptions are not proposed as the *only* correct approaches, but rather as methods that have proven moderately successful, that are practical, and whose strengths and weaknesses are known.

REFERENCES

1. Cournand AF: Nobel Lecture, December 11, 1956. *In* Nobel Lectures, Physiology and Medicine 1942–1962. Amsterdam, Elsevier Publishing Co., 1964. p 529.
2. Cournand A: Cardiac catheterization. Development of the technique, its contributions to experimental medicine, and its initial application in man. Acta Med Scand Suppl 579:1–32, 1975.
3. Forssmann W: Die Sondierung des rechten Herzens. Klin Wochenschr 8:2085, 1929.
4. Klein O: Zur Bestimmung des zerkulatorischen minutens Volumen nach dem Fickschen Prinzip. Munch Med Wochenschr 77:1311, 1930.
5. Cournand AF, Ranges HS: Catheterization of the right auricle in man. Proc Soc Exp Biol Med 46:462, 1941.
6. Richards, DW: Cardiac output by the catheterization technique in various clinical conditions. Fed Proc 4:215, 1945.
7. Cournand AF, et al: Measurement of cardiac output in man using the technique of catheterization of the right auricle or ventricle. J Clin Invest 24:106, 1945.
8. Dexter L, et al: Studies of congenital heart disease. II. The pressure and oxygen content of blood in the right auricle, right ventricle, and pulmonary artery in control patients, with observations on the oxygen saturation and source of pulmonary "capillary" blood. J Clin Invest 26:554, 1947.
9. Dexter L, Burwell CS, Haynes FW, Seibel RE: Oxygen content of pulmonary "capillary" blood in unanesthetized human beings. J Clin Invest 25:913, 1946.
10. Hellems HK, Haynes FW, Dexter L: Pulmonary "capillary" pressure in man. J Appl Physiol 2:24, 1949.
11. Lagerlöf H and Werkö L: Studies on circulation of blood in man. Scand J Clin Lab Invest 7:147, 1949.
12. McMichael J, Sharpey-Schafer EP: The action of intravenous digoxin in man. Q J Med 13:1123, 1944.
13. Lenègre J, Maurice P: Premiers recherches sur la pression ventriculaire droits. Bull Mem Soc Med d'Hôp Paris 80:239, 1944.
14. Stead EA Jr, Warren JV: Cardiac output in man: analysis of mechanisms varying cardiac output based on recent clinical studies. Arch Intern Med 80:237, 1947.
15. Stead EA Jr, Warren JV, Brannon ES: Cardiac output in congestive heart failure: analysis of reasons for lack of close correlation between symptoms of heart failure and resting cardiac output. Am Heart J 35:529, 1948.
16. Bing RJ, et al: Catheterization of coronary sinus and middle cardiac vein in man. Proc Soc Exp Biol Med 66:239, 1947.
17. Bing RJ, et al: Measurement of coronary blood flow, oxygen consumption, and efficiency of the left ventricle in man. Am Heart J 38:1, 1949.
18. Vandam LD, Bing RJ, Gray FD Jr: Physiologic studies in congenital heart disease. IV. Measurements of circulation in 5 selected cases. Bull Johns Hopkins Hosp 81:192, 1947.
19. Bing RJ, Vandam LD, Gray FD Jr: Physiological studies in congenital heart disease. I. Procedures. Bull Johns Hopkins Hosp 80:107, 1947.
20. Burchell HB: Cardiac catheterization in diagnosis of various cardiac malformations and diseases. Proc Mayo Clin 23:481, 1948.
21. Wood EH, et al: General and special techniques in cardiac catheterization. Proc Mayo Clin 23:494, 1948.
22. Burwell CS, Dexter L: Beri-beri heart disease. Trans Assoc Am Physicians 60:59, 1947.
23. Harvey RM, et al: Some effects of digoxin upon heart and circulation in man: digoxin in left ventricular failure. Am J Med 7:439, 1949.
24. Zimmerman HA, Scott RW, Becker ND: Catheterization of the left side of the heart in man. Circulation 1:357, 1950.
25. Limon-Lason R, Bouchard A: El Cateterismo Intracardico; Cateterizacion de las Cavidades Izquierdas en el Hombre. Registro Simultaneo de presion y Electrocadiograma Intracavetarios. Arch Inst Cardiol Mexico 21:271, 1950.
26. Seldinger SI: Catheter replacement of the needle in percutaneous arteriography: a new technique. Acta Radiol 39:368, 1953.
27. Ross J Jr: Transseptal left heart catheterization: a new method of left atrial puncture. Ann Surg 149:395, 1959.
28. Cope C: Technique for transseptal catheterization of the left atrium: preliminary report. J Thoracic Surg 37:482, 1959.
29. Sones FM Jr, Shirey EK, Prondfit WL, Westcott RN: Cine-coronary arteriography. Circulation 20:773, 1959 (abstract).
30. Sones FM Jr: Cine Coronary Arteriography. *In* Hurst JW, Logue RB (eds): The Heart. 2nd edition. New York, McGraw Hill Book Co., 1970. p 377.
31. Ricketts JH, Abrams HL: Percutaneous selective coronary cine arteriography. JAMA 181:620, 1962.
32. Judkins MP: Selective coronary arteriography: a percutaneous transfemoral technique. Radiology 89:815, 1967.
33. Swan HJC, et al: Catheterization of the heart in man with use of a flow directed balloon-tipped catheter. N Engl J Med 283:447, 1970.
34. Grüntzig A, et al: Coronary transluminal angioplasty. Circulation 56:II–319, 1977 (abst).
35. Grüntzig A, Senning A, Siegenthaler WE: Nonoperative dilatation of coronary artery stenoses. Percutaneous transluminal coronary angioplasty. N Engl J Med 301:61, 1979.
36. Sigwart U, Puel J, Mirkovich V, Joffre F, Kappenberger L: Intravascular stents to prevent occlusion and restenosis after transluminal angioplasty. N Engl J Med 316:701, 1987.
37. Simpson JB, Selmon MR, Robertson GC, Cipriano PR, Hayden WG, Johnson DE, Fogerty TJ: Transluminal atherectomy for occlusive peripheral vascular disease. Am J Cardiol 61:96G–101G, 1988.
38. Spears JR: Percutaneous laser treatment of athero-

sclerosis: an overview of emerging techniques. Cardiovasc Intervent Radiol 9:303, 1986.

39. Spears JR, et al: Percutaneous coronary laser balloon angioplasty: preliminary results of a multicenter trial. J Am Coll Cardiol 13:61A, 1989.

40. Warren JV: Fifty years of Invasive Cardiology. Werner Forssmann (1904–1979). Am J Med 69:10, 1980.

41. St. John Sutton MG, et al: Valve replacement without preoperative cardiac catheterization. N Engl J Med 305:1233, 1981.

42. Robert WC: Reasons for cardiac catheterization before cardiac valve replacement. N Engl J Med 306:1291, 1982.

43. Rahimtoola SH: The need for cardiac catheterization and angiography in valvular heart disease is not disproven. Ann Intern Med 97:433, 1982.

44. Alpert JS, Sloss LJ, Cohn PF, Grossman W: The diagnostic accuracy of combined clinical and noninvasive evaluation: comparison with findings at cardiac catheterization. Cathet Cardiovasc Diagn 6:359, 1980.

45. Green GS, McKinnon CM, Rosch J, Judkins MP: Complications of selective percutaneous transfemoral coronary arteriography and their prevention. Circulation 45:552, 1972.

46. Anderson KO, Masur FT: Psychologic preparation for cardiac catheterization. Heart Lung 18:154–163, 1989.

47. Friesinger GC, et al: Intersociety Commission for Heat Disease Resources: Report on Optimal Resources for Examination of the Heart and Lungs: Cardiac catheterization and radiographic facilities. Circulation 68:893A–930A, 1983.

48. Conti CR: Presidents' Page: Cardiac catheterization laboratories: Hospital-based, free-standing or mobile? J Am Coll Cardiol 15:748, 1990.

49. Fierens E: Outpatient coronary arteriography. A report on 12,719 studies. Cathet Cardiovasc Diagn 10:27, 1984.

50. Mahrer PR, Young C, Magnusson PT: Efficacy and safety of outpatient catheterization. Cathet Cardiovasc Diagn 13:304, 1987.

51. Pink S, Fiutowski L, Gianelly RE: Outpatient cardiac catheterizations: analysis of patients requiring admission. Clin Cardiol 12:375–378, 1989.

52. Block PC, Ockene I, Goldberg RJ, Butterly J, Block EH, Degon C, Beiser A, Colton T: A prospective randomized trial of outpatient versus inpatient cardiac catheterization. N Engl J Med 319:1251, 1988.

2

Angiography: Principles Underlying Proper Utilization of Cineangiographic Equipment and Contrast Agents

DONALD S. BAIM and SVEN PAULIN

Although the physician performing cardiac catheterization procedures has had rigorous training in cardiac anatomy, physiology, and pathophysiology, he or she usually has *not* had formal instruction in the principles underlying the optimal use of radiologic equipment and contrast agents. This forces operators not fortunate enough to enjoy close collaboration with a knowledgeable radiologic colleague to adopt a "learn as you go" approach to understanding this increasingly complex area. Crises may develop when it becomes necessary to choose new equipment or provide the technical expert with appropriate observations about malfunctions of existing equipment. Moreover, such a laboratory may suffer from failing to devote adequate attention to monitoring the optimal function of its image chain, and the radiation safety of its patients and personnel. Accordingly, we include this chapter in the hope of heightening the awareness of the catheterizing physician of some essential radiographic principles, the equipment components now available for cardiac angiography, generally accepted programs for radiographic quality assurance and radiation protection, and the various intravascular contrast agents. Those seeking more detailed technical information are referred to the summary by the Inter-Society Commission for Heart Disease Resources[1] or the excellent text of Moore.[2]

THE ANGIOGRAPHIC ROOM

The modern cardiac catheterization laboratory (Fig. 2–1) consists of a patient support table, equipment for the monitoring of intracardiac pressures and electrocardiographic activity, and an imaging chain. The last is used to provide fluoroscopy to facilitate placement of cardiac catheters and cineangiography to record permanently details about the anatomic and functional state of cardiac chambers, great vessels and the coronary circulation.

The imaging chain consists of a generator/cine pulse system, an x-ray tube, an image intensifier, an optical distributor, a 35-mm cine camera, a television camera and monitor, and a floor or ceiling-suspended gantry to allow complex angulation of the x-ray beam (Fig. 2–2). These modern gantries permit the use of a flat table-top with free-floating horizontal movement for panning, and adjustable table height. This represents a distinct improvement in both patient comfort and avail-

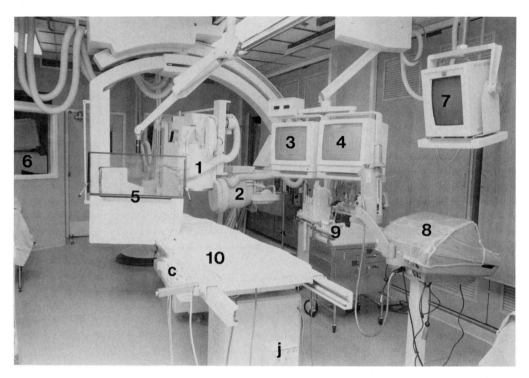

Fig. 2–1. Biplane cineangiographic room showing (1) AP plane image intensifier, cine camera, TV camera and x-ray tube (partially hidden below table), attached to a floor-mounted parallelogram gantry to allow complex angulation; (2) Lateral plane image chain attached to a ceiling-suspended gantry that can be moved into place when biplane imaging is desired; (3) and (4) TV monitors for AP and lateral image chains; (5) Movable radiation shield to protect operators from scatter dose to eyes and thyroid; (6) Physiologic pressure recorder located behind lead-glass window to protect the cardiovascular technician from scatter radiation; (7) Remote display of physiologic data; (8) Power injector for contrast delivery during ventriculography; (9) Emergency cart containing defibrillator, airway management and drug supplies; (10) Patient support table with (c) control box for table and gantry movement, magnification mode and beam-restricting "cones"; and (j) junction box for connection of pressure transducers to physiologic recorder. The generator and image chain electronics are concealed behind the louvered doors seen along the right hand wall of the room.

able imaging angulation compared to earlier systems in which the image chain was stationary and the patient was rolled from side to side in a cradle. A second complete imaging chain may be used to provide simultaneous viewing of cardiac structures from a separate angle (i.e., a biplane system). Biplane imaging is commonly used in laboratories that study a high percentage of congenital cases, or whose operators prefer biplane imaging for certain procedures such as left ventriculography, transseptal puncture, or coronary angioplasty.

To house this bulky and expensive equipment and support personnel, the room should have a floor space of at least 500 square feet (47 square meters) with a ceiling height of at least 10 feet (3 meters). The walls should be shielded with 1 mm of lead up to a height of 7 feet to provide radiation protection for personnel in surrounding work areas, and any observation windows should be of lead-treated glass to provide similar radiation shielding. Many recently designed rooms segregate equipment, such as generator controls and pressure recorders, and personnel not involved in direct patient contact activities within a shielded "control area" contiguous with the room itself. The bulky components of the generator and associated electronics (racks) are best placed in ventilated closets along the walls of the room, which must be positioned in such a way that the high-voltage cable runs are short (less than 40 feet [13 meters]) and the racks themselves are easily accessible to service personnel for diagnostic and repair activities.

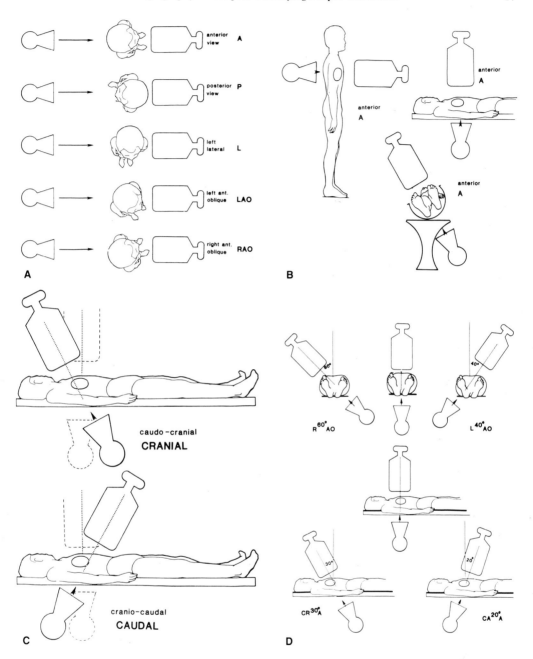

Fig. 2–2. (A) Principle of radiographic nomenclature for different projections around the patient's long axis. The object's (patient's) surface facing the observer determines the identification for a specific view. (B) The terminology for radiographic projections relates to the patient's body and not to the orientation in space. Thus, all three illustrated situations—standing, recumbent, recumbent in turned cradle—represent posteroanterior projections. (C) Angulations in relation to the patient's long axis. In accordance with nomenclature principles based on direction of x rays, the upper illustration represents a cranial and the lower a caudal projection or view. (D) Angulations in cranial or caudal direction can occur in combination with any of the conventional projections. The center row illustrations represent the true posteroanterior view with 0 degree angulation. Degree of angulation can be expressed numerically in elevated position following the corresponding symbols as exemplified in illustrations to left and right.

THE GENERATOR

The generator is basically a step-up transformer that converts three-phase 480 volt line current into the high voltage (70 to 120 kV) and current (300 to 800 mA) needed to power the x-ray tube for the generation of an x-ray beam. The transformer is submerged in a large tank of oil for cooling and insulation. Satisfactory performance can be obtained using either the "constant potential" or the somewhat less expensive 12-pulse design.[1,2]

To be useful in a cardiac study, the generator must be combined with a cine pulse system, which chops the generator output into the brief (4 to 6 ms) pulses required to freeze motion without blurring of the rapidly-moving coronary arteries. Such pulsing is best performed in the secondary or high voltage side of the system, using either a grid-controlled x-ray tube or vacuum switching tubes (triodes or tetrodes) to transiently interrupt generator current. The cine pulse system must be capable of handling sufficient power (at least 40 kW) if the 60 to 100 kW power capacity of the generator is to be delivered to the x-ray tube effectively.

A final portion of generator function is automatic exposure control, which compensates for changes in the transmission of x-rays to the image intensifier as the beam is "panned" through structures of differing attenuation. When the sensing photocell (located above the output phosphor of the image intensifier) detects a drop in light, the exposure control increases the number of x rays striking the image intensifier by increasing one of three factors: *kV or kilovolts* refers to the electrical potential, which increases the penetrating power of each x-ray photon; *mA or milliamperes* refers to the electrical current through the x-ray tube, which relates to the number of x-ray photons generated; *ms or milliseconds* refers to the duration of each x-ray pulse, which also increases the total number of photons in each x-ray pulse. Most automatic exposure systems vary predominantly the kV, because a comparatively small (6 to 8 kV) change will produce the same increase in film blackening as a doubling of the mA of ms. Doubling mA might exceed the power-handling capacity of the cine pulse system and/or x-ray tube, and increase patient dose; doubling the ms would cause significant motion blurring and also increase patient dose. On the other hand, optimal imaging of iodine-based contrast agents is best achieved with comparatively low photon energies because iodine absorption of x-rays is greatest at 33 keV [the K-shell binding energy] and falls off progressively with increasing kV. Attempting to compensate for an underpowered generator or cine pulse system by using high (100 to 120) kV thus tends to result in poor, low-contrast angiographic images.

THE X-RAY TUBE

The x-ray tube consists of an evacuated glass or metal housing that contains a tungsten filament (housed in a cathodal focusing cup) and an anode disc (tungsten alloy 100 to 120 mm in diameter) which rotates at more than 10,000 rpm during cineangiography (Fig. 2–3). Electrons boil off the filament by thermionic emission, and are accelerated toward the

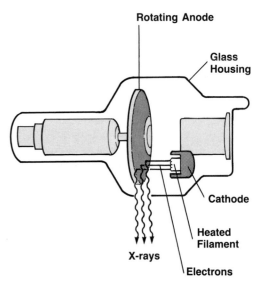

Fig. 2–3. Schematic illustration of an x-ray tube. Electrons liberated from the heated filament of the cathode are accelerated toward the slanted surface of the rapidly rotating anode. On impact with the target material, the electron flow generates x-ray photons leaving the x-ray tube in the direction of the tube window.

anode by the kV and mA supplied by the generator, where their rapid decelerative interaction with the tungsten atoms results in the emission of x-ray photons. The dimensions of the filament and the target angle (or bevel) of the anode at the point where the electron beam strikes determine the apparent focal spot of the x-ray tube—the dimensions of the x-ray source as viewed from the image intensifier. More than one focal spot may be included in a single tube. The smaller (usually 0.6 mm) focal spot more closely resembles a point source, and thus minimizes geometric unsharpness of the image, but it also concentrates the intense electron beam on a small area of the anode. Rapid rotation and beveling of the anode spread the electron beam impact over a larger area, so that a small apparent focal spot can be maintained while the surface temperature remains well below the melting point of tungsten (3370°C) (Fig. 2–4). Shallow target angles increase the area of electron impact, but target angles below 6 to 9 degrees fail to provide adequate beam coverage for a 9-inch field, due to a "heel effect" by which the anode absorbs part of the generated x-ray beam. Moreover, the small focal spot in most x-ray tubes is quite limited in terms of power handling capacity (35 kW), forcing the automatic exposure control to resort to a low mA–high kV technique,

which provides film blackening at the expense of poor image contrast. In cineangiography of larger patients or studies performed in extreme angulation, it is thus preferable to select the larger (usually 1.0 mm) focal spot for its higher power handling capacity (100 kW) and consequent lower kV technique, despite a slight associated loss of image sharpness.

In addition to the problem of instantaneous power (kW) loading, x-ray tubes are limited by cumulative heart load. Less than 1% of the electrical energy delivered to the tube is converted to x-rays, with the rest retained as heat. The heat load is expressed as heat units (HU) = $1.35 \times kV \times mA \times sec$. A typical single-frame cine exposure delivers roughly 200 HU, and a 10-second run of such exposures at 30 frames per second, 60,000 HU. The anode of most tubes can absorb only 400,000 HU before reaching a temperature at which the anode bearings seize and the tube self-destructs. Heat input, however, is counterbalanced by heat transfer to the oil-filled tube housing, which can absorb roughly 1,500,000 HU before reaching sufficient temperature to rupture its oil seals. This margin can be extended by using forced air, water, or oil to conduct heat away from the housing more rapidly, particularly if the laboratory is intended for rapid sequence performance of studies involving multiple cine runs.

Although not part of the x-ray tube per se, beam filtration and collimation are important aspects of the radiation beam. The energies of the photons in an x-ray beam are not uniform, but are distributed over a range which extends up to the kV responsible for their generation. The lowest energy photons in this distribution contribute to patient exposure, but do not have adequate penetrating power to participate in film blackening. Thus, Federal Department of Health, Education and Welfare regulations require that they be filtered out by passing the beam through the equivalent of 2.5 to 3.0 mm thick aluminum before it leaves the x-ray tube housing. The x-ray beam must also be limited spatially by a lead collimator which restricts the beam size so that it just covers the input phosphor of the image intensifier. Additional

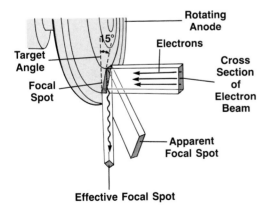

Fig. 2–4. Illustration of relationship between anode target angle, electron beam dimension, and effective focal spot, which by definition is specified in the direction perpendicular to the electron beam. The apparent size of a focal spot depends upon the direction from which it is viewed.

adjustable lead "cones" are also provided to further limit the beam to the region of the cine film frame, and their use is essential to reduce patient and operator radiation exposure and the unsharpness caused by scatter of radiation that strikes the patient outside of the imaging field.

THE IMAGE INTENSIFIER

Before the image intensifier was introduced, x-ray shadows were observed only on a fluorescent zinc cadmium sulfide screen, which was so dim that it had to be viewed in a darkened room after prior dark adaptation of the operator with red goggles. The image intensifier (developed in the 1950s) consists of a large glass vacuum bottle with a fluorescent phosphor at each end (cesium iodide at the input, and zinc cadmium sulfide at the output) (Fig. 2–5). It increases the brightness of the viewed image by a multiple of 4000 to 10,000. This brightness gain results from minification because the output phosphor surface area is smaller than that of the input phosphor, and electron amplification by which the electrons that come from the photocathode just beneath the input phosphor are accelerated by application of a 25 to 35 kV field so that they strike the output phosphor with greater energy.

The image intensifier also contains an electrostatic lens to focus the electrons during their flight. Although single mode image intensifiers are still available, most imaging systems include a means to vary the focus potential to

change the image magnification (dual or triple mode image intensifiers). Such intensifiers include a 9 inch (23 cm) mode that covers virtually the entire input phosphor area and is well suited to studies such as left ventriculography, which require imaging of a large area without a high degree of spatial resolution. The 6 or 7 inch (15 or 17 cm) mode displays a magnified image of the central portion of the input phosphor, optimally enhancing spatial resolution during coronary angiography. Triple mode tubes usually contain a third, 4.5 or 5 inch (11 or 12 cm) mode, which provides still greater magnification during special procedures such as percutaneous transluminal coronary angioplasty (PTCA); however, its use for routine cineangiography overtaxes the generator and tube capacity and requires careful panning by the operator if the whole coronary tree is to be imaged.

The qualities of the image intensifier are central to the performance of the image chain. Certain desirable characteristics such as gain, quantum detection efficiency, spatial resolution, and contrast tend to be mutually exclusive, so that all available image intensifiers involve some performance trade-offs. Moreover, an image intensifier's performance degrades rapidly, giving it a useful life of only 3 to 5 years in a busy laboratory before loss of gain and contrast require replacement. Despite these limitations, image intensifiers are currently available with on-line resolution in excess of a 4-line pair per mm in the 6 to 7 inch mode, and excellent balances of desirable characteristics. Regardless of test specifications, however, no image intensifier should be accepted until its satisfactory performance has been confirmed by clinical evaluation.

CINE CAMERA AND ASSOCIATED OPTICS

It is customary to record catheterization images on 35 mm movie film, at a speed of 60 frames per second for left ventriculography, and 30 frames per second for coronary angiography. In cineangiography, film advancement within the camera triggers the generator

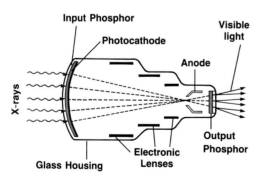

Fig. 2–5. Image intensifier in cross-sectional view. The path of x rays, electrons released by the photocathode and accelerated toward the anode to hit the small output phosphor, is illustrated.

to produce an x-ray exposure, so that a smooth and reliable camera operation is essential.

The camera is coupled to the output phosphor of the image intensifier by an optical system consisting of matched collimator and camera lenses designed to maximize light transmission and spatial resolution, and minimize image unsharpness due to veiling glare. The lens is also equipped with an adjustable F-stop and an interchangeable system of different-sized apertures which restrict light transmission in order to balance intensifier output, film characteristics, and processing parameters. The focal length of the optical system determines framing mode—the way in which the round output phosphor is represented on the rectangular cine frame (Fig. 2–6). We currently employ maximal (or total) overframing, using the cones to block the areas of the circle that lie outside the rectangular cine frame. Compared to maximum *horizontal* overframing, maximal overframing increases image magnification and restricts the field of view slightly. This compromise, however, works well in conjunction with the 9-inch and 7-inch intensifier modes described above.

THE TELEVISION CHAIN

Currently, 35 mm film remains the standard diagnostic and archival recording medium for cardiac examinations, but there has been an increasing effort to improve the quality of the simultaneously-obtained television images, and retain them for subsequent review or archival storage. This may facilitate precise catheter manipulation and on-line evaluation of interim results during interventional procedures (i.e., PTCA).

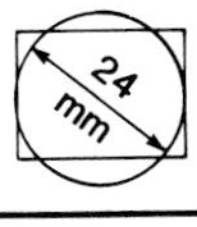

The television camera and the 35 mm cine camera are both mounted on a *distributor* that contains a partially silvered mirror. During cineangiography, this mirror allows 90% of the light to pass to the cine camera, while diverting 10% of the light to the television camera. During fluoroscopy, however, essentially all light from the image intensifier is sent to the television camera. This design forces the television camera to adapt to a wide range of input light levels, beyond its usual operating range. In part, this is compensated for electronically by an automatic gain control within the television circuitry, but current installations are increasingly using a motor-driven iris shutter on the television input lens, which can close as needed to reduce light overload during cine runs.

Television systems vary as to the type of image tube used. Compared to the standard Vidicon (which uses an antimony trisulfide target), most catheterization systems use either a Plumbicon (lead monoxide target), Saticon (selenium arsenic tellurium target), or Primicon (selenium tellurium arsenic target), to maximize image contrast and minimize image carryover or "lag" so that less than 10% of the image signal persists into the third video field.

Another important variable is the scanning format. Interlaced scan systems (like broadcast TV) alternately sweep the even and odd numbered lines from the overall raster. This may result in degradation of the television image

Framing Mode		Film Area Used
Exact Framing	18mm / 24mm / 18mm (circle)	58%
Mean Diameter Overframing	21mm (circle)	73%
Maximum Horizontal Overframing	24mm (circle)	88%
Total Overframing	30mm (circle)	100%

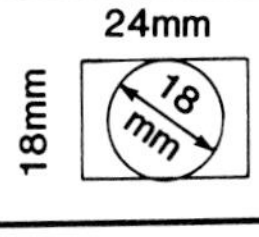

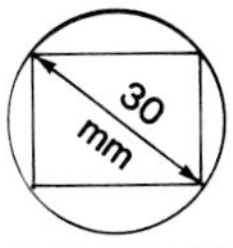

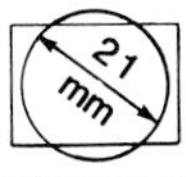

Fig. 2–6. Relationship of framing method to field size reduction in cinefluoroscopy. (Modified from Friesinger GC, et al: Report of Inter-Society Commission for Heart Disease Resources. Circulation 68(4):893A, 1983.)

during 30 fps cineangiography, due to misregistration of anatomic details between the odd and even scan lines, and "flicker" resulting from the collection of one set of lines at a time when the x-ray beam is "off." These limitations may be overcome by use of a progressive scanning television format, in which all scan lines are acquired in numerical sequence each time the x-ray tube is pulsed.[3] A scan converter then picks off the even and odd numbered scan lines for display on a standard interlaced monitor.

The other scan variable is the number of scan lines that make up the image. High line systems (up to 1023 horizontal lines, compared to the standard 525-line system) theoretically improve vertical resolution on the TV monitor, but the associated increase in amplifier bandwidth results in the introduction of more electronic noise.[4] Computer systems that perform on-line digital processing of the television image (manipulating contrast, noise, and background) are now becoming available for use in the catheterization laboratory although they remain complex and expensive.[5]

As the intrinsic quality of the television image has been improved, more effort has been devoted to recording that image for review during the procedure. Recording may involve videotape. Recorders using a 1-inch format provide adequate bandwidth, a low signal-to-noise ratio, and digital time base correction to make reliable slow motion and freeze frame viewing possible. A second type of recording is an electronic frame storage, which can capture and display a single video frame for reference ("roadmapping") during an interventional procedure. The reference image can be displayed using either a separate TV monitor or the main television monitor when live image collection is not taking place. More elaborate systems can collect a series of such frames during cine, replaying them at any speed as a "video loop."

In some systems, the quality of the video images has become good enough that videotaped or electronically stored images approach the quality of cine film.[5] This is particularly true of the digitally processed systems that may ultimately replace cine film.

CINE FILM SELECTION, PROCESSING, AND VIEWING

The ultimate quality of the recorded image depends nearly as much on the selection of cine film and processing parameters, as it does on the other elements of the image chain. Cine film emulsions are generally slower than those of standard photographic films, but virtually any cine film can be used in a given system with correct selection of F-stop, aperture, and processing parameters. The selection of a cine film thus depends more on other important features such as contrast, latitude, and grain size.

Film characteristics are best explored by plotting the characteristic curve (or H and D curve, after Hurter and Driffield), using a sensitometer to perform calibrated test strip exposures, and densitometer to measure the resulting film optical density (Fig. 2–7). Relevant parameters include the base-plus-fog measured as the optical density of the film at step 0 (not exposed to light) and the relative speed index. The latter is measured as the interpolated step producing a specified increment in optical density above base-plus-fog. Two

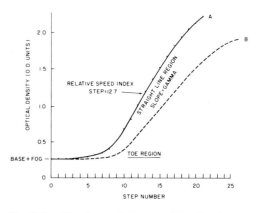

Fig. 2–7. Film characteristic curves (H + D), showing the relationship between light exposure (increasing step number on the horizontal axis), and film blackening (increasing optical density on the vertical axis). Measurements are shown for two different films (A and B), including the base + fog, relative speed index, and gamma (see text). Film B is less sensitive to light, but has a lower contrast and a wider latitude.

indices of contrast are also measured: the gamma and the average gradient, which have to do with how steeply optical density rises with increasing exposure.

In general, more diagnostic information can be recovered from films with lower contrast because their greater latitude allows distinction of more shades of gray and hence more anatomic detail between the extremes of black and white. Appropriate latitude is thus preferable to the steep edge gradients produced by some higher contrast films.

It must be emphasized that the characteristics of cine film described above also depend markedly on how the film is processed, including differences in the precise chemistry, temperature, agitation, and immersion time used in the automatic processor. Processing variables and the cine camera aperture should be matched carefully by the technical representative of the film-supplying company. It is then up to laboratory personnel to ensure that these parameters remain stable from day to day, as monitored by routine sensitometry and limited densitometry. Measurements should include the base-plus-fog, the optical density (OD) of a "speed step" (whose OD is known to be near 1.0), and the "contrast index" (the difference in OD between the speed step and the next higher numbered step). Base-plus-fog should not vary more than 0.02, and speed and contrast index should not vary by more than 0.1 from the initial values. Even slight variations beyond these levels should alert personnel to a potential problem with the processor, which must be corrected before clinical films are run if adequate film quality is to be ensured.

Documented stability of film and processing characteristics also make it possible to perform daily checks on the x-ray equipment itself, by measuring the optical density that results from filming a known attenuator (2.3 mm Cu) using a consistent geometry and exposure mode (selected magnification, focal spot, pulse width, and camera speed). System stability is documented by day-to-day reproducibility of the optical density at the center of the frame of the resulting film, which averages 0.90 OD

units in most laboratories. The daily routine may also involve imaging a resolution phantom to monitor image intensifier and camera focus. More detailed assessment of system function should be performed by technical representatives at least twice a year, with correction of adjustments (aperture, processing parameters) and any equipment defects (dose, image intensifier focus, contrast, etc.) by appropriate service personnel. Without these routine surveillance measures, significant deterioration may occur in imaging performance before it becomes apparent to the operators.[6]

Perceived film quality also depends to some extent on the system used to view films. Suitable systems are available for private viewing or projection of the image on a conventional movie screen. The larger format requires use of a high-output illumination system (arc lamp or halogen bulb). Either claw-advance or rotating prism systems can provide a high resolution flicker-free image of film during forwards or backwards transport at frame rates up to 60 frames per second. Like all elements of the image chain, film projectors require regular maintenance and cleaning to deliver optimal performance.

RADIATION SAFETY

The potential hazards of radiation must never be far from the operator's mind because the catheterization laboratory exposes both patients and personnel to the highest radiation levels of any commonly performed x-ray study.[1]

The primary unit of radiation exposure is the roentgen (R), defined in terms of the amount of ionization that the beam produces in air. This can be measured using ionization chambers, photographic film (i.e., a film badge), or thermoluminescent dosimeter salts that emit light in proportion to previous radiation exposure when heated. A more relevant unit is the *rad* or radiation absorbed dose, which deals with how much heating the radiation beam produces in each gram of a specified material. A new unit termed the gray [one gray = 100 rads] has recently been introduced, but is not widely used in the cardiology literature. For soft tissues, the absorbed dose generally equals 0.9 rad for every R of exposure; denser tissues such as bone absorb 4 rad for every R. To take into account the different degrees of damage produced by different types of radiation (i.e., alpha particles), absorbed doses are often expressed in *rem* (radiation equivalent in man). This is largely a semantic distinction for diagnostic x-rays because the rad and the rem are equivalent for this type of radiation.

There is no absolutely "safe" radiation exposure, i.e., a dose that poses no risk. The average person receives about 200 millirem (mrem) per year, about half from natural and half from man-made sources including medical x rays. While radiation increases the risk of genetic damage, gonadal doses of 20 to 200 rems are required to significantly increase the incidence of mutations. The somatic risk, which includes carcinogenesis (particularly thyroid cancer and leukemia) and tissue damage such as cataract formation, is thus of more practical concern.

The most important factor in radiation exposure is the imaging dose. Cineangiographic systems are usually set to deliver 30 micro R per cine frame (54 milliR per minute) to the face of the image intensifier in the 6-to-7-inch mode. The corresponding dose during fluoroscopy is roughly 10 times lower (3 to 5 mR per minute). Lower radiation flux produces poor images due to "quantum mottle,"[2] but higher doses do not substantially improve image quality. They require high mA and kV, which may overtax the generator and x-ray tube and paradoxically worsen the image, while increasing radiation exposure of both the patient and operator.[6] Patient input dose may be reduced by coning the image to the size of the cine frame, keeping the image intensifier as close as possible to the patient's chest, and avoiding unnecessary fluoroscopy or cineangiographic time.

The patient's dose comes from his position within the direct radiation beam.[1,7] In fact, most of the incident radiation beam is absorbed by the patient, with less than 1% of the beam passing through the patient to strike the image intensifier. To provide the input phosphor doses described above, the patient typically receives a skin input dose of 30 R per minute during cineangiography and 3 R/minute during fluoroscopy, for a total skin dose of nearly 50 R during the typical examination (the equivalent of 100 to 250 chest x-rays). Gonadal dose from secondary scatter is minimal, but should be decreased further by avoidance of imaging over the pelvis and use of a pelvic or gonadal shield in younger patients.

The remaining portion of the incident beam is scattered back into the procedure room mostly from the point where the beam enters the patient. During a standard catheterization, the head of the primary operator receives a dose of approximately 20 mrem, about half from fluoroscopy and half from cineangiography.[7] At that rate, an operator could perform no more than 250 cases per year without exceeding the Federal guidelines of 5,000 mrem per year, monitored by a film badge worn on the left collar outside the lead apron to record thyroid and lens dose. Performance of more complex procedures such as PTCA involves greater fluoroscopy time and operator radiation dose,[8] which would further reduce the number of cases that a single operator could perform each year.

In fact, the operator can use several methods to reduce his scatter dose, other than the measures described above to reduce patient dose. The operator can stand as far from the beam as possible to take advantage of the inverse square law. This is particularly important during angulated shots such as the left lateral or LAO cranial projections, which place him in close proximity to the beam entry point (Fig. 2–8). Keeping one's distance is easier with the femoral than the brachial approach, which thus carries about twice the exposure to the operator's head.

It is also advisable to use additional shielding to reduce exposure of radiation-sensitive areas, analogous to the use of a lead apron to shield one's torso. Shielding equivalent to 0.5 mm of lead attenuates exposure by a factor of nearly 50 (i.e., to less than 1 mrem per case),

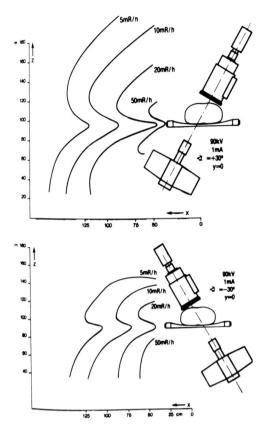

Fig. 2–8. Isoexposure curves representing radiation exposure to the operator during cardiac catheterization using U-arm or C-arm systems. The upper panel represents a 30-degree LAO view; the lower panel shows a 30-degree RAO view. The operator is standing to the patient's right, and the patient's feet are toward the reader. Radiation is highest at the level of the table and patient due to radiation scatter. (Reprinted from Balter S, Sones FM Jr, Brancato R: Radiation exposure to the operator performing cardiac angiography with U-arm systems. Circulation 58:925, 1978, with permission.)

and is available in thyroid collars and wraparound leaded eye glasses. Our preference, however, has been for a movable rectangular lead-acrylic shield (United Shielding Technologies, Lawrence, MA) that can be positioned between the point at which the x-ray beam enters the patient's body and the operator's head (see Fig. 2–1). It protects both thyroid and eye as effectively as separate shields, can be covered with a sterile plastic bag to allow placement within the sterile field, and is less cumbersome than separate eye and thyroid shields.

INTRAVASCULAR CONTRAST AGENTS

Shortly after the classic papers by Roentgen in the 1890s, the search began for effective and nontoxic contrast agents to define vascular anatomy. Although early experimentation involved a number of heavy metals (bismuth, barium, thorium), modern contrast systems are based exclusively on iodine, which by virtue of its high atomic number and chemical versatility has proved an excellent agent for intravascular opacification.

Inorganic iodine (sodium iodide) caused marked toxic reactions, compared to the organic iodide (Selectan), which was introduced in 1929 and contained one iodine atom per benzoic acid ring. In the 1950s a series of substituted triiodobenzoic acid derivatives (three iodine atoms per ring) were developed.[9] These compounds differ from each other in terms of the specific side chains used in positions 1, 3, and 5 (Fig. 2–9), which influence solubility and toxicity.

The most widely used ionic contrast agents (Renografin [Squibb], Hypaque [Winthrop], and Angiovist [Berlex]) are mixtures of the meglumine and sodium salts of *diatrizoic* acid. Functionally similar agents are based on iothalmic acid (Conray [Mallinckrodt]) or metrizoic acid (Isopaque). They have a sodium concentration roughly equal to blood, and pH titrated between 6.0 and 7.0, and a low concentration (0.1 to 0.2 mg/ml) of calcium disodium EDTA.[9] Higher or lower sodium concentrations may contribute to ventricular arrhythmias during coronary injection. Each of these agents contain 3 atoms of iodine for every 2 ions, including the sodium or meglumine cation. Solutions have an iodine concentration of 320 to 370 mgI/ml, as required for left ventricular and coronary contrast injections, are thus markedly hypertonic with an osmolality roughly 6 times that of blood. This contributes to the general effects observed after their administration (Table 2–1).[10]

One modification of ionic contrast came with the introduction of low osmolality contrast materials (LOCM) such as ioxglate (Hex-

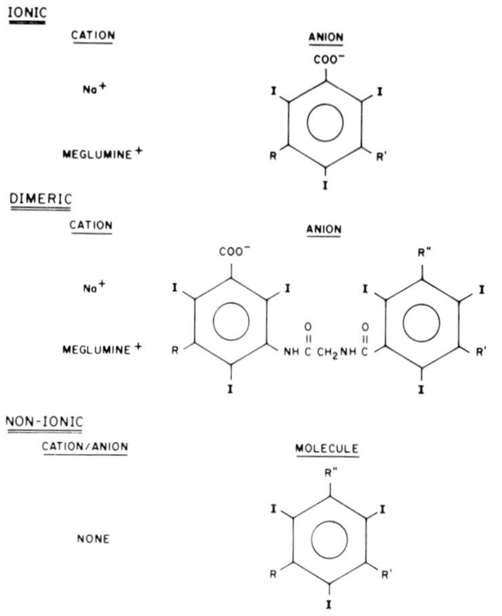

IONIC

EXAMPLES	IODINE (mg I/ml)	OSMOLALITY (mOsm/Kg water)	VISCOSITY (cps) 20°C	37°C
DIATRIZOATE (RENOGRAFIN, HYPAQUE, ANGIOVIST)	370	2076	14	8.4
IOTHALMATE (CONRAY)	325	1797	4	2.8
METRIZOATE (ISOPAQUE)	—	—	—	—

DIMERIC

EXAMPLE				
IOXAGLATE (HEXABRIX)	320	600	15.7	7.5

NON-IONIC

EXAMPLES				
IOPAMIDOL (ISOVUE)	370	796	20.4	9.4
IOHEXOL (OMNIPAQUE)	350	844	20.4	10.4
METRIZAMIDE (AMIPAQUE)	370	—	—	16.0
IOVERSOL (OPTIRAY)	320	702	9.9	5.8

Fig. 2–9. Structures and properties of current available contrast agents. The traditional (HOCM or high-osmolar contrast media) are Na$^+$/meglumine salts of substituted tri-iodobenzoic acid, having 4–6 times the osmolality of blood. Two types of new low-osmolality contrast media (LOCM) are also shown: the Na$^+$/meglumine salt of an ionic *dimer*, and the four new, true *non-ionic* agents, each of which has an osmolality 2 to 3 times that of blood. R, R′, and R″ refer to specific side branch molecules in the different agents. See text for details.

abrix [Mallinckrodt]).[11] Although ioxglate is still ionic, existing as a mixture of meglumine and sodium salts, its unique dimeric structure includes 6 molecules of iodine (3 atoms of iodine for every 1 ion) making it a low osmolality contrast agent. For an iodine concentration of 320 mgI/ml, Hexabrix has an osmolality roughly three times that of blood, significantly reducing the undesirable side effects related to hypertonicity.

Table 2–1. *Side Effects of Contrast Agents*

Effects related to hypertonicity (virtually eliminated by use of LOCM)
Arteriolar vasodilatation (hypotension, sensation of heat)
Increased intravascular volume
Electrophysiologic changes (ST-T wave alterations, bradycardia, prolonged PR/QT interval)
Nausea and vomiting
Depression of myocardial function

Other adverse effects (only partially reduced by use of LOCM)
Anaphylaxis
Renal toxicity

Another modification has been the development of true non-ionic, low osmolality contrast agents. They are water-soluble in a non-charged form, without an associated cation.[12] Examples include iopamidol (Isovue [Squibb]), iohexol (Omnipaque [Winthrop]), metrizamide (Amipaque [Winthrop]), and ioversol (Optiray [Mallinckrodt]), which contain 3 atoms of iodine for every molecule. With calcium disodium EDTA as a stabilizer and tromethamine (1.2–3.6 mg/ml) as a buffer, an iodine content of 320 to 370 mgI/ml can be achieved with an osmolality roughly three times that of blood. These agents appear to have a slightly lower incidence of side effects than Hexabrix.[11–13] Both Hexabrix and the true non-ionic contrast agents, however, are considerably more expensive than conventional contrast agents: the 200 ml of contrast consumed in the average diagnostic catheterization would cost $150 to 200, compared to roughly $20 for the same amount of ionic contrast. The exact degree to which they protect against *serious* side effects such as anaphylaxis and renal failure remains controversial.[14–15]

There has been some suggestion that blood remaining in contact with non-ionic contrast, as in a carelessly filled injection syringe, is more likely to clot than blood in similar contact with a conventional ionic agent.[16] Finally, these agents have a fairly high viscosity at room temperature, making it difficult to perform adequate coronary injections through standard diagnostic catheters unless the contrast is prewarmed to 37°C.

Given this diversity in contrast agents, operators must choose a contrast agent based on: (1) adequate opacification, (2) side effect profile, and (3) cost. In our laboratory, we currently use Angiovist as our routine contrast agent, but resort to a low-osmolar agent in roughly 20 to 25% of cases based on specific indications: severe hemodynamic dysfunction not responding to pharmacotherapy; history of prior allergic reaction to ionic contrast; internal mammary injection; or baseline renal insufficiency with a creatinine above 2.5 mg/dl.[17–18] With this strategy, the incidence of *severe* contrast reaction (wheezing, prolonged hypotension, or frank anaphylactoid reaction) remains well below 0.05%. Some laboratories, however, now use the more expensive low-osmolality contrast agents routinely in the hope of improving patient comfort and further lowering side effects.[19] This practice is likely to become more common as the cost of the newer non-ionic agents falls more into line with that of the ionic compounds.

REFERENCES

1. Friesinger GC, et al: Optimal resources for examination of the heart and lungs: cardiac catheterization and radiologic facilities. Circulation 68:893A, 1983.
2. Moore RJ: Imaging Principles of Cardiac Angiography. Bethesda, Aspen Publishers, 1990.
3. Holmes DR, Bove AA, Wondrow MA, Gray JE: Video x-ray progressive scanning: new technique for decreasing x-ray exposure without decreasing image quality during cardiac catheterization. Mayo Clin Proc 61:321, 1986.
4. Gray JE, Wondrow MA, Smith HC, Holmes DR: Technical considerations for cardiac laboratory high-definition video systems. Cathet Cardiovasc Diagn 10:73, 1984.
5. Gurley et al: Comparison of simultaneously performed digital and film-based angiography in assessment of coronary artery disease. Circulation 78:1411, 1988.
6. Levin DC, Dunham LR, Stueve R: Causes of cine image quality deterioration in cardiac catheterization laboratories. Am J Cardiol 52:881, 1983.
7. Miller SW, Castronovo FP: Radiation exposure and protection in cardiac catheterization laboratories. Am J Cardiol 55:171, 1985.
8. Dash H, Leaman DM: Operator radiation exposure during percutaneous transluminal coronary angioplasty. J Am Coll Cardiol 4:725, 1984.
9. King BF, et al: Low-osmolality contrast media: A current perspective. Mayo Clin Proc 64:976, 1989.
10. Moore RD et al: Frequency and determinants of adverse reactions induced by high-osmolality contrast media. Radiology 170:727, 1989.
11. Piao ZE et al: Hemodynamic abnormalities during coronary angiography: comparison of hypaque-76, hexabrix, and omnipaque-350. Cathet Cardiovasc Diagn 16:149, 1989.
12. Mancini GBJ et al: Hemodynamic and electrocardiographic effects in man of a new nonionic contrast agent (Iohexol): Advantages over standard ionic agents. Am J Cardiol 51:1218, 1983.
13. Wisneski JA, Gertz EW, Dahlgren M, Muslin A: Comparison of low osmolality ionic (ioxaglate) versus nonionic (iopamidol) contrast media in cardiac angiography. Am J Cardiol 63:489, 1989.
14. Bettmann MA: Radiographic contrast agents—a perspective (editorial). N Engl J Med 317:891, 1987.
15. Powe NR et al: Contrast medium-induced adverse reactions: Economic outcome. Radiology 169:163, 1988.
16. Grollman JH et al: Thromboembolic complications in coronary angiography associated with the use of non-ionic contrast medium. Cathet Cardiovasc Diagn 14:159, 1988.
17. Lasser EC et al: Pretreatment with corticosteroids to alleviate reactions to intravenous contrast material. N Engl J Med 317:845, 1987.
18. Schwab SJ et al: Contrast nephropathy: a controlled trial of a non-ionic and an ionic radiographic contrast agent. N Engl J Med 320:149, 1989.
19. Palmer FJ: The RACR survey of intravenous contrast media reactions final report. Aust Radiol 32:426, 1988.

3

Complications of Cardiac Catheterization: Incidence, Causes, and Prevention

WILLIAM GROSSMAN

In support of the principle that if anything can go wrong it will, there is an extensive literature describing a wide array of complications that have been associated with cardiac catheterization.* Although many reports detail the complications of coronary angiography or other specific subtypes of cardiac catheterization, relatively few reports deal with complications of all types of cardiac catheterization procedures. Two multicenter studies are of particular interest in this regard: (1) the Cooperative Study on Cardiac Catheterization,[1] which represented a prospective study of all catheterization procedures (n = 12,367) in 16 laboratories over a 24-month period, and; (2) the Registry report from the Society for Cardiac Angiography,[2] which represented the experience of 66 laboratories that studied 53,581 patients over a period of 14 months. The Cooperative Study involved a small group of major medical centers at a time when the caseload involved primarily valvular heart disease; coronary angiography was a part of the

catheterization procedure in only 27% of the patients in that report. In contrast, the Registry report from the Society for Cardiac Angiography,[2] based on self-reporting from a mixture of academic and private laboratories, covered a period when suspected or known coronary artery disease was the commonest indication for catheterization: 41,204 of the 53,581 patients (77%) were studied by coronary angiography and did not have valvular, congenital, or other types of coronary disease.

The Society for Cardiac Angiography has updated its Registry report from 1982 with a summary of data on an additional 222,553 patients who underwent coronary angiography between July 1, 1984 and December 31, 1987.[3] Although this report represents the largest published series on complications, the Committee limited its analysis to patients who underwent coronary angiography, whereas in the earlier Registry report[2] nearly one fourth of the patients did not undergo coronary angiography and presumably had been referred for catheterization primarily for evaluation of valvular, myocardial or congenital heart disease. The updated Registry report[3] also excluded patients who had undergone coronary angioplasty, valvuloplasty or intracoronary

*The term *cardiac catheterization* will be taken to include catheterization and related angiography (e.g., left ventriculography, coronary angiography), whether the procedure is purely diagnostic or includes a therapeutic or "interventional" component.

thrombolytic therapy as part of their catheterization procedure. Nevertheless, within the confines of these limitations, some valuable lessons can be learned from the enormous experience summarized in the report.

None of these multicenter studies[1-3] included significant numbers of interventional catheterization procedures, such as PTCA or valvuloplasty. In addition, many of the technical aspects of cardiac catheterization as well as adjunctive medical therapy have changed substantially in the years since the first two studies[1,2] were conducted (e.g., widespread use of sheaths, non-ionic contrast agents, aspirin and anti-thrombolytic drugs, etc.). In this regard, a report[4] from our laboratory assessed complications in 2883 consecutive cardiac catheterization procedures performed during an 18-month period. Procedures performed during the study period included 1609 diagnostic catheterizations, 933 percutaneous transluminal coronary angioplasties, 199 percutaneous balloon valvuloplasties, and 32 other procedures performed by the catheterization team (intra-aortic balloon placements, right ventricular endomyocardial biopsies, and pericardiocentesis). For diagnostic catheterizations, major complications defined as those with permanent sequelae (death, myocardial infarction, and stroke) occurred in 0.25% of patients. Comparable figures for the Cooperative Study[1] and the two Registry reports[2,3] are 0.65% and 0.26% and 0.23% respectively. A meaningful comparison among these studies is difficult because there were substantial differences in the patient populations among the three reports. Both the Cooperative Study[1] and the first Registry report[2] included catheterization procedures in infants, who are at higher risk of death during cardiac catheterization, while the Boston study included only adult patients. On the other hand, in the Registry reports[2,3] approximately 28% of the patients studied had either minimal or no cardiac disease, and these patients tend to have a low incidence of myocardial infarction, stroke, or death.

A list of the principal complications of cardiac catheterization, both diagnostic and therapeutic, is given in Table 3–1. Specific complications and their causes and prevention are discussed in the remainder of this chapter. As an exception, complications related to radiographic contrast agents are discussed in Chapter 2.

DEATH

Death occurred in 75 of 53,581 cases (0.14%) in the first Registry report,[2] and was much more common in infants under 1 year of age (1.7%). In the second Registry report[3] death occurred in 218 or 0.1% of 222,553 patients undergoing diagnostic coronary angiography. A subset analysis of these 218 deaths[5] showed that death from cardiac catheterization was more likely in patients over 60. It was increased by a factor of 10 in patients with NYHA functional class IV symptoms compared to those with class I and II symptoms, and by a factor of 10 in patients with left main coronary disease compared to those with single-vessel disease. A 10-fold increase in risk was also seen in the subset with LV ejection fraction under 30% compared with those who had ejection fractions over 50%. Patient gender and operator's choice of approach (brachial vs. femoral) did not significantly affect mortality. Patients with valvular heart disease generally may be expected to have a greater risk of death during cardiac catheterization, especially if there is associated coronary artery disease and heart failure. The VA Cooperative Study on Valvular Heart Disease has published its findings on complications of cardiac catheterization and angiography in 1559 preoperative catheterizations performed in patients with valvular heart disease.[6] Death occurred in three patients (0.2%), one with mitral regurgitation and two with aortic stenosis. Based on these and other reports, features that increase the risk of death are listed in Table 3–2.

The mortality rate associated with coronary angiography has improved considerably in the last 20 years. Previously, this rate was in excess of 1% in many laboratories,[7,8] but with improvement in technique and widespread use

Table 3–1. *Complications of Cardiac Catheterization in 2,801 Cases*[4]

	Diagnostic Catheterization (n = 1,609)	PTCA (n = 993)	Balloon Valvuloplasty n = 199
Death	2 (0.12%)	3 (0.3%)	3 (1.5%)
Myocardial infarction	0	3 (0.3%)	1 (0.5%)
Neurologic events			
Transient	2 (0.1%)	0	1
Persistent (stroke)	2 (0.1%)	1 (0.1%)	1 (0.5%)
Emergency CABG	0	12 (1.2%)	0
Cardiac perforation			
observed, no intervention	1	0	0
pericardiocentesis	0	0	1
heart surgery	0	0	5 (2.5%)
Arrhythmias requiring countershock or temporary pacemaker	5 (0.3%)	6 (0.6%)	5 (2.5%)
Local vascular problem requiring repair	26 (1.6%)	15 (1.5%)	15 (7.5%)
Vasovagal reactions	33 (2.1%)	7 (0.7%)	4 (2.0%)
Allergic			
Hives	32	5	0
Hypotension/anaphylaxis	1	1	0

Of the diagnostic catheterizations, associated procedures included temporary pacemaker insertion (n = 193), intra-aortic balloon counterpulsation (n = 38) and endomyocardial biopsy (n = 36). Sixty-one of the 199 balloon valvuloplasties involved transseptal catheterization. CABG = coronary artery bypass graft surgery. Mean patient age was 62 ± 13 years.

of heparinization, the death rate with coronary angiography has fallen to its current low level of 0.1 to 0.3%, depending on case mix.

Similarly, the older literature often showed a difference in mortality between brachial and femoral approaches to coronary angiography,[8,9] with the femoral approach having a greater risk. However, recent studies[2,3] show comparable risk for both brachial and femoral techniques, probably reflecting in part the value of systemic heparinization with the percutaneous femoral approach.[10,11]

In cardiac catheterization laboratories today, deaths are most common in the subset of patients with *left main coronary artery disease* undergoing left heart catheterization and cor-

Table 3–2. *Patient Characteristics Associated with Increased Mortality from Cardiac Catheterization*

1. *Age:* Infants (<1 year old) and the elderly (>60 years old) are at increased risk of death during cardiac catheterization.

2. *Functional Class:* Mortality in Class IV patients is more than 10 times greater than in Class I–II patients.

3. *Severity of Coronary Obstruction:* Mortality for patients with left main disease is more than 10 times greater than for patients with single vessel disease.

4. *Valvular Heart Disease:* Especially when combined with coronary disease is associated with a higher risk of death at cardiac catheterization than coronary artery disease alone.

5. *Left Ventricular Dysfunction:* Mortality for patients with LV ejection <30% is more than 10 times greater than if ejection fraction is ≥50%.

6. *Severe Non-Cardiac Disease:* Patients with renal insufficiency, insulin-requiring diabetes, advanced cerebrovascular and/or peripheral vascular disease, and severe pulmonary insufficiency appear to have an increased incidence of death and other major complications from cardiac catheterization.

onary arteriography. Bourassa has emphasized this, and in his institution the mortality rate in such patients was 6% in a series reported in 1976.[12] In the first Registry report of the Society for Cardiac Angiography,[2] 22 of the 2452 patients with ≥50% obstruction of the left main coronary artery died in association with cardiac catheterization. This considerably lower death rate (0.86%) was nevertheless more than 20 times higher than the death rate for patients with 1 vessel coronary disease (0.03%) in that series.

Prevention of a fatal outcome in patients with one or more of the "risk factors" listed in Table 3–2 requires that catheterization and cardiac surgical schedules should be coordinated so that patients at highest risk can be moved from the catheterization laboratory directly to the operating room. During the procedure itself, keeping the volume of radiographic contrast to a minimum or using nonionic or low-osmolar contrast agents (see Chapter 2) especially in patients known to have depressed left ventricular contractile function (ejection fraction by echocardiogram or radionuclide scan ≤30%) and increased pulmonary capillary pressure (≥30 mm Hg), is important. If physiologic measurements (e.g., pressures and output) routinely precede angiography, such high risk patients will be identified more easily and can be "pretreated" with intravenous furosemide, oxygen, and a vasodilator (e.g., intravenous nitroglycerin, sodium nitroprusside) prior to performing angiographic studies. We have found that a *tilting* cardic catheterization table, which allows rapid transition to Trendelenburg position (for hypotension) or reverse-Trendelenburg (for pulmonary congestion/edema), is valuable in helping to get very sick patients through cardiac catheterization and angiography.

Careful entry of the coronary catheter into the left coronary ostium is important in all patients, but it is mandatory in those suspected of having left main coronary artery disease in whom preformed catheters are being used. Meticulous attention to *all the details* of technique is important in preventing deaths in the cardiac catheterization laboratory, since even a minor complication (e.g., vasovagal reaction, arrhythmia) may be fatal in a patient with limited cardiac reserve. Despite all such measures, it seems likely that a certain irreducible mortality rate will be associated with cardiac catheterization in patients with the characteristics enumerated in Table 3–2.

MYOCARDIAL INFARCTION

Myocardial infarction as a complication of the procedure has been reported in 0.09%,[12] 0.45%,[9] 0.61%,[13] 0.06%,[3] 0%,[4] and 2.6%[7] of patients undergoing diagnostic cardiac catheterization and angiography.

Factors predisposing to myocardial infarction are *unstable angina* (including crescendo pattern and angina at rest), *recent subendocardial infarction,* and *insulin-requiring diabetes mellitus.* Documentation of myocardial infarction when it is less than transmural in extent may be difficult following cardiac catheterization, since intramuscular injections (e.g., lidocaine) and the soft tissue trauma of the catheterization may lead to increases in serum enzyme levels (LDH, GOT, total CPK) often used to assess the presence or absence of myocardial infarction.[14,15] Such elevations of enzyme levels may be seen with either brachial or femoral approaches. In a study of CPK isoenzymes following uncomplicated cardiac catheterization, although total CPK was increased in nearly all patients, none had elevation of CPK-MB activity.[16] Thus, an increase in serum CPK-MB activity is necessary for the diagnosis of myocardial infarction following cardiac catheterization.

Prevention of myocardial infarction involves the same principles discussed under prevention of death, particularly (1) the use of heparin during coronary angiography; (2) immediate recognition and treatment of vagal reactions, arrhythmia, angina, or hypotension; (3) full medical therapy prior to and during catheterization in patients with unstable angina (adequate use of beta-adrenergic blocking agents, aspirin and/or heparin, oxygen, nitrates, and control of blood pressure); and (4) intraaortic balloon counterpulsation in patients who remain unstable despite full medical therapy.

CEREBROVASCULAR COMPLICATIONS

Cerebrovascular complications occurred in 0.2% of diagnostic catheterizations from our laboratory (0.1% transient, 0.1% persistent),[4] 0.23% of studies in the survey of Adams et al.[9] and 0.07% of studies in the Registry report.[3] Neuro-ophthalmologic complications of cardiac catheterization are most commonly caused by artery-to-artery emboli,[17,18] although they can result from thrombus formation on guidewires or catheters.

Prevention of cerebrovascular complications can be accomplished largely by systemic anticoagulation, paying meticulous attention to proper technique of catheter flushing, wiping guidewires free of blood before insertion, and restricting the time for use of guidewires to two minutes at a stretch (after which the wire is removed and wiped, and the catheter aspirated and flushed before re-entry of the wire) even in the patient who has received systemic heparinization. In addition, it is probably wise to avoid advancing the left heart catheter out to the left ventricular apex in patients with suspected left ventricular aneurysm or recent myocardial infarction and possible mural thrombus. Patients with known cerebrovascular disease, diminished or absent carotid pulsations, bruits over the carotids, subclavian, or vertebrobasilar arteries are probably at increased risk for cerebrovascular complications of catheterization. Careful avoidance of unnecessary catheter or guidewire entry into the carotid and vertebrobasilar arteries should reduce the risk of stroke in these patients.

LOCAL BRACHIAL AND FEMORAL COMPLICATIONS

Local arterial complications of cardiac catheterization are a frequently discussed problem.[1–4,10,19–30] Machleder, Sweeney, and Barker reported a 5.4% brachial re-exploration

rate.[22] In a report from Judkins' laboratory,[13] local femoral complications occurred in 16 out of 445 consecutive cases (3.6%). Sones reported 2% to 3% segmental occlusion at the site of arteriotomy.[31] Judkins has emphasized that serious femoral complications are related to the presence of preexisting iliofemoral disease, and that in such patients it is best to avoid a percutaneous femoral approach.[13] Nearly all laboratories have noted that women have a higher incidence of both femoral and brachial arterial thrombosis following cardiac catheterization.[12,24]

A much lower rate of vascular complications (0.46%) was noted in the Registry report,[3] perhaps reflecting technical improvements in recent years.

Brachial Approach. The types of local complication differ with the brachial and femoral approaches. With the brachial approach, arterial thrombosis accounts for the great majority of local complications. This is often related to formation of a thrombus in the proximal arterial segment during the catheterization procedure and failure to effectively remove it prior to arterial repair. Prevention of this complication can be accomplished by routinely using a Fogarty catheter prior to arterial repair,[30] followed by instillation of a heparin solution into the proximal and distal arterial segments to prevent thrombus formation during closure of the arteriotomy. Brachial arterial thrombosis may also develop secondary to an intimal flap that is not properly "tacked down" or removed at the time of arterial repair and creates a small pocket of stasis where a thrombus can form. Occasionally, arterial spasm developing in the hours immediately following catheterization and successful arterial repair will result in secondary arterial thrombosis and convert an initially bounding radial pulse into one that is weak or absent six hours postcatheterization.

Prevention of brachial artery thrombosis can best be accomplished by meticulous attention to the details of arterial repair, which are discussed in Chapter 4. In my practice, adequate heparinization includes systemic administration of heparin (5000 units intravenously) shortly after initial arterial entry and local administration of heparin (1000 to 1500 units into both proximal and distal arterial segments) at the time of arterial repair. Inspection of the arteriotomy site, trimming of any free intimal flaps, and avoidance of arterial narrowing (as frequently occurs with a purse-string closure) will minimize arterial thrombosis. I do not reverse anticoagulation with protamine at the end of a brachial catheterization; if the arterial repair has been done properly, there should not be any local bleeding.

Correction of brachial arterial thrombosis requires re-exploration of the arm incision with repeat brachial arteriotomy, Fogarty catheter thrombectomy, and arterial repair. Although this is usually done by a vascular surgeon in the operating room, cardiologists experienced with the brachial approach may carry out such corrective procedures in the catheterization laboratory. Two recent reports[25,26] describe successful treatment of brachial artery thrombosis by percutaneous transluminal angioplasty from the femoral artery.

Other potential local complications of brachial arterial catheterization include injury to the median nerve during cutdown and isolation of the artery, delayed dehiscence of arterial sutures with late arterial bleeding, bacterial arteritis, and local cellulitis-phlebitis associated with the cutdown itself. Injury to the median nerve is rare and should not occur if the dissection is careful. Rarely, postcatheterization bleeding within the brachial wound may lead to hematoma formation and compression of the nerve. This responds to prompt evacuation of the hematoma. Mild injury to the median nerve results in numbness and weakness of the thenar aspect of the hand, which almost always returns to normal within 3 to 4 weeks, although occasionally some neurologic symptoms may require up to 6 months for complete resolution. Local cellulitis-phlebitis is most likely to occur if (1) there is extensive soft tissue dissection during the brachial cutdown; (2) large veins are used and tied off; (3) the catheterization procedure is long; (4) seroma or hematoma forms in the incision; (5) nonviable tissue (e.g., fat deprived of its blood

supply) is left in the incision; and (6) there is poor surgical technique or violation of sterile procedure. The routine use of a potent germicidal agent (e.g., 1% povidone-iodine solution) for wound irrigation prior to skin closure substantially reduces the incidence of infection. Prophylactic antibiotics are not necessary in the routine case, but I recommend their use in any situation in which a high probability of wound infection exists (e.g., a long procedure in which a known breach of sterile technique occurred). In such instances, oxacillin 500 mg p.o. every six hours for five days beginning at the time of wound closure (initial loading dose given intravenously) is generally adequate.

Femoral Approach. With regard to the femoral approach, potential local complications include arterial or venous thrombosis, distal embolization, false aneurysm, arteriovenous fistulae, hematoma with vascular and neural compression, and delayed hemorrhage.[1–4,9–11,13,19,20,23,24,28,29,32,33]

In general, femoral arterial thrombosis requires urgent surgical intervention. Failure to accomplish this may result in propagation of thrombus into smaller distal branches of the femoral arterial tree, making ultimate restoration of normal perfusion to the limb impossible and necessitating amputation. Distal embolization represents a difficult problem, which is fortunately rare with the routine use of anticoagulants.

False aneurysm, which represents pulsating encapsulated hematoma in communication with a ruptured artery, generally develops when there has been improper groin compression following removal of the arterial catheter. Auscultation generally reveals a systolic bruit over the puncture site, which, combined with the finding of a pulsatile mass, makes the diagnosis of false aneurysm almost certain.[19] These aneurysms are painful and almost invariably rupture, although rupture may not occur until several days (or even weeks) following catheterization. Surgical intervention is necessary to correct the problem in all cases. An example of a false aneurysm of the femoral artery is shown in Figure 3–1.

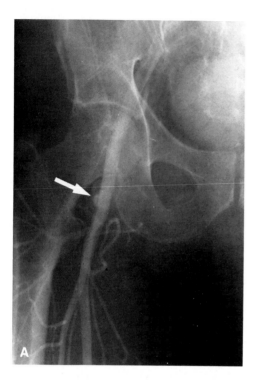 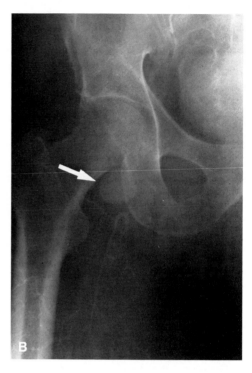

Fig. 3–1.   False aneurysm of right femoral artery (arrows) which developed 4 to 5 days following percutaneous retrograde femoral arterial catheterization complicated by a significant postcompression local hematoma after groin compression. (A) Arterial injection. (B) Residual contrast seen in the aneurysm during the washout phase.

Pseudoaneurysm and arteriovenous fistula often represent the result of an inappropriately low femoral puncture,[20] inadequate control during catheter removal, or impaired clotting function (see Chapter 5). Diagnosis of femoral arterial complications has recently been aided by the use of color flow echocardiographic imaging,[21] but the important first step is careful examination of the groin 1 to 2 days after the procedure.

Delayed hemorrhage may result from false aneurysm, but more commonly it results from either poor clot formation or premature ambulation. Patients with defective platelet function (e.g., those with uremia) or who are receiving systemic anticoagulants may exhibit delayed bleeding or hemorrhage.[23] Premature activity, particularly if it is associated with a substantial rise in blood pressure, may dislodge the platelet-fibrin plug from the arterial puncture site and cause arterial bleeding. Most laboratories require at least 6 hours of bed rest following femoral arterial catheterization, and many require 12 to 18 hours of bed rest.

Femoral venous thrombosis is a potential complication of right heart catheterization from the femoral venous approach, and I have seen an instance of pulmonary embolism in one such case. Iliac vein thrombosis may be more common in pediatric practice, especially when repeated venous catheterization procedures may be done in cyanotic, polycythemic patients. Thrombosis of the lower portion of the inferior vena cava, iliac, or femoral veins was reported in 22 children out of a total of 1043 (2.1%) who had undergone serial cardiac catheterizations.[33]

Local infection is rare with the percutaneous femoral approach.

Local arterial complications can be minimized by paying meticulous attention to the details of arterial entry and repair. It is generally acknowledged that the incidence of thrombosis is related to the duration of the procedure (especially the "arterial time"), the number of catheters used, and the presence of underlying atherosclerotic disease. Claudication of the arm or leg following cardiac catheterization is not unheard of, and if distal arterial pulses are feeble or absent following catheterization, surgical exploration should be performed.

PERFORATION OF THE HEART OR GREAT VESSELS

Perforation of the heart or intrathoracic great vessels has been reported with cardiac catheterization. In the Cooperative Study,[1] 100 patients (0.8%) had perforation of the heart or great vessels. Seventy-six of these were cardiac perforations (0.6%), and the most common sites were the right atrium (33 cases), right ventricle (21 cases), left atrium (10 cases), and left ventricle (12 cases). Thirty of the 33 right atrial perforations were related to transseptal catheterization; thus, the right ventricle is the commonest site of cardiac perforation in patients undergoing catheterization by techniques other than transseptal. In our experience, the risk of cardiac perforation is greatest in elderly women ($\geq$65 years) undergoing right heart catheterization. Stiff catheters (such as NIH or Gorlin pacing catheters) should be avoided in these patients, and inexperienced individuals (e.g., trainees with less than four months' experience in right heart catheterization) should defer to senior personnel in such cases. Perforation of the subclavian artery, iliac artery, abdominal aorta, or great veins has been reported and is generally associated with excessive catheter manipulation. In many such instances, catheter manipulation was continued despite resistance to passage or complaints by the patient of pain related to the catheter passage.

Eshagy and co-workers[34] reported mediastinal and retropharyngeal hemorrhage as a complication of retrograde brachial left heart catheterization in two patients. Both patients were receiving anticoagulants prior to catheterization (prothrombin times were 42 and 23 seconds), and in both cases there was difficulty in catheter manipulation from the subclavian artery to the ascending aorta. Treatment with maintenance of an adequate airway, correction of hypoprothrombinemia, and blood replacement was successful in both cases.

Perforation of the heart is the main hazard of transseptal catheterization because the procedure actually entails controlled perforation of the interatrial septum. Unintentional perforation of the aorta, atrial wall, coronary sinus, or right atrial appendage may occur, leading to cardiac tamponade. Balloon valvuloplasty is associated with an increased incidence of cardiac perforation.[4] For balloon mitral valvuloplasty, this may be associated with transseptal catheterization. With aortic valvuloplasty, guidewire perforation of the left ventricle has been observed to occur,[4] and may lead to cardiac tamponade. Perforation of the heart is the major complication of endomyocardial biopsy and will be discussed in Chapter 24.

VASOVAGAL REACTIONS

Vasovagal or so-called vagal reactions are common and may be serious. In our experience,[4] mild vasovagal reactions occurred in 41 (1.4%) of 2883 diagnostic or therapeutic catheterization procedures, and moderate or severe vasovagal reactions were rare (0.1%). They are frequently (but not always) incited by *pain* in a tense, anxious patient and consist of nausea, hypotension, and bradycardia. In older patients the entire picture of a vagal reaction may be present *without the bradycardia*. The mechanism of the reaction is presumed to be sudden peripheral vasodilatation involving arterioles and venules, unaccompanied by a compensatory increase in cardiac output.[35] Vagal reactions respond dramatically to intravenous atropine, 0.5 to 1.0 mg (*and* to cessation of catheter manipulation) if they are recognized promptly. Elevation of the legs is a helpful adjunct to the treatment of vagal hypotension in the supine patient and generally results in partial correction of hypotension within 10 to 15 seconds; by this time the atropine is usually taking effect. If the hypotension and bradycardia of a vagal reaction are permitted to persist for any period of time, serious arrhythmias or irreversible shock may develop, particularly in patients with ischemic heart disease or aortic stenosis.

ARRHYTHMIA AND CONDUCTION DISTURBANCE

Major arrhythmias occurred in 1.2% of cardiac catheterizations in the Cooperative Study,[1] and included ventricular fibrillation (59 cases, 0.4%), ventricular tachycardia (12 cases, 0.10%), asystole or marked bradycardia (37 cases, 0.30%), complete heart block (7 cases, 0.06%), and supraventricular arrhythmia (35 cases, 0.28%), among other arrhythmias. In studies reflecting the current predominance of patients with coronary artery disease in catheterization laboratories, ventricular fibrillation was reported in 1.28% (600 instances in a total of 46,904 cases) of patients undergoing coronary angiography in the survey of Adams and co-workers.[9] Ventricular fibrillation, tachycardia, or asystole occurred in 0.77% of 5,250 patients undergoing left heart catheterization and coronary arteriography at the Montreal Heart Institute between 1970 and 1974.[12] In the most recent Registry report from the Society of Cardiac Angiography,[3] arrhythmias requiring treatment occurred in 0.47% of patients. There is some evidence that ventricular fibrillation during coronary angiography is associated with prolongation of the precatheterization QT interval.[36] As a related observation, administration of atropine intravenously has been reported[37] to reduce the incidence of sustained ventricular arrhythmias during coronary angiography, perhaps related to altered autonomic tone.

Arrhythmias may occur with either right or left heart catheterization. Balloon-flotation right heart catheterization is by no means free of risk of serious arrhythmias. In a prospective study of 150 bedside pulmonary artery catheterizations using balloon-flotation catheters,[38] ventricular salvos (3 to 5 consecutive ventricular depolarizations) occurred in 30% of insertions, nonsustained ventricular tachycardia (5 to 30 ventricular premature beats in a row) occurred in 22% of insertions, "sustained" ventricular tachycardia (>30 beats in sequence) occurred in 3%, and 2/150 insertions were complicated by ventricular fibrillation. A new right bundle branch block was noted in 5% of insertions and lasted an average of 9.5 hours.

In general, serious ventricular arrhythmias occur in two situations: (1) with excessive catheter manipulation within the left or right ventricular chambers, especially in a patient with resting ventricular irritability, or (2) suddenly, following coronary artery contrast injection, especially of the right coronary artery. Those that occur in the second situation give the impression of being idiosyncratic reactions because the patients may have normal coronary anatomy. Their incidence may be reduced by injecting the smallest amount of radiographic contrast agent sufficient to opacify the arterial tree.

Complete heart block has been reported from several laboratories as a complication of cardiac catheterization.[39,40] It is most commonly seen during right heart catheterization in a patient with preexisting left bundle branch block (LBBB), when the sudden development of transient right bundle branch block (RBBB) during passage of a catheter from the right ventricle to the pulmonary artery leaves the patient with no mechanism for conduction of atrial impulses to the ventricles. Unless an adequate ventricular escape focus takes over, profound hypotension and asystole may occur. The availability of either a standby external or internal pacemaker is mandatory in such cases,[40] and we commonly use a pacing catheter (e.g., 7 Fr balloon-tipped catheters with distal electrodes [Baim-Turi, USCI, Billerica, MA]) for right heart catheterizations in patients with preexisting LBBB. A study from our laboratory, however, shows that *prophylactically* inserted pacing catheters are both costly and infrequently needed.[41] Left bundle branch block can develop during retrograde left ventricular catheterization, and if this occurs in the setting of pre-existing right bundle branch block, complete heart block with asystole may ensue. Withdrawal of the left or right heart catheters to the aorta or right atrium, respectively, is usually followed by restoration of a normal conduction pattern. I am aware, however, of one case in which a Sones catheter in the left ventricle was used to rhythmically tap the ventricular endocardium, thereby producing a regular series of ventricular ectopic beats and maintaining blood pressure while a pacing catheter was being readied for advancement to the right ventricle.

Atrial arrhythmias that occur during cardiac catheterization are generally atrial fibrillation or flutter. Again, a common precipitating cause is excessive catheter manipulation in the right atrium, where multiple atrial extrasystoles commonly precede the development of atrial fibrillation or flutter. Both arrhythmias usually revert spontaneously to sinus rhythm, but external cardioversion may be necessary in some cases. In patients requiring a right heart or coronary sinus catheterization who are felt to have a higher risk for developing atrial fibrillation (e.g., a history of paroxysmal atrial fibrillation, frequent atrial extrasystoles at rest, increased left or right atrial pressures), a single dose of quinidine or procainamide 1 to 2 hours before the scheduled catheterization procedure may help prevent atrial fibrillation.

PHLEBITIS, INFECTIONS, FEVER

Phlebitis, fever, or local infection occurs in fewer than 1% of cardiac catheterizations, and some of the causes and predisposing factors have been discussed previously. The phlebitis, usually minor, almost always responds to hot soaks and elevation of the affected limb. Fever is rare and usually transient; it may represent pyrogen reaction, allergy to contrast agent, or systemic reaction to local phlebitis or infection. Bacterial endocarditis as a complication of cardiac catheterization is rare. As mentioned previously, although some laboratories routinely use antibiotic prophylaxis, most do

not, and I do not favor routine use of antibiotics before catheterization. Paying careful attention to sterile technique and cleansing the brachial wound with copious quantites of sterile saline followed by 1% aqueous iodine-povidone solution will minimize the incidence of these complications.

PYROGEN REACTIONS

Pyrogen reactions are not commented upon in most reported series of cardiac catheterization. The Cooperative Study mentions two cases.[1] Pyrogen reactions result from the introduction of foreign protein, endotoxin, or other antigenically active substances into the blood. A series of cases occurring within a single laboratory should raise suspicion of contamination in the catheter or instrument sterilization procedures. In one such epidemic,[42] an increase in the incidence of fever and chills in association with cardiac catheterization was traced to contamination of the hospital distilled water reservoir with acinetobacteria calcoaceticus and a pseudomonas species. Sterilization killed the bacteria but left endotoxin coated on the internal lumen of the catheters, and when this was flushed into the circulation during catheterizaton and angiography, a pyrogen reaction resulted. Endotoxin may be detected with either the limulus lysate assay or a rabbit pyrogen test.[42]

A typical pyrogen reaction consists of rigors with subsequent development of fever and may follow intravascular injections or angiograms by intervals ranging from 1 to 60 minutes. The rigors can be severe, and temperatures in excess of 102°F may be seen. In my experience the clinical manifestations of these reactions have often responded dramatically to small intravenous doses of morphine (e.g., 2 to 4 mg IV), repeated as necessary. Catheterization should be discontinued with the development of such reactions, since the source of the pyrogenic material is rarely immediately obvious. Careful cleaning and preparation of catheters and instruments are generally all that is required to minimize the occurrence of these reactions, should there be a strong reason to consider catheter reuse. The almost universal practice of using disposable catheters, stopcocks, and other equipment, however, has virtually eliminated the problem of pyrogen reactions.

HYPOTENSION

Hypotension during cardiac catheterization is generally a consequence of one of the complications already discussed (such as vagal reaction or myocardial infarction). However, hypotension may develop following left ventriculography because of the vasodepressor properties of the contrast agent (dilation of systemic arterioles and venules) as well as its myocardial depressant properties. Such hypotension is usually transient and passes within 30 seconds. On occasion it may persist longer and usually responds to elevation of the legs and expansion of intravascular volume with half-normal saline solution.

Postcatheterization hypotension may develop in the patient who has received large amounts of radiographic contrast agent at catheterization, in whom postcatheterization diuresis (the hyperosmolar contrast material acts as an osmotic diuretic) combines with continued vasodepressor effect to cause relative hypovolemia. The hypotension of such patients is associated almost invariably with *normal* or *increased warmth of the skin,* suggesting that paresis of vasomotor regulation persists as long as contrast agent remains in the circulation. Such postcatheterization hypotension virtually always has a major orthostatic component and usually responds promptly to fluid administration and the supine or Trendelenberg position. In my experience, women of asthenic build with a history of chronic "low blood pressure" are particularly susceptible to this complication and may exhibit blood pressures of 70 to 80 mm Hg during the first 6 hours following catheterization and angiography. The administration of colloid-containing solutions (Plasmanate, dextran) may be helpful in cases that fail to respond to increased rate of crystalloid administered intravenously. The hypotension usually resolves

after the radiographic contrast agent is "washed out" of the circulation by way of the kidneys.

Other causes to be considered in the patient with postcatheterization hypotension include delayed cardiac tamponade caused by gradual leak from unrecognized cardiac perforation produced at the time of catheterization and blood loss because of hemorrhage from the arterial puncture site or from an internal vascular perforation.

ELECTRICAL HAZARDS

Electrical hazards have been reported in association with cardiac catheterization, including fatal ventricular fibrillation.[43] With the present standard use of isolation transformers and equipotential environment, such events are rare.

OTHER COMPLICATIONS

Pulmonary edema developing during cardiac catheterization is rare and usually related to (1) a new untoward cardiac event (e.g., acute myocardial infarction); (2) the stress of angiographic contrast material; (3) the recumbent position; or (4) other factors in a patient with already compromised left ventricular function. The Cooperative Study[1] described four patients who experienced this complication. Bourassa reports this complication in four patients (0.1%) following coronary angiography at the Montreal Heart Institute.[12] This complication usually responds promptly to (1) helping the patient to sit up, (2) administering an intravenous diuretic (e.g., 20 to 40 mg furosemide), and (3) oxygen by mask. If there is not prompt evidence of major improvement (within three minutes), consideration of more aggressive therapy (e.g., sodium nitroprusside if the arterial systolic pressure is 120 mm Hg or more, and intra-aortic balloon counterpulsation if there is associated hypotension) is in order.

Pulmonary artery perforation and pulmonary hemorrhage associated with use of the flow-directed balloon-tipped catheter have been reported from several laboratories.[44–48] Several of these cases were fatal. Overinflation of the balloon and excessive time in "wedge" (balloon inflated) position appear to have been factors. This complication seems to be more likely to occur in women, elderly persons, and those with pulmonary hypertension. Giving careful attention to the instructions in Chapter 7 of this textbook will prevent this complication. Other complications reported in association with the flow-directed balloon-tipped catheter include arrhythmias (discussed above), ruptured chordae of the tricuspid valve,[49] pulmonary thromboembolism,[50] and intracardiac knotting of the catheter.[51] Again, careful adherence to proper technique (Chapter 7) should prevent (or at least minimize) the occurrence of such complications with this catheter.

Coronary artery dissection is a rare complication of cardiac catheterization.[52–54] This seems to be more common with the right coronary artery and may result from vigorous injection of a jet of contrast agent against an atherosclerotic plaque, or from excessive force of catheter tip entry into the coronary ostium.

Morise and co-workers have reported 3 cases of coronary artery dissection secondary to coronary angiography and have reviewed 39 additional cases reported in the literature.[54] Their 3 patients were young women (37, 40, and 42 years old), without significant atherosclerotic coronary narrowing. From their cases and review of the literature they concluded that catheter-induced coronary dissection can occur with either brachial or femoral approach and is more likely to occur in the right coronary artery and in women under age 45 with minimal atheromatous disease. Most left coronary dissections result in infarction.

Cholesterol embolization leading to renal failure has occurred from retrograde femoral arterial catheterization of the aorta.[55,56] Characteristically, the renal insufficiency develops slowly (weeks to months) and progressively following the catheterization, and renal biopsy specimens show intravascular cholesterol crystals. Evidence of peripheral embolization, such as livido reticularis or ischemia of the toes, may be present: again, these may develop only after a considerable time interval (weeks) following catheterization. Eosinophilia is often present and episodic hypertension is also a frequent finding. The prognosis is not good, and renal insufficiency commonly progresses to complete and permanent renal failure.

Systemic or pulmonary embolization of vegetations is a potential hazard of cardiac catheterization in patients with endocarditis of the left- or right-sided cardiac valves. Although often discussed, there is little if any evidence that catheter-induced dislodgement of vegetations occurs. Welton and co-workers reviewed their experience with 35 patients who underwent catheterization for severe heart failure (30 patients) and persistent sepsis or recurrent embolization (5 patients) during active endocarditis. Catheterization-induced embolization did not occur in any of these 35 patients.[57] They concluded that catheterization can be performed safely and yields important information in patients with active endocarditis who are being considered for surgical intervention.

Pulmonary embolism can occur after cardiac catheterization, and a study comparing the incidence of new focal pulmonary embolism after brachial and femoral catheterization has been reported.[58] Using ventilation-perfusion scans before and one day after catheterization, an 8.3% incidence of new perfusion defects was seen after retrograde femoral catheterization (combined left and right heart), but no new defects occurred with brachial catheterization.

Severe protamine reactions that simulate anaphylaxis have been reported in association with cardiac catheterization.[59] These reactions tend to occur immediately after administration of protamine intravenously, which is used for reversing systemic heparinization after percutaneous femoral catheterization. The reactions consist of profound hypotension with dyspnea, wheezing, and circulatory collapse. Death may ensue, although most patients respond to epinephrine and supportive measures. In one study, protamine reactions were much more likely to occur in diabetics who had been receiving NPH insulin, occurring in 27% of these patients.[59] A more recent study[60] has failed to confirm this observation, however, and found it safe to administer protamine sulfate to diabetics with prior exposure to protamine if the dose administered at catheterization was 50 mg or less. Until this issue is clarified, patients who have been receiving NPH insulin, as well as those with a history of allergy to fish, should not receive protamine if at all possible.

Catheter entanglement in a cardiac valve prosthesis is a dreaded complication of left or right heart catheterization. Certain prosthetic valves (e.g., Starr-Edwards caged-ball valves, porcine xenograft valves) can be crossed safely retrograde or antegrade with a variety of catheters or guidewires. Tilting disc valves such as the Bjork-Shiley valve or St. Jude valve, however, should *not* be crossed lest the catheter or guidewire become trapped between the disc and the small orifice. When this happens, prosthetic valve dysfunction may be severe and can lead to death[61] if immediate surgery is not undertaken to remove the trapped catheter.

GENERAL CONSIDERATIONS

Caseload. At least one report has found an inverse correlation between the *caseload* of a cardiac catheterization laboratory and its incidence of major complications.[9] With regard to coronary angiographic procedures, the mortality rate in institutions performing fewer than 100 procedures per year was eight times higher than in institutions performing more than 400 procedures per year.[9] These data were interpreted to mean that greater caseload per physician leads to greater skill and technical proficiency and fewer complications. This important conclusion, which has influenced the ICHD report on optional resources for cardiac catheterization and angiography,[62] has been challenged by a study of eight cardiac catheterization laboratories in the State of Washington.[63] That study found an extremely low rate of major complications in association with coronary angiography, even though the

caseload/laboratory (average 50 to 250 cases/year) and caseload/angiographer (average 65 cases/year) was low. These authors suggest that skill can be maintained even without a large caseload and that the low complication rates of some laboratories with high volume may primarily reflect liberal indications for the procedure and relatively small numbers of patients with high-risk conditions (e.g., left main coronary disease, unstable angina, overt left ventricular failure). This complex and important issue cannot be resolved on the basis of current data.

Speed. The *speed* with which a catheterization procedure is accomplished is also widely regarded as a determinant of the risk of complications. Unfortunately, there are few data on this subject. The Cooperative Study[1] analyzed the duration of catheterization procedures in 16 participating laboratories and found that there was a bell-shaped curve with the most common duration being 2.0 to 3.0 hours (5022 cases, 41% of total procedures, median = 2.5 hours), with 4207 procedures (34%) lasting 1.0 to 2.0 hours, and 2054 procedures (17%) lasting between 3 and 4 hours. Procedures accomplished under 1 hour and those that took longer than 5 hours accounted for 1.9% and 2.8% of total cases, respectively. Data compiled in our laboratory show that the average time required (from the administration of xylocaine to that of protamine, using the femoral approach) is 67 minutes for a procedure including right and left heart catheterization, left ventricular angiography, and coronary angiography. No attempt was made in the Cooperative Study[1] to relate duration of procedure to major complications. Duration of a cardiac catheterization procedure may be prolonged by factors that tend to be associated with a high risk of complication. For example, the elderly patient with extensive atherosclerosis and arterial tortuosity may have a long procedure because of technical difficulties associated with catheter passage in such patients. There may also be an increased risk of complications in such patients because they frequently have more extensive disease and diminished reserve. In this instance the high risk is not necessarily caused by the increased duration of the procedure: the two are ''true, true; unrelated.'' Similarly, a young patient with normal vessels and minimal cardiac disease may have a rapid catheterization procedure, but speed of the procedure in this instance cannot fairly be credited with the low risk. In my view, duration of the procedure is an important ''independent'' risk factor only when it can clearly be related to lack of skill or inexperience of the operator or when severe cardiac decompensation requires that the patient spend minimal time in the supine position.

Pseudocomplications. Finally, a word relevant to ''pseudocomplications'' of cardiac catheterization is in order.[64,65] Patients suffering from serious cardiac disease experience major cardiac events (myocardial infarction, ventricular arrhythmia, systemic embolus) as part of the natural history of their disease. If one of these events happens to occur during or within 24 hours of a scheduled cardiac catheterization, is it fair to always regard it as a complication of the procedure? Hildner and co-workers[64,65] examined events that occurred from 24 hours before to 72 hours after scheduled catheterizations. The incidence of ''pseudocomplications'' or events occurring in the 24 hours prior to catheterization was 0.81%, including 0.24% deaths. During the same period there was a 0.81% incidence of catheterization procedure-related complications with no deaths. Thus it is clear that the incidence of complications after cardiac catheterization is influenced by rate of occurrence of unexpected major cardiac events and the natural history of the patient's basic cardiac disease.

REFERENCES

1. Braunwald E, Swan HJC (eds): Cooperative study on cardiac catheterization. Circulation 37 (Suppl. III):1, 1968.
2. Kennedy JW, et al: Complications associated with cardiac catheterization and angiography. Cathet Cardiovasc Diagn 8:5, 1982.
3. Johnson W, et al: Coronary angiography 1984–1987: A report of the Registry of the Society for Cardiac Angiography and Interventions. I. Results and complications. Cathet Cardiovasc Diagn 17:5, 1989.
4. Wyman RM, et al: Current complications of diagnostic and therapeutic cardiac catheterization. J Am Coll Cardiol 12:1400, 1988.
5. Lozner E, et al: Coronary arteriography 1984–1987: A report of the Registry of the Society for Cardiac Angiography and Interventions. 2. An analysis of 218 deaths related to coronary angiography. Cathet Cardiovasc Diagn 17:11, 1989.
6. Folland ED, et al: Complications of cardiac catheterization and angiography in patients with valvular heart disease. Cathet Cardiovasc Diagn 17:15, 1989.
7. Walson WJ, Lee GB, Amplatz K: Biplane selective coronary arteriography via percutaneous transfemoral approach. Am J Roentgen 100:332, 1967.
8. Takaro T, Hultgren HN, Littman D, Wright EC: An analysis of deaths occurring in association with coronary arteriography. Am Heart J 86:587, 1973.
9. Adams DF, Fraser DB, Abrams HL: The complications of coronary arteriography. Circulation 48:609, 1973.
10. Freed MD, Keane JF, Rosenthal A: The use of heparinization to prevent arterial thrombosis after percutaneous cardiac catheterization in children. Circulation 50:565, 1974.
11. Judkins MP, Gander MP: Prevention of complications of coronary arteriography. Circulation 49:599, 1974.
12. Bourassa MG, Noble J: Complication rate of coronary arteriography. A review of 5250 cases studied by percutaneous femoral technique. Circulation 53:106, 1976.
13. Green GS, McKinnon CM, Rosch J, Judkins MP: Complications of selective percutaneous transfemoral coronary arteriography and their prevention. Circulation 45:552, 1972.
14. Burckhardt D, Vera CA, LaDue JS, Steinberg I: Enzyme activity following angiography. Am J Roentgen 102:406, 1968.
15. Michie DD, Conley MA, Carretta RF, Booth RW: Serum enzyme changes following cardiac catheterization with and without selective coronary arteriography. Am J Med Sci 260:11, 1970.
16. Roberts R, Ludbrook PA, Weiss ES, Sobel BE: Serum CPK isoenzymes after cardiac catheterization. Br Heart J 37:144, 1975.
17. Kosmorsky G, Hanson MR, Tomsak RL: Neuro-ophthalmologic complications of cardiac catheterization. Neurology 38:483, 1988.
18. Oliva A, Scherokman B: Two cases of occipital infarction following cardiac catheterization. Stroke 19:773, 1988.
19. Skillman JJ, Kim D, Baim DS: Vascular complications of percutaneous femoral cardiac interventions. Arch Surg 123:1207, 1988.
20. Altin RS, Flicker S, Naidech HJ: Pseudo-aneurysm and arteriovenous fistula after femoral artery catheterization: Associated with low femoral punctures. Am J Radiol 152:629, 1989.
21. Sheikh KH, et al: Utility of color flow imaging for identification of femoral arterial complications of cardiac catheterization. Am Heart J 117:623, 1989.
22. Machelder HI, Sweeney JP, Barker JF: Pulseless arm after brachial artery catheterization. Lancet 1:407, 1972.
23. Bristow JD, et al: Late, heparin-induced bleeding af-

ter retrograde arterial catheterization. Circulation 37:393, 1968.

24. Kloster FE, Bristow JD, Griswold HE: Femoral artery occlusion following percutaneous catheterization. Am Heart J 79:175, 1970.

25. Angelini P, Bush HS: Brachial artery injury as a complication of cardiac catheterization: Percutaneous transluminal angioplasty and streptokinase as a treatment alternative. Cathet Cardiovasc Diagn 15:245, 1988.

26. Maouad J, Guermonprez JL: Percutaneous femoral angioplasty of a right brachial artery occluded after Sones coronary angiography. Cathet Cardiovasc Diagn 14:165, 1988.

27. Nicholas GG, DeMuth WE: Long term results of brachial thrombectomy following cardiac catheterization. Ann Surg 183:436, 1976.

28. Takahashi O: The effects of transfemoral cardiac catheterization on limb blood flow in children. Chest 71:159, 1977.

29. Rosengart R, Nelson RJ, Emmanoulides GC. Anterior tibial compartment syndrome in a child: an unusual complication of cardiac catheterization. Pediatrics 58:456, 1976.

30. Baker LD, Leshin SJ, Mathur VS, Messer JV: Routine Fogarty thrombectomy in arterial catheterization. N Engl J Med 279:1203, 1968.

31. Sones FM Jr: Cine coronary arteriography. *In* Hurst JW, Logue RB, (eds): The Heart. 2nd ed. New York, McGraw-Hill Book Company, 1970, p 377.

32. Stanger P: Complications of cardiac catheterization of neonates, infants and children. Circulation 50:595, 1974.

33. Mathews RA, et al: Iliac venous thrombosis in infants and children after cardiac catheterization. Cathet Cardiovasc Diagn 5:67, 1979.

34. Eshagy B, et al: Medastinal and retropharyngeal hemorrhage: a complication of cardiac catheterization. JAMA 226:427, 1973.

35. Weissler AM, Warren JV: Vasodepressor syncope. Am Heart J 57:786, 1959.

36. Arrowood JA, Mullan DF, Kline RA, Engel TR, Kowey PR: Ventricular fibrillation during coronary angiography: the precatheterization QT interval. J Electrocardiol 20:255, 1987.

37. Lehmann KG, Chen YC: Reduction of ventricular arrhythmias by atropine during coronary angiography. Am J Cardiol 63:447, 1989.

38. Sprung CL, et al: Advanced ventricular arrhythmias during bedside pulmonary artery catheterizations. Am J Med 72:203, 1982.

39. Gupta PK, Haft JI: Complete heart block complicating cardiac catheterization. Chest 61:185, 1972.

40. Sprung CL, et al.: Risk of right bundle branch block and complete heart block during pulmonary artery catheterization. Crit Care Med 17:1, 1989.

41. Harvey JR, Wyman RM, McKay RG, Baim DS: Use of balloon flotation pacing catheters for prophylactic temporary pacing during diagnostic and therapeutic catheterization procedures. Am J Cardiol 62:941, 1988.

42. Reyes MP, et al: Pyrogenic reactions after inadvertent infusion of endotoxin during cardiac catheterizations. Ann Intern Med 93:32, 1980.

43. Starmer CF, McIntosh HD, Whalen RE: Electrical hazards and cardiovascular function. N Engl J Med 284:181, 1971.

44. Golden MS, Pinder T Jr, Anderson WT, Cheitlin MD: Fatal pulmonary hemorrhage complicating use of a flow-directed balloon-tipped catheter in a patient receiving anticoagulant therapy. Am J Cardiol 32:865, 1973.

45. Chun CHM, Ellestad MH: Perforation of the pulmonary artery by a Swan-Ganz catheter. N Engl J Med 284:1041, 1971.

46. Pope LA, et al: Fatal pulmonary hemorrhage after use of the flow-directed balloon-tipped catheter. Ann Intern Med 90:344, 1979.

47. Foote GA, Schabel SI, Hodges M: Pulmonary complications of the flow-directed balloon-tipped catheter. N Engl J Med 290:927, 1974.

48. McDaniel DD, et al: Catheter-induced pulmonary artery hemorrhage. J Thorac Cardiovasc Surg 82:1, 1981.

49. Smith WR, Glauser FL, Jemison P: Ruptured chordae of the tricuspid valve: The consequence of flow directed Swan Ganz catheterization. Chest 70:790, 1976.

50. Goodman DJ, Rider AK, Billingham ME, Schroeder JS: Thromboembolic complications with the indwelling balloon tipped pulmonary arterial catheter. N Engl J Med 291:777, 1974.

51. Lipp H, O'Donoghue K, Resnekov L: Intracardiac knotting of a flow-directed balloon-tipped catheter. N Engl J Med 284:220, 1972.

52. Meller J, Friedman D, Dack S, Herman MV: Coronary artery dissection—a complication of cardiac catheterization without sequelae: case report and review of the literature. Cath Cardiovasc Diagn 2:301, 1976.

53. Haas JM, Peterson CR, Jones RC: Subintimal dissection of the coronary arteries: a complication of selective coronary arteriography and the transfemoral percutaneous approach. Circulation 38:678, 1968.

54. Morise AP, Hardin NJ, Bovill EG, Grundel WD: Coronary artery dissection secondary to coronary arteriography. Cathet Cardiovasc Diagn 7:283, 1981.

55. Colt HG, et al: Cholesterol emboli after cardiac catheterization. Eight cases and a review of the literature. Medicine (Baltimore) 67:389, 1988.

56. Gaines DA, et al: Cholesterol embolization: a lethal complication of vascular catheterization. Lancet 1(8578):168, 1988.

57. Welton DE, et al: Value and safety of cardiac catheterization during active infective endocarditis. Am J Cardiol 44:1306, 1979.

58. Gowda S, Bollis AM, Haikal AM, Salem BI. Incidence of new focal pulmonary emboli after routine cardiac catheterization comparing the brachial to the femoral approach. Cathet Cardiovasc Diagn 10:157, 1984.

59. Stewart WJ, McSweeney SM, Kellet MA, Faxon DB, Ryan TJ: Increased risk of severe protamine reactions in NPH insulin dependent diabetics undergoing cardiac catheterization. Circulation 70:788, 1984.

60. Reed DC, Gascho JA: The safety of protamine sulfate in diabetics undergoing cardiac catheterization. Cathet Cardiovasc Diagn 14:19, 1988.

61. Kober G, Hilgermann R: Catheter entrapment in a

Bjork-Shiley prosthesis in aortic position. Cathet Cardiovasc Diagn 13:262, 1987.

62. Friesinger GC, et al: Optimal resources for examination of the heart and lungs. Cardiac catheterization and radiographic facilities. Circulation 68:893A, 1983.

63. Hansing CE, et al: Cardiac catheterization experience in hospitals without cardiovascular surgery programs. Cathet Cardiovasc Diagn 3:207, 1977.

64. Hildner FJ, Javier RP, Ramaswamy K: Pseudocomplications of cardiac catheterization. Chest 63:15, 1973.

65. Hildner FJ, Javier RP, Tolentino A, Samet P: Pseudocomplications of cardiac catheterization: update. Cathet Cardiovasc Diagn 8:43, 1982.

Part II

Techniques of Cardiac Catheterization

4

Cardiac Catheterization by Direct Exposure of Artery and Vein

WILLIAM GROSSMAN

After the question of indications and contraindications has been settled and the properly premedicated patient arrives at the laboratory, the catheterization protocol is transformed into action. This chapter and Chapters 5 and 7 will deal with techniques predominantly used in the catheterization of adults and older children. Special considerations in infants and smaller children will be discussed in Chapter 6.

In our laboratory the patient is usually transferred from the stretcher to a flat carbon-fiber table top that is comfortably padded. Electrocardiogram (ECG) leads are placed, and the patient is then draped. The pertinent areas (antecubital fossae, groins) are scrubbed with 1% povidone-iodine solution or another suitable antiseptic solution.

Before proceeding to the actual catheterization, it is our policy to obtain a full 12-lead ECG at this point and to place an intravenous line in the arm opposite that through which the catheterization is planned. These tasks can be accomplished by the catheterization laboratory nurse or a properly trained technician. The intravenous line can be used for administering drugs (such as heparin or atropine) during catheterization and fluids following catheterization. The ECG should be examined by the physician who will perform the catheteriza-

tion, and the procedure is aborted if any significant changes (e.g., evidence of new myocardial infarction, arrhythmia) have developed since the last previous ECG.

The remainder of this chapter will provide a detailed description of cardiac catheterization by direct surgical exposure and cannulation of brachial artery and vein. *Percutaneous* catheterization of brachial vessels is described, along with percutaneous femoral catheterization, in Chapter 5.

INCISION, ISOLATION OF VESSELS, AND CATHETER INSERTION

With the direct brachial approach I favor a single cutdown in the right antecubital fossa through which both right and left heart catheterizations are performed. The brachial artery is identified by palpation (Fig. 4–1), and local anesthesia is induced (I use 2% lidocaine), first through a short 25- or 27-gauge needle to raise an intradermal bleb, and then through a long (1½-inch) 22-gauge needle to infiltrate the subcutaneous, deep fascial, and periosteal tissues.

When inducing local anesthesia, it is important to remember that *slow injection* is less painful and produces better tissue infiltration. We use liberal amounts of lidocaine, 5 to 15

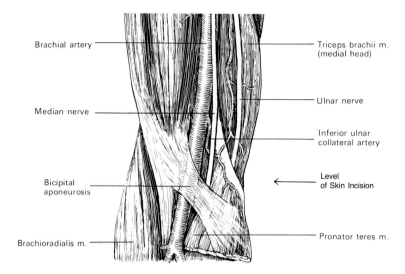

Brachial artery

Median nerve

Bicipital
aponeurosis

Brachioradialis m.

Triceps brachii m.
(medial head)

Ulnar nerve

Inferior ulnar
collateral artery

Level
of Skin Incision

Pronator teres m.

Fig. 4–1. Anatomy of antecubital fossa illustrating course of the brachial artery. The artery is best sought at or slightly above the antecubital skin crease, medial to the bicipital aponeurosis. Care must be taken not to disturb the median nerve, which usually lies medial to the brachial artery. (From Clemente, C.: Gray's Anatomy of the Human Body, 30th American ed. Philadelphia, Lea & Febiger, 1985.)

ml initially, repeating frequently so that 15 to 20 ml are commonly administered in the course of a catheterization. If anesthetization is done properly, the catheter insertion site ought to be virtually painless throughout the procedure.

Next, a transverse incision is made with a number 15 surgical blade just proximal to the flexor crease. If right and left heart catheterizations are contemplated, the incision is wide and made over the palpable brachial artery; if right heart study alone is planned, the incision is narrow and made directly over a previously identified *medial* vein. Those who ignore this latter dictum soon learn that the large plump veins of the lateral antecubital fossae usually drain into the cephalic system, through which it may be difficult to navigate the catheter into the right atrium. The medial veins drain into either the basilic or brachial venous systems, both of which join the axillary vein by direct continuation and are thus easy routes to the superior vena cava and right atrium (Fig. 4–2).

The operator should stand between the patient's arm and chest during the cutdown, so that his line of vision within the incision is angled from medial to lateral. This is important because the brachial artery usually lies below the bicipital aponeurosis and will be visualized only as the aponeurosis is lifted and retracted laterally. Standing at the outside (lateral) aspect of the arm makes it more likely that the first structure seen and isolated by the operator will be the median nerve, and this must be avoided.

The tissues are separated by blunt dissection with a curved Kelly forceps (this and the other instruments that I use in a brachial catheterization are shown in Fig. 4–3) and an appropriate vein is brought to the surface, separated from adjacent nerves and fascia, and tagged proximally and distally with 3-0 or 4-0 silk. The brachial artery is similarly brought to the surface with a curved Kelly forceps, isolated from adjacent nerves, veins, and fascia, and tagged proximally and distally with moistened umbilical tape or silicone elastomer surgical tape* (Fig. 4–4).

Before proceeding with the right heart catheterization, we usually elect to place an arterial monitor line in the left radial or right femoral artery, using percutaneous technique (see Chapter 5 for details of technique of percutaneous entry). A 4F or 5F catheter-introducer,

*Retract-o-tape. Med-Pro Division, Quest Medical, Inc., Dallas, TX.

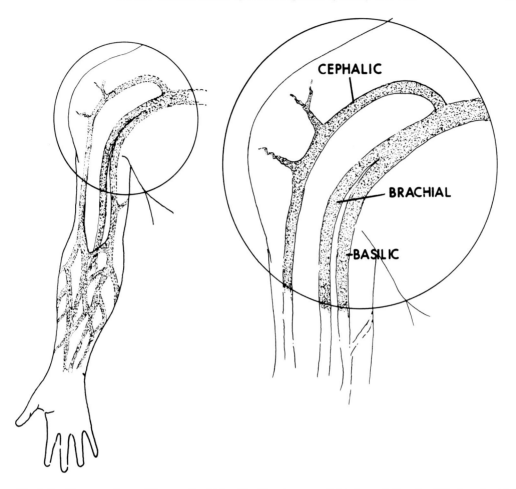

Fig. 4–2. Venous anatomy of the arm. Brachial and basilic veins are medial to the cephalic vein within the antecubital fossa. Note that the brachial and basilic veins continue directly into the axillary and subclavian system, whereas the cephalic system frequently joins the subclavian vein at a right angle. Passage of a catheter from the cephalic system to the right atrium may thus be quite difficult; the medial veins provide the straightest pathway.

advanced over an appropriate J guide wire, is adequate to monitor arterial pressure during the catheterization procedure. The usefulness of such an arterial monitor line cannot be overstated. It need not be kept sterile, can be used during the catheterization to obtain arterial blood samples during the Fick cardiac output determinations, to withdraw arterial blood during indicator-dilution studies, and to monitor arterial pressure nearly continuously. Although catheterization can be done without such a line, the presence of an arterial monitor line can be of great value, especially if trouble develops (e.g., hypotension, arrhythmias, perforation).

After placing the arterial monitor line and isolating the brachial artery and basilic or brachial vein, it is time to proceed with the right heart catheterization. An appropriate catheter is selected (see next section) such as a Goodale-Lubin or Cournand, and flushed vigorously with heparinized solution (concentration, 3000 IU heparin per liter of 5% dextrose in water or normal saline solution). A 7 Fr balloon flotation catheter is a suitable alternative, although it offers lower-frequency fidelity than the stiffer woven Dacron catheters. A transverse incision is made in the vein with small scissors, and the catheter is introduced with the aid of either curved tissue forceps without

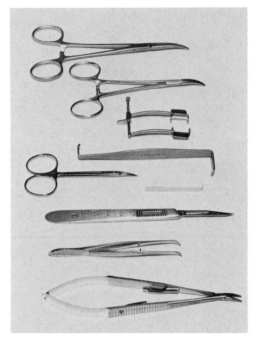

Fig. 4–3. Instruments that I use in cardiac catheterization by the brachial approach. From top to bottom: curved Kelly forceps (V. Mueller, SU 2722); curved mosquito forceps; ophthalmic retractor (V. Mueller, OP-160, XSAQ) used to hold skin margins open; hand-held retractor (V. Mueller, SU 3720); iris scissors (V. Mueller, OP 5005); plastic introducer (Becton-Dickinson); scalpel (No. 11 blade for arteriotomy, No. 15 for skin); small curved forceps without teeth (Miltex, 18-784) and Castro-Viejo needle holder (V. Mueller, XHMQ, OP-7380) both for use in arterial repair.

teeth or a small plastic catheter introducer.* I occasionally place the vein over a ''bridge'' formed by straight forceps to enable better control and to diminish oozing during passage of the catheter (Fig. 4–4).

Once the catheter has been introduced and passed a short distance, blood is aspirated, and the catheter is again flushed with heparinized solution. The catheter may then be connected directly, or by means of flexible plastic tubing to either the side port of a Morse manifold† (at whose end port is a pressure transducer) (see Chapter 9). We have chosen the latter system because of its better frequency-re-

*Catheter Introducer, Becton Dickinson and Company, Rutherford, NJ.

†NAMIC, Medical Products Division, Hudson Falls, NY.

sponse characteristics and the resultant superior quality pressure tracings. The interposed manifold allows entry of heparinized flush solution, and by turning the stopcock the operator can have intermittent pressure monitoring and catheter flush.

After passage of the right heart catheter, which will shortly be discussed in detail, the brachial artery is cleaned and incised transversely with a number 11 surgical blade (Fig. 4–4). An appropriately selected left heart catheter (see the following section), which has been flushed as described, is then inserted and passed retrograde a short distance before it is aspirated, flushed with heparinized solution, and connected to a pressure measurement, intermittent flush system similar to that described for the right heart catheter. When the catheter is flushed manually, the barrel of the flush syringe should *always* be vertical, with the hub facing downward. The catheter should be aspirated first until there is a free return of blood, and only 2 to 3 ml of flush solution need be injected, although the syringe should contain more than this. These precautions will greatly reduce the hazard of air embolism. Many laboratories routinely administer heparin solution (e.g., 3000–5000 IU heparin) into the *distal* brachial artery; this may reduce the incidence of arterial thrombosis. In my own practice, I do not give heparin locally into the artery; instead, I administer 5000 IU of heparin intravenously after the arterial catheter has been passed to the central aorta.

CATHETER SELECTION

Right Heart Catheters. Usually these are utilized for measurement of right atrial, right ventricular, pulmonary artery, and pulmonary capillary wedge pressures. For the latter purpose, only an end-hole catheter is adequate, although the catheter may in addition have side holes in close proximity to the tip. I use either a ***Goodale-Lubin*** or ***Cournand catheter***‡ as the initial right heart catheter, although many prefer a flow-directed balloon-flotation cath-

‡Bard, Inc, USCI Division, Billerica, MA.

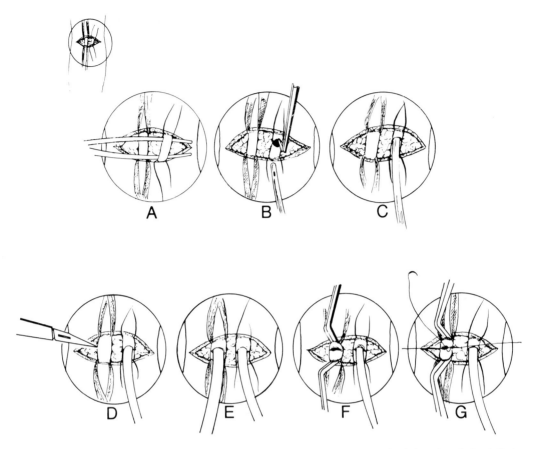

Fig. 4–4. Catheterization by direct exposure of brachial artery and vein. (A) Artery and vein have been isolated. Both are tagged proximally and distally; the artery with moist umbilical or silicone-elastomer tape, the vein with 3-0 silk. The vein has been placed over a "bridge" formed by a straight forceps to enable better control. (B) The vein has been incised with a small scissors, and the catheter is about to be inserted with the aid of a plastic catheter introducer (see text). (C) Passage of the right heart catheter. (D) Incision of the brachial artery with a number 11 surgical blade. The cutting edge of the blade is facing upwards, and the point approaches the artery from the side and at an angle of ~10 to 20 degrees to the horizontal to avoid perforating the posterior wall. (E) Passage of the left heart catheter. (F) In preparation for arterial repair, concentrated heparinized saline solution is "locked" in the vessel by placing bulldog clamps as far above and below the arteriotomy as possible (see text). (G) Closure of the arteriotomy by continuous or running stitch. Stay sutures are placed at each end of the arteriotomy (see text).

eter, (e.g., ***Swan-Ganz catheter***) for routine right heart catheterization (see Chapter 7).

Another right heart catheter used by some operators is the standard ***Lehman catheter**** (not to be confused with the Lehman ventriculography catheter), which is similar to the Cournand catheter but has a larger lumen. If atrial pacing is planned, a 7F ***Pacewedge dual-pressure bipolar pacing catheter*** or a ***Mansfield Atri-Pace I***† is effective for combined coronary sinus sampling and pacing.

*Elecath, Electrocatheter Corp., Rahway, NJ.
†Mansfield Scientific, Mansfield, MA

Passage of the right heart catheter occasionally is accompanied by transient right bundle branch block. Should this occur in a patient with pre-existing left bundle branch block, bilateral or complete heart block will develop and may require emergency ventricular pacing. A Swan-Ganz balloon-tipped catheter may be used in patients with left bundle branch block, as it is less likely to cause trauma to the right bundle. Alternatively, a pacing catheter may be used so that immediate ventricular pacing can be instituted should complete heart block develop.

For right-sided angiography, a closed-end catheter that has multiple side holes and is easy to pass to the pulmonary artery should be chosen, and for this purpose I frequently use the **Eppendorf catheter**.* Other frequently employed right heart angiographic catheters include the **Grollman pigtail catheter**† and the **Berman angiographic catheter**‡ for pulmonary angiography.

Left heart catheters utilized when the direct brachial approach is employed include both open-end and closed-end multiple side-hole catheters, which are used for both pressure measurement and angiography. The **Sones** catheter is commonly used as a left heart catheter, and it can be most helpful at times in crossing a tight aortic valve when other catheters have failed. It has a tendency to recoil during ventriculography, and it may produce myocardial staining when used by an inexperienced operator. However, with proper positioning and a low injection rate (i.e., 7 to 10 cc/sec), excellent left ventriculograms can be obtained routinely.

The polyurethane Sones catheter, marketed by Cordis Corporations§ (see Chapter 13), is particularly easy to manipulate into the ascending aorta, coronary arteries, and left ventricle, and is my first choice for left heart catheterization by the brachial approach. This catheter has a variety of curves (I generally use the type II), and in 7 and 8 Fr size tapers to a 5 Fr external diameter near its tip. It has an end-hole and four side-holes within 7 mm of the tip. The catheter will accept an 0.035-inch guide wire, which is often helpful in navigating through a tortuous subclavian artery into the ascending aorta. It is an excellent catheter for crossing a tight aortic valve, with or without the added help of a straight guide wire.

I occasionally use a closed-end, multiple side-hole catheter for left ventriculography and initial hemodynamic measurements. In this regard, the polyurethane 7F or 8F NIH catheter

made by Cordis Corporation is easy to use and to advance into the left ventricle. The Eppendorf catheter (USCI) is similar to the NIH catheter and may be used for ventriculography. Some operators prefer to use a pigtail catheter from the brachial approach, inserting this catheter over a protruding J-guide wire to straighten its tip during arterial entry. The catheters I use most frequently for right and left heart catheterization are shown in Figure 4–5.

When high-fidelity artifact-free tracings are needed, a micromanometer-tipped catheter may be chosen, such as the **Mikro-tip**‖ (see

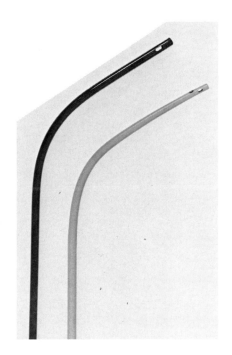

Fig. 4–5. Catheters that I use routinely when doing right and left heart catheterization. The Goodale-Lubin catheter (left) has an end-hole and 2 side-holes and is ideal for right heart catheterization, including measurement of pulmonary capillary wedge pressure. The polyurethane Sones catheter (right) tapers to a 5F tip with an end-hole and 4 side-holes; it is useful for coronary angiography and also for left ventriculography (at low flow rates).

---

*Bard, Inc., USCI Division, Billerica, MA.
†Cook, Inc., Bloomington, IN.
‡Arrow International, Reading, PA.
§80 cm Cordis Son-II, Sones technique, Cordis Corporation, Miami, FL.

‖Millar Instruments, Houston, TX.

Chapter 9). The Mikro-tip catheter is available in modifications with multiple side holes through which angiography can be performed. It is also available with a "pigtail" end for percutaneous placement.

Other left heart catheters include the *Gensini** (usually employed with percutaneous technique; see Chapter 5), the Lehman ventriculography catheter,† the *Rodriguez-Alvarez‡* catheter, and the *Shirey catheter§* (which may be used for a retrograde approach to the left atrium).

ADVANCING THE RIGHT HEART CATHETER

Both right and left heart catheters should be advanced as soon as possible after introduction into the vascular system because letting them sit in the bloodstream at body temperature results in loss of catheter stiffness and diminishes catheter control. The right heart catheter is advanced under fluoroscopic control to the superior vena cava. If there is difficulty entering the superior vena cava, it is sometimes helpful to try the following maneuvers: have the patient take a deep breath; raise the right arm and shoulder toward the head (ask the patient to shrug his right shoulder); turn the patient's head to the extreme left; remove the patient's pillow. If the catheter tip consistently points in a cephalad direction, try to *gently* form a loop proximal to the tip, which then may buckle and prolapse into the superior vena cava. In the last suggestion, the word *gently* must be emphasized; a catheter should *never* be forcibly advanced against a resistance. On occasion, a guide wire may be helpful in passing from the subclavian vein into the superior vena cava. If these maneuvers do not meet with prompt success, try a different catheter. Each catheter has a slightly different bend, and generally one will be just right for a given patient.

A word of caution is offered here concerning *venous spasm*, which may develop in any patient but is especially common in women. If

*Bard Inc., USCI Division, Billerica, MA
†Bard Inc., USCI Division, Billerica, MA
‡Bard Inc., USCI Division, Billerica, MA
§Bard Inc., USCI Division, Billerica, MA

spasm develops, do not try to advance the catheter, but instead withdraw it for a distance of 10 to 20 cm and then briskly move it to and fro in short (approximately 5-cm) strokes. This will commonly "break" the spasm, and the catheter may then be freely advanced to the right heart. *If spasm persists, a smaller catheter must be used.* Right heart catheterization in adults can be accomplished with size 5 or 6 French catheters, and a percutaneous femoral venous approach can be used if this is not successful. Persisting in the presence of spasm produces pain, vagal reactions, and hypotension, and a minor problem can thus be converted into a catastrophe. The same approach, by the way, applies equally to *arterial spasm.*

When the catheter tip has been advanced to the superior vena cava (SVC), I generally draw a blood sample for oximetry. If the SVC blood oxygen saturation is substantially lower than the pulmonary artery oxygen saturation, a full oximetry run should be done (Chapter 12). Such an oxygen "step up" may be the only clue to unsuspected atrial septal defect. To accomplish all these tasks successfully requires 1 to 2 minutes. The catheter tip is next advanced to the right atrium, where pressure is recorded before advancing the catheter to the pulmonary artery.

Advancing from Right Atrium to Pulmonary Artery. In navigating from the right atrium to right ventricle and pulmonary artery, the J-loop technique should be tried first. The catheter is advanced so that its tip catches on the lateral right atrial wall and the catheter looks like the letter J on fluoroscopy (Fig. 4–6). The catheter is next rotated counterclockwise so that the tip of the J sweeps the anterior right atrial wall (thus avoiding the coronary sinus, whose ostium lies posterior to the tricuspid valve) and jumps across the tricuspid valve into the right ventricle. At this point, the technician monitoring the patient's ECG frequently notes extrasystoles and calls these off to the operator; this is a sign that the catheter has entered the right ventricle. Because the catheter usually still retains its J curve (woven Dacron catheters have a "memory" and will retain an imposed shape for a short time after the imposing force has been removed), its tip will now be pointing toward the right ventricular outflow tract and can easily be advanced

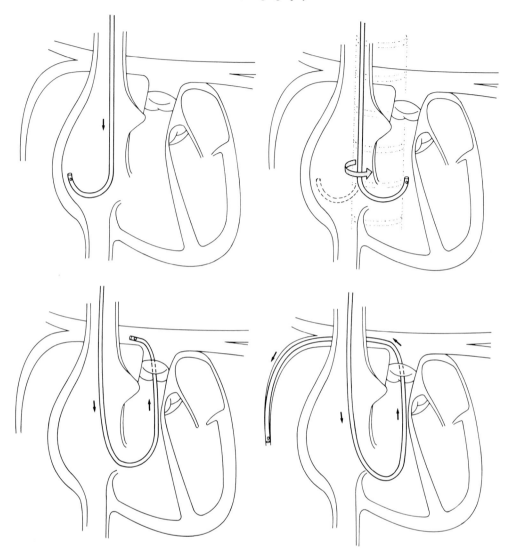

Fig. 4–6. Advancing the right heart catheter. In navigating from right atrium to pulmonary artery, the J-loop technique should be tried first. Upper left: The catheter is advanced so that its tip catches on the lateral right atrial wall and forms the letter J. Upper right: It is then rotated counterclockwise so that the catheter tip sweeps the anterior right atrial wall (thus avoiding the coronary sinus) and jumps across the tricuspid valve into the right ventricle. Lower left: The catheter tip, pointing towards the right ventricular outflow tract, can be easily advanced into the pulmonary artery. Lower right: The patient takes a deep breath, and the catheter is advanced to the "wedge" position (see text).

into the pulmonary artery. Right ventricular pressure may be recorded during the transit, or subsequently during the catheter pull-back.

If the catheter tip meets any resistance during its transit through the right ventricular outflow tract, *do not advance it*. Pull back until the tip is free, and again gently try to advance to the pulmonary artery. It is easy to perforate the right ventricular outflow tract and end up

in the pericardial space. In this regard, it should be pointed out that older women (e.g., over 65 years of age) seem particularly susceptible to this complication, and we therefore use 7 Fr (or smaller) catheters routinely in these patients.

With the catheter now in the pulmonary artery, pressure is again measured and blood is sampled for oximetry.

Advancing to Pulmonary Capillary Wedge Position. Next, the catheter is advanced to the "wedge" position. This can be done simply by having the patient take a deep breath and hold it while the catheter is advanced until its tip will go no farther (Fig. 4–6) and does not pulsate with the heart. Having the patient cough at this time will frequently advance the catheter tip into a true "wedge" position. The catheter loop may need to be pulled back slightly at this point to avoid coiling up in the right ventricle and atrium.

The pressure waveform is examined, and if it has the appearance of a true wedge pressure (Fig. 4–7), it is recorded. If there is any doubt that a true wedge position has been achieved, blood is sampled from the catheter. The pressure is confirmed as a true wedge pressure only if completely (95% or more) oxygen-saturated blood can be aspirated gently from the catheter.[1] In patients who are hypoxemic, a wedge blood oxygen saturation of 90% or more may be accepted, especially if the oxygen saturation of pulmonary artery blood is much lower (e.g., 70% or lower). When mitral stenosis is not expected to be present, the wedge pressure

may be "confirmed" simply by its typical waveform and by its match against simultaneous left ventricular diastolic pressure. If an unexpected diastolic gradient is detected between left ventricular and pulmonary wedge pressures, the wedge position should be confirmed by blood sampling. As mentioned, blood oxygen saturation from a true wedge position should be 95% or more, unless the catheter is wedged in a lung segment with poor aeration (e.g., atelectatic lobe, pneumonia, pulmonary edema). If a Swan-Ganz catheter is used to obtain pulmonary capillary wedge pressure, it is often necessary to aspirate and discard the 5 to 15 ml of pulmonary artery blood that lie between the balloon and the pulmonary capillary bed before bright red pulmonary capillary blood can be sampled.

Over the years there has been continued debate about the validity and usefulness of pulmonary capillary wedge pressure (sometimes called pulmonary artery wedge pressure) as a measure of pulmonary venous and left atrial pressure.[2–10] Most studies[2–7,10] have reported excellent agreement between mean left atrial and pulmonary capillary wedge pressure. The

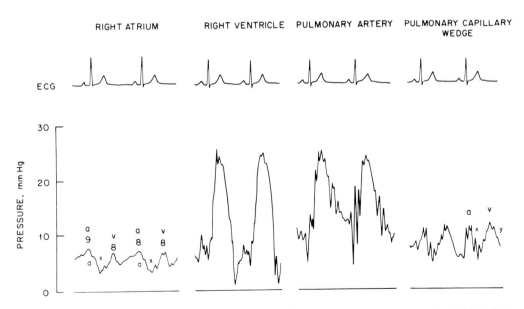

Fig. 4–7. Normal right heart pressures as measured through a 7Fr Goodale-Lubin catheter in a patient with moderate coronary artery disease, normal left ventricular function, and normal cardiac output. Both right atrial and pulmonary capillary wedge pressures show distinct "*a*" and "*v*" waves. See text for details.

phasic pressure waveform of the wedge pressure is commonly somewhat damped compared to a matched left atrial waveform, with "a" and "v" wave peaks being smaller in the wedge tracing. The timing of "a" and "v" waves is delayed in the wedge tracing compared to left atrial pressure (Fig. 4–8). Lange et al[10] found this time delay to average 70 ± 15 milliseconds (mean ± SD), and reported a significant improvement in accuracy of mitral valve gradient and valve area calculations when appropriate adjustment was made for this time delay (see Chapter 11 for details). In Lange's study, wedge pressure was measured with an 8F Goodale-Lubin catheter, which almost certainly maximized the fidelity of waveform transmission from the left atrium. Use of smaller lumen balloon-tipped catheters increases somewhat the likelihood of excessive damping of the waveform and longer transmission time delay. In both of the studies[8,9] that found wedge pressure unreliable compared with left atrial pressure for the accurate assessment of transmitral gradient, the wedge pressure was measured with smaller-lumen balloon-tipped catheters, without oximetric confirmation. *In my opinion, pulmonary capillary wedge pressure provides an accurate*

Simultaneous LA-PCW Pressures

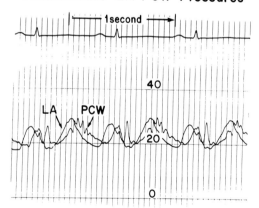

Fig. 4–8. Simultaneous left atrial (LA) and pulmonary capillary wedge (PCW) pressures in a patient undergoing transseptal catheterization. Note that the "a" and "v" waves are delayed by 50 to 70 milliseconds in the PCW tracing compared to the LA tracing. See text for details. Modified from Lange et al (J Am Coll Cardiol 13:825, 1989) with permission.

estimate of left atrial pressure, whether measured with Cournand, Goodale-Lubin, or balloon-tipped catheters, if appropriate attention is paid to: (a) accurate assessment of pressure waveform, (b) oximetric confirmation, and (c) correction for time delay. Accurate assessment of pressure waveform requires a proper pressure measurement technique with high natural frequency and optimal damping, as discussed in Chapter 9. With regard to the pressure measurement technique, a "trick" that is sometimes helpful is a maneuver called "developing the wedge pressure." Many operators have noticed that the wedge pressure waveform often appears damped at first but improves immediately following a slow, gentle saline flush or brief infusion through the lumen of the wedged catheter. This may, in some instances, be related to clearing the catheter of blood, platelet aggregates, or microthrombi that are causing damping of the pressure waveform, but it seems equally likely that *vasodilatation of the pulmonary capillary bed* is playing a role. Similar improvement in pulmonary capillary wedge waveform may also be seen after sublingual or intravenous administration of nitroglycerin.

When using a Cournand, Goodale-Lubin, or Lehman (end-hole) catheter to obtain a wedge pressure, it is our practice to leave the catheter in the wedge position, flushing *intermittently* at three-minute intervals (continuous flushing in the wedge position frequently causes the patient to develop violent coughing), and proceed with the left heart catheterization. We perform cardiac output determinations with right heart pull-back to the pulmonary artery only after simultaneous pulmonary capillary wedge and left ventricular pressures have been recorded. A different practice must be followed when the Swan-Ganz or other balloon catheter is used as a right heart catheter. *These catheters must never be left in the wedge (balloon-up) position for any significant period of time. Failure to observe this rule may cause pulmonary infarction and/or rupture of the pulmonary artery,* as is discussed in Chapter 7.

The Cournand catheter is somewhat stiffer

than the Goodale-Lubin, and may be easier to control in the right heart and to advance to wedge position. Stiffer right heart catheters (such as the Cournand and Gorlin catheters) may also be more dangerous, particularly in elderly women, in whom perforation of the heart can easily occur (see Chapter 3). One way of temporarily stiffening a Goodale-Lubin or other catheter is to advance a 0.038- or 0.045-inch guide wire (soft end first) to within 2 to 3 inches of the catheter's tip. This maneuver commonly gives the added stiffness necessary to get from the pulmonary artery to the wedge position. The guide wire should not remain in the catheter for more than 2 to 3 minutes, after which it is removed and the catheter is carefully aspirated and flushed. This maneuver should *not* be used in attempting to manipulate the catheter from the right atrium to the right ventricle and pulmonary artery because it will increase the risk of cardiac perforation.

ADVANCING THE LEFT HEART CATHETER

After the right heart catheter has been advanced to the pulmonary artery or wedge position, an appropriately selected left heart catheter is inserted into the brachial artery as described previously. This catheter is then advanced into the ascending aorta just above the aortic valve. If there is difficulty navigating from the subclavian or innominate arteries into the ascending aorta, the operator may try all the maneuvers suggested for guiding the right heart catheter into the superior vena cava. These include having the patient take a deep breath, shrug his right shoulder, turn his head to the extreme left, remove his pillow, and extend his right arm by manual traction on the wrist. It has been my impression that passage of a left heart catheter from the subclavian artery to the central aorta is easier when the patient is lying on a flat-topped table, as opposed to the cradle-type table. The cradle often forces the shoulders forward and distorts the arterial anatomy, such that more bends and

curves need to be negotiated in navigating from brachial artery to central aorta.

As with right heart catheterization, *if the catheter does not pass easily after a relatively brief attempt at manipulation, resist the temptation to become more vigorous.* When using an end-hole catheter (e.g., the Sones catheter) a soft J-tipped spring guide wire may be advanced through the catheter tip to lead the way. The 0.035-inch-diameter guide wire can be used with the Cordis Sones catheter, and larger sizes with the pigtail or Gensini catheters. If the ascending aorta cannot be entered easily with a standard J-tipped guidewire, I use a Wholey wire*, which is useful for negotiating tortuous arterial systems. On rare occasions, the ascending aorta cannot be entered by way of the right brachial artery, necessitating a percutaneous femoral approach or left brachial artery cutdown.

Once in the ascending aorta, central aortic pressure is measured and recorded simultaneously with arterial monitor pressure. The catheter is then advanced across the aortic valve into the left ventricle. This usually can be accomplished by producing to-and-fro excursions of the catheter while gradually rotating it through 360 degrees, so that the catheter tip moves up and down on the aortic valve over its entire plane.

As mentioned previously, the Cordis polyurethane Sones catheter is used routinely as a left heart catheter in our laboratory when the brachial approach is employed. This soft-tipped catheter may be advanced directly (tip first) into the left ventricle, or it may be prolapsed across the aortic valve, loop first, as illustrated in Figure 4–9.

On occasion, it may be difficult to enter the left ventricle, particularly when dealing with severe aortic stenosis. In this circumstance, one should try several catheters of different types (we have had good results with the Sones catheter which occasionally will pass a tight aortic valve easily), or utilize a straight-tipped guide wire approach before abandoning the attempt. When crossing a stenotic aortic valve

*Wholey Hi-torque modified J 260 cm, Advanced Catheter Systems, Inc., Temecula, CA

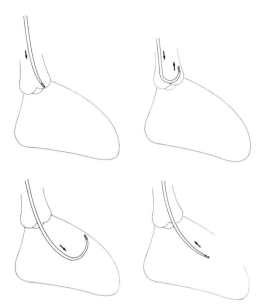

Fig. 4–9. Illustration of technique for retrograde catheterization of the left ventricle using the Sones catheter. The catheter is advanced (upper left) to touch the aortic valve. Further advancement usually produces a loop (upper right) in the ascending aorta, which prolapses readily (lower left) into the left ventricle. The catheter is then withdrawn (lower right) to eliminate the loop and obtain a proper axial orientation for left ventriculography.

retrograde, it is often helpful to view the aortic root and valve in left anterior oblique projection. This view shows the calcified leaflets well and may demonstrate the location of the orifice that will provide a target for repeated to-and-fro excursions of the catheter tip or straight-tipped guide wire. If a guide wire is used, the catheter is advanced over the guide wire into the ventricular chamber, and following removal of the guide wire, the catheter is then aspirated vigorously and flushed. With a guide wire–facilitated entrance into the left ventricle, *there is a danger that the guide wire tip may pass under endocardial trabeculations,* so that the catheter subsequently advanced over the guide wire is not free in the ventricular chamber. This can lead to serious myocardial staining during power injection of contrast, but should be detectable from appearance of the catheter tip and from the washout of contrast after a test injection. Success in crossing a tight aortic valve depends on experience, luck, and sheer determination.

A special-purpose left heart catheter was developed by Dr. Earl Shirey for retrograde catheterization of the left atrium. The Shirey catheter* is a tapered, multiple side-hole woven Dacron catheter that resembles the Sones catheter. It can be prolapsed loop-first into the left ventricle, so that its tip faces the aortic and mitral valves (Fig. 4–10) rather than the left ventricular apex. Withdrawal of the redundant loop frequently guides the catheter tip into the left atrium.

Once the left ventricle has been entered and a stable position is found, it is advisable to immediately obtain simultaneous recordings of critical pressures, such as left ventricular, peripheral arterial (through the arterial monitor line), and pulmonary capillary wedge pressures. Although these pressures will be recorded again during the cardiac output determinations, arrhythmias or other unanticipated problems may develop, greatly altering the basal physiologic state and possibly requiring catheter withdrawal. In such circumstances, the operator will sorely regret not having measured the pressures earlier.

After completion of hemodynamic and cardiac output measurements (Chapter 8), most

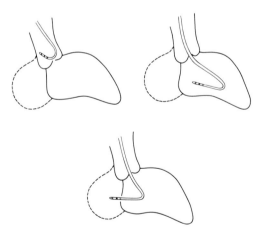

Fig. 4–10. Diagrammatic illustration of retrograde catheterization of the left atrium using the Shirey catheter. It can be prolapsed loop-first into the left ventricle (upper left), so that its tip faces the aortic and mitral valves (upper right) rather than the left ventricular apex. Withdrawal of the redundant loop frequently guides the catheter tip into the left atrium (lower panel).

*USCI, Billerica, MA.

cardiac catheterization procedures today proceed to left ventriculography and coronary angiography. The details of these techniques as applied to both brachial and femoral approaches will be discussed in Chapters 13 and 14.

REPAIR OF VESSELS AND AFTERCARE

After the completion of diagnostic studies, the left heart catheter is removed and the brachial arteriotomy is repaired. Repair may be done in many ways (purse-string, interrupted, continuous), but I will describe only my own approach.

The proximal and distal portions of the artery are checked for vigorous and free bleeding, and an arterial ("Fogarty") embolectomy catheter* is employed.[11] The use of a Fogarty catheter routinely in all brachial catheterizations has resulted in a low incidence of diminished radial pulse and arterial insufficiency. Although I perform the procedure routinely, it should be pointed out that other brachial operators reserve it for instances in which proximal flow or distal pulsation (after repair) are impaired.

When good proximal flow has been established, 10 to 15 ml of a concentrated solution of heparinized saline (3000 IU of heparin in 30 ml normal saline) are infused into the proximal artery through the Sones catheter; this solution is "locked" in the vessel by immediately placing a vascular bulldog type clamp† as far above the arteriotomy as possible (Fig. 4–4). The same procedure is then repeated for the distal segment (i.e., use of Fogarty catheter, administration of heparin, placement of bulldog clamp). At this point, a stay suture is placed at each end of the arteriotomy, which is then closed using a continuous or running stitch (Fig. 4–4) with fine nonwettable suture material such as 6-0 Tevdek.‡ The stay suture

at one end of the incision is the start of the running stitch, and the stitch is completed by tying to the other stay suture. The advantage of a continuous suture is that it tightens as the artery expands after the clamps are removed.

I prefer to use a special needle holder (Castro-Viejo type), with a delicate hold and release mechanism when doing the arterial repair. Needle holders of this type (Fig. 4–3) are commonly used in ophthalmologic and vascular surgery and aid in the fine control of suture placement.

After suturing the artery, the distal bulldog clamp is removed first, and the forearm is massaged from the wrist toward the elbow, to milk out any air within the lumen of the artery before releasing the proximal bulldog clamp. The proximal clamp is then removed, and any minor leaks are controlled by direct finger pressure, which must be sufficiently gentle that the radial pulse can be palpated. If leaking does not stop within a few minutes of such finger pressure, an additional suture or two may be required. It is important that the radial pulse be palpable and essentially of the same amplitude as before the arteriotomy. If it is absent or greatly diminished, the artery should be reopened and a Fogarty catheter again passed *proximally and distally.* When this is unsuccessful, prompt consultation should be obtained with an experienced vascular surgeon (if possible while the wound is still open), who usually will be able to identify and correct the problem. The operator should carefully watch the vascular surgeon and learn from him exactly what the problem was, how it was corrected, and how it might have been prevented.

After successfully repairing the arteriotomy, the vein utilized in the right heart catheterization may be tied off or repaired like the arteriotomy, depending on the needs of the individual case. The wound is then flushed out with copious quantities of fresh sterile saline solution followed by 10% povidone-iodine solution.§ Currently, we close the wound using a subcuticular stitch of an absorbable suture (4-0 Dexon Plus‖ on a cutting needle), thereby

---

*Arterial embolectomy catheter; 3 French, 40 cm. Shiley Laboratories, Irvine, CA.

†DeBakey peripheral vascular bulldog clamps with 45-degree to 60-degree angled jaws. V. Mueller, Chicago, IL.

‡Tevdek, Deknatel Company, Queens Village, NY.

§Pharmadine, Sherwood Pharmaceutical, Mahwah, NJ.

‖Davis and Geck, Inc., Manati, Puerto Rico.

avoiding the need for suture removal. Alternatively, the skin may be closed with interrupted mattress sutures of 4-0 nylon. These sutures must then be removed 7 to 10 days later. Antibiotic ointment is placed on the suture line and covered with a firm dressing (although not so firmly that it diminishes the radial pulse).

The patient is usually instructed to drink 1 to 2 quarts of water or juice over the next 6 to 8 hours, to compensate for the diuretic action of the angiographic contrast material, as well as to help wash this myocardial and vascular depressant out of his vascular system. If there is any question about the patient's ability to drink the required fluid, an equivalent amount should be administered intravenously. We have rarely seen pulmonary congestion from this regimen, but have frequently seen hypotension when this instruction was not followed or was countermanded by a well-meaning but uninformed house officer. In patients with poor left ventricular function and/or pulmonary capillary wedge pressures ≥ 25 mmHg, or in whom little or no radiographic contrast was used, the fluid orders should be correspondingly reduced.

Brachial artery catheterization may be done on an outpatient basis, in which case the patient can usually be discharged to home after 4 to 6 hours of observation if he or she is stable. For hospitalized patients (e.g., those with unstable angina), in a typical case our postcatheterization orders might read:

1. Resume all previous medications.
2. Blood pressure (specify arm), pulse, and inspection of dressings every 15 minutes $\times 4$, then 1 hour $\times 4$, then every 4 hours.
3. Call intern *and* catheterization laboratory (specify phone number) for any problems (such as bleeding, loss of pulse, or hypotension).
4. Encourage p.o. fluids: 1–2 L over 6–8 hours.
5. Pain medication (e.g., Tylenol, meperidine).

There is no need for the patient to be kept flat or motionless in bed following the procedure. The patient may sit up, eat, and (if no groin procedure has been done) get out of bed (with assistance) to go to the bathroom. The operator should see the patient later in the afternoon in order to check the dressing, peripheral pulses, and general condition of the patient. This may also be a suitable time to discuss with the patient and his family the results of the investigation and recommendations for further treatment (e.g., surgical procedures) if any. In a patient in whom the catheterization was done as an outpatient procedure, the patient may be discharged to home following check of the radial pulse and antecubital fossa incision.

In less than 2% of cases, a radial pulse has been absent by the time we have seen the patient on late afternoon rounds. In such cases, I usually administer one aspirin and watch the patient overnight, with a plan to bring the patient to the catheterization laboratory the next morning for re-exploration by me and the Cardiology Fellow who had done the catheterization with me. In about one third of the cases there is a strong pulse the next morning, and the absence of a pulse on evening rounds is attributed to spasm or a transient thrombus. In two thirds of the cases, the radial pulse is still weak or absent, and these patients come to the laboratory where under local (2% xylocaine) anesthesia, I reopen the incision, take down the arterial repair, pass a Fogarty catheter in both directions (usually getting a sizeable thrombus) and remove any intimal fronds or flaps that are visible. Heparin is administered systemically (5000 IU) and locally into the proximal and distal segments of the artery, and the artery is repaired using 6-0 Tevdek in a continuous suture, as before. This approach is recommended only for operators who have extensive experience with the brachial approach and use of the Fogarty catheter. For those with limited brachial experience, or when the initial arterial repair was difficult, prompt consultation with an experienced vascular surgeon is indicated. The word ''prompt'' is worth emphasizing because patients with a weak or absent radial pulse 18 to 24 hours after brachial catheterization almost always have a localized thrombus. These thrombi propagate over the ensuing days and weeks, often eventuating in severe claudication. When seen late (e.g., more than 1 week postcatheterization), these thrombi may be impossible to remove, necessitating venous bypass surgery to relieve arm ischemia.

It is important to emphasize that the complications of a catheterization should be managed *by the physicians who have done the catheterization*. Not only are these individuals the ones most likely to understand the genesis of a specific problem, but this is clearly the best method of continuing education to ensure the prevention of future complications.

REFERENCES

1. Rapaport E, Dexter L: Pulmonary "capillary" pressure. *In* Methods in Medical Research. Year Book Publishers 7:85, 1958.
2. Dexter L, Burwell CS, Haynes FW, Seibel RE: Oxygen content of pulmonary "capillary" blood in unanesthetized human beings. J Clin Invest 25:913, 1946.
3. Dexter L, et al: Studies of congenital heart disease: II. The pressure and oxygen content of blood in the right auricle, right ventricle and pulmonary artery in control patients, with observations on the oxygen saturation and source of pulmonary "capillary" blood. J Clin Invest 26:554, 1947.
4. Hellens HK, Haynes FW, Dexter L: Pulmonary "capillary" pressure in man. J Appl Physiol 2:24, 1949.
5. Werko L, Varnauskas E, Eliasch H, et al: Further evidence that the pulmonary capillary venous pressure pulse in man reflects cyclic changes in the left atrium. Circ Res 1:337, 1953.
6. Connolly DC, Kirklin JW, Wood EH: The relationship between pulmonary artery wedge pressure and left atrial pressure in man. Circ Res 2:434, 1954.
7. Batson GA, Chandrasekhar KP, Payas Y, Rickards DF: Measurement of pulmonary wedge pressure by the flow directed Swan-Ganz catheter. Cardiovasc Res 6:748, 1972.
8. Schoenfeld MH, Palacios IF, Hutter AM, Jacoby SS, Block PC: Underestimation of prosthetic mitral valve areas: Role of transseptal catheterization in avoiding unnecessary repeat mitral valve surgery. J Am Coll Cardiol 5:1387, 1985.
9. Hosenpud JD, McAnulty JH, Morton MJ: Overestimation of mitral valve gradients obtained by phasic pulmonary capillary wedge pressure. Cathet Cardiovasc Diagn 9:283, 1983.
10. Lange RA, Moore DM Jr, Cigarroa RG, Hillis LD: Use of pulmonary capillary wedge pressure to assess severity of mitral stenosis: Is true left atrial pressure needed in this condition? J Am Coll Cardiol 13:825, 1989.
11. Baker LD, Leshin SJ, Mathur VS, Messer JV: Routine Fogarty thrombectomy in arterial catheterization. N Engl J Med 279:1203, 1968.

5

Percutaneous Approach, Including Transseptal Catheterization and Apical Left Ventricular Puncture

DONALD S. BAIM and WILLIAM GROSSMAN

In contrast with the direct brachial technique, the percutaneous approach to left and right heart catheterization involves achieving vascular access by means of needle puncture,[1] obviating surgical isolation of the vessel during either the introduction or subsequent withdrawal of the cardiac catheter. Once the needle has been positioned within the vessel lumen, a flexible guide wire can be advanced through the needle and well into the central vasculature.[2] When this needle is withdrawn, the guide wire remains in its intravascular position and provides a means of introducing the desired catheter. Whereas some catheters may be inserted directly over the guide wire, it is now more common to place an introducing sheath over the guide wire,[3,4] and then advance the catheter through this sheath. With appropriate skill and knowledge of regional anatomy, the percutaneous technique can be adapted to catheter insertion from a variety of entry sites. Venous catheterization can be performed via the femoral, internal jugular, subclavian, or median antecubital vein, whereas arterial catheterization can be performed via the femoral,[3,4] brachial,[5] or axillary[6] or radial[7] artery. At the termination of the procedure, the catheters and introducing

sheaths are withdrawn, and bleeding from the puncture sites is controlled by the application of direct pressure.

CATHETERIZATION VIA FEMORAL ARTERY AND VEIN

Patient Preparation

After palpation of the femoral arterial pulse within the inguinal skin crease, a safety razor is used to shave an area approximately 10 cm in diameter surrounding this point. Although most catheterizations can be performed quickly and easily from a single groin (usually the right), we have found it expedient to routinely prepare both groins, in case difficulties in catheter advancement force a switch to the other groin once the procedure has begun. The shaved area is scrubbed with a povidone-iodine/detergent mixture and then painted with povidone-iodine solution. The latter is blotted dry using a sterile towel and the patient is draped from clavicles to below the feet, leaving exposed only the sterile prepared groin areas. Most laboratories now use disposable paper drapes with adhesive-bordered apertures for this purpose, frequently packaged together with other disposable supplies (syringes, needles, bowels, etc.) in a custom kit available from any of several vendors.

Selection of Puncture Site

The adjacent femoral artery and vein (Fig. 5–1) are the most commonly used vessels for percutaneous diagnostic cardiac catheterization. Vessel puncture should be achieved between 1 and 3 cm below the inguinal ligament, which can be easily palpated as it courses from the anterior superior iliac spine to the pubic tubercle. While some operators rely on the location of the inguinal skin crease rather than the inguinal ligament for the selection of the puncture site, skin crease position can be misleading in obese patients, but the iliac spine and ligament continue to be reliable anatomic landmarks. The femoral artery typically lies at the midpoint of the inguinal ligament and can be palpated over a several centimeter span distal to the ligament. The femoral vein lies approximately one fingerbreadth *medial* to the artery, along a parallel course.

Most difficulties in entering the femoral artery and vein—and most vascular complications—arise as the result of inadequate identification of these landmarks prior to attempted vessel puncture. Punctures of the artery at or above the inguinal ligament make catheter advancement difficult and predispose to inadequate compression, hematoma formation, and/or retroperitoneal bleeding following catheter removal. Punctures of the artery more than 3 cm below the inguinal ligament increase the chance that the femoral artery will have divided into its profunda and superficial femoral branches. Puncture in the crotch between these two branches fails to enter the arterial lumen, and puncture of either one of the branches increases the risk of a thrombotic occlusion due to smaller vessel caliber. Because the superficial femoral artery frequently overlies the femoral vein, low venous punctures may pass inadvertently through the superficial femoral artery, leading to excessive bleeding and possible arteriovenous fistula formation.

Local Anesthesia

Adequate local anesthesia is absolutely necessary for a successful catheterization. It can-

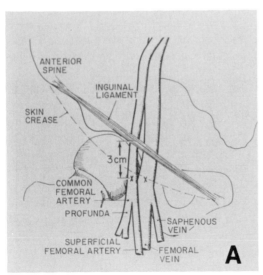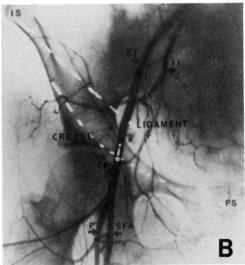

Fig. 5–1. Regional anatomy relevant to percutaneous femoral arterial and venous catheterization: (A) Schematic diagram show the right femoral artery and vein coursing underneath the inguinal ligament, which runs from the anterior superior iliac spine to the pubic tubercle. The arterial skin nick (indicated by X) should be placed approximately 3 cm below the ligament and directly over the femoral arterial pulsation, and the venous skin nick should be placed at the same level but approximately one fingerbreadth more medial. Although this level corresponds roughly to the skin crease in most patients, anatomic localization relative to the inguinal ligament provides a more constant landmark (see text for details). (B) Corresponding radiographic anatomy as seen during abdominal aortography.

not be overemphasized that poor anesthetization leads to poor patient cooperation and makes a long morning in the catheterization laboratory for both patient and operator. Once the inguinal ligament and femoral artery have been identified, the femoral artery is palpated along its course using the three middle fingers of the left hand, with the uppermost finger positioned just below the inguinal ligament. Without moving the left hand, a linear intradermal wheal of 1 or 2% lidocaine is raised slowly by tangential insertion of a 25- or 27-gauge needle along a course overlying both the femoral artery and vein at the desired level of entry.

With the left hand remaining in place, transverse skin punctures are made over the femoral artery and vein, using the tip of a No. 11 scalpel blade. The smaller needle is then replaced by a 22-gauge 1½-inch needle, which is used to infiltrate the deeper tissues along the intended trajectory for arterial and venous entry. As this needle is advanced, small additional volumes of lidocaine are infiltrated by *slow* injection. Each incremental infiltration should be preceded by aspiration so that intravascular boluses can be avoided. If the anesthetic track passes through the artery or vein, infiltration should be suspended until the tip of the needle has passed out of the back wall of the vessel and then continued to the full length of the needle or to the point where the needle tip contacts the periosteum. Approximately 10 to 15 ml 1% xylocaine administered in this fashion usually provides adequate local anesthesia. The patient should be warned that he may experience some burning as the anesthetic is injected but that the medication will abolish any subsequent sharp sensations.

Once local anesthesia has been achieved, the small skin nicks can be enlarged and deepened, using the tips of a curved "mosquito" forceps. This procedure decreases the resistance that is encountered during subsequent advancement of the Seldinger needle and catheter and increases the likelihood that any vascular bleeding will become manifest as oozing through the puncture rather than hidden in the formation of a deep hematoma.

Femoral Vein Puncture

Femoral venous puncture is usually performed prior to arterial puncture. This provides secure venous access for the administration of fluids or drugs and shortens the arterial catheter time by allowing completion of the right heart catheterization before introduction of the arterial catheter. With the left hand palpating the femoral artery along its course below the inguinal ligament, the Seldinger needle (Fig. 5–2) is introduced through the more medial skin nick. This 18-gauge thin-walled needle consists of a blunt, tapered external cannula through which a sharp solid obturator projects. The needle should be grasped so that the index and middle fingers lie below the lateral flanges of the needle, and the thumb rests on the top of the solid obturator as the needle is advanced along the sagittal plane angled approximately 45 degrees cephalad (Fig. 5–3). While this needle can occasionally be advanced up to its hub, the tip of the needle will usually stop more superficially as it encounters the periosteum of the pubic tubercle. The periosteum is well innervated and may be quite tender if the initial lidocaine infiltration failed to reach this level. Accordingly, forceful contact with the periosteum is neither necessary nor desirable. If the patient experiences significant discomfort, some operators will remove the obturator from the Seldinger needle and infiltrate additional lidocaine into the deep tissues through the outer cannula.

At this point, it is hoped that the Seldinger needle has transfixed the femoral vein. The obturator is removed, and a 10-ml syringe is attached to the hub of the cannula. The syringe and cannula are then depressed so that the syringe lies closer to the anterior surface of the thigh (Fig. 5–3) and the needle is more parallel (rather than perpendicular) to the vein. Gentle suction is applied to the syringe, and the whole assembly is slowly withdrawn toward the skin surface. In doing so, it is helpful to control the needle with both the left hand (which also rests on the patient's leg for support) and the right hand (which also controls the aspirating syringe). As the tip of the cannula is withdrawn

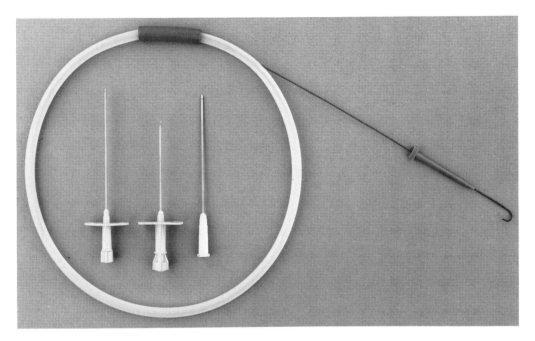

Fig. 5–2. Percutaneous needles and guide wire. Left, a Seldinger needle with its sharp solid obturator in place. Center, a Potts-Cournand needle, which differs in the fact that its obturator is hollow and therefore allows the operator to see blood flashback as the artery is punctured. Right, 18-gauge thin-wall needle used for internal jugular vein puncture. The percutaneous needles are surrounded by an 0.038 inch, 145 cm J guide wire.

into the lumen, venous blood will flow freely into the syringe. With the left hand stabilizing the needle, the right hand is used to remove the syringe and to advance a 0.035- or 0.038-inch J guide wire into the hub of the needle. In doing so, the wire tip may be straightened by hyperextension of the wire shaft in the right hand or by leaving the tip of the wire within the plastic introducer supplied by the manufacturer. The wire should slide through the needle and 10 to 15 cm into the vessel with no perceptible resistance. Fluoroscopy should then show the tip of the guide wire just to the left (patient's right) of the spine.

If difficulty is encountered in advancing the guide wire, it should never be overcome by the application of force. Fluoroscopy may simply reveal that the tip of the wire has entered a small lumbar branch and that it can be drawn back slightly and redirected or gently prolapsed up the iliac vein. When resistance to advancement is encountered at or just beyond the tip of the needle, however, even greater care is required. This resistance may simply

be caused by apposition of the tip of the needle to the back wall of the vein, which can be corrected by further depression of the needle hub, with or without slight withdrawal of the needle shaft. If this maneuver fails to allow free advancement of the wire, however, the wire should be removed and the syringe should be reattached to the needle hub to ensure that free flow of venous blood is present before additional wire manipulation is attempted— the wire should not be reintroduced unless free flow is obtained. If the wire still cannot be advanced, the needle cannula should be withdrawn, and the puncture site should be compressed for 1 to 3 minutes. The anatomic landmarks should be reconfirmed, and puncture reattempted. In some cases, venous puncture during a Valsalva maneuver may help by distending the femoral vein and making clean puncture more likely.

At this point, the needle is removed, leaving the wire within the vein and secured at the skin entry site by the left hand. The protruding wire is wiped with a moistened gauze pad, and its

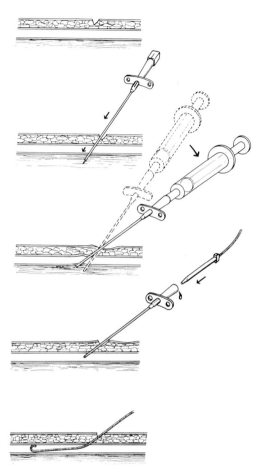

Fig. 5–3. Seldinger technique for venous puncture. A skin nick has been created overlying the desired vein, which is punctured through and through by a Seldinger needle with its solid obturator in place. In the center panel, the obturator is removed and the needle cannula is attached to a syringe. Depression of the syringe toward the surface of the skin tents the vessel slightly and facilitates axial alignment of the cannula at the moment that slow withdrawal brings the tip of the cannula back into the vessel lumen. This is recognized by the sudden ability to withdraw venous blood freely into the syringe, which is then removed from the needle cannula to permit advancement of the J guide wire (shown here with a plastic straightener in place). Once the guide wire has been advanced safely into the vessel, the needle cannula can be removed.

free end is threaded into the lumen of a sheath and dilator combination adequate to accept the intended right heart catheter. Our laboratory routinely uses a sheath equipped with a back-bleed valve and sidearm connector (Fig. 5–4, USCI "Hemaquet" or Cordis sheath) to control bleeding around the catheter shaft and to provide a means of administering extra fluid during the right heart catheterization. Whichever device is used, it is important to ensure that one has control of the proximal end of the guide wire, which is held in a fixed position as the dilator is introduced through the skin. The sheath and dilator are rotated as they are advanced progressively through the soft tissues. If excessive resistance is encountered, it may be necessary to remove the dilator from the sheath and to introduce the dilator alone before attempting to introduce the combination. If inspection shows that initial attempts have created significant burring at the end of the sheath, a new sheath should be obtained.

Catheterizing Right Heart from Femoral Vein

Once the sheath is in place, the wire and dilator are removed, and the sheath is flushed by withdrawal of blood and administration of heparinized saline solution. In our laboratory we usually connect the sidearm of the venous sheath to a one-liter bag of normal saline solution, using a sterile length of intravenous extension tubing. The desired venous catheter is then flushed, attached to the venous manifold, introduced through the sheath, and advanced up the vena cava. We previously used a 7 Fr Swan-Ganz catheter because of its ease of passage, low risk of injury to the right heart chambers, and its ability to perform thermodilution measurements of cardiac output. Conventional woven Dacron (Goodale-Lubin or Cournand) catheters were reserved for instances when thermodilution outputs were not desired or when greater catheter control was needed. More recently, we have begun using a stiffer, balloon-tipped catheter (PWP monitoring catheter, USCI) to combine the safety of the Swan-Ganz catheter with the catheter control and frequency response previously found only in the woven Dacron catheters.

Deviation of the catheter tip from its paraspinous position during advancement suggests entry into a renal or hepatic vein, which can be corrected by slight withdrawal and rotation of the catheter. Once the catheter is

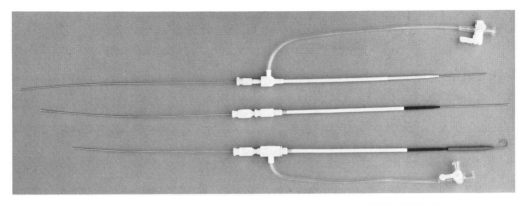

Fig. 5–4. Vascular sheaths. Center, conventional sheath and dilator assembly (USCI "888"). Two arterial-venous introducers equipped with backbleed valves and sidearm attachment; top, a Cordis sheath; bottom, a USCI Hemaquet. Each device is inserted over a conventional guide wire as a unit, following which the inner Teflon dilator is removed to permit catheter introduction. The two side-arm sheaths also permit fluid infusion and an additional site for pressure monitoring with the catheter in place.

above the diaphragm and within the right atrium, it is rotated counterclockwise to face the lateral wall of the right atrium (Fig. 5–5). Additional counterclockwise rotation and gentle advancement allow passage of the catheter tip into the superior vena cava, which is contiguous with the posterolateral wall of the right atrium. In contrast, anterior orientation of the catheter tip at this point may result in its entrapment in the right atrial appendage and inability to reach the superior vena cava. Once in position, a baseline superior vena caval blood sample is obtained for measurement of oxygen saturation and comparison with the subsequently measured pulmonary arterial blood O_2 saturation, to screen for unsuspected left-to-right shunts. The catheter is then flushed with heparinized saline solution and withdrawn to the right atrium for pressure measurement.

The principles of advancing a catheter from the femoral vein to the pulmonary artery apply to either the Swan-Ganz or stiffer woven Dacron catheters. With the tip of the catheter positioned at the lower portion of the lateral right atrial border, clockwise rotation causes the catheter tip to sweep the anterior and anteromedial wall of the right atrium, along which the tricuspid valve is located (Fig. 5–5). As the catheter tip passes over the tricuspid orifice, slight advancement causes it to enter

the right ventricle where pressure is again recorded. If the right atrium is enlarged, greater curvature of the catheter may be necessary: a large J loop may be formed by engaging the tip of the catheter against the lateral right atrial wall or in the ostium of the hepatic vein just below the diaphragm. This larger loop can then be rotated clockwise in the atrium as described above, and usually enters the right ventricle.

Simple advancement of the catheter in the right ventricle causes the tip to move toward the apex of that chamber and usually does *not* result in catheterization of the pulmonary artery. To achieve this latter end, the catheter must be withdrawn slightly so that its tip lies horizontally and just to the right (patient's left) of the spine. In this position, clockwise rotation causes the tip of the catheter to point upwards (and slightly posteriorly) in the direction of the right ventricular outflow tract (Fig. 5–5). The catheter should be advanced only when it is in this orientation to minimize the risk of ventricular arrhythmias or injury to the right ventricle. Advancement may be facilitated if performed as the patient takes a deep breath. If these maneuvers fail to achieve access to the pulmonary artery due to enlargement of the right atrial and ventricular chambers, the catheter may be withdrawn to the right atrium and formed into a large "reverse loop," which allows the tip of the catheter to

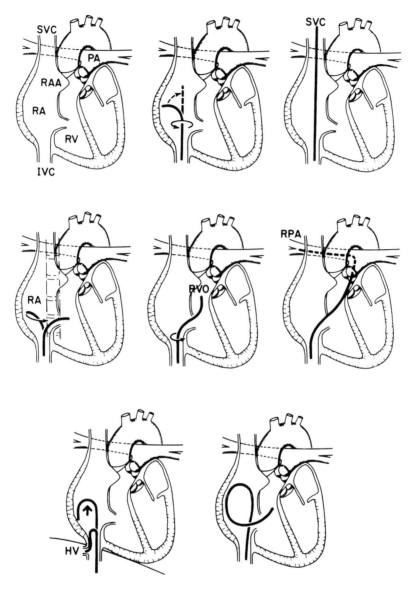

Fig. 5–5. Right heart catheterization from the femoral vein, shown in cartoon form. Top panel, the right heart catheter is initially placed in the right atrium (RA) aimed at the lateral atrial wall. Counterclockwise rotation aims the catheter posteriorly and allows advancement into the superior vena cava (SVC). Although not evident in the figure, clockwise catheter rotation into an anterior orientation would lead to advancement into the right atrial appendage (RAA), precluding SVC catheterization. Center row, the catheter is then withdrawn back into the right atrium and aimed laterally. Clockwise rotation causes the catheter tip to sweep anteromedially and cross the tricuspid valve. With the catheter tip in a horizontal orientation just beyond the spine, it is positioned below the right ventricular outflow tract (RVO). Additional clockwise rotation causes the catheter to point straight up, allowing for advancement into the main pulmonary artery and from there into the right pulmonary artery (RPA). Bottom row, two maneuvers useful in catheterization of a dilated right heart. A larger loop with a downward directed tip may be required to reach the tricuspid valve and can be formed by catching the catheter tip in the hepatic vein (HV) and advancing the catheter quickly into the right atrium. The reverse loop technique (bottom, right) gives the catheter tip an upward direction, aimed toward the outflow tract.

cross the tricuspid valve in an upward orientation more likely to enter the outflow tract (Fig. 5–5, bottom right). When manipulated appropriately, the catheter tip should cross the pulmonic valve and advance to a wedge position without difficulty. Having the patient take a deep breath and cough during advancement is often of assistance in achieving a wedge position. While catheters advanced from the leg are more likely to seek the left pulmonary artery than catheters advanced from above, either pulmonary artery can be catheterized by appropriate manipulation or careful introduction of a curved J guide wire. Following measurement of the wedge pressure, the catheter is withdrawn to the proximal left or right pulmonary artery, and a second blood saturation is obtained.

Attempts to perform right heart catheterization occasionally result in entry into other structures. If a woven Dacron catheter is advanced in the right atrium with a posteromedial orientation, it may cross a patent foramen ovale and enter the left atrium. This can be recognized by a change in the pressure waveform, position of the catheter tip across the spine, and the ability to withdraw fully oxygenated blood from the catheter tip. Although more unusual, it is also possible for a woven Dacron catheter to enter the ostium of the coronary sinus, inferiorly and posteriorly to the tricuspid orifice. There will be continued presence of a right atrial waveform, but blood sampling will disclose a far lower oxygen saturation (20 to 30%) than was present in the superior vena cava. The most important points about these side trips off the beaten path to the right ventricle are that the operator should recognize that the tip of the catheter is *not* in the right ventricle (i.e., one should not attempt to get to the pulmonary artery) and should decide where the catheter is (by pressure monitoring, saturation analysis, or injection of a small amount of contrast agent) before withdrawing the catheter to the right atrium and proceeding with the right heart catheterization.

Unsuspected anatomic abnormalities can frequently be detected by an unusual catheter position or course. In Figure 5–6, the appearance of the right heart catheter course in three such congenital abnormalities (persistent left superior vena cava, patent ductus arteriosus and anomalous pulmonary venous return) is depicted. The commonest abnormality, atrial septal defect, is sometimes hard to detect by catheter position alone because the catheter appearance in the left atrium or ventricle may be indistinguishable (in the anteroposterior view) from its course during usual right heart catheterization. Measurement of pressure and blood oxygen saturation, together with hand injection of radiographic contrast and use of oblique and lateral views, should allow the operator to sort out the anatomy.

In patients with elevated right heart pressures, those undergoing specialized procedures (endomyocardial biopsy, coronary sinus catheterization), or those in whom prolonged post-procedure monitoring with a balloon-flotation catheter is desired, the right internal jugular vein offers an excellent alternative to the femoral vein. The technique for jugular puncture is described in Chapter 32, and the method of advancing the right heart catheter to the pulmonary artery is identical to that described in Chapter 4. On occasion, percutaneous right heart catheterization is performed from the subclavian or median basilic vein, using a similar technique.

Femoral Artery Puncture

The femoral artery is punctured by inserting the Seldinger needle through the more lateral skin nick. Again, the needle is inserted at approximately 45 degrees, along the axis of the femoral artery as palpated by the three middle fingers of the left hand. The experienced operator may feel the transmitted pulsations as the tip of the needle contacts the wall of the femoral artery, but it is customary to advance the needle completely through the artery until the periosteum is encountered. If a single wall puncture is desired, the operator may prefer a Potts-Cournand needle (Fig. 5–2), in which the obturator has a small lumen that transmits a flashback of arterial blood as the vessel is entered. Once the obturator is removed, the

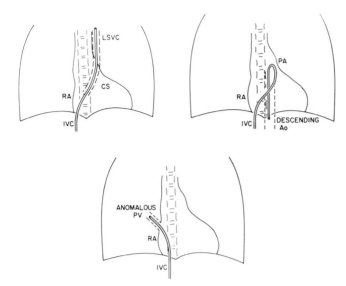

Fig. 5–6. Unsuspected anatomic abnormalities frequently can be detected by an unusual catheter course or position. Upper left panel, the course of a catheter passed from the femoral vein to inferior vena cava (IVC), right atrium (RA), coronary sinus (CS), and up into an anomalous left superior vena cava (LSVC). Upper right panel, the catheter crossing from pulmonary artery (PA) to descending aorta (Ao) by way of a patent ductus arteriosus. Bottom panel, the catheter entering an anomalous pulmonary vein draining into the right atrium.

hub of the needle may be depressed slightly toward the anterior surface of the thigh. Arterial pressure makes it unnecessary to attach a syringe to the cannula, so that both hands can be used to stabilize the needle as it is slowly withdrawn. When the needle comes back into the lumen of the femoral artery as evidenced by vigorous pulsatile flow of arterial blood, a 0.035- or 0.038-inch J guide wire should then be advanced carefully into the needle. It should move freely up the aorta, located to the right (patient's left side) of the spine on fluoroscopy, up to the level of the diaphragm.

If wire motion ceases to be free after several centimeters, or if the patient complains of *any* discomfort during wire advancement, subintimal position of the wire is a distinct possibility. The wire should be withdrawn slightly under fluoroscopic control, and the needle should be removed as the left hand is used to stabilize the wire and control arterial bleeding. After the wire is wiped with a moist gauze pad, a small (5 Fr) dilator can be cautiously introduced up to the point where the wire had advanced without difficulty. The wire is then withdrawn from the dilator, which is aspirated to ensure free flow of blood and flushed carefully. A small bolus of contrast medium is then injected gently under fluoroscopic monitoring. This injection usually discloses the anatomic reason for difficult wire advancement—either

iliac tortuosity, stenosis, or dissection. If dissection is present, retrograde left heart catheterization should be relocated to the other femoral artery or to the brachial artery, and the patient should be observed for signs of progressive dissection or arterial compromise, both of which are fortunately rare with retrograde guide wire dissections. If tortuosity or stenosis is the problem, more specialized guide wires (a large 15 mm, floppy or movable core J, or a steerable wire [e.g., a Wholey wire*]) may be carefully reintroduced through the dilator in an attempt to reach the descending aorta.

When difficulty in advancing the guide wire is encountered at or just beyond the tip of the needle and is not corrected by slight depression or slight withdrawal of the needle, the guide wire should be withdrawn to ensure that vigorous arterial flow is still present before any further wire manipulation is attempted. If flow is not brisk or if the wire still cannot be advanced, the needle should be removed and the groin should be compressed for 5 minutes. The operator should verify the correctness of the anatomic landmarks and attempt repuncture of the femoral artery. If the second attempt is unsuccessful in allowing wire advancement, a third attempt on the same vessel is unwise.

*Advanced Cardiovascular Systems, Temecula, CA.

Catheterizing Left Heart from Femoral Artery

Once the guide wire has been advanced to the level of the diaphragm, the needle cannula is removed. The left hand is used to stabilize the wire and control arterial bleeding while the wire is wiped with a moistened gauze pad to remove any adherent blood. If the catheter is to be introduced directly into the artery, it is customary to pre-dilate the soft tissues by brief introduction of a Teflon arterial dilator one Fr size smaller than the intended catheter, before inserting the left heart catheter itself. In our laboratory, however, essentially all left heart catheterizations from the femoral approach are performed using a 7 Fr sheath equipped with a backbleed valve and sidearm tubing, as described above. This is introduced over the guide wire (the proximal end of which is held in a straightened, fixed position) with a rotational motion, following which the guide wire and dilator are removed, and the sheath is aspirated, flushed, and connected by its sidearm to a manifold for monitoring arterial pressure. This sheath should be reflushed immediately after each catheter is introduced or withdrawn and every 5 minutes during the catheterization to avoid encroachment of blood and potential thrombus formation within the sheath. The desired left heart catheter is then flushed and loaded with a 145 cm J guide wire. The tip of the catheter is straightened manually to facilitate introduction into the backbleed valve. The soft end of the guide wire is then advanced carefully through the catheter, out the end of the sheath, and to the level of the diaphragm before the catheter itself is advanced. If the back end of the wire is extended straight down the patient's leg and held fixed to the leg, this will ensure that the wire remains in constant position within the aorta during catheter advancement. The guide wire is then removed and the catheter is connected to the arterial manifold and double flushed (withdrawal and discarding of 10 ml of blood, followed by vigorous injection of heparinized saline solution). Full intravenous heparinization (5000 U) is established immediately after the left heart cath-

eter is inserted, providing therapeutic anticoagulation lasting at least 40 minutes in most patients.[8]

While the above technique is commonly used, it may lead to vascular injury during attempted readvancement of the guide wire out the end of the previously inserted sheath. We have therefore modified our technique to use a short-exchange length (175 cm) Newton J (Cook, Inc.) as the initial wire placed through the Seldinger needle. The tip of the guide wire is then left at the diaphragm while the dilator is removed from the sheath and the left heart catheter is introduced, thereby avoiding the need to renegotiate complex iliofemoral anatomy with the guide wire. Similarly, all subsequent left heart catheters may be introduced by reinserting this wire to the level of the diaphragm as one catheter is removed and the second is reintroduced, rather than withdrawing one catheter and inserting the second catheter and wire through the sheath de novo. Of course, if the left heart catheterization is being performed without the aid of a sheath, it is mandatory to leave the tip of the wire in the abdominal aorta during the removal of the first catheter and the introduction of a second catheter in order to retain access to the vessel.

The initial left heart catheter in most cases is a pigtail catheter with multiple side holes. This catheter can be advanced to the ascending aorta without difficulty, at which point the ascending aortic and femoral arterial (sheath side arm) pressure are recorded simultaneously (Fig. 5–7).[3,4] The systolic peak in the femoral waveform may be slightly delayed and accentuated compared to the ascending aortic pressure trace, but the diastolic and mean pressures should be virtually identical. The pigtail catheter is then advanced across the aortic valve and into the left ventricle. If the aortic valve is normal and the pigtail is oriented correctly, it will usually cross the valve directly. In many cases, however, it may be necessary to advance the pigtail down into one of the sinuses of Valsalva so as to form a secondary loop (Fig. 5–8). As the catheter is withdrawn slowly, this loop will open to span the full

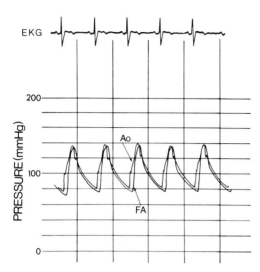

Fig. 5–7. Central aortic pressure (Ao) measured through a 7.3 French pigtail catheter (Cook) and femoral artery (FA) pressure measured from the sidearm of an 8 French arterial sheath (Cordis). Only minimal damping of the femoral artery pressure is seen, blunting its systolic overshoot, which frequently exceeds central aortic systolic pressure (see Chapter 9). With larger (7.5 French and 8 French) catheters, more damping may occur in the sidearm pressure. Catheter and sidearm are connected to small volume-displacement transducers without intervening tubing.

diameter of the aorta and then fall across the valve (Fig. 5–8).

If significant aortic stenosis is present, the pigtail must be advanced across the valve with the aid of a straight 0.038-inch guide wire. Approximately 6 cm of the guide wire is advanced beyond the end of the pigtail catheter, and the catheter is withdrawn slightly until the tip of the guide wire is leading (Fig. 5–8). The position of the tip of the guide wire within the aortic root can then be controlled by rotation of the pigtail catheter and adjustment of the amount of wire that protrudes; less wire protruding directs the wire tip more toward the left coronary ostium, whereas more wire protruding directs the wire more toward the right coronary ostium. With the wire tip positioned so that it is directed toward the aortic orifice, the tip of the wire usually quivers in the systolic jet. Wire and catheter are then advanced as a unit until the wire crosses into the left ventricle. If the wire buckles in the sinus of Valsalva instead of crossing the valve, the

catheter-wire system is withdrawn slightly and readvanced with or without subtle change in the length of protruding wire or the orientation of the pigtail catheter. Alternatively, some operators prefer to leave the pigtail catheter fixed and move the guide wire independently in attempts to cross stenotic aortic valves. During attempts to cross the aortic valve, the wire should be withdrawn and cleaned and the catheter should be double-flushed vigorously every three minutes despite systemic heparinization. If promising wire positions are not obtained, the process should be repeated using a different catheter: an angled pigtail or left Amplatz catheter if the aortic root is dilated or a Judkins right coronary catheter if the aortic root is unusually narrow. Other catheters have been proposed for this purpose, but we have found these standard catheters to suffice in virtually all cases.[9]

When the tip of the guide wire is across the aortic valve, additional wire should be inserted before the catheter itself is advanced; otherwise the catheter may be diverted into the sinus of Valsalva and flip the wire out of the left ventricle. Once the catheter is in the left ventricle, the wire is immediately withdrawn and the catheter is aspirated vigorously, flushed and hooked up for pressure monitoring, so that a gradient can be measured even if the catheter is rapidly ejected from the left ventricle or must be withdrawn because of arrhythmias. When using a left Amplatz catheter to cross a stenotic valve, however, we prefer to cross the valve with a full exchange-length (260 cm) guide wire. Once the tip of this wire has entered the left ventricle, it is left in position as the Amplatz catheter is removed and a conventional pigtail catheter is substituted before an attempt is made to measure LV pressure.

At the termination of the left heart catheterization, heparin is usually reversed by the administration of protamine (1 ml = 10 mg of protamine for every 1000 U of heparin). The operator should be watchful for potential adverse reactions to protamine, characterized by hypotension and vascular collapse, as discussed in Chapter 3. Protamine reactions appear to be more common in insulin-dependent

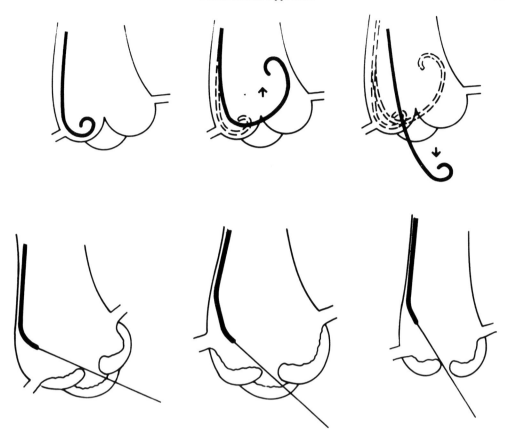

Fig. 5–8. Crossing the aortic valve with a pigtail catheter. Although a correctly oriented pigtail catheter will frequently cross a normal aortic valve directly, it may also come to rest in the right or noncoronary sinus of Valsalva (top row, left). Further advancement of the catheter enlarges the loop to span the aortic root (top row, center) and positions the catheter so that slow withdrawal causes it to sweep across the aortic orifice, and fall into the left ventricle (top row, right). To cross a stenotic aortic valve, the pigtail catheter must be led by a segment of straight guide wire (bottom row, left). Increasing the length of protruding guide wire straightens the catheter curve and causes the wire to point more toward the right coronary ostium; reducing the length of protruding wire restores the catheter curve and causes the wire to point more toward the left coronary. Once the correct length of wire and the correct rotational orientation of the pigtail catheter have been found, repeated advancement and withdrawal of both the catheter and guide wire as a unit will allow the wire to cross the valve. In a dilated aortic root, an angled pigtail provides more favorable wire positions (bottom row, center). In a small aortic root (bottom row, right), a Judkins right coronary catheter may be preferable.

diabetics and patients with previous protamine exposure, who are more likely to have elevated levels of IgG or IgE antiprotamine antibodies.[10] Although severe protamine reactions in these patients are uncommon, we prefer a trial of groin compression *without* protamine administration (unless needed) in insulin-dependent diabetics.[11]

After administration of protamine, the arterial catheter and sheath are removed, and firm manual pressure is applied using three fingers of the left hand positioned sequentially up the femoral artery beginning at the skin puncture. With the fingers in this position, there should be no ongoing bleeding into the soft tissues or through the skin puncture. It should be possible to apply sufficient pressure to obliterate the pedal pulses, and then release just enough pressure to allow them to barely return. This pressure is then gradually reduced over the next 10 to 15 minutes, at the end of which time pressure is removed completely. The venous sheath is usually removed 5 minutes after compression of the arterial puncture has begun, with gentle pressure applied over the venous puncture using the right hand. After procedures using larger arterial sheaths (i.e., PTCA or balloon valvuloplasty), we tend to perform more prolonged compression (30 to 45 minutes) using a mechanical device (Compressar, Instromedix, Beaverton, OR), but continuous presence of a trained person is required to ensure that the device is providing adequate control and is not compromising distal perfusion. The puncture site and surrounding area are then inspected for hematoma formation and active oozing, and the quality of the distal pulse is assessed before application of a bandage.

It is our policy to keep the patient at bed rest with the leg straight for at least 4 to 6 hours following percutaneous femoral catheterization, with a sandbag in place over the puncture site for the first few hours after catheter removal. In patients at higher risk for rebleeding (those with hypertension, obesity, or aortic regurgitation) application of a pressure bandage in addition to the sandbag may be of value. Although the patient should be instructed not to move the leg for several hours following the catheterization procedure, this does not mean that the patient must lie flat during this time. Elevation of the head and chest to 30 to 45 degrees by the electrical or manual bed control, without muscular effort by the patient, will greatly increase the patient's comfort and will not increase the risk of local bleeding. The only reason to insist that the patient lie completely flat is if there is significant orthostatic hypotension. Before ambulation, the puncture site should again be inspected for recurrent bleeding, hematoma formation, development of a bruit suggestive of pseudoaneurysm or A-V fistula formation, or loss of distal pulses.

Relative Contraindications to Femoral Artery Catheterization

As discussed in Chapter 1, the choice of catheterization approach (femoral or brachial) is usually a function of operator, institution, and patient preference. Catheter insertion and manipulation in patients with peripheral vascular disease (femoral bruits or diminished lower extremity pulses), abdominal aortic aneurysm, marked iliac tortuosity, prior femoral arterial graft surgery, or gross obesity, however, may present technical challenges even for experienced operators. Recognition of these factors may favor the use of the brachial approach (if a skilled operator is available), even though in the final analysis there are relatively few patients who absolutely cannot be catheterized from the femoral approach.

The choice of approach should also take into account potential difficulties in catheter removal. Hemostasis is usually obtained easily after removal of a percutaneous arterial catheter, but it should be emphasized that patients with a wide pulse pressure (e.g., severe aortic incompetence or systemic hypertension), gross obesity, or ongoing anticoagulation have more problems with bleeding after femoral catheterization than do patients without these factors.

Complications of percutaneous retrograde arterial catheterization are fortunately infrequent and usually not life-threatening. These complications, as well as their causes and prevention, are discussed in Chapter 3.

BRACHIAL OR AXILLARY ARTERY CATHETERIZATION

The techniques described above for percutaneous insertion of a femoral catheter also can be used successfully from the brachial, axillary or even the radial artery, with or without an introducing sheath. The smaller caliber of these vessels, potential difficulties in controlling the catheterization site at the end of the procedure, and the tendency for hematomas at these locations to be poorly tolerated make them less desirable than femoral catheterization unless the latter is unsuccessful or contraindicated and an operator experienced in the conventional direct brachial approach (described in Chapter 4) is not available.

TRANSSEPTAL LEFT HEART CATHETERIZATION

With refinements and improvements in techniques for retrograde left heart catheterization, the use of transseptal puncture for access to the left atrium and left ventricle[13,14] had become an infrequent procedure in most adult cardiac catheterization laboratories.[15] In these laboratories, transseptal puncture was reserved for situations in which direct left atrial pressure recording was desired (pulmonary venous disease), in which it was important to distinguish true idiopathic hypertrophic subaortic stenosis (IHSS) from catheter entrapment, in which retrograde left heart catheterization had failed (e.g., due to severe peripheral arterial disease or aortic stenosis) or was dangerous due to the presence of a certain type of mechanical prosthetic valve (e.g., Bjork-Shiley or St. Jude valves). The infrequency with which the procedure was performed made it difficult for most laboratories to maintain operator expertise and to train cardiovascular fellows in transseptal puncture and gave the procedure an aura of danger and intrigue. With the advent of percutaneous mitral valvuloplasty (Chapter 29) and the availability of improved equipment, however, transseptal catheterization has again become a relatively common procedure.[16]

The goal of transseptal catheterization is to cross from the right atrium to the left atrium through the fossa ovalis. In approximately 10% of patients, this maneuver is performed inadvertently during right heart catheterization with a woven Dacron catheter because of the presence of a probe-patent foramen ovale, but in the remainder, mechanical puncture of this area with a needle and catheter combination is required to enter the left atrium. Although puncture of the fossa ovale itself is quite safe, the danger of the transseptal approach lies in the possibility that the needle and catheter will puncture an adjacent structure. To minimize this risk, the operator must have a detailed familiarity with the regional anatomy of the atrial septum (Fig. 5–9). As viewed from the feet with the patient lying supine, the plane of

the atrial septum runs from 1 o'clock to 7 o'clock. The area of the fossa ovalis is bounded anteriorly and superiorly by the aortic root and posteriorly by the posterior free wall of the right atrium. The fossa ovalis is located superiorly and posteriorly to the ostium of the coronary sinus and well posterior of the tricuspid annulus and right atrial appendage. The fossa ovalis is approximately 2 cm in diameter and is bounded superiorly by a ridge—the limbus.

Transseptal catheterization is performed *only* from the right femoral vein. We use a 70 cm curved Brockenbrough needle, (USCI, Billerica, MA) which tapers from 18 gauge to 21 gauge at the tip (Fig. 5–10). It is usually inserted into a matching catheter or 8 Fr Mullins sheath and dilator[17] (USCI), with an obturator (Bing stylet) protruding slightly beyond the tip of the needle to avoid abrasion or puncture of the catheter wall during needle advancement. The hub of this needle is equipped with a metal flange, which indicates the orientation of the needle curve and serves as a reference point for monitoring the position of the needle tip relative to the tip of the catheter. Before insertion, a sterile ruler may be used to measure the distance between the needle flange and the catheter hub under two conditions: first, with the tip of the Bing stylet at the tip of the catheter, and second, with the tip of the Brockenbrough needle itself at the tip of the catheter (Fig. 5–11). Alternatively, current high-quality fluoroscopy can be used to visually monitor advancement of the needle to the catheter tip.

Venous entry is performed as described above, except that no sheath is used. An 0.032 inch 145 cm J guide wire is advanced well up into the vena cava, the introducing needle is then removed, and the protruding guide wire is wiped with a moistened gauze pad. The previously calibrated transseptal catheter (usually a 70 cm, 8 Fr Teflon Brockenbrough catheter with six side holes and an end hole, and a 2.5 or 3.0 cm distal curve) or 8 Fr Mullins sheath is then inserted into the superior vena cava over the guide wire. Once the catheter is

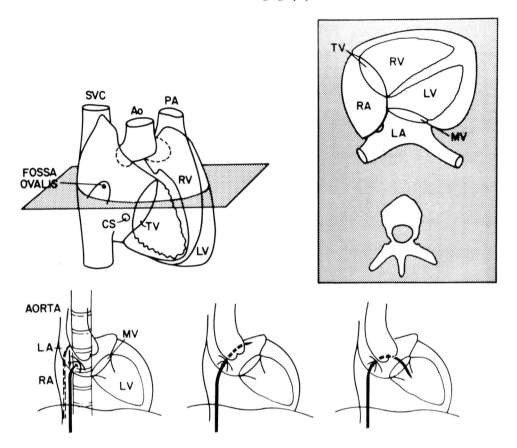

Fig. 5–9. Regional anatomy for transseptal puncture. Upper left, the position of the fossa ovalis is shown relative to the superior vena cava (SVC), aortic root (Ao), coronary sinus (CS), and tricuspid valve (TV). Upper right, a cross section through the fossa (looking up from below) demonstrating the posteromedial direction of the interatrial septum (bold line) and the proximity of the lateral free wall of the right atrium. Bottom row, the appearance of the transseptal catheter as it is withdrawn from the SVC in a posteromedial orientation. As the catheter tip slides over the aortic root (bottom left, dotted position) it appears to move rightward on to the spine. Slight further withdrawal leads to more rightward movement into the fossa (solid position). Puncture of the fossa with advancement of the catheter into the left atrium (bottom row, center), and advancement into the left ventricle with the aid of a curved tip occluder (right). (Redrawn from Ross J Jr: Considerations regarding the technique for transseptal left heart catheterization. Circulation 34:391, 1966.)

in position, the guide wire is removed, and the catheter or sheath is vigorously double flushed.

The next step is the advancement of the Brockenbrough needle and Bing stylet up to, but not beyond, the tip of the catheter. As the needle and its stylet are advanced into the catheter with stylet in place, the patient may experience a slight sensation of pressure. The progress of the needle tip should be monitored fluoroscopically, looking for any sign of perforation of the catheter by the needle. It is essential to allow the needle to rotate freely during advancement so that it may follow the curves of the catheter; the hub of the needle should never be grasped and rotated at this point. As the tip of the Bing stylet approaches the tip of the catheter (indicated by measurement of the distance between the needle flange and the catheter hub or by fluoroscopic observation), the stylet should be removed and the needle itself should be advanced to the tip of the catheter, again monitored by fluoroscopy and ruler measurement. The needle is connected to a pressure manifold, using a three-way stopcock and a short length of pressure tubing, and double flushed. The superior

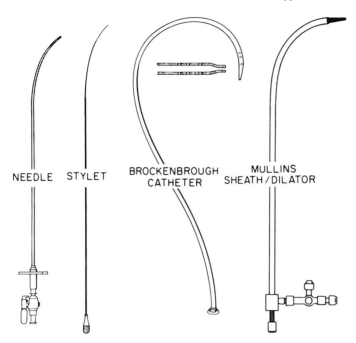

NEEDLE   STYLET   BROCKENBROUGH
CATHETER

MULLINS
SHEATH/DILATOR

Fig. 5–10. Equipment for transseptal puncture. The Brockenbrough needle and Bing stylet (left and left center, respectively) can be used in conjunction with either the traditional Brockenbrough catheter (right center) or the Mullins sheath/dilator system (right).

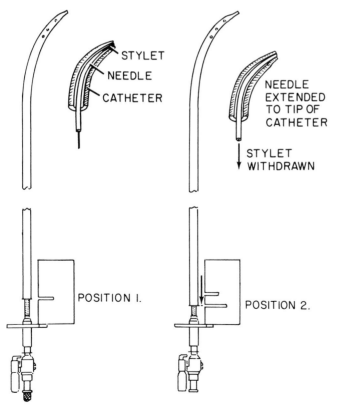

STYLET
NEEDLE
CATHETER

NEEDLE
EXTENDED
TO TIP OF
CATHETER

STYLET
WITHDRAWN

POSITION I.

POSITION 2.

Fig. 5–11. The Brockenbrough system with the needle and stylet inserted into the catheter. Ruler measurement of the distance from the catheter hub to the needle flange is shown with the tip of the stylet at the tip of the catheter (position 1) and with the stylet withdrawn and the needle tip extended to the tip of the catheter (position 2). (Redrawn from Ross J Jr: Considerations regarding the technique for transseptal left heart catheterization. Circulation 34:391, 1966.)

vena caval pressure should then be recorded through the needle, and the needle rotated so that the direction indicator points anteriorly.

Under continuous fluoroscopic and pressure monitoring, the needle and catheter are held in constant relationship as they are withdrawn slowly, using both hands, firmly controlling the direction indicator with the right hand. During this withdrawal from the superior vena cava, the direction indicator is slowly but firmly rotated clockwise until the arrow is oriented posteromedially (4 o'clock when looking from below) as the tip of the catheter enters the right atrium. The needle and catheter are maintained in their posteromedial orientation and continue to be withdrawn slowly; this withdrawal will cause the catheter tip to slip over the bulge of the ascending aorta and move rightward (toward the patient's left) so as to overlie the vertebrae in the anterior projection (Fig. 5–9). Slight further withdrawal is associated with a second rightward movement as the catheter tip "snaps" into the fossa ovalis. If the foramen is patent, the catheter may cross into the left atrium spontaneously at this point, as indicated by a change in atrial pressure waveform and the ability to withdraw oxygenated blood from the needle. Otherwise, the catheter is advanced slightly to engage the limbus at the superior portion of the foramen ovale. This engagement, evident both fluoroscopically and tactilely, is essential to successful transseptal puncture. Once the operator is satisfied with the position of the catheter, the Brockenbrough needle is advanced abruptly so that its point emerges from the tip of the catheter and perforates the atrial septum. Successful entry into the left atrium is confirmed by both the recording of a left atrial pressure waveform *and* the withdrawal of oxygenated blood, or a puff of contrast. Once the operator is confident that the needle tip is across the interatrial septum, the needle and catheter are advanced as a unit a *short* distance into the left atrium, taking care to control their motion so that the protruding needle does not injure left atrial structures. Once the catheter is across the atrial septum, the needle is withdrawn and the catheter is double-flushed vig-

orously and connected to a manifold for pressure recording.

The main risk during transseptal catheterization is inadvertent puncture of the aortic root, coronary sinus, or posterior free wall of the right atrium, rather than the fossa ovalis. As long as the patient is not anticoagulated and perforation is limited to the 21-gauge tip of the Brockenbrough needle (i.e., perforation is recognized and the catheter itself is not advanced), this is usually benign. However, if the 8F catheter itself is advanced into the pericardium or aortic root, potentially fatal complications may occur, underscoring the need for the operator to monitor closely the location of the transseptal apparatus by fluoroscopic, pressure, and oxygen saturation at each stage of the procedure. If the pressure waveform during attempted septal puncture becomes damped, this may indicate puncture into the pericardium or simply incomplete penetration of a thickened interatrial septum. Injection of a small amount of contrast through the needle can be useful in this case by staining the atrial septum and allowing confirmation of an appropriate position in the LAO and RAO projection before more forceful needle advancement is attempted.[18]

If the initial attempt at transseptal puncture is unsuccessful, the operator may wish to repeat the catheter positioning procedure by removing the transseptal needle from the catheter, withdrawing the catheter slightly, and reinserting the 0.032 inch guide wire into the superior vena cava. *One should never attempt to reposition the catheter-needle combination in the superior vena cava in any other way, since perforation of the right atrium or atrial appendage is a distinct possibility during such maneuvers.*

Once the catheter is safely in the left atrium, additional manipulation may be required to enter the left ventricle. If the tip of the catheter has entered an inferior pulmonary vein (as evident by its projection outside the posterior heart border in the right anterior oblique projection), the left ventricle can be approached by torquing the catheter 180 degrees in a counterclockwise direction so that its tip moves anteriorly as it is withdrawn slightly. As the catheter tip moves anteriorly and downward, further advancement will usually allow it to cross the mitral valve and enter the left ventricle. If not, it may be necessary to insert a curved tip occluder into the catheter through an o-ring sidearm adaptor to tighten the tip curve and facilitate advancement into the ventricle. By converting the Brockenbrough catheter from an end- and side-hole to a side-hole only device, the tip occluder also minimizes the chance for left ventricular staining and perforation during contrast ventriculography. However, contrast angiography at 8 to 10 ml/sec for 40 to 50 ml total injection (as with the Sones catheter) can usually be accomplished safely without a tip occluder, if desired. Following the completion of hemodynamic and angiographic evaluation, the Brockenbrough catheter is withdrawn in the usual manner during continuous pressure recording.

The technique using the Mullins sheath[17] in place of the Brockenbrough catheter is similar, except that care must be taken to advance both the dilator and the 8 Fr sheath into the left atrium without injuring the opposite left atrial wall. Slight counterclockwise rotation and repeated puffs of contrast to define location of the catheter tip may be helpful in this regard. Once the sheath is secure in the left atrium, the needle and dilator are withdrawn and the sheath is flushed carefully. Either a specially curved pigtail catheter (in patients with a normal mitral valve) or a CO_2-inflated balloon flotation catheter (in patients with mitral stenosis) may then be inserted through the sheath and passed into the left ventricle. The variant of the Mullins sheath which we use has a sidearm connection and backbleed valve, allowing ongoing measurement of left atrial pressure around the left ventricular catheter.

Complications of transseptal catheterization are generally infrequent (''needle tip'' perforation less than 3%, tamponade less than 1%, and death less than 0.5%) in experienced hands, but complications may be significantly more common early in an operator's experience or in high-risk patients. The technique should be avoided in patients with distorted anatomy due to congenital heart disease, marked left or right atrial enlargement, significant chest or spine deformity, inability to lie flat, ongoing anticoagulation, or left atrial thrombus/tumor.

APICAL LEFT VENTRICULAR PUNCTURE

Historically, a variety of direct puncture techniques were used to enter the cardiac chambers before the introduction of percutaneous left and right heart catheterization. These techniques included transbronchial[19] and transthoracic[20] approaches to the left atrium, the suprasternal puncture technique of Radner[21] and apical left ventricular puncture.[22,23] Of these, only the last has survived, albeit as an infrequent (roughly 1 per year in our laboratory) way to measure left ventricular pressure in a patient where retrograde and transseptal catheterization of the LV are precluded by the presence of mechanical aortic and mitral prostheses.

The site of the apical impulse is located by palpation and confirmed by fluoroscopy of a hemostatic clamp placed at the intended puncture site. Alternatively, the left ventricular apex can be located using echocardiography,[24] and may be found to lie significantly more lateral than the palpated ''apical'' impulse in patients with right ventricular enlargement. After liberal local anesthesia, an 18- or 19-gauge needle is introduced and directed along the long axis of the left ventricle, aimed roughly toward the second right costochondral junction and slightly posteriorly. According to the technique of Semple,[23] an outer Teflon catheter was advanced into the left ventricle (and sometimes out through the aortic valve) over the puncture needle, but we have used a more familiar technique in which the apex is punctured with the same 3-½ inch long, 18-gauge thin-wall needle that we use for internal jugular puncture. An 0.035″ 65 cm-long J guide wire is then advanced into the left ventricle under fluoroscopic guidance, allowing the advancement of a 4 Fr dilator followed by a 4 Fr pigtail catheter to allow pressure meas-

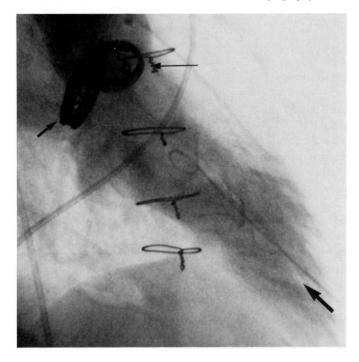

Fig. 5–12. Apical left ventricular puncture. In this patient with Björk-Shiley aortic and mitral valve prostheses (arrow, upper left), percutaneous puncture of the left ventricular apex was performed to allow left ventricular pressure measurement and contrast ventriculography using a 4 Fr angiographic pigtail catheter shown entering the LV apex (arrow, lower right). This catheter was advanced into the left ventricle over an 0.035 inch guide wire, following apical puncture with an 18 gauge thin-wall needle (see text for details).

urement and/or left ventricular angiography (Fig. 5–12).

Although one recent series describes excellent results in more than 100 such procedures, complications occurred in 3% and included cardiac tamponade (uncommon in postoperative patients), hemothorax, pneumothorax, intramyocardial injection, ventricular fibrillation, and reflex hypotension due to vagal stimulation. We thus reserve this technique for patients in whom it is essential to enter the left ventricle, and in whom neither retrograde nor anterograde (transseptal) approaches are feasible.

REFERENCES

1. Seldinger SI: Catheter replacement of the needle in percutaneous arteriography, a new technique. Acta Radiol 39:368, 1953.
2. Judkins MP, Kidd HJ, Frische LH, Dotter CT: Lumen-following safety J-guide for catheterization of tortuous vessels. Radiology 88:1127, 1967.
3. Barry WH et al: Left heart catheterization and angiography via the percutaneous femoral approach using an arterial sheath. Cathet Cardiovasc Diagn 5:401, 1979.
4. Hillis LD: Percutaneous left heart catheterization and coronary arteriography using a femoral artery sheath. Cathet Cardiovasc Diagn 5:393, 1979.
5. Fergusson DJG, Kamada RO: Percutaneous entry of the brachial artery for left heart catheterization using a sheath: Further experience. Cathet Cardiovasc Diagn 12:209, 1986.
6. Velix B, et al: Selective coronary arteriography by percutaneous transaxillary approach. Cathet Cardiovasc Diagn 10:403, 1984.
7. Campeau L: Percutaneous radial artery approach for coronary angiography. Cathet Cardiovasc Diagn 16:3, 1989.
8. Dehmer GJ et al: Anticoagulation with heparin during cardiac catheterization and its reversal by protamine. Cathet Cardiovasc Diagn 13:16, 1987.
9. Feldman T, Carroll JD, Chiu YC: An improved catheter design for crossing stenosed aortic valves. Cathet Cardiovasc Diagn 16:279, 1989.
10. Weiss ME et al: Association of protamine IgE and IgG antibodies with life-threatening reactions to intravenous protamine. N Engl J Med 320:886, 1989.
11. Click RL, Homburger HA, Bove AA: Complement activation from protamine sulfate administration after coronary angiography. Cathet Cardiovasc Diagn 16:221, 1989.
12. Smith DC, Willis WH: Transfemoral coronary arteriography via a prosthetic aortic bifurcation graft. Cathet Cardiovasc Diagn 14:121, 1988.
13. Ross J Jr: Considerations regarding the technique for transseptal left heart catheterization. Circulation 34:391, 1966.
14. Brockenbrough EC, Braunwald E: A new technique for left ventricular angiocardiography and transseptal left heart catheterization. Am J Cardiol 6:1062, 1960.
15. Schoonmaker FW, Vijay NK, Jantz RD: Left atrial and ventricular transseptal catheterization review: losing skills? Cathet Cardiovasc Diagn 13:233, 1987.
16. O'Keefe JH et al: Revival of the transseptal approach

for catheterization of the left atrium and ventricle: Mayo Clin Proc 60:790, 1985.

17. Mullins CE: Transseptal left heart catheterization: experience with a new technique in pediatric and adult patients. Ped Cardiol 4:239, 1983.

18. Croft CH, Lipscomb K: Modified technique of transseptal left heart catheterization. J Am Coll Cardiol 5:904, 1985.

19. Morrow AG, Braunwald E, Lanenbaum HL: Transbronchial left heart catheterization: modified technique and its physiologic evaluation. Surg Forum 8:390, 1958.

20. Bjork VD: Direct pressure measurement in the left atrium, the left ventricle and the aorta. Acta Chir Scand 107:466, 1954.

21. Radner S: Extended suprasternal puncture technique. Acta Med Scand 151:223, 1955.

22. Brock R, Milstein BB, Ross DN: Percutaneous left ventricular puncture in the assessment of aortic stenosis. Thorax 11:163, 1956.

23. Semple T, McGuiness JB, Gardner H: Left heart catherization by direct ventricular puncture. Brit Heart J 30:402, 1968.

24. Vignola PA, Swaye PS, Gosselin AJ: Safe transthoracic left ventricular puncture performed with echocardiographic guidance. Cathet Cardiovasc Diagn 6:317, 1980.

25. Morgan JM et al: Left heart catheterization by direct ventricular puncture: withstanding the test of time. Cathet Cardiovasc Diagn 16:87, 1989.

6

Cardiac Catheterization in Infants and Children

JOHN F. KEANE, JAMES E. LOCK, and STANTON B. PERRY

Since the last edition of this text, several important changes have occurred in pediatric catheterization, including:
1. A major increase in the number of patients undergoing cardiac catheterization;
2. A shift in the types of lesions studied;
3. Their increasing management by catheter-based techniques (see Chapter 30).

At the Children's Hospital, Boston,[1] the number of studies done yearly has increased from 630 to 1100, mostly because of a rapid expansion in interventional therapeutic procedures which now account for some 38% of all of our cardiac catheterizations. Electrophysiologic studies have also increased and now account for 16% of the total catheterization laboratory volume. Another recent change is that almost 20% of studies (including some interventional procedures) are now performed on an outpatient basis. Furthermore, the remarkable advances in two-dimensional echocardiographic and color-flow Doppler techniques have allowed patients with some types of congenital heart disease (e.g., babies with total anomalous pulmonary venous return and children with ostium primum defects) to undergo operation without prior catheterization.[2,3] On the other hand, lesions such as patent ductus arteriosus (PDA) and secundum atrial defect (ASD), which were formerly re-ferred for surgery based on noninvasive data only, now come to the catheterization laboratory for definitive closure by interventional technique. It is also apparent that, because of advances in cardiac surgery, patients are living longer and adults who have had prior surgical repair of complex congenital defects are now being evaluated in increasing numbers by ourselves and our colleagues in adult cardiology.[4]

In this chapter, our standard catheterization methodology for acquiring physiologic and anatomic data is presented, followed by brief descriptions of some specialized pediatric procedures, such as ASD creation, transseptal puncture, subclavian vein catheterization, coronary angiography, pulmonary vein wedge angiography, and endomyocardial biopsy. Details of interventional techniques for the treatment of PDA, ASD, ventricular septal defect (VSD), stenotic valves, and collateral vessels are presented in Chapter 30.

GENERAL CATHETERIZATION PROTOCOL

Pre-Catheterization Preparations

As in any cardiac catheterization procedure, all available data including clinical, echocardiographic and previous catheterization information are assembled and examined in detail so that a study protocol can be formulated. If an intervention is likely, an intravenous line is placed, nursing assistance is available throughout the study and arrangements are made for general anesthesia standby (for umbrella closures and infant valve dilations). Premedication in the first year of life generally consists of chloral hydrate (50 mg/kg p.o.). Demerol Compound, which contains chlorpromazine (Thorazine, 6.25 mg/ml), promethazine HCl (Phenergan 6.25 mg/ml), and meperidine (Demerol, 25 mg/ml) is used in older children with the dose based on weight and cyanosis.[1,7] Older patients are held N.P.O. after midnight, and infants are given clear liquids up to 3 hours before the procedure.

Catheterization Study

Although most lesions today have been identified by physical examination or noninvasive techniques before beginning the study, it remains vitally important to set out with an open mind rather than simply trying to prove the existence of what one already thinks is present.

Catheters are introduced percutaneously in the femoral vessels in the great majority of cases, using the smallest catheters that are adequate to obtain the necessary information. The initial phase is aimed at gathering physiologic data. A right heart catheterization is performed, measuring oxygen saturation in the superior vena cava and recording pressures and saturations in the midlateral right atrium (RA), inflow and outflow portions of the right ventricle, main, right and left pulmonary arteries (PA), and pulmonary capillary wedge (PCW) position. Next the catheter is withdrawn to the RA and the atrial septum explored and, if it is traversed, pressure and saturation are recorded in left atrium (LA), left ventricle (LV) and at least one pulmonary vein (PV). The catheter is then withdrawn to the RA while recording pressure and repositioned in a distal branch of the PA. If the atrial septum is not traversed, an arterial catheter is placed and used to record pressure and sample blood for O_2 saturation

and blood gas determination in the descending and then ascending aorta. At this point, heparin (100 IU/kg) is administered intravenously to a maximum of 5000 IU. The arterial catheter is advanced to the LV, oxygen saturation is measured and pressure is recorded simultaneously with PCW pressure. Oxygen consumption is measured using a flow-through metabolic rate meter (Waters Inc., Rochester, MN), as right and left heart chamber pressures and saturations are recorded during catheter withdrawal for use in computation of pulmonary and systemic flow and resistance values. In the absence of intracardiac shunting, cardiac output may also be assessed by thermodilution.[5]

The next phase of the study consists of biplane cineangiography with particular emphasis on appropriate patient positioning for optimum visualization of the patient's specific cardiac anatomy. If no other data collection or procedures are contemplated, the renal shadows are viewed under fluoroscopy,[6] the catheters are removed, and bleeding at the entry site is controlled by a minimum of 15 minutes of local pressure without administration of protamine sulfate.

Exceptions to the Above Protocol

While this protocol is applicable to the majority of patients, some exceptions should be noted:

1. Premedication: Infants in the first month of life generally do not receive premedication. In patients of all ages with a presumed diagnosis of tetralogy of Fallot (TOF), particularly those with cyanosis or a history of cyanotic spells, morphine sulfate (0.1 mgm/kg) is used. In other cyanotic conditions, Demerol Compound is administered in doses related to weight and degree of cyanosis.[1] Overall, Demerol Compound continues to be the premedication used in most of our patients.[7]

2. Vessel entry in newborn: In the newborn infant, the umbilical artery can be cannulated up to 10 days of age, providing alternative access to aorta and LV. The umbilical vein can also be used for vascular access within the first

3 days of life. While this entry site is often satisfactory for ultimate access to the left heart chambers, it is often more difficult to enter the right ventricle and the pulmonary artery from the umbilical venous as compared to the femoral venous approach.

3. Neonates: These babies are frequently critically ill, unstable, acidotic, cyanotic and intubated. They require constant and meticulous attention and control of many parameters, including body temperature, throughout the study. The catheterization procedure should be kept as brief and focused as possible. Most of our major complications occur in these babies, with a mortality rate associated with cardiac catheterization of 2.7% in the first week of life, compared to 0.8% in those over 1 year of age.

Equipment Used in Catheterization

1. Catheters: Based on issues of patient safety, teaching responsibilities and cost, balloon-tipped flow-directed transvenous catheters are used initially in all age groups. These may be either end-hole or side-hole (angiographic) in type, and range from 4 to 8 Fr in size. Acute bends may be hand-shaped just before insertion, especially with the smaller catheters. Deflector wires (Cook, Bloomington, IN) may be used within these catheters to help attain access to desired sites, e.g., LV from LA. For arterial studies, ultra-thin walled Teflon pigtail catheters (UMI, Ballston, Spa, NY) ranging from 3.2 to 7 Fr in size are used,[8,9] providing satisfactory contrast flow rates up to 35 ml/second through a 6 Fr, 80 cm catheter. Using a Y adaptor (USCI, Billerica, MA) satisfactory pressures and angiograms are obtainable even with a 0.035 inch guide wire in place through a 7 Fr pigtail.

2. Contrast Material: While we use Renovist (E.R. Squibb and Sons, Princeton, NJ) predominantly, use of less toxic but more expensive non-ionic or dimeric contrast materials is increasing (see Chapter 2). These low-osmolar contrast agents are indicated particularly when ventricular end diastolic pressures are elevated. For any contrst agent we make every effort not to exceed a total dose of 5 ml/kg for the entire angiographic study.

3. X-ray equipment: Because of contrast agent constraints and the necessity of acquiring as much anatomic information as possible from each injection, biplane equipment is essential for pediatric catheterization. Cineangiography has completely replaced earlier full-size cutfilm systems in our institution, and a recently added system for simultaneous biplane cine with digital enhancement capability appears to offer additional promise. Given the range in patient age and size, a wide range of image intensifier modes is necessary, from 5 inches for neonates to 14 inches for older patients, in whom it is often necessary to image the pulmonary arteries and larger cardiac chambers.

Precise patient positioning is essential to provide optimum visualization of anatomy.[10,11] The most common views used are the long axial oblique (for VSD, Figs. 6–1, 6–2, subaortic stenosis), four-chamber or hepatoclavicular (for endocardial cushion defect) and the "sitting up" or cranial angled view (for central PA anatomy, Fig. 6–3).

SPECIAL PROCEDURES

Atrial Septostomy

Balloon Atrial Septostomy

Since the introduction of this technique by Rashkind and Miller in 1966,[12] balloon septostomy has remained the standard initial therapy for infants with d-transposition of the great arteries. In this congenital anomaly, the pulmonary and systemic circuits run in parallel rather than in series, resulting in severe hypoxia and acidosis shortly after birth. In this setting, septostomy allows bidirectional mixing at the atrial level, resulting in an immediate rise in arterial oxygen saturation with alleviation of acidosis. This procedure is also of value in neonates with left atrial outflow obstruction (such as mitral atresia) when an initial atrial septal opening frequently narrows within weeks of birth.

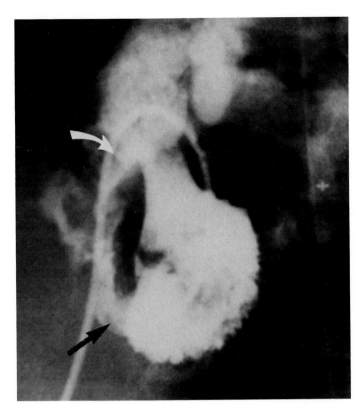

Fig. 6–1. Long axial oblique (analogous to LAD cranial) view of left ventricular cineangiogram in an infant with membranous (white arrow) and apical (black arrow) ventricular septal defects.

While the principles of atrial septostomy have changed little since the original description, recent equipment modifications have made the procedure easier and more effective. Vascular entry is obtained either by way of the umbilical vein or percutaneously from a femoral vein. The septostomy catheter we use most commonly is the 5 Fr Miller catheter (American Edwards Laboratories, Santa Ana, CA), which requires a 7 Fr sheath for insertion to allow passage of the unrecessed balloon. When using the umbilical venous approach, it is important to use a sheath with a valve (backflow adaptor) to avoid air embolism. The catheter tip is advanced to the mid LA, using biplane fluoroscopy. Alternatively, this procedure can be carried out at the bedside under two-dimensional echocardiographic guidance. The balloon is held against the atrial septum and inflated rapidly (to a maximum of 4 ml). The catheter is then advanced 1 or 2 mm before being pulled briskly to the inferior vena cava/RA junction, advanced to the RA, and then rapidly deflated. This sequence is usually repeated at least twice to ensure that an adequate atrial septal opening has been created. A successful outcome is associated with a rapid rise in arterial blood O_2 saturation, evidence of bidirectional shunting at the atrial level, and abolition of the interatrial pressure gradient. Complications are extremely rare, but tears of pulmonary veins and atrial walls have occurred.

Blade Atrial Septostomy

Balloon septostomy is generally not adequate to open the septum primum after 1 month of age. An alternative catheter, equipped with a retractable blade at its tip, was developed by Park et al.[13] The blade lengths available are 9.4, 13.4, and 20 mm (Cook, Bloomington, IN). The catheter is advanced via a percutaneously placed femoral vein sheath. The blade is opened carefully in the LA under biplane fluoroscopic monitoring and then withdrawn slowly across the atrial septum. This procedure is then followed by a balloon septostomy to enlarge the resulting opening. If O_2 saturation

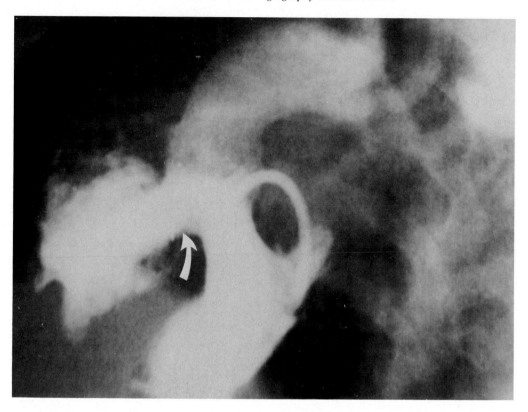

Fig. 6–2. Long axial oblique view of left ventricular cineangiogram in infant with large single malalignment ventricular septal defect (arrow).

and pressure measurement suggest inadequate mixing, this is repeated using a larger blade and/or balloon catheter until the mean residual left-to-right atrial gradient is less than or equal to 3 mmHg.[14]

Transseptal Left Heart Catheterization

The availability of biplane fluoroscopy has significantly reduced the complication rate associated with this technique. In addition, introduction of the long Mullins sheath (USCI, Billerica, MA) has made transseptal catheterization easier and has broadened the indications for this procedure.[15] Current indications include LA access for balloon mitral valvotomy, ASD creation, pulmonary vein wedge angiography, pressure measurements in mitral stenosis and for LV catheterization in the presence of an aortic valve prosthesis. In approximately 150 patients to date (including new-borns), we have not encountered any fatal complications related directly to this procedure.

For pediatric patients, available equipment includes a 6 Fr long sheath and a shorter needle. The appropriate Mullins sheath is introduced percutaneously by way of the right femoral vein, although we have occasionally used the left femoral vein after additional prebending of the distal needle. We prefer to attach the needle lumen to a syringe of contrast rather than a pressure transducer to allow precise location of the needle tip following its initial extrusion. Availability of two-dimensional echocardiographic visualization during the procedure is also helpful when atrial septal location is unusual.

Subclavian Vein Catheterization

This procedure, used by our adult colleagues for many years, is now being used

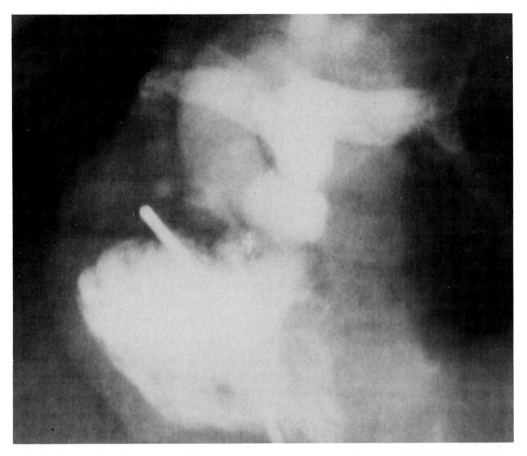

Fig. 6–3. ''Sitting up'' view (cranial angulation) of right ventricular cineangiogram in infant with tetralogy of Fallot, outlining the central pulmonary arteries, with faint spacification of ascending aorta via a ventricular septal defect.

increasingly in infants and children.[16] This has come about in part because thrombosis of iliac veins or infrarenal inferior vena cava has occurred in some patients after prior catheterization, and also because recent palliative surgical procedures, such as the bidirectional Glenn procedure, involve anastomosis of the cephalad end of the superior vena cava with the isolated pulmonary arteries. Subclavian vein catheterization may be performed at any age. We prefer the left subclavian vein only because later catheter manipulation seems easier. The patient is first positioned in a slight Trendelenberg position, a small rolled-up towel then placed lengthwise under the thoracic spine and the patient's arm positioned at his or her side. Lidocaine is injected down to and into the periosteum of the clavicle and first rib. A 19-gauge short bevelled thin-walled needle is used to enter the skin at the junction of the medial and middle thirds of the clavicle in adults and 1 to 2 cm lateral to that point in infants and children.[17] The needle is advanced toward the suprasternal notch, while maintaining an orientation that is both perpendicular to the spine and parallel to the floor as the needle tip passes between the clavicle and first rib under gentle, continuous aspiration by a syringe. Once venous blood returns freely, a preformed guide wire is inserted and advanced to the heart and an appropriate-sized sheath with a backstop valve is then inserted. At the conclusion of the study, the sheath is removed and bleeding controlled with at least 5 minutes of gentle pressure on the first rib.

Although we have rarely entered the sub-

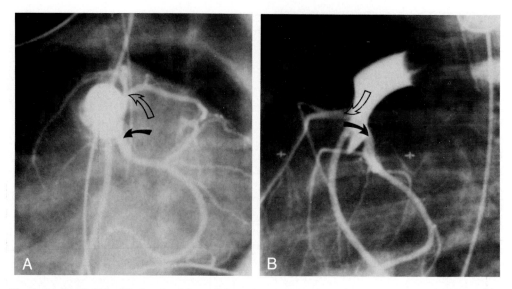

Fig. 6–4. A, "Laid back" view (caudal angulation) of aortic cineangiogram during distal balloon occlusion in an infant with D transposition of the great arteries, outlining locations of origin of right (open arrow) and left (solid arrow) coronary arteries. B, lateral view of same cine.

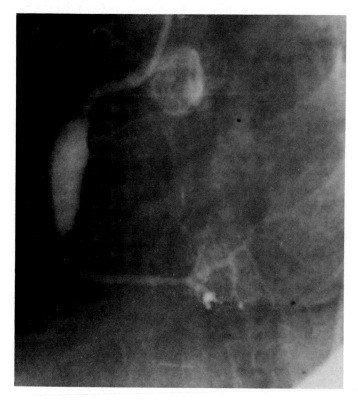

Fig. 6–5. Selective right coronary artery cineangiogram, lateral view, using a 5F Judkins (R)-2 cm catheter in a child with coronary artery aneurysm due to Kawasaki disease. (Reprinted with permission from Lock JE, Keane JF, Fellows KE in *Diagnostic and Interventional Catheterization in Congenital Heart Disease*. Boston, Martinus Nijhoff Publishing, 1986, p. 89.)

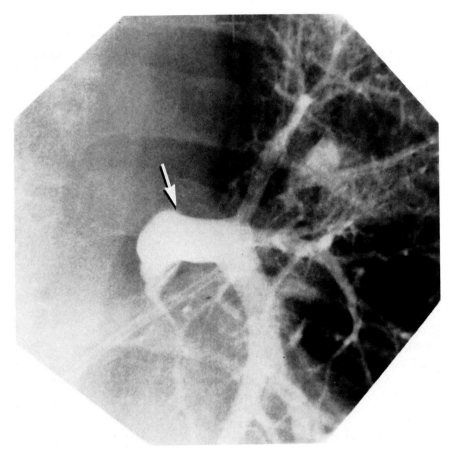

Fig. 6–6. Pulmonary vein wedge angiogram in 5-year-old with tricuspid and pulmonary atresia and Glenn shunt. Retrograde filling of large proximal left pulmonary artery (arrow) and hypoplastic main pulmonary artery following injection in left upper lobe pulmonary vein.

clavian artery with the needle, we have not encountered any complications to date in some 100 procedures, even in infants as small as 3 to 5 kg.

Selective Coronary Arteriography

In general, ventriculography and aortography are sufficient to identify abnormalities of the major proximal coronary arteries as seen in such conditions as tetralogy of Fallot, d-transposition of the great vessels (Fig. 6–4), or double-outlet right ventricle. Nevertheless, there is an increasing list of indications for selective coronary injections, including Kawasaki's disease (Fig. 6–5), coronary artery fistulae and pulmonary atresia with intact ventricular septum.

Borrowing from the enormous experience of our adult colleagues in this field, investigators have miniaturized catheters for use in pediatric patients, including infants. We use a variety of such catheters ranging from 4.5 Fr to 7.3 Fr, in Judkins or Amplatz configurations (Cook, Bloomington, IN) with varying secondary loop sizes. We use standard adult techniques and angiographic views (see Chapter 13), but appropriately smaller doses of contrast material.

Pulmonary Vein Wedge Angiography

There are patients who, as the result of a congenital defect or prior cardiac surgery, have complete occlusion of a proximal pulmonary artery. Although an injection in the aorta or even in a collateral vessel frequently outlines the size and location of the isolated artery, it is essential before any surgical attempts at flow-reconstruction to identify unequivocally the presence or absence of such pulmonary arteries.

With this in mind, a balloon-tipped end-hole catheter is placed across the atrial septum and into a pulmonary vein in the appropriate lung. With the balloon inflated, 0.3 ml/kg of nonionic contrast agent (which causes less coughing than conventional ionic high osmolar agents) is injected by hand and followed immediately by an equal volume of saline from a separate syringe. The parenchymal vessels are usually well outlined by this method, with the mediastinal segment also backfilling, if present (Fig. 6–6). On occasion, the main and contralateral pulmonary arteries may also fill if they are in continuity. It is important to use biplane cineangiography for these injections to identify accurately how far into the mediastinum the vessel extends.

Endomyocardial Biopsy

The technique of endomyocardial biopsy has improved considerably in recent years (see Chapter 23). The availability of small bioptomes such as the soft 5 Fr model made by Cordis Corp. (Miami, FL) and preformed long sheaths have made biopsy a rather safe procedure even in infants.[18,19] The number of biopsies at our institution has increased markedly in recent years, mostly because of cardiac transplantation. The great majority of procedures involve right ventricular biopsy, although left-sided specimens can be obtained if necessary.

Because the procedure is repeated frequently in patients with a cardiac transplant, a different venous percutaneous access site is usually used with each procedure. The vessels used commony are the internal jugular, subclavian, and femoral veins for right-sided biopsies. If left ventricular samples are required, the approach is transatrial in infants and retrograde from a femoral artery in older patients.

REFERENCES

1. Lock JE: Evaluation and Management Prior to Catheterization. In: *Diagnostic and Interventional Catheterization in Congenital Heart Disease* by Lock JE, Keane JF, Fellows KE. Boston, Martinus Nijhoff Publishing, 1987, p. 1.
2. Lipshultz SE, Sanders SP, Mayer JE, et al: Are routine preoperative cardiac catheterization and angiography necessary before repair of ostium primum atrial septal defect? J Am Coll Cardiol 11:373, 1988.
3. Huhta JC, Glasgow P, Murphy DJ Jr, et al: Surgery without catheterization for congenital heart defects: management of 100 patients. J Am Coll Cardiol 9:823, 1987.
4. Flanagan MF, Leatherman GF, Carls A, et al: Changing trends of congenital heart disease in adults: a catheterization laboratory perspective. Cathet Cardiovasc Diagn 12:215, 1986.
5. Freed MD, Keane JF: Cardiac output by thermodilution in infants and children. J Pediatr 92:39, 1978.
6. Nussbaum AR, Newman B, Freed MD, et al: Nonutility of cineurograms in children with congenital heart disease. Am J Cardiol 60:684, 1987.
7. Ruckman RN, Keane JF, Freed MD, et al: Sedation for cardiac catheterization: a controlled study. Pediatr Cardiol 1:263, 1980.
8. Keane JF, Fellows KE, Lang P, Fyler DC: Pediatric arterial catheterization using a 3.2 French catheter. Cathet Cardiovasc Diagn 8:201, 1982.
9. Keane JF, Freed MD, Fellows KE, Fyler DC: Pediatric cardiac angiography using a 4 French catheter. Cathet Cardiovasc Diagn 3:313, 1977.
10. Elliott LP, Bargeron LM Jr, Bream PR, et al: Axial cineangiography in congenital heart disease. Section II: Specific lesions. Circulation 56:1084, 1977.
11. Fellows KE, Keane JF, Freed MD: Angled views in cineangiocardiography of congenital heart disease. Circulation 56:485, 1977.
12. Rashkind WJ, Miller WW: Creation of an atrial septal defect without thoracotomy. A palliative approach to complete transposition of the great arteries. JAMA 196:991, 1966.
13. Park SC, Neches WH, Zuberbuhler JR, et al: Clinical use of blade atrial septostomy. Circulation 58:600, 1978.
14. Perry SB, Lang P, Keane JF, et al: Creation and maintenance of an adequate interatrial communication in patients with left atrioventricular valve atresia or stenosis. Am J Cardiol 58:622, 1986.
15. Mullins CE: Transseptal left heart catheterization: Experience with a new technique in pediatric and adult patients. Pediatr Cardiol 4:239, 1983.
16. Linos DA: Subclavian vein: A golden route. Mayo Clinic Proc 55:315, 1980.
17. Keane JF, Lock JE: Vessel entry and catheter manipulation. In: *Diagnostic and Interventional Catheterization in Congenital Heart Disease* by Lock JE, Keane JF, Fellows KE. Boston, Martinus Nijhoff Publishing, 1987, p. 14.
18. Lurie PR, Fujita M, Neustein HB: Transvascular endomyocardial biopsy in infants and small children: Description of a new technique. Am J Cardiol 42:453, 1978.
19. Rios B, Nihill MR, Mullins CE: Left ventricular endomyocardial biopsy in children with the transseptal long sheath technique. Cathet Cardiovasc Diagn 10:417, 1984.

7

Balloon-Tipped Flow-Directed Catheters

PETER GANZ, H.J.C. SWAN, and WILLIAM GANZ

Diagnostic catheterization of the right side of the heart with semirigid cardiac catheters requires fluoroscopic guidance and substantial skill. Abnormal positions of the heart chambers and of the great vessels associated with cardiac dilatation or with congenital malformation present difficulties even to experienced laboratory cardiologists. These problems have been largely overcome by the introduction of balloon-tipped flow-directed catheters,[1,3] which allow for rapid and relatively safe catheterization of the pulmonary artery without fluoroscopy. It was through the application of these catheters in the intensive care unit that the many pitfalls in the clinical assessment of hemodynamic disturbances became apparent. It was learned in patients with acute myocardial infarction that the value of central venous pressure (or jugular venous pressure) is limited by the fact that it reflects the functional state of the right ventricle, which frequently does not parallel that of the left ventricle.[4] Although S3 gallop sounds may be useful in the clinical recognition of chronic ventricular failure, their presence or absence has limited predictive value in estimating left ventricular filling pressure in myocardial infarction.[5,6] Similarly, serious discrepancies have been noted between radiologic evidence of heart failure and the level of pulmonary wedge pressure when rapid hemodynamic changes take place.[7,8] These observations have been extended to critically ill medical[9] and surgical[10] patients without acute myocardial infarction. Balloon-tipped catheters have made an important contribution in extending the applicability of hemodynamic monitoring to the bedside. Information derived from right heart catheterization is often pivotal in the evaluation of hemodynamic disorders, in directing treatment, and in monitoring the results of therapy in critically ill patients.

BASIC FEATURES AND CONSTRUCTION

An inflated balloon at the tip of the catheter is carried by the circulation and guides the catheter from the right atrium into the pulmonary artery or to other sections of the vascular bed in patients with congenital cardiac malformations. The inflated balloon protrudes beyond the tip of the catheter and protects the tip from impinging on the myocardium, thereby preventing it from damaging the endocardium and producing arrhythmias or heart block.

The most widely used catheter* is con-

*Swan-Ganz Flow-Directed Catheter, Edwards Laboratories, Santa Ana, CA.

structed from polyvinyl chloride and has a soft pliable shaft that softens further at body temperature (Fig. 7–1). A balloon is fastened 1 to 2 mm from the tip. The standard catheter is 110 cm long and is color-coded according to size from 5, 6 to 7 Fr in external diameter. As the deflated balloon extends slightly outside the shaft, the venous sheath used to introduce the catheter may have to be 0.5 Fr larger than the stated catheter size.

Most catheters have a preformed J curvature at the distal end to facilitate passage from the superior vena cava through the right ventricle. A catheter with an "S" tip has also been designed for femoral vein insertion. Catheters intended for long-term use are available with heparin coating to reduce thromboembolic complications. Triple-lumen catheters are available with distal and proximal ports (the third lumen being for balloon inflation), which allow simultaneous measurement of right atrial and pulmonary artery or pulmonary capillary wedge pressures. The proximal port terminates either 20 or 30 cm proximal to the catheter tip, facilitating location in the right atrium under varying conditions of cardiac size and anatomy. Additional lumens may carry thermistor wires for thermodilution, cardiac output

studies, pacing electrodes, venous position monitoring, or blood oxygen saturation studies. The catheters are all radiopaque and can be readily visualized by fluoroscopy or plain-film chest roentgenography.

TECHNIQUE OF FLOW-DIRECTED CATHETERIZATION

Before insertion, the integrity of the balloon must be tested by inflating under sterile liquid (e.g., saline solution) to the volume specified by the manufacturer, while observing for gas leakage. The antecubital, femoral, internal jugular, and subclavian veins may be used as insertion sites, the latter two being used particularly outside the catheterization laboratory. After entry into the selected vein, the catheter is advanced until the tip is in or near the right atrium. This usually occurs after advancement of 15 cm from the jugular or subclavian vein, 40 cm from the right and 50 cm from the left antecubital area, and about 30 cm when a femoral vein is used. An increase in respiratory fluctuation of the intravascular pressure monitored from the catheter confirms intrathoracic location of the catheter tip. At this time, the balloon is inflated to its specified volume (this

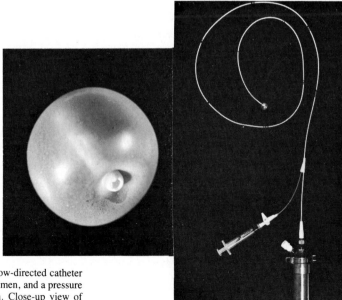

Fig. 7–1.   Standard balloon-tipped, flow-directed catheter with inflated balloon, closed inflation lumen, and a pressure transducer attached to the large lumen. Close-up view of the inflated balloon.

volume is printed on the catheter by most manufacturers).

Air may be used for balloon inflation, but carbon dioxide should be used when there is any possibility that the catheter may enter the left heart or the arterial circulation. Release of carbon dioxide into the arterial circulation in the event of balloon rupture is free of the hazard of serious consequences because the solubility of CO_2 in blood is about 20 times that of air at normal body temperature. The balloon may have to be refilled every few minutes, because carbon dioxide slowly diffuses through the wall of the latex balloon.

The catheter-tip pressure and surface electrocardiogram are monitored as the catheter proceeds through the right ventricle and pulmonary artery into a "wedge" position (Fig. 7–2). That the catheter is truly in the wedge position can be recognized by several methods: (1) ascertaining fluoroscopically that the catheter stops "bobbing" with each cardiac cycle; (2) demonstrating clearcut A and V waves in the wedge tracing (in sinus rhythm); (3) documenting a fall in pressure from mean pulmonary artery to mean wedge; and (4) demonstrating a wedge oxygen saturation equal to or greater than that in a systemic artery (e.g., 95% or more). Because the wedge pressure is obtained from a large pulmonary artery, it is necessary to discard 5 to 15 ml of "pulmonary artery" blood before fully oxygenated capillary blood is sampled. This "dead space" blood is sitting in the pulmonary artery between the catheter tip and the capillary network and must be withdrawn before oxygenated blood from the pulmonary capillary can reach the catheter. When the balloon is deflated, the catheter recoils to its original position.

As the catheter softens with time, the contractions of the right ventricle may diminish the transcardiac catheter loop and advance the catheter tip into a smaller branch of the pulmonary artery. In such cases, inflation of the balloon to full capacity will cause overdistension with potential damage to the pulmonary arterial wall and/or falsely high pulmonary wedge pressure reading (due to compression of the catheter lumen). To avoid damage to the vessel wall and recording inaccurate pressures, *it is imperative that inflation of the balloon for obtaining wedge pressure be per-*

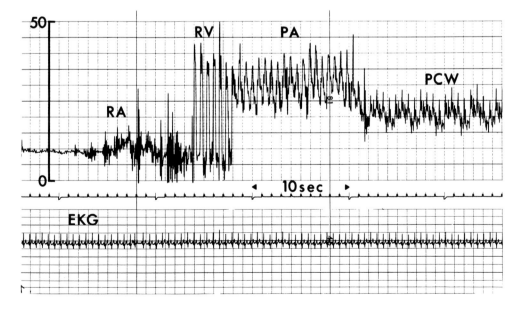

Fig. 7–2. Pressures recorded during insertion of a balloon-tipped, flow-directed catheter. RA = right atrial pressure, RV = right ventricular pressure, PA = pulmonary arterial pressure, PCW = pulmonary capillary wedge pressure. The scale at the left calibrates pressures from 0 to 50 mm Hg.

formed gradually under continuous monitor-ing of the pulmonary artery pressure and that the inflation of the balloon be stopped when the change from pulmonary artery to pulmo-nary wedge pressure configuration is noted.

To avoid damage to the vessel wall by in-flation of the balloon in a small distal pul-monary artery branch or by the action of an unprotected catheter tip, the capacity of mon-itoring catheter tip position was recently de-veloped. These new position-monitoring ("PA WATCH") catheters have a special lumen opening at 10 cm from the tip. When the cath-eter is in a proper position, the position-mon-itoring lumen transmits right ventricular pres-sure wave forms. When this lumen transmits pulmonary artery pressure wave forms, the catheter has migrated distally and may be in an unsafe position. In such a case, the catheter is slowly pulled back just enough to see ap-pearance of right ventricular pressure wave forms. Excessive pullback into the right ven-tricle may result in inability to reach the wedge position following inflation of the balloon. The initial insertion of position monitoring cathe-ters remains unchanged: after reaching the wedge position, the balloon is deflated. If the position-monitoring lumen transmits right ven-tricular pressure, the catheter is in proper po-sition; if it transmits pulmonary artery pres-sure, the catheter is slowly pulled back until a right ventricular pressure wave form is noted.

Position-monitoring modalities are as fol-lows:

1. The pulmonary artery pressure and the right ventricular pressure from the position monitoring lumen are monitored continu-ously. Distal migration can be recognized immediately and corrected.
2. Pulmonary artery pressure is monitored continuously and the position-monitoring lumen is checked intermittently (half-hourly, hourly, or continuously for a limited critical period).
3. Before cardiopulmonary bypass, the cath-eter is pulled back 5 cm and refloated fol-lowing the cardiopulmonary bypass.

Passage of the balloon flotation catheter is more difficult in patients with right-sided chamber enlargement, especially in face of low cardiac output. Deep inspiration, use of the Valsalva maneuver, and stiffening of the catheter by slow perfusion with 5 to 10 ml of sterile cold saline solution or by inhibition of an appropriate guide wire may facilitate pas-sage into the pulmonary artery.

Because femoral vein insertion of the stand-ard J-curved balloon catheter points the tip of the catheter at the right ventricular apex, gentle rotation under fluoroscopy is often required to orient the tip into the right ventricular outflow tract. If difficulty in positioning the catheter persists, a suitable guide wire may be inserted to stiffen the catheter. It is preferable not to advance the guide wire beyond the catheter tip to avoid damaging intracardiac structures. On occasion, it is useful to form a 270-degree loop against the lateral wall of the right atrium, directing the tip of the catheter at the outflow tract, but taking care not to form a knot. Spe-cial S-shaped catheters are available for fem-oral vein insertion.

MEASUREMENT OF PULMONARY ARTERY AND WEDGE PRESSURES

In a series of comparisons in the catheteri-zation laboratory and in the animal laboratory, there was no noteworthy difference between the pressures recorded from the tip of the flow-guided catheter after occlusion of a pulmonary artery branch by the inflated balloon and those obtained by conventional end-hole catheters advanced more peripherally to the true wedge position. True wedge pressure is usually con-firmed by visual inspection of the pressure waveform and its diastolic tracking of a si-multaneously measured LV pressure. If there is any doubt about the waveform, or if an unexpected diastolic gradient is present, the wedge position may be confirmed by blood sampling. If this is not possible, the operator should attempt to wedge the catheter with the balloon deflated, or use another right-heart catheter.

The pulmonary capillary wedge pressure

provides information about two important determinants of cardiopulmonary function. First, the level of this pressure is a factor in the genesis of pulmonary congestion by regulating the transfer of fluid from the pulmonary capillaries into the interstitial space and the alveoli. Second, the pulmonary wedge pressure accurately reflects the mean left atrial pressure and therefore, in the absence of mitral valvular disease, closely approximates left ventricular mean diastolic pressure, an index of left ventricular preload. In the absence of pulmonary vascular disease, generally the pulmonary arterial end diastolic pressure is only 1 to 3 mm Hg higher than the mean pulmonary wedge pressure; it can therefore serve as an indicator of the mean wedge pressure in patients without pre-existing pulmonary hypertension and avoid the need for frequent balloon inflations. Differences between the pulmonary arterial end diastolic and pulmonary wedge pressure in excess of 5 mm Hg suggest a primary pulmonary vascular disorder. In patients with severe mitral regurgitation and large V waves in the left atrial and pulmonary capillary pressures, the mean wedge pressure may exceed pulmonary artery end diastolic pressure as the V wave is averaged into the mean wedge but not into the pulmonary artery diastolic pressure.

The balloon should be kept inflated only for the minimum time necessary. As soon as the wedge pressure reading has been taken, the balloon should be deflated. Leaving the balloon inflated, particularly if the catheter tip happens to be in a distal pulmonary artery branch, may lead to erosion of the pulmonary artery wall with consequent pulmonary artery perforation and massive hemoptysis.

MEASUREMENT OF CARDIAC OUTPUT BY THERMODILUTION

Flow-directed thermodilution catheters allow for rapid determinations of cardiac output by injection of a known amount of cold sterile solution into the right atrium and measurement of the resultant change in blood temperature in the pulmonary artery by the catheter thermistor.[11,12] (See Chapter 8.)

TEMPORARY VENTRICULAR PACING AND RECORDING OF INTRACAVITARY ELECTROGRAMS

Rapid insertion of bipolar balloon-tipped flow-directed catheters into the right ventricle usually can be accomplished by electrocardiographic monitoring without fluoroscopy. A unipolar electrocardiogram can be recorded from the distal tip electrode by connection to the V lead of the electrocardiogram (ECG). Entry of the catheter into the right atrium is indicated by a large atrial complex. At this point, the balloon is inflated. Once the catheter has entered the right ventricle, the balloon is immediately deflated to avoid flotation into the right ventricular outflow tract. Entry of the catheter into the right ventricle is indicated by a marked decrease in the amplitude of the atrial complex and a marked increase in the amplitude of the ventricular complex. The catheter is gradually advanced several centimeters into the right ventricle until elevation of the ST segment is observed, indicating endocardial contact. The catheter is available in two modifications: the first is designed for insertion from the femoral vein and is J curved distally for stable placement in the apex. The second type, designed for insertion via the superior vena cava, is straight.

Flow-directed catheters are now available that, in addition to recording pulmonary artery, pulmonary capillary wedge and right atrial pressures, and thermodilution cardiac outputs, allow for atrial and ventricular pacing and intracavitary ECG monitoring.* The unique feature of these catheters entails a bend at the site of the ventricular electrodes which forces the electrodes against the endocardium for firm contact. When used in patients during cardiac surgery, atrial pacing could be achieved in 85% of patients, ventricular pacing in 94%, and sequential pacing in 82%.[13] The

*Swan-Ganz Pacing TD Catheter, Edwards Laboratories, Santa Ana, CA.

stated percentages would be expected to decrease with time in awake mobile patients. These catheters have been used for A-V sequential pacing for hemodynamic reasons and for diagnosis or overdrive of arrhythmias. Modifications of the standard flow-directed thermodilution catheter* are now available that allow for atrial or atrioventricular pacing in case of need. Special lumens opening at 27 cm and 19 cm from the tip can be used for insertion of pacing probes into the right atrium and right ventricle, respectively.

The intracardiac electrograms are relatively insensitive to muscle tremor and to electrical interference and can be used for initiation of intraaortic balloon pumping even in face of electrocautery.[14] The availability of stable atrial and ventricular complexes should facilitate computer analysis of cardiac rhythm disturbances. Catheters with a fiberoptic lumen are now available for study of the oxygen saturation of blood.

APPLICATIONS IN ADULTS

Cardiac Catheterization Laboratories

Catheterization of the right ventricle and pulmonary artery with the balloon-tipped flow-guided catheter can frequently be accomplished in the same time as or less time than that required for semirigid nonfloating catheters and at a lower risk of serious arrhythmias. For these reasons, catheterization with flow-directed balloon-tipped catheters has become routine in most cardiac catheterization laboratories.[1,15]

A special application of the balloon-tipped flow-directed catheter has included its use in transseptal left-heart catheterization.[16] Unlike with conventional methods, it is easier to advance the catheter into the left ventricle and also into the aorta. Balloon-tipped catheters have also been used to occlude temporarily a patent ductus arteriosus or an atrial septal defect, thus defining the size and hemodynamic importance of the shunt.[17] The use of the cath-

*AV-Paceport, Baxter, Santa Ana, CA.

eter for balloon-wedge angiography is discussed below.

Coronary Care Units

The hemodynamic status of patients with acute myocardial infarction cannot always be defined correctly by the clinical evaluation.[18] Catheterization of the pulmonary artery permits rapid and accurate assessment of cardiac performance. With the data derived from measurements of cardiac output and pulmonary capillary wedge pressure, one can define hemodynamic subsets that determine both the prognosis and the appropriate therapeutic intervention.[18]

Recording pressures from the right atrium, right ventricle, pulmonary artery, and pulmonary wedge position and sampling blood from the right heart chambers for oxygen saturation also may allow the physician to recognize right ventricular infarction[19,20] and specific complications of acute myocardial infarction such as acute mitral regurgitation, ventricular septal rupture,[21] or cardiac tamponade.[22]

Intensive Care Units

Right-heart catheterization is used widely to monitor patients without acute myocardial infarction who are critically ill from a variety of other causes.[9,10] In a group of medical patients who were not responding to initial therapy, the information provided by right heart catheterization prompted a change in therapy in almost 50% of the cases.[9] Hemodynamic monitoring is essential to detect left ventricular failure in patients with adult respiratory distress syndrome.[23]

Interpretation of hemodynamic data may pose difficulty in patients on mechanical ventilators. Intrathoracic pressure becomes positive during the forced inspiration driven by the ventilator and falsely elevates intravascular pressure. These effects are usually obvious on examination of the phasic wedge tracing, which shows obliteration of the normal A and V wave pattern when the capillary bed is compressed by the increased intra-alveolar pressure. It has been recommended that pressures be recorded at end-expiration for patients on ventilators.[24,25] The additional effects of positive end-expiratory pressure (PEEP) on the measured intraluminal pressures will depend in part upon pulmonary compliance; patients with decreased compliance may not have intrapleural (and thus intrapericardial) pressures elevated significantly by PEEP. In such cases, an elevated measured-LV filling pressure would likely be accurate. When large disparity is found in intravascular filling pressures on vs off PEEP, it is better to rely more on the thermodilution cardiac output determinations and their response to volume-loading or volume-reduction (e.g., diuresis) as a means of assessing adequacy of left heart filling pressure. On occasion when the accurate determination of filling pressure is deemed important, esophageal balloons or intrapleural catheters have been employed for measurement of intrapleural (and thus intrapericardial) pressure,[26] which is then subtracted from the measured pulmonary wedge pressure.

Surgery and Anesthesiology

The clinical outcome in patients undergoing major operations, such as abdominal aortic surgery, is greatly influenced by the risk of cardiac decompensation. Major stresses on the cardiovascular system involve sudden shifts in intravascular volume, third space accumulation of fluid, and alterations in systemic vascular resistance due to anesthesia. A safer perioperative course with the ability to modulate hemodynamic variables has been reported with the use of pulmonary artery catheterization.[27]

APPLICATIONS IN CHILDREN AND INFANTS

Smaller (4 Fr size) and more flexible catheters, including catheters for measurement of cardiac output by thermodilution, are available for pediatric use. The following indications for the use of the flow-directed balloon-tipped catheters have been reported.

1. Catheterization of children in whom the exact anatomy and position of the cardiac chambers before catheterization are not known.
2. Manipulation of the catheter into chambers and vessels not readily accessible by conventional means, for instance, entry into the pulmonary artery from the left or common ventricle and entry into the aorta from the right or common ventricle in transposition of the great vessels.[28-31]
3. Passage of the catheter through an interatrial communication into the left atrium, left ventricle, and aorta to avoid retrograde arterial catheterization and an arteriotomy.
4. Obtaining pulmonary arterial wedge pressure in patients in whom wedge pressure might otherwise be difficult to obtain. Obtaining pulmonary arterial wedge arteriograms and visualization of the relevant pulmonary vein by rapid washout of contrast medium following sudden deflation of the balloon, particularly in partial or total anomalous venous connection.
5. In patients liable to have arrhythmias initiated by catheter manipulation, as in patients with Wolff-Parkinson-White syndrome or Ebstein's anomaly.

Caution must be exercised when the catheter is in the aorta or any large artery because the arterial flow may carry the inflated balloon distally until it occludes a major vessel, such as the carotid artery or descending aorta. This complication can be avoided by continuous pressure monitoring and partial deflation of the balloon in order to maintain its position.

SIGNIFICANCE OF LARGE PULMONARY V WAVES

The phasic contour of the pulmonary wedge tracing may yield important diagnostic information. The V wave in the left atrial and pulmonary wedge tracing normally represents filling of the left atrium during systole against a closed mitral valve. An abnormally large V wave is sometimes defined as being 10 mm Hg greater than mean pulmonary wedge pressure.[32,33] The most common cause of large V waves is mitral regurgitation. It has been pointed out that large V waves are not specific for mitral regurgitation and that its other important causes include left ventricular failure, mitral stenosis, and ventricular septal defects.[32,33] To understand the mechanisms of large V waves, the major determinants of their height have to be considered:

1. The size of the V wave is in part determined by the amount of blood entering the left atrium during systole. Increased blood enters the left atrium retrograde in mitral regurgitation, or antegrade from shunts that increase pulmonary venous return as in ventricular septal defects.

2. The pressure-volume relationship of the left atrium is curvilinear (Fig. 7–3), with the result that changes in volume produce little change in pressure when the left atrial pressure is low, but a similar change in volume is associated with a large change in pressure at the high pressure end of the curve. Thus, atrial inflow during systole results in large V waves when the left atrial

pressure is elevated as in left ventricular failure or mitral stenosis. Conversely, large V waves may be absent in patients with severe mitral regurgitation who are hypovolemic. Patients with acute mitral regurgitation may have particularly steep pressure-volume curves, signifying noncompliance of the small left atrium, and such patients often exhibit giant V waves (i.e., peak V wave more than twice the mean wedge pressure). The value of the V wave in diagnosing mitral regurgitation is discussed in Chapter 31.

PULMONARY WEDGE ANGIOGRAPHY

Injection of contrast medium into the pulmonary vascular bed through a catheter with the balloon inflated in the wedge position yields a standstill, high-resolution angiogram.[34,35] By injecting distal to the inflated balloon, it is possible to evaluate an entire segment of lung.[34] Finding of an elevated pulmonary vascular resistance by hemodynamic criteria in patients considered for cardiac surgery may not distinguish increased vascular reactivity from structural morphologic damage. Pulmonary wedge angiography has been used to evaluate the extent of structural pulmonary vascular disease, especially in patients with congenital heart disease. Wedge angiograms have shown progressively more abrupt tapering of the pulmonary arteries in patients who have both increasingly abnormal pulmonary hemodynamics and increasingly severe structural changes in lung biopsy tissue. Methods for quantifying such pulmonary artery taper have been described.[34] The degree of filling of small peripheral arteries that become obliterated in this disease process also can be estimated.

Pulmonary wedge angiography has also been used to diagnose pulmonary emboli,[36,37] and this is discussed in detail in Chapter 15. When performed at the bedside with portable x-ray equipment, some studies have suggested a high incidence of false negatives and false positives. This is not surprising in view of the

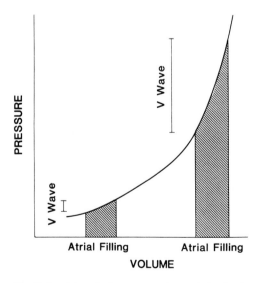

Fig. 7–3. A hypothetic pressure-volume relation for the left atrium is depicted. At the low pressure end of the curve, inflow of blood (during ventricular systole), represented by the hatched bars, results in a relatively small increase in pressure, i.e., a small V wave; at the high pressure end of the curve, an identical inflow of blood results in a larger V wave.

small portion of the lung vasculature visualized through the use of relatively low-resolution x-ray equipment. The predictive power of this method is likely to be improved when there has been the prior suggestion of multiple embolic events by radionuclide methods or when a high-resolution wedge angiogram is performed on a specific segment of the lung to further clarify the findings from routine pulmonary angiography.

COMPLICATIONS

The flexibility of the flotation catheters and the protective function of the inflated balloon tend to minimize serious complications. The simplicity of the procedure itself, however, has led on more than one occasion to underestimation of potential hazards of this invasive method and to unnecessary complications. Fortunately, several prospective studies that examined complications associated with the placement and maintenance of pulmonary catheters found the morbidity and mortality rate to be quite low and generally outweighed by the information obtained.[31-41]

Rupture of Balloon

If rupture of the balloon occurs, the catheter's flotation properties are lost. Injection of 1 to 2 ml of air into the right heart chambers or the pulmonary artery has not been reported to have adverse consequences. This does not apply to children and patients with congenital heart disease in whom the possibility of a right-to-left shunt exists. In these patients, carbon dioxide must be used as the inflation medium. Rupture of the balloon is often recognized fluoroscopically in the catheterization laboratory and can be frequently confirmed by the appearance of blood at the inflation port following gentle aspiration.

Arrhythmias

Although the protective effect of the inflated balloon and the flexibility of the catheter minimize the incidence of serious arrhythmias,

sustained ventricular tachycardia was reported in 3% and ventricular fibrillation in 2% of 119 critically ill patients undergoing bedside pulmonary artery catheterization.[42] Ventricular ectopy was more frequent among patients predisposed to ectopy or with prolonged catheterization time. A new right bundle branch block developed in 5% of patients and persisted for a mean of 10 hours. Caution must be exercised therefore in the catheterization of patients with pre-existent left bundle branch block. Prophylactic use of lidocaine appears effective in reducing the incidence of catheter-induced advanced ventricular arrhythmias.[43]

Pulmonary Complications

An ideal position of the catheter is with its tip in the right or left main branches of the pulmonary artery. Flotation catheters, even when the balloon is deflated, have a tendency to advance into a distal branch. Inadvertent wedging in a small branch of the pulmonary artery for prolonged periods may result in the development of segmental pulmonary infarction. This can be avoided by carefully monitoring the catheter tip pressure and, if necessary, by determining the position of the catheter by radiologic means. Ideally, the catheter should be in a proximal position from which it moves forward into wedged position following inflation of the balloon. Supervising personnel should be instructed clearly as to the significance of an apparently damped pressure from the pulmonary artery.

Perforation or Rupture of Pulmonary Artery

Inadvertent injection of a large amount of fluid under high pressure into the balloon inflation port may cause rupture of the pulmonary artery. Therefore, it is advisable to keep the inflation syringe constantly attached to the inflation lumen.

An instance of pulmonary artery rupture has been reported in a patient with mitral stenosis and pulmonary hypertension.[44] In this case, the catheter was distally in a smaller branch.

Upon inflation of the balloon to full capacity, the pulmonary arterial wall was exposed to significant distending forces, which together with the weakening of the arterial wall by long-standing pulmonary hypertension, resulted in rupture of the artery. The pressure gradient between the pulmonary artery and pulmonary wedge pressure advancing the catheter tip may have been a contributory factor.

Several other cases of fatal pulmonary hemorrhage have been reported in association with use of the flow-directed balloon-tipped catheter in relation to balloon inflation or tip perforation.[45] As pointed out in Chapter 3, these complications can be avoided if the guidelines of technique described previously are observed strictly. The new position monitoring (PA watch) catheter will allow us to prevent any significant distal migration.

As a rule, we recommend that inflation of the balloon always be performed gradually and under visual inspection of the pulmonary arterial pressure tracing and that the inflation be stopped immediately when a change from pulmonary arterial to pulmonary wedge waveform is noted on the pressure tracing. Furthermore, the balloon should remain inflated only for the shortest possible time, particularly in patients with pulmonary hypertension.

Knotting

Knotting caused by coiling of the catheter is more frequent with smaller, more flexible catheters. To minimize the likelihood of knotting in the absence of fluoroscopy, advancement of the catheter should be discontinued if the right ventricle is not reached within the expected distance from the insertion site or if the pulmonary artery is not reached within 15 cm from the right ventricle. Nonsurgical techniques for untying knots have been developed.[46,47]

Thrombotic Complications

It has been demonstrated that a small thrombus may form on pulmonary artery catheters in most patients.[48] Coating of catheters by heparin appears to reduce greatly the incidence of such adherent thrombi.[48]

Infections

Whenever a foreign body enters the vascular system, it may introduce infection. The likelihood of bacterial contamination increases with repeated catheter manipulations. A sterile protective sleeve that has been introduced allows repositioning of the catheter with minimal bacteriologic risk.[49]

SIGNIFICANCE

Balloon-tipped, flow-directed cardiac catheters permit the measurement of many parameters of cardiovascular function at the bedside, without the requirement of fluoroscopy or a special facility for their placement, and at low risk of significant arrhythmias. Variables that may be measured easily include: right atrial, right ventricular, pulmonary artery and pulmonary wedge pressures, right ventricular and right atrial cavity potentials, cardiac output by the thermodilution technique, and oxygen saturation of mixed venous blood.

Catheterization using the balloon-tipped catheters permits entry into chambers or vessels hardly accessible by conventional means in complex cardiac anomalies. Significantly, this easy and safe way of monitoring physiologic variables enables the physician to use direct data routinely in the management of his patient. The catheters can be used for urgent atrial, ventricular, or atrioventricular pacing.

REFERENCES

1. Swan HJC, et al: Catheterization of the heart in man with use of a flow-directed balloon-tipped catheter. N Engl J Med 283:447, 1970.
2. Buchbinder N, Ganz W: Hemodynamic monitoring: Invasive techniques. Anesthesiology 45:145, 1976.
3. Swan HJC, Ganz W: Measurement of right atrial and pulmonary arterial pressures and cardiac output: Clinical application of hemodynamic monitoring. Adv Intern Med 27:453, 1982.
4. Forrester JS, Diamond G, McHugh TJ, Swan HJC: Filling pressures in the right and left sides of the heart in acute myocardial infarction. A reappraisal of cen-

tral-venous pressure monitoring. N Engl J Med 285:190, 1971.

5. Riley CP, Russell RO, Rackley CE: Left ventricular gallop sound and acute myocardial infarction. Am Heart J 86:598, 1973.

6. Carabello B, Cohn PF, Alpert JS: Hemodynamic monitoring in patients with hypotension after myocardial infarction. The role of the medical center in relation to the community hospital. Chest 74:5, 1978.

7. McHugh TJ, et al: Pulmonary vascular congestion in acute myocardial infarction: Hemodynamic and radiologic correlations. Ann Intern Med 76:29, 1972.

8. Kostuk W, Barr JW, Simon AL, Ross JR: Correlations between the chest film and hemodynamics in acute myocardial infarction. Circulation 48:624, 1973.

9. Connors AF, McCaffree DR, Gray BA: Evaluation of right-heart catheterization in the critically ill patient without acute myocardial infarction. N Engl J Med 308:263, 1983.

10. Eisenberg P, et al: Clinical evaluation compared to pulmonary artery catheterization in the hemodynamic assessment of critically ill patients. Crit Care Med 12:549, 1984.

11. Ganz W, et al: A new technique for measurement of cardiac output by thermodilution in man. Am J Cardiol 27:392, 1971.

12. Forrester JS, et al: Thermodilution cardiac output determination with a single flow-directed catheter. Am Heart J 83:306, 1972.

13. Zaidan JR, Freniere S: Use of a pacing pulmonary artery catheter during cardiac surgery. Ann Thorac Surg 35:633, 1983.

14. Lichtenthal PR, Collins JT: Multipurpose pulmonary artery catheter. Ann Thorac Surg 36:493, 1983.

15. Steele P, Davies H: The Swan-Ganz catheter in the cardiac laboratory. Br Heart J 35:647, 1973.

16. Kotoda K, Hasegawa T, Mizuno A, Saigusta M: Transseptal left-heart catheterization with Swan-Ganz flow-directed catheter. Am Heart J 105:436, 1983.

17. Sakurai T, et al: Balloon catheter test in patients with atrial septal defect and patent ductus arteriosus. Jpn Heart J 21:779, 1980.

18. Forrester JS, et al: Medical therapy of acute myocardial infarction by application of hemodynamic subjects. N Engl J Med 2985:1356, 1404, 1976.

19. Cohn JN, Guiha NH, Broder MI, Limas CJ: Right ventricular infarction: Clinical and hemodynamic features. Am J Cardiol 33:209, 1974.

20. Lorell B, et al: Right ventricular infarction: Clinical diagnosis and differentiation from cardiac tamponade and pericardial constriction. Am J Cardiol 43:465, 1979.

21. Meister SG, Helfant RH: Rapid bedside differentiation of ruptured interventricular septum from acute mitral insufficiency. N Engl J Med 287:1024, 1972.

22. Reddy PS, Curtiss EI, O'Toole JD, Shaver JA: Cardiac tamponade: Hemodynamic observations in man. Circulation 58:265, 1978.

23. Unger KM, Shibel EM, Moser KM: Detection of left ventricular failure in patients with adult respiratory distress syndrome. Chest 67:8, 1975.

24. Gooding JM, Laws HL: Interpretation of pulmonary capillary wedge pressure during different modes of ventilation. Respir Care 22:161, 1977.

25. Berryhill RE, Benumof JL, Rauscher LA: Pulmonary

vascular pressure reading at the end of exhalation. Anesthesiology 49:365, 1978.

26. Milic-Emili J, et al: Improved technique for estimating pleural pressure from esophageal balloons. J Appl Physiol 19:207, 1964.

27. Cohen JL, et al: Hemodynamic monitoring of patients undergoing abdominal aortic surgery. Am J Surg 146:174, 1983.

28. Kelly DT, Krovetz LJ, Rowe RD: Double-lumen flotation catheter for use in complex congenital cardiac anomalies. Circulation 44:910, 1971.

29. Stanger P, Heymann MA, Hoffman JIE, Rudolph AM: Use of Swan-Ganz catheter in cardiac catheterization of infants and children. Am Heart J 83:749, 1972.

30. Black JFS: Floating a catheter into the pulmonary artery in transposition of the great arteries. Am Heart J 84:761, 1972.

31. Jones SM, Miller GAH: Catheterization of the pulmonary artery in transposition of the great arteries using a Swan-Ganz flow-directed catheter. Br Heart J 35:298, 1973.

32. Fuchs RM, Heuser RR, Yin FCP, Brinker JA: Limitations of pulmonary wedge V waves in diagnosing mitral regurgitation. Am J Cardiol 49:849, 1982.

33. Pichard AD, et al: Large V waves in the pulmonary wedge pressure tracing in the absence of mitral regurgitation. Am J Cardiol 50:1044, 1982.

34. Rabinovitch M, et al: Quantitative analysis of the pulmonary wedge angiogram in congenital heart defects. Circulation 63:152, 1981.

35. Bell ALL, et al: Wedge pulmonary arteriography. Its application in congenital and acquired heart disease. Radiology 73:566, 1959.

36. Dougherty JE, LaSala AF, Fieldman A: Bedside pulmonary angiography utilizing an existing Swan-Ganz catheter. Chest 77:43, 1980.

37. LePage JR, Garcia RM: The value of bedside wedge pulmonary angiography in the detection of pulmonary emboli: A predictive and prospective evaluation. Radiology 144:67, 1982.

38. Boyd KD, et al: A prospective study of complications of pulmonary artery catheterizations in 500 consecutive patients. Chest 84:245, 1983.

39. Davies MJ, Cronin KD, Domaingue CM: Pulmonary artery catheterization. An assessment of risks and benefits in 220 surgical patients. Anaesth Intens Care 10:9, 1982.

40. Elliott CG, Zimmerman GA, Clemmer TP: Complications of pulmonary artery catheterization in the care of critically ill patients. Chest 76:647, 1979.

41. Sise MJ, et al: Complications of the flow-directed pulmonary artery catheter: A prospective analysis in 219 patients. Crit Care Med 9:315, 1981.

42. Sprung CL, et al: Advanced ventricular arrhythmias during bedside pulmonary artery catheterization. Am J Med 72:203, 1982.

43. Sprung CL, et al: Prophylactic use of lidocaine to prevent advanced ventricular arrhythmias during pulmonary artery catheterization. Prospective double-blind study. Am J Med 75:906, 1983.

44. Lapin ES, Murray JA: Hemoptysis with flow-directed cardiac catheterization. JAMA 29:1246, 1972.

45. Kelly TF Jr, et al: Perforation of the pulmonary artery

with Swan-Ganz catheters: Diagnosis and surgical management. Ann Surg 193:686, 1981.

46. Cho SR, et al: Percutaneous unknotting of intravascular catheters and retrieval of catheter fragments. AJR 141:397, 1983.

47. Sumesnil JG, Proulx G: A new nonsurgical technique for untying tight knots in flow-directed balloon catheters. Am J Cardiol 15:395, 1984.

48. Hoar PF, et al: Heparin bonding reduces thrombogenicity of pulmonary artery catheters. N Engl J Med 305:993, 1981.

49. Bessette MC, Quintin L, Whalley DG, Wynands JE: Swan-Ganz contamination: A protective sleeve for repositioning. Can Anaesth Soc J 28:86, 1981.

Part III

Hemodynamic Principles

8

Blood Flow Measurement: The Cardiac Output

WILLIAM GROSSMAN

The maintenance of blood flow commensurate with the metabolic needs of the body is a fundamental requirement of human life. In the absence of major disease of the vascular tree (e.g., arterial obstruction), the maintenance of appropriate blood flow to the body depends largely upon the heart's ability to pump blood in the forward direction. The quantity of blood delivered to the systemic circulation per unit time is termed the *cardiac output,* generally expressed in liters/minute.

ARTERIOVENOUS DIFFERENCE AND EXTRACTION RESERVE

Because the extraction of nutrients by metabolizing tissues is a function not only of the rate of delivery of those nutrients (the cardiac output) but also of the ability of each tissue to extract those nutrients from the circulation, tissue viability can be maintained despite a fall in cardiac output as long as there is increased extraction of required nutrients. The extraction of a given nutrient (or of any substance) from the circulation by a particular tissue is expressed as the *arteriovenous difference* across that tissue, and the factor by which the arteriovenous difference can increase at constant flow (due to changes in metabolic demand) may be termed the *extraction reserve.* For example, arterial blood in man is normally 95%

saturated with oxygen; that is, if 1 L of blood has the *capacity* to carry approximately 200 ml of oxygen when fully saturated, arterial blood will usually be found to contain 190 ml of oxygen per liter (190/200 = 95%). Venous blood returning from the body normally has an average oxygen saturation of 75%; that is, mixed venous blood generally contains 150 ml of oxygen per liter of blood (150/200 = 75%). Thus, the normal arteriovenous difference for oxygen is 40 ml/L (190 ml/L − 150 ml/L).

The normal extraction reserve for oxygen[1] is 3, which means that, given adequate metabolic demand, the body's tissues can extract 120 ml of oxygen (3 × 40 ml) from each liter of blood delivered. Thus, if arterial saturation remains constant at 95%, full utilization of the extraction reserve will result in a mixed venous oxygen content of 70 ml/L (190 ml/L − 120 ml/L), or a mixed venous oxygen saturation of 35% (70/200 = 35%). This is essentially the value found for mixed venous (i.e., pulmonary artery) oxygen saturation in normal men studied at maximal exercise. The relation between cardiac output and arteriovenous O_2 difference is illustrated in Figure 8–1.

LOWER LIMIT OF CARDIAC OUTPUT

The value of 3 for the oxygen extraction reserve predicts that, in progressive cardiac

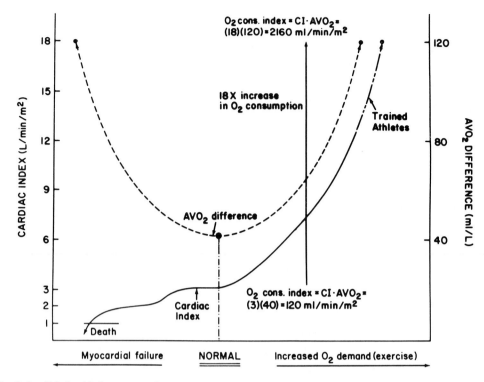

Fig. 8–1. Relationship between arteriovenous oxygen (AVO_2) difference (broken line) and cardiac index (solid curve) in normal subjects at rest (center) and during exercise (right), and in the patient with progressively worsening myocardial failure (left). See text for discussion.

decompensation, to meet the basal oxygen requirements of the body, oxygen extraction increases as cardiac output falls until arteriovenous oxygen difference has tripled and cardiac output has fallen to one third of its normal value (Fig. 8–1). Because the extraction reserve has now been fully used, further reduction of cardiac output will result in tissue hypoxia, anaerobic metabolism, acidosis, and eventually, circulatory collapse. This prediction seems quite accurate; clinical investigators have observed for many years that a fall in resting cardiac output to below one third of normal (i.e., a cardiac index ≤ 1.0 L/min/M^2) is incompatible with life.

UPPER LIMIT OF CARDIAC OUTPUT

Several studies have indicated that the largest increase in cardiac output that can be achieved by a trained athlete at maximal exercise is 600% of the resting output. If a nor-

mal 70 kg man has a cardiac output of 5 L/min or 3.0 L/min/M^2, his maximal cardiac output might be as high as 30 L/min (18/L/min/M^2). Because cardiac output increases approximately 600 ml for each 100 ml increase in oxygen requirements of the body, an increase in cardiac output of 25 L/min with maximal exercise would suggest an increase in total body oxygen requirements of 4167 ml/min, which is approximately an 18-fold increase over the normal resting value of 250 ml/min. The 18-fold increase in total body oxygen requirements is met by the combined sixfold increase in oxygen "delivery" (i.e., cardiac output), and threefold increase in oxygen extraction (oxygen reserve). These relations are illustrated in Figure 8–1.

FACTORS INFLUENCING CARDIAC OUTPUT IN NORMAL SUBJECTS

The range of the "normal" cardiac output is difficult to define with precision because it

BSA

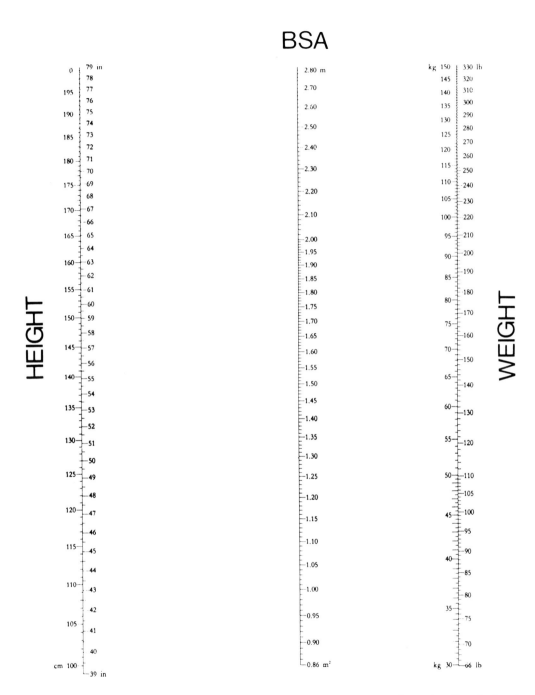

Fig. 8–2. Nomogram for calculation of body surface area, given the weight and height of the patient. From the formula of Dubois.[4]

is influenced by several variables. Obviously, body size is important, and the ranges of normal values for cardiac output of 2-year-old children, 10-year-old children, and 50-year-old men are so different that they show only minimal overlap. For this reason, normalization of the cardiac output for differing body size is considered fundamental by all students of this subject, although there is disagreement about the best way to accomplish this normalization. Because cardiac output seems to be predominantly a function of the body's oxygen consumption or metabolic rate,[1,2] and because metabolic rate was thought to correlate best with body surface area,[3,4] it has become customary to express cardiac output in terms of the *cardiac index* (L/min)/(body surface area, M²). Body surface area is not measured directly but is instead calculated from one of the experimentally developed formulae, such as that of Dubois.[4]

Body surface area (M²)
$$= 0.007184 \times \text{Weight}^{0.425} \times \text{Height}^{0.725}$$
$$\text{(kg)} \qquad \text{(cm)}$$

Despite the shortcomings and weaknesses of this approach to normalization of the cardiac output,[1,5] the method has gained nearly universal acceptance by clinicians over the past 40 years, and will be employed throughout this book. A chart to aid calculation of body surface area (if weight and height are known) appears in Figure 8–2.

Although expression of cardiac output as the *cardiac index* greatly narrows the range of normal values among our groups of 2-year-old children, 10-year-old children, and 50-year-old men, it does not completely abolish the differences in these ranges. In fact, the normal cardiac output appears to vary with age, steadily decreasing from approximately 4.5 L/min/M² at age 7 years to 2.5 L/min/M² at age 70 years.[1,6] This is not surprising, because it is well known that the body's metabolic rate is affected greatly by age, being highest in childhood and progressively diminishing to old age.

In addition to age, cardiac output is affected by posture, decreasing approximately 10% when rising from lying to sitting position and approximately 20% when rising (or being tilted) from lying to standing position. Also, body temperature, anxiety, environmental heat and humidity, and a host of other factors influence the normal resting cardiac output,[1] and these must be considered in interpreting any value of cardiac output measured in the clinical setting.

TECHNIQUES FOR DETERMINATION OF CARDIAC OUTPUT

Of the numerous techniques devised over the years to measure cardiac output, two have won general acceptance in cardiac catheterization laboratories: the Fick oxygen technique and the indicator dilution technique. Both techniques resemble each other in that they are based on the theoretic principle enunciated by Adolph Fick in 1870.[7] The principle, which was never actually applied by Fick, states that ***the total uptake or release of any substance by an organ is the product of blood flow to the organ and the arteriovenous concentration difference of the substance.*** For the lungs the substance released to the blood is oxygen, and the pulmonary blood flow can be determined by knowing the arteriovenous difference of oxygen across the lungs and the oxygen consumption per minute.

Fick's principle is illustrated in Figure 8–3. In this figure, a train is passing by a hopper that is delivering marbles to the boxcars at a rate of 20 marbles/min. If the boxcars each contain 16 marbles before passing under the hopper and 20 marbles after passing under the hopper, each boxcar is picking up 4 marbles, and must be taking only ⅕ of a minute to pass under the hopper, because it would pick up 20 marbles in each full minute under the hopper. If each boxcar takes ⅕ of a minute to pass by the hopper, the train is moving at a speed sufficient to deliver 5 boxcars/min to any point down the line. This could have been calculated as shown in Figure 8–3:

Train's speed
(boxcars/min)
= Marble delivery rate/"A-V" marble
difference
(marbles/min)   (marbles/boxcar)
= (20 marbles/min)(4 marbles/boxcar)
= 5 boxcars/min

If one boxcar is 1 L of blood and each marble is 10 ml of oxygen, then we have an arteriovenous O_2 difference of 40 ml/L, an oxygen consumption of 200 ml/min, and a cardiac output of 5 L/min.

Fick Oxygen Method

In the Fick oxygen method, pulmonary blood flow should be determined by measuring the arteriovenous difference of oxygen across the lungs and the rate of oxygen uptake by blood from the lungs. If there is no intracardiac shunt and pulmonary blood flow is equal to systemic blood flow, the Fick oxygen method also measures systemic blood flow. Thus, *cardiac output = oxygen consumption ÷ arteriovenous oxygen difference.*

In actual practice, the rate at which oxygen is taken up from the lungs by blood is not measured, but rather the uptake of oxygen from room air by the lungs is measured, because in a steady state, these two measurements are equal. Furthermore, arteriovenous oxygen difference across the lungs is not meas-

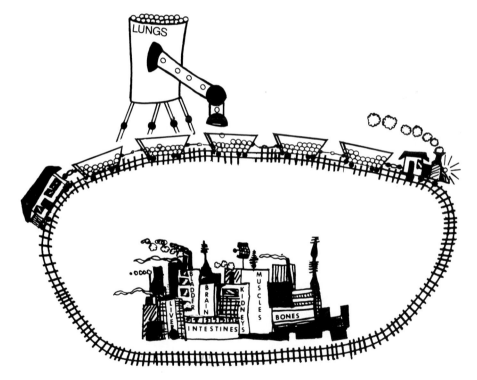

Fig. 8–3. Illustration of Fick's principle. A train, representing the circulation, passes by a hopper (the lungs) that delivers marbles (oxygen) to the train's boxcars at a rate of 20 marbles/min. Because the boxcars each contain 16 marbles before and 20 marbles after passing under the hopper, each boxcar is picking up 4 marbles, and must be taking only ⅕ minute to pass under the hopper, since it would pick up 20 marbles in each full minute under the hopper. If each boxcar takes only ⅕ minute to pass by the hopper, the train is moving at a speed sufficient to deliver 5 boxcars/min to any point down the line. This could have been calculated as

Train's speed = Marble delivery rate/"A-V" marble difference
(boxcars/min)   (marbles/min)   (marbles/boxcar)
= (20 marbles/min)/(4 marbles/boxcar)
= 5 boxcars/min

If one boxcar is 1 L of blood and each marble is 10 ml oxygen, then we have an arteriovenous oxygen difference of 40 ml/L, an O_2 consumption of 200 ml/min, and a cardiac output of 5 L/min. (Illustration kindly provided by Jennifer Grossman, age 11.)

ured directly. Generally, pulmonary arterial blood (true mixed venous blood) is sampled, but pulmonary venous blood is not sampled. Instead, left ventricular or systemic arterial blood is sampled and assumed to have an oxygen content representative of mixed pulmonary venous blood. Actually, because of bronchial venous and thebesian venous drainage, the oxygen content of systemic arterial blood is commonly 2 to 5 ml/L of blood lower than pulmonary venous blood as it leaves the alveoli.

Oxygen Consumption

Two different methods for measurement of oxygen consumption are widely used today: the polarographic method and the Douglas bag method.

Polarographic O_2 Method. In our laboratory, oxygen consumption is currently measured using the metabolic rate meter (MRM) made by Waters Instruments (Rochester, Minnesota). The instrument contains a polarographic oxygen sensor cell (gold and silver/silver chloride electrodes), a hood or face mask, and a blower of variable speed connected to a servocontrol loop with the oxygen sensor (Fig. 8–4). This device is convenient and accurate and represents a significant advance over the older, standard procedure of collecting expired air for 3 minutes in a Douglas bag and measuring volume (Tissot spirometer) and oxygen content. The principle of operation for the MRM involves using a variable-speed blower to maintain a unidirectional flow of air from the room through the hood and via a connecting hose to the polarographic oxygen-sensing cell. As illustrated in Figure 8–4, room air enters the hood at a rate, $\dot{V}_R$ (ml/min), which is determined by the blower's discharge rate, $\dot{V}_M$ (ml/min), as well as the patient's ventilatory rate ($\dot{V}_i$, inhaled air in ml/min; $\dot{V}_E$, exhaled air). The blower speed, $\dot{V}_M$, is controlled by a servoloop designed to maintain the oxygen content of air flowing past the polarographic cell constant at a predetermined value. In a steady state, the average value of $\dot{V}_M$ together with the oxygen content of room air and of air flowing past the polarographic

cell can be used to calculate the patient's oxygen consumption, as follows:

The patient's oxygen consumption, $\dot{V}_{O_2}$ is given by:

$$\dot{V}_{O_2} = (F_R O_2 \cdot \dot{V}_R) - (F_M O_2 \cdot \dot{V}_M)$$
[Equation 1]

where $F_R O_2$ and $F_M O_2$ are the fractional contents of oxygen in room air and in air flowing past the polarographic cell, respectively.

As can be seen from Figure 8–4,

$$\dot{V}_M = \dot{V}_R - \dot{V}_i + \dot{V}_E,,$$

which can be rewritten as

$$\dot{V}_R = \dot{V}_M + \dot{V}_i - \dot{V}_E$$

Substituting this in Equation 1 gives:

$$\dot{V}_{O_2} = F_R O_2(\dot{V}_M + \dot{V}_i - \dot{V}_E) - F_M O_2 \cdot \dot{V}_M$$

$$= F_R O_2(\dot{V}_M) - F_M O_2(\dot{V}_M) + F_R O_2(\dot{V}_i) - F_R O_2(\dot{V}_E$$

$$= \dot{V}_M(F_R O_2 - F_M O_2) + F_R O_2(\dot{V}_i - \dot{V}_E)$$

Since the fractional content of oxygen in room air ($F_R O_2$) is 0.209, oxygen consumption is given by:

$$\dot{V}_{O_2} = \dot{V}_M(0.209 - F_M O_2) + 0.209(\dot{V}_i - \dot{V}_E)$$
[Equation 2]

Thus, in a steady state (where $\dot{V}_i - \dot{V}_E$ is constant), oxygen consumption can be determined by measurement of the volume rate of air moved by the blower motor ($\dot{V}_M$) and the fractional O_2 content of air moving past the polarographic sensor. In the MRM, a servo-controlled system adjusts $\dot{V}_M$ to keep $F_M O_2$ at a constant predetermined value. In practice, $F_M O_2$ is set at 0.199, so that Equation 2 becomes

$$\dot{V}_{O_2} = \dot{V}_M(0.209 - 0.199) + 0.209(\dot{V}_i - \dot{V}_E)$$

$$\dot{V}_{O_2} = 0.01 \, \dot{V}_M + 0.209(\dot{V}_i - \dot{V}_E).$$

For practical purposes, the respiratory quotient (RQ) is assumed to be 1.0; accordingly, $\dot{V}_i = \dot{V}_E$ and $\dot{V}_{O_2} = 0.01 \, \dot{V}_M$. If the RQ is actually 0.9 (e.g., the patient releases 0.9 liters of CO_2 for each liter of O_2 consumed), the error in $\dot{V}_{O_2}$ resulting from the assumption of

SERVO UNIT

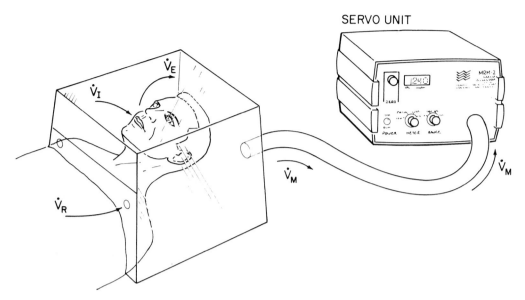

Fig. 8–4. Measurement of O_2 consumption by a polarographic cell technique using the Waters Instruments metabolic rate meter (MRM). A transparent hood fits snugly over the patient's head, resting on his pillow. Air enters the hood through holes in a plastic sheet at a flow rate V_R. The patient's inspiratory (V_I) and expiratory (V_E) flow rates subtract and add to V_R to yield V_M, the flow rate leaving the hood and entering the servo-unit. A blower motor in the servo-unit adjusts V_M to keep the O_2 sensed by a polarographic cell constant. See text for details.

an RQ of 1.0 is 1.6%, and if RQ is 0.8 the error would be 3.2%. The MRM O_2 consumption monitor has a calibrated blower motor in addition to the servocontrol polarographic sensor, and gives a readout of oxygen consumption in liters/minute by digital scale (MRM-2) or by meter and paper (MRM-1). The MRM-2 model is calibrated to be highly accurate in the oxygen consumption range from 10 to 1000 ml O_2/min and is thus best suited for measurement of resting O_2 consumption in the catheterization laboratory. The MRM-1 model, which is calibrated in the 150 to 5000 ml O_2/min range, is best suited for exercise studies.

The metabolic rate meter is relatively easy to use. In our experience it is accurate, although a fair amount of attention to detail is required to obtain reproducible readings consistently. A study by Lange et al.,[8] however, found that values of oxygen consumption measured by a metabolic rate meter (MRM-2, Waters Instruments, Rochester, MA) were significantly lower than those measured using the standard Douglas bag technique (see below).

Douglas Bag Method. In addition to the MRM O_2 device, it is valuable to have as backup the older, standard volumetric technique for measuring O_2 consumption which involves the collection of expired air for subsequent analysis. In this method, a timed sample (usually 3 minutes) of the patient's expired air is collected in a Douglas bag.* In making this collection, the patient's nose is first firmly clipped† shut so that no air can escape through it. Once the clip is in place, the patient is asked to hold a special mouthpiece between his lips and breathe entirely through the mouthpiece, great care being taken that no air escapes around it. A technician holds the mouthpiece for the patient in a steady and comfortable position with one hand and may use the other hand to hold the patient's lips firmly around the mouthpiece. The mouthpiece is attached to the Douglas bag by a two-way valve‡ that

*60-Liter Douglas type gas bag, Warren Collins, Inc., Boston, MA.

†Rubber-tipped nose clip, Warren Collins, Inc., Boston, MA.

‡Two-way valve with rubber fittings, Warren Collins, Inc., Boston, MA.

has a sidearm open to room air. The valve and sidearm function in such a way that the patient inspires air from the room but expires completely into the Douglas bag. The Douglas bag has a built-in three-way valve that allows the operator to open and then seal off the bag after the timed sample of expired air has been collected. An equilibration period of at least 30 seconds of breathing quietly through the mouthpiece should be allowed before beginning the timed air collection. This permits the patient to adjust to the technique and washes out the dead space in the valve and connecting tubing interposed between the patient and the Douglas bag.

Contents of the bag should be analyzed as soon as possible following the collection, because some diffusion occurs through the walls of the bag. The bag, however, may be placed aside until completing the cardiac catheterization, although it is helpful to know the oxygen consumption before the catheterization is completed and the catheters are removed from the patient's vascular system.

In calculating the oxygen consumption using the Douglas bag to collect expired air, it is helpful to have a flow sheet such as the one reproduced in Figure 8–5. Calculation of the oxygen consumption is done in two steps. First, one measures the oxygen content of room air and that of the patient's expired air. This may be done with a Beckman oxygen analyzer,* which enables one to determine the oxygen content of a gas sample in millimeters of mercury partial pressure, or a Lex-O_2-Con† oxygen analyzer, which precisely measures oxygen content of air by a fuel-cell technique. Corrected barometric pressure is determined each day from a barometer and thermometer located in the catheterization laboratory. Barometric pressure is corrected for temperature with the aid of a standard table (Table 8–1). The values for barometric pressure, temperature, and corrected barometric pressure are entered at the top of the flow sheet (Fig. 8–5, a, b, and c).

The volume of expired air in the Douglas bag may be measured with a Tissot spirometer‡ or gas meter,§ and this is corrected to standard temperature and pressure (STP) by means of standard tables. (Tables for correcting gas volumes to STP, "dry" or saturated, are available in a number of texts of standard tables, such as Documenta Geigy—Scientific Tables. Ardsley, NY, Geigy Pharmaceuticals, 1962, pp. 300–309). Some spirometers give volume readings directly; others require that the volume be calculated from the difference in height of the spirometer before and after the introduction of the expired air (steps 4 and 5, Fig. 8–5). The total volume originally present in the Douglas bag equals the Tissot spirometer volume plus the small volume of air removed for analysis in the Beckman oxygen analyzer (step 6, Fig. 8–5). The total volume of expired air is corrected to STP by standard tables (step 7, Fig. 8–5) and is divided by the number of minutes of collection time to obtain the minute ventilation (step 8, Fig. 8–5).

The oxygen difference, milliliters of oxygen consumed per liter of air (step 3, Fig. 8–5), is multiplied by the minute ventilation (step 8, Fig. 8–5) to obtain the oxygen consumption in milliliters/minute (step 9, Fig. 8–5). The latter is divided by the body surface area (Fig. 8–2), yielding the oxygen consumption index in milliliters of oxygen consumed per minute per square meter of body surface area (step 10, Fig. 8–5). The normal basal oxygen consumption in man is usually between 110 and 150 ml O_2 per minute square meter of body surface area.

Arteriovenous Oxygen Difference

The arteriovenous oxygen difference across the lungs must be measured to calculate cardiac output by Fick's principle, and this can be accomplished by the following method. From appropriately positioned catheters, systemic arterial and mixed venous (pulmonary arterial) blood samples are obtained during the

---

*Model C2 oxygen analyzer, Beckman Instruments, Fullerton, CA.

†Lexington Instruments, Lexington, MA.

‡Respiratory gasometer, Tissot type, Arthur Thomas & Co., Philadelphia, PA.

§Wet test meter. Precision Scientific Company, Chicago, IL.

Name: _____ Date: _____

BSA: _____ Height: _____ Weight: _____ No.: _____

    (a) Barometric pressure   _____ mm Hg

    (b) Barometric temperature   _____ ° C

    (c) Corrected barometric pressure _____ mm Hg (Table 8-1)

    (d) pO_2 room air   _____ mm Hg

    (e) pO_2 expired air   _____ mm Hg

    (f) Tissot: initial   _____ cm

    (g) Tissot: final   _____ cm

    (h) Sample volume   _____ L

    (i) Correction factor   _____ (standard tables)

    (j) Collection time   _____ min

OXYGEN DIFFERENCE

Step 1. O_2 content in room air:

$$\frac{pO_2 \text{ room air (d)} \times 100}{\text{corrected barometric pressure (c)}} = \text{_____} \text{ ml } O_2/100 \text{ ml air}$$

Step 2. O_2 content of expired air:

$$\frac{pO_2 \text{ expired air (e)} \times 100}{\text{corrected barometric pressure (c)}} = \text{_____} \text{ ml } O_2/100 \text{ ml air}$$

Step 3. $\big[O_2$ room air $- O_2$ expired air$\big] \times 10 = \text{_____}$ ml O_2 consumed/L air
       (step 1)   (step 2)

MINUTE VENTILATION

Step 4. Tissot initial (f) − Tissot final (g) = _____ cm

Step 5. Tissot volume:

    Difference (step 4) × 1.329* = _____ L

Step 6. Total volume:

    Tissot volume (step 5) + sample (h) = _____ L

Step 7. Total volume (step 6) × correction factor (i) = _____ L

Step 8. $\dfrac{\text{Ventilation volume (step 7)}}{\text{Collection time (j)}} = \text{_____}$ L/min

Step 9. Oxygen consumption:

    O_2 difference × minute ventilation = _____ ml/min
      (step 3)   (step 8)

Step 10. Oxygen consumption index:

    $\dfrac{O_2 \text{ consumption (step 9)}}{\text{Body surface area}} = \text{_____}$ ml/min/m^2

---

*Correction factor for each instrument. In this case 1.0L of gas produces an excursion of 1.329 cm on the meter scale.

Fig. 8–5. Oxygen consumption calculation.

Table 8–1. *Millimeters to be Subtracted from Barometer Readings to Reduce Them to 0°C*

Temp. °C.	Barometric pressure in mm Hg				
	740	750	760	770	780
11.0	1.33	1.35	1.36	1.38	1.40
11.5	1.39	1.41	1.42	1.44	1.46
12.0	1.45	1.47	1.49	1.51	1.53
12.5	1.51	1.53	1.55	1.57	1.59
13.0	1.57	1.59	1.61	1.63	1.65
13.5	1.63	1.65	1.67	1.69	1.71
14.0	1.69	1.71	1.73	1.76	1.78
14.5	1.75	1.77	1.79	1.82	1.84
15.0	1.81	1.83	1.86	1.88	1.91
15.5	1.87	1.89	1.92	1.94	1.97
16.0	1.93	1.96	1.98	2.01	2.03
16.5	1.99	2.02	2.04	2.07	2.09
17.0	2.05	2.08	2.10	2.13	2.16
17.5	2.11	2.14	2.16	2.19	2.22
18.0	2.17	2.20	2.23	2.26	2.29
18.5	2.23	2.26	2.29	2.32	2.35
19.0	2.29	2.32	2.35	2.38	2.41
19.5	2.35	2.38	2.41	2.45	2.48
20.0	2.41	2.44	2.47	2.51	2.54
20.5	2.47	2.50	2.54	2.57	2.61
21.0	2.53	2.56	2.60	2.63	2.67
21.5	2.59	2.63	2.66	2.70	2.73
22.0	2.65	2.69	2.72	2.76	2.79
22.5	2.71	2.75	2.78	2.82	2.86
23.0	2.77	2.81	2.84	2.88	2.92
23.5	2.83	2.87	2.91	2.95	2.99
24.0	2.89	2.93	2.97	3.01	3.05
24.5	2.95	2.99	3.03	3.07	3.11
25.0	3.01	3.05	3.09	3.13	3.17
25.5	3.07	3.11	3.15	3.20	3.24
26.0	3.13	3.17	3.21	3.26	3.30
26.5	3.19	3.23	3.28	3.32	3.36
27.0	3.25	3.29	3.34	3.38	3.42
27.5	3.31	3.35	3.40	3.45	3.49
28.0	3.37	3.41	3.46	3.51	3.55
28.5	3.43	3.48	3.52	3.57	3.62
29.0	3.49	3.54	3.58	3.63	3.68
29.5	3.55	3.60	3.65	3.69	3.74
30.0	3.61	3.66	3.71	3.75	3.80
30.5	3.67	3.72	3.77	3.82	3.87
31.0	3.73	3.78	3.83	3.88	3.93
31.5	3.79	3.84	3.89	3.94	3.99
32.0	3.85	3.90	3.95	4.00	4.05
32.5	3.91	3.96	4.01	4.07	4.12
33.0	3.97	4.02	4.07	4.13	4.18
33.5	4.03	4.08	4.14	4.19	4.25
34.0	4.09	4.14	4.20	4.25	4.31
34.5	4.15	4.20	4.26	4.31	4.37
35.0	4.21	4.26	4.32	4.38	4.43
35.5	4.26	4.32	4.38	4.44	4.50
36.0	4.32	4.38	4.44	4.50	4.56

period when O_2 consumption is being measured. The samples are drawn into heparinized syringes and quickly capped. If the patient has received heparin systemically, the syringes for collection of these blood samples need not be heparinized. If the samples will be analyzed immediately by oximetry, plastic syringes may be used. O_2 may diffuse through the walls of plastic syringes, however, and glass syringes are considered preferable by some if there will be a delay in oximetric analysis of the blood. In a test in our laboratory, no appreciable increase in O_2 saturation of venous blood could be detected over 2 hours (capped plastic 15-ml syringe filled with venous blood sitting at room temperature was sampled every 15 minutes for oximetry). The samples should be drawn simultaneously and as close to the midpoint of the oxygen consumption determination as possible. Care must be taken to avoid contamination of the blood samples with air bubbles.

Oxygen content (in milliliters of oxygen per liter of blood) can be determined by a variety of methods, the most classic of which (and the one that serves as a standard for all others) is the manometric technique of Van Slyke and Neill.[9] The major drawback of the Van Slyke technique is that 15 to 30 minutes are required to run a single blood sample. Reflectance oximetry of heparinized blood samples is simple and quick and measures the percentage of hemoglobin present as oxyhemoglobin. This percentage, multiplied by the theoretic *oxygen carrying capacity* of the patient's blood, yields the calculated *oxygen content* of that sample (Fig. 8–6). A formula for approximating the theoretic oxygen carrying capacity in man is:

Hemoglobin (gm/dl) × 1.36 (ml O_2/gm hemoglobin) × 10 = theoretic O_2 carrying capacity (ml O_2/L blood)

In several textbooks, the constant is given as 1.34, but studies on crystalline human hemoglobin suggest that the correct number may be 1.36.[10,11] Whatever its correct value, the formula is only an approximation. To the extent that some hemoglobin may be bound to carbon monoxide (cigarette smokers) or that abnormal hemoglobins (e.g., HgbS) may be present, the approximation will be incorrect. Newer methods have been introduced that utilize an oxygen-sensing cell for direct measurement of oxygen content.*

Figure 8–6 is a flow sheet that may be used to calculate oxygen content of blood samples and arteriovenous oxygen difference when the spectrophotometric oximeter method is used. Oxygen contents of arterial and mixed venous blood samples are calculated as the percentage of oxyhemoglobin saturation of these samples multiplied by the oxygen carrying capacity (steps 2 to 5, Fig. 8–6). The arteriovenous oxygen difference (step 3 minus step 5, Fig. 8–6) may then be divided into the oxygen consumption to yield the cardiac output.

Arterial blood may be taken from a systemic artery, the left ventricle, the left atrium, or the pulmonary veins. Theoretically, pulmonary venous blood is preferable to peripheral arterial blood for the arteriovenous oxygen difference calculations. Except in the presence of a right-to-left intracardiac shunt, pulmonary venous oxygen content may be approximated by systemic arterial oxygen content, ignoring the small amount of venous admixture result-

*Lex-O₂-Con, Lexington Instruments, Waltham, MA.

ing from bronchial and thebesian venous drainage. If arterial desaturation (e.g., arterial blood oxygen saturation <95%) is present, a central right-to-left shunt should be excluded before accepting systemic arterial oxygen content as representative of that of pulmonary venous blood. Techniques for detecting and quantifying such shunts are described in Chapter 12.

The most reliable site for obtaining mixed venous blood is the pulmonary artery. Because of streaming and incomplete mixing, using blood from more proximal sites such as the right atrium or vena cavae as representative of mixed venous blood is much less accurate.[12,13] Right ventricular blood is closer to true mixed venous blood, and may be substituted for pulmonary arterial blood if necessary.

Sources of Error. The techniques described for cardiac output measurement by application of Fick's principle assume that a steady state exists; that is, that the cardiac output and oxygen consumption are constant during the period of measurement. Therefore, strict quiet, calm, and decorum must be maintained in the catheterization laboratory during this time, to encourage the achievement of a steady state condition. Potential errors in the determination of cardiac output by the Fick oxygen technique

Step 1. Theoretic oxygen-carrying capacity:

Hemoglobin (gm/dl) × 1.36 (ml of O_2/gm of Hb) × 10 = _____ ml O_2/L blood

Step 2. Saturation of arterial (BA, FA, Ao) blood = _____ %

Step 3. Oxygen content of arterial blood:

Theoretic capacity × % saturation = _____ ml/L
    (step 1)   (step 2)

Step 4. Saturation of mixed venous (PA) blood = _____ %

Step 5. Oxygen content of mixed venous blood:

Theoretic capacity × % saturation = _____ ml/L
    (step 1)   (step 4)

Step 6. AV O_2 difference:

Arterial O_2 content − venous O_2 content = _____ ml/L
    (step 3)   (step 5)

Fig. 8–6. Calculation of oxygen content and AV oxygen difference when using the reflectance oximetry method.

may come from a number of sources, among which are the following:

(1) *Incomplete collection of the expired air sample when the Douglas bag method is used* may result in underestimation of oxygen consumption and, therefore, of cardiac output. Malfunction of the rubber fittings within the unidirectional air-flow valves in the patient's mouthpiece is a common problem. The technician should observe these valves to see that they open freely and close snugly with inspiration and expiration, respectively. Having the patient take deep, slow breaths will help proper function of the valves, whose inertia may not allow adequate response to rapid, shallow respirations.

Perforated ear drums, an air leak around the mouthpiece (e.g., from loose dentures), or incomplete clamping of the nostrils are also common causes of incomplete air collection. If the patient's ear drums are perforated, rubber ear plugs should be used. Careful attention given by the technician collecting the expired air sample to holding the patient's lips firmly around the mouthpiece and to proper placement of the nose clamp will obviate some of these problems.

These problems are obviated with the use of the MRM technique with either hood or face-mask method. With these methods, however, it is essential that a tight seal be obtained with the hood or face mask, so that room air entering the hood or face mask must flow across the patient's face before exiting through the tube connected to the polarographic sensor (Fig. 8–4), and all the patient's expired air is evacuated towards the sensor.

(2) *Changes in mean pulmonary volume* can result in a major error in oxygen consumption and cardiac output calculations. It is clear from the foregoing descriptions that the Douglas bag expired air method, as well as the MRM method, do not measure the amount of oxygen entering the blood each minute; instead, they measure (at best) the amount of oxygen entering the lungs each minute. Because the lungs could act as a reservoir, oxygen *consumption* by the body is not necessarily measured by these techniques. For example, if a patient progressively increases his pulmonary volume by 300 ml/min, by the end of a three-minute collection of expired air he will have taken into his lungs 900 ml of air (or 180 ml of oxygen) more than that necessary for his steady state metabolic oxygen requirements. This extra 180 ml of oxygen, which is now in his "pulmonary reservoir," will falsely elevate the estimate of his actual oxygen consumption and cardiac output. If his actual oxygen consumption is 250 ml/min, then his "measured" oxygen consumption will be $250 + (180/3) = 310$ ml/min, and this will result in a 24% error in the cardiac output calculation. In practice, the error probably occurs more often in the opposite direction, since when patients first have their nose clamps placed and start breathing into the mouthpiece or when they are first placed in the MRM hood, they may become somewhat "claustrophobic" and tend to breathe faster and deeper (during the equilibration period) than they do later during the actual expired air collection. This obviously results in an *artifactual underestimation of oxygen consumption* and cardiac output.

(3) As can be seen from Figure 8–5, the Douglas bag method assumes that the patient's minute ventilation (step 8) can be calculated from the measurement of the volume of expired air, and this assumption in turn requires that the volume of air entering the lungs per minute equals the volume of air leaving the lungs per minute (in a steady state). This is not quite true, even in a steady state, however, because the ratio of carbon dioxide molecules produced to oxygen molecules consumed does not equal unity. In fact, this ratio (the respiratory quotient) varies depending on the diet and metabolic state of the patient. Thus, a small error is introduced into the measurement of the oxygen consumption as calculated here because *the volume of carbon dioxide expired is not exactly equal to the volume of oxygen taken up.* A correction for this, assuming a respiration quotient of 0.8, is performed in some catheterization laboratories.

An example of the error introduced by neglecting the respiratory quotient follows: Suppose a patient breathes in 5.00 L of air/min, and that the inspired air contains 20% oxygen and 80% nitrogen. From the 5000 ml of air, the patient extracts 250 ml of oxygen (his oxygen consumption) but returns only 200 ml of carbon dioxide, as would be expected if his respiratory quotient is 0.8. The expired air collection will then contain 4000 ml nitrogen, 750 ml of oxygen, and 200 ml of carbon dioxide, for a total volume of 4950 ml expired air. If analyzed as indicated in Figure 8–5, the calculations will indicate that oxygen difference between inspired and expired air is 48.5 ml/L, since inspired air contained 20% oxygen while expired air contained 15.15% oxygen (750 ml O_2/4950 ml air). By neglecting the respiratory quotient, it will be assumed that minute ventilation was 4.950 L/min, and therefore the oxygen consumption was 4.950 L air/min $\times$ 48.5 ml O_2/L air = 240 ml O_2/min. Since the true oxygen consumption in this example was 250 ml/min, we can see that neglecting the respiratory quotient leads to an underestimation in both the oxygen consumption and cardiac output calculations (in this case by approximately 4%).

(4) *Incorrect timing of the expired air collection* may be a problem when the Douglas bag technique is used, and it is best to use either a hand-held stop watch or some other precision timing device. Some laboratories use a 5-minute period for collection of expired air to minimize errors related to inaccuracies of timing, or the problem of beginning and ending at different phases of the respiratory cycle.

(5) *The spectrophotometric determination of blood oxygen saturation* may introduce inaccuracies related to carboxyhemoglobin or other abnormal hemoglobins, as discussed previously. This method may also be inaccurate if indocyanine green dye is present in the circulation. Therefore, indicator dilution curves should be done only after all samples for spectrophotometric oximetry have been taken. Reflectance oximetry, as performed on whole blood is accurate in the range of blood oxygen saturations from 45 to 98% but may not be reliable when blood O_2 saturation is less than 40%, as is the case in pulmonary artery blood

from patients with very low cardiac output or during strenuous exercise.

(6) *Improper collection of the mixed venous blood sample* (e.g., air bubbles) is a common source of error. Partial contamination of pulmonary arterial blood with pulmonary capillary wedge blood may result in a falsely high mixed venous oxygen content. If the mixed venous blood sample is taken from the right atrium, inferior vena cava, coronary sinus, or similar sites, a falsely low or high value for arteriovenous difference may result. Also, care must be taken not to dilute the blood sample with too much heparinized saline solution.

The average error in determining oxygen consumption has been estimated to be approximately 6%.[13] The error for arteriovenous oxygen difference has been estimated at 5%.[14,15] Narrow arteriovenous oxygen differences are more prone to introduce error than wide arteriovenous oxygen differences. Thus, *the Fick oxygen method is most accurate in patients with low cardiac output*, in whom the arteriovenous oxygen difference is wide. The total error in determination of the cardiac output by the Fick oxygen method has been established to be about 10%.[16]

Does oxygen consumption actually need to be measured? To avoid the technical difficulties and expense associated with measurement of oxygen consumption, some laboratories *assume* that O_2 consumption can be predicted from the body surface area, with or without a correction for age and sex. Thus, some laboratories assume that resting O_2 consumption is 125 ml/M^2, or 110 ml/M^2 for older patients. The validity of such an assumption has been addressed in a study from the University of Texas at Dallas.[17] Cardiac output was determined by the indicator dilution technique, and O_2 consumption was calculated by dividing cardiac output by arteriovenous oxygen difference, which was measured directly. In the 108 patients studied, O_2 consumption index averaged 126 $\pm$ 26 ml/min/M^2 (mean $\pm$ standard deviation), but there was wide variability as indicated by the standard deviation, and the authors concluded that O_2 consumption varies greatly among adults at the time of cardiac catheterization. In another study from Bristol Royal Infirmary in the U.K.,[18] direct measurement of O_2 consumption was compared with assumed values in 80 patients (aged 38 to 78 years). Large discrepancies were evident, with over half the values differing by more than $\pm 10\%$, and several by $\pm 25\%$ or more. Thus, assumed values for O_2 consumption are likely to introduce considerable error.

Indicator Dilution Methods

The indicator dilution method is merely a specific application of Fick's general principle. In the Fick oxygen method, the "indicator" is oxygen, the site of injection is the lungs, and the injection procedure is that of continuous infusion. Stewart was the first to use the so-called indicator dilution method for measuring cardiac output; he used the continuous infusion technique and reported his first studies in 1897.[19]

There are two general types of indicator dilution method: the continuous infusion method and the single injection method. The single injection method is the most widely used and is discussed here in detail. The fundamental requirements for this method include the following:

1. A bolus of nontoxic indicator substance, which mixes completely with blood and whose concentration can be measured accurately, is injected.
2. The indicator substance is neither added to nor subtracted from the blood during passage between injection and sampling site.
3. Most of the indicator must pass the site of sampling before recirculation begins.
4. The indicator substance must go through a portion of the central circulation where all the blood of the body becomes mixed.

For the single-injection method, theoretical considerations may be summarized as follows. An injection of a specified amount of an indicator (I) into a proximal vessel or chamber (e.g., the vena cava or right atrium for the thermodilution method, and the pulmonary artery for the indocyanine green dye method) is

followed by continuous measurement of the indicator concentration (C) in blood as a function of time (t) at a point downstream from the injection (e.g., pulmonary artery for thermodilution technique, radial or femoral artery for indocyanine green dye method). Because all of the injection indicator, I, must pass the downstream measurement site,

$$I = \dot{Q} \int_0^\infty C(t)dt$$

where $\dot{Q}$ is the volume flow (ml/min) between the sites of injection and measurement. Thus $\dot{Q}$ (which is the cardiac output in the methods to be described) may be calculated as:

$$\dot{Q} = \frac{I}{\int_0^\infty C(t)dt}$$

Numerous indicators have been successfully used, and the history of this subject is reviewed thoroughly by Guyton.[1] Indocyanine green has enjoyed long-standing acceptance in clinical practice, although thermodilution (in which "cold" is the indicator) is now more widely used.

Indocyanine Green Method. Typically, indocyanine green solution is prepared with a concentration of 5 mg/ml, and 1.0 ml is injected on the right side of the circulation as a bolus (commonly into the pulmonary artery). Samples are taken from a peripheral systemic artery (e.g., the brachial, radial, or femoral artery). Sampling is done by continuous withdrawal of arterial blood at a constant rate (at least 15 ml/min) through a densitometer cuvette capable of measuring the concentration of indocyanine green dye in the blood. Injection must be made as a precise bolus, and the catheter through which the injection is made must be flushed immediately to ensure that the total amount of indicator has been delivered into the circulation and is not partially sitting in the catheter, stopcocks, or connecting tubing. The densitometer records a concentration curve such as that in Figure 8–7, which is calibrated by passing known concentrations of dye in blood through the densitometer cuvette.

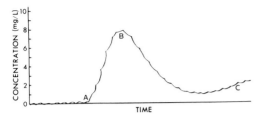

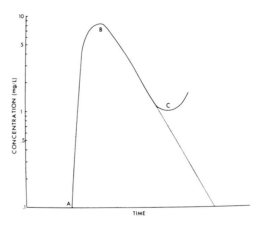

Fig. 8–7. Indicator dilution concentration curve in a patient with normal cardiac output: 1.0 ml of indocyanine green dye solution (5.0 mg/ml), was injected into the pulmonary artery at time zero. Blood was withdrawn continuously from the brachial artery through a densitometer cuvette, and the time-concentration curve from the densitometer was recorded. First appearance (A) is followed by a steep rise to peak concentration (B), and the subsequent gradual decline of the indicator curve, which is interrupted by a secondary rise (C) due to recirculation of the indicator substance.

Fig. 8–8. Replotting of the indicator-dilution curve from Figure 8–7 on semilog paper. Note that the downslope of the curve to the point of recirculation is essentially a straight line. It can be shown mathematically[20] that the true or "first pass" curve is given by such a semilogarithmic replot of the concentration curve, and by extrapolating the early linear part of the concentration decline, as illustrated here by the dotted line. See text for details.

Note the lag between injection (time zero) and the point of first appearance of green dye in the arterial blood (A), the steep rise to a peak (B), and the subsequent gradual decline of the indicator dilution curve which is interrupted by a secondary rise (C) due to recirculation of the indicator substance.

The problem of isolating data related only to the first pass of the indicator has been attacked by several investigators, but the method originally proposed by Kinsman, Moore, and Hamilton[20] is perhaps the best known. This method depends on replotting the curve on semilog paper, as shown in Figure 8–8. Note that the downslope of the curve to the point of recirculation is essentially a straight line. Kinsman et al. showed mathematically that the true or "first pass" curve will be obtained by plotting the concentration decline on a semilog scale and extrapolating the early linear part of the plot. Therefore, the dotted line of Figure 8–8 completes the true curve, which could then be replotted in Figure 8–7.

To calculate the cardiac output, we use a special application of Fick's principle: $\dot{Q} = I/(\overline{C} \times t)$, where Q is the flow rate (in this case, the cardiac output), I is the amount of indicator injected, $\overline{C}$ is the average concentration of indicator during the first pass, and t is the total duration of the curve. The product $\overline{C} \times t$ is easily measured as the area under the first pass curve, determined by planimetry. This may be

further simplified by the use of any number of available computer methods in which the semilog replotting, area computation, and cardiac output calculation are all accomplished electronically.

Practical Aspects of Indocyanine Green Dye Curves. A typical cardiac output determination may be accomplished as follows. Catheters are placed in the pulmonary artery and brachial or femoral artery, and hemodynamic measurements are recorded. The arterial catheter is connected by short stiff plastic tubing to a densitometer cuvette, which is then connected to a 30- to 50-ml syringe mounted in a constant withdrawal pump. A precise bolus of 1.0 ml of a solution containing 5.0 mg of indocyanine green/ml is loaded into the right heart catheter (if its capacity is greater than 1.5 ml, as is true for 7 Fr and 8 Fr Goodale-Lubin or Cournand catheters) and the arterial withdrawal pump is turned on. As blood passes through the densitometer cuvette (e.g., at a withdrawal rate of 20 ml/min), the densitometer is carefully adjusted until a stable zero reading is obtained. At that moment, the green dye bolus is flushed into the circulation with approximately 10 ml of heparinized saline solution. The densitometer concentration curve is recorded at a slow paper speed (e.g., 10 mm/sec) until the curve has been recorded through part or all of its recirculation phase.

The arterial blood in the withdrawal syringe may be returned to the patient if desired, using strictly aseptic precautions. Alternatively, the contents of the syringe may be used in obtaining the calibration curve after the catheterization. This is obtained by adding indocyanine green dye to the patient's blood in varying amounts and plotting the known concentration *increments* (they are not necessarily absolute concentrations because there may be some green dye in the blood used for making the calibration samples) against the densitometer deflections that result when each sample is passed through the densitometer. The slope of the resultant calibration line (D_s, which is mg green dye/L/mm deflection), the area of the first pass curve (A, which is mm deflection × sec), and the amount of injected indicator (I, which in this case was 5.0 mg) are then used to calculate cardiac output, as follows:

$$\text{Cardiac Output (L/min)} = \frac{I}{A \times D_s} \times 60 \text{ (sec/min)}$$

Sixty is inserted to convert the output from liters/second to liters/minute. As can be seen, this equation is obtained by substitution in the fundamental indicator dilution equation given earlier in this chapter.

One can see from this example that, because I and D_s are likely to be constant from patient to patient, cardiac output will be an inverse function of the area of the indicator dilution curve. Low outputs are associated with curves of large area, and high outputs are associated with curves of small area.

The indicator-dilution technique using indocyanine green dye can be carried out without right heart catheterization. A study from the University of Texas at Dallas[21] examined the reliability, advantages, and limitations of a left-sided indicator-dilution technique for measuring cardiac output in 40 patients. Indocyanine green (5 mg) was injected into the left ventricle through a pigtail catheter while blood was withdrawn from the side-port extension of the arterial sheath through which the pigtail catheter had been inserted. The results were compared with standard indicator dilution technique using indocyanine green (pulmonary artery to systemic artery) or thermodilution (right atrium to pulmonary artery). There was excellent agreement between the left-sided indicator dilution technique and standard methods, with r = 0.98 and a small standard error.

Indocyanine green dye injections are not completely benign, and severe allergic reactions have been described.[22] These reactions appear to be more common in patients with renal failure.[22]

Sources of Error. Firm adherence to certain principles and procedures helps one to obtain accurate cardiac output determinations with the indicator dilution technique. For the *indocyanine green dye technique,* these principles include:

1. The indocyanine green dye solution should be freshly prepared each day and shielded from the light until ready for use (it is unstable with time and exposure to light).

2. The indicator must be introduced into the circulation as a single bolus over as brief an injection interval as possible.

3. The exact amount of dye injected must be known, and loss of indicator in stopcocks or other parts of the injecting system should be prevented.

4. To be certain that the indicator is completely mixed with the blood, injection of indicator should be either proximal to or directly into a "mixing chamber" (ventricle).

5. The dilution curve obtained must have an exponential downslope of sufficient length to allow accurate extrapolation of the first-pass curve. Guyton suggests that it is unreasonable to use the semilog plot method for extrapolating the downslope of an indicator dilution curve if recirculation of the indicator begins before the halfway mark on the recorded downslope.[1] With severe valvular regurgitation or very low output states, the first-pass curve may be so prolonged that recirculation begins before the downslope of the primary curve has been inscribed, making accurate determination of cardiac output impossible by

this method. For this reason, the green dye technique is least accurate in low-output states, and most accurate in high-output states, in contrast to the Fick oxygen method, for which the reverse is true.

In addition to low-output states, intracardiac shunts that lead to "early recirculation" (see Chapter 12) of indicator invalidate this method of calculating cardiac output.

6. The withdrawal rate of the arterial sample must be constant. Air bubbles in the withdrawal tubing or syringe alter the rate of blood withdrawal and may result in artifactual alteration in the shape of the dilution curve. All connections, therefore, must be airtight and well flushed with saline.

Thermodilution Method. A thermal indicator method for measuring cardiac output was first introduced by Fegler[23] in 1954, but was not applied to the clinical situation until the work of Branthwaite[24] and Ganz et al.[25,26] In the initial report by Ganz et al.,[25] two thermistors were used: one in the superior vena cava at the site at which the cold dextrose solution was injected into the bloodstream, and a second "downstream" thermistor in the pulmonary artery. These two thermistors allowed accurate measurement of the temperature of the injectate (T_I) as well as the temperature of blood (T_B) downstream from the injectate. Using the basic indicator dilution equation, the cardiac output by thermodilution (CO_{TD}) in ml is given as:

$$CO_{TD} = \frac{V_I(T_B - T_I)(S_I \cdot C_I/S_B \cdot C_B)60 \ (sec/min)}{\int_0^\infty \Delta T_B(t)dt}$$

where V_I = volume of injectate (ml); S_B, S_I, C_B, and C_I are the specific gravity and specific heat of blood and injectate, respectively. When 5% dextrose is used as an indicator, ($S_I \cdot C_I/S_B \cdot C_B$) equals 1.08. Most commercially used thermodilution systems use a single thermistor only, placed at the downstream site, and assume that the temperature of the injectate (measured in a bowl before injection) increases by a predictable amount ("catheter warming") during injection. The calculated cardiac output by the thermodilution equation is multiplied

by an empiric correction factor (0.825) to correct for the catheter warming.[26,27] The thermodilution method for measuring cardiac output has several advantages over the indocyanine green dye method, and these include:

1. It does not require withdrawal of blood.
2. It does not require an arterial puncture.
3. An inert and inexpensive indicator is used.
4. There is virtually no recirculation, making computer analysis of the primary curve simple.

Sources of Error. 1. The method is unreliable in the presence of significant tricuspid regurgitation.

2. The baseline temperature of blood in the pulmonary artery usually shows distinct fluctuations associated with respiratory and cardiac cycles. If these fluctuations are large, they may approach the magnitude of the temperature change produced by the "cold" indicator injection.

3. Loss of injected indicator ("cold") between injection and measuring sites (vena cava and pulmonary artery) is not usually a problem, but in low-flow, low-output states, loss of indicator may occur because of warming of blood by the walls of the cardiac chambers and surrounding tissues. This concern is supported by the study of Grondelle et al.[28] who found that thermodilution cardiac output measurements overestimated cardiac output consistently in patients with low output (<3.5 L/min) and this overestimation was greatest, averaging 35%, in patients whose cardiac outputs were <2.5 L/min. This is what might be expected from the equation for calculation of cardiac output by thermodilution, since the change in pulmonary artery blood temperature (ΔT_B) will be reduced if cold is lost by warming of the injectate during slow passage through the vena cava, right atrium, and right ventricle. Because ΔT_B is the denominator in the equation for cardiac output calculation, reduction in ΔT_B will result in a rise in calculated cardiac output.

4. The empiric correction factor of 0.825 may be inadequate to correct for deviations in

true injectate temperature from the temperature of the injectate bowl or reservoir, due to warming in the syringe, by the hand of the individual injecting the dextrose solution from the syringe, or by catheter warming.

In general, indicator dilution cardiac output determinations have an error of 5% to 10% when performed carefully. The values obtained correlate well with those calculated by the Fick oxygen method.

REFERENCES

1. Guyton AC, Jones CE, Coleman TG: Circulatory Physiology: Cardiac Output and Its Regulation. Philadelphia, WB Saunders, 1973, pp 4–80.
2. Dexter L, et al: Effect of exercise on circulatory dynamics of normal individuals. J Appl Physiol 3:439, 1951.
3. Berkson J, Boothby WB: Studies of metabolism of normal individuals. Comparison of estimation of basal metabolism from linear formula and surface area. Am J Physiol 116:485, 1936.
4. Dubois EF: Basal Metabolism in Health and Disease. Philadelphia, Lea & Febiger, 1936.
5. Holt JP, Rhode EA, Kines H: Ventricular volumes and body weight in mammals. Am J Physiol 215:704, 1968.
6. Brandfonbrener M, Landowne M, Shock NW: Changes in cardiac output with age. Circulation 12:556, 1955.
7. Fick A: Uber die Messung des Blutquantums in den Herzventrikeln. Sitz der Physik-Med ges Wurtzberg 1870, p 16.
8. Lange RA, Dehmer GJ, Wells, PJ, et al: Limitations of the metabolic rate meter for measuring oxygen consumption and cardiac output. Am J Cardiol 64:783, 1989.
9. Van Slyke DD, Neill JM: The determination of gases in blood and other solutions by vacuum extraction and manometric measurements. J Biol Chem 61:523, 1924.
10. Bernhart FW, Skeggs L: The iron content of crystalline human hemoglobin. J Biol Chem 147:19, 1943.
11. Diem K, (ed): Documenta Geigy—Scientific Tables. 6th ed. Ardsley, NY, Geigy Pharmaceuticals, 1962, p 578.
12. Dexter L, et al: Studies of congenital heart disease. II: The pressure and oxygen content of blood in the right auricle, right ventricle, and pulmonary artery in control patients. J Clin Invest 26:554, 1947.

13. Barratt-Boyes BG, Wood EH: The oxygen saturation of blood in the venae cavae, right heart chambers, and pulmonary vessels of healthy subjects. J Lab Clin Med 50:93, 1957.
14. Selzer A, Sudrann RB: Reliability of the determination of cardiac output in man by means of the Fick principle. Circ Res 6:485, 1958.
15. Thomassen B: Cardiac output in normal subjects under standard conditions. The repeatability of measurements by the Fick method. Scand J Clin Lab Invest 9:365, 1957.
16. Visscher MB, Johnson JA: The Fick principle: analysis of potential errors in its conventional application. J Appl Physiol 5:635, 1953.
17. Dehmer GJ, Firth BG, Hillis LD: Oxygen consumption in adult patients during cardiac catheterization. Clin Cardiol 5:436, 1982.
18. Kendrick AH, West J, Papouchado M, Rozkovec A: Direct Fick cardiac output: Are assumed values of oxygen consumption acceptable? Eur Heart J 9:337, 1988.
19. Stewart GN: Researches on the circulation time and on the influences which affect it. IV: The output of the heart. J Physiol 22:159, 1897.
20. Kinsman JM, Moore JW, Hamilton WF: Human studies on the circulation. I: Injection method. Physical and mathematical considerations. Am J Physiol 89:322, 1929.
21. vandenBerg E, Pacifico A, Lange RA, Wheelan KR, Winniford MD, Hillis LD: Measurement of cardiac output without right heart catheterization: Reliability, advantages and limitations of a left-sided indicator dilution technique. Cathet Cardiovasc Diagn 12:205, 1986.
22. Benya R, Quintana J, Brundage B: Adverse reactions to indocyanine green: A case report and a review of the literature. Cathet Cardiovasc Diagn 17:231, 1989.
23. Fegler G: Measurement of cardiac output in anesthetized animals by a thermodilution method. Q J Exp Physiol 39:153, 1954.
24. Branthwaite MA, Bradley RD: Measurement of cardiac output by thermal dilution in man. J Appl Physiol 24:434, 1968.
25. Ganz W, et al: A new technique for measurement of cardiac output by thermodilution in man. Am J Cardiol 27:392, 1971.
26. Forrester JS, et al: Thermodilution cardiac output determination with a single flow-directed catheter. Am Heart J 83:306, 1972.
27. Weisel Rd, Berger RL, Hechtman HB: Measurement of cardiac output by thermodilution. N Engl J Med 292:682, 1975.
28. Grondelle AV, et al: Thermodilution method overestimates low cardiac output in humans. Am J Physiol 245 (Heart Circ Physiol 14):H690, 1983.

9

Pressure Measurement

WILLIAM GROSSMAN

The measurement of dynamic blood pressure has been of interest to physiologists and physicians since 1732, when Reverend Stephen Hales measured the blood pressure of a horse by using a vertical glass tube.[1] Methodology has advanced impressively since Reverend Hales' day, but with increased technical capability has come greater complexity of instrumentation, so that few physicians today have a firm understanding of the instruments on which they rely.

THE INPUT SIGNAL: WHAT IS A PRESSURE WAVE?

Force is transmitted through a fluid medium as a pressure wave, and an important objective of the cardiac catheterization procedure is to assess accurately the forces and therefore the pressure waves generated by various cardiac chambers. For example, a ventricular pressure wave may be considered *a complex periodic fluctuation in force per unit area,* with one cycle consisting of the time interval from the onset of one systole to the onset of the subsequent systole. The number of times the cycle occurs in one second is termed the *fundamental frequency* of cardiac pressure generation. Thus, a fundamental frequency of two corresponds to a heart rate of 120 beats/minute. Definitions of terms relevant to the theory and practice of pressure measurement are listed in Table 9–1.

Considered as a complex periodic wave form, the pressure wave may be subjected to a type of analysis developed by the French physicist Fourier, whereby any complex wave form may be considered the mathematical summation of a series of simple sine waves of differing amplitude and frequency (Fig. 9–1). Even the most complex wave form can be represented by its own Fourier series, in which the sine wave frequencies are usually expressed as *harmonics,* or multiples of the fundamental frequency. Thus, at a heart rate of 120 beats/minute, the fundamental frequency is 2 Hz and the first 5 harmonics are sine waves whose frequencies are 2, 4, 6, 8 and 10 Hz. The practical consequence of this analysis is that, to record pressure accurately, a system must respond with equal amplitude for a given input throughout the range of frequencies contained within the pressure wave. If components in a particular frequency range are either suppressed or exaggerated by the transducer system, the recorded signal will be a grossly distorted version of the original physiologic wave form. For example, the dicrotic notch of the aortic pressure wave contains frequencies above 10 cycles per second. If the pressure measurement system were unable to respond to frequencies greater than 10 cycles per second, the notch would be slurred or absent.

PRESSURE MEASURING DEVICES

The manometer used by Starling, Wiggers, and others[2] was a modification of that devised

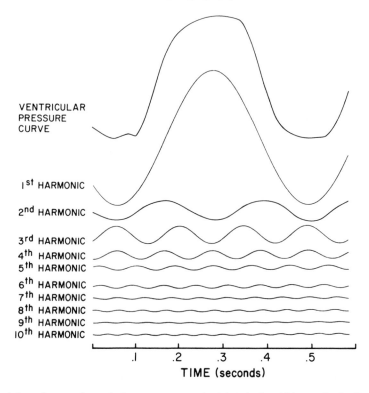

Fig. 9–1. Resolution of a normal ventricular pressure curve (top) into its first 10 harmonics by Fourier analysis. If components in a particular frequency range (e.g., the third harmonic, which in this case is 7 cycles per second) were either suppressed or exaggerated by the transducer system, the recorded signal would be a grossly distorted version of the original physiologic signal. (Adapted from Wiggers.[2])

by Hürthle[3] in 1888 and is illustrated in Figure 9–2. A rubber tambour was coupled with a writing lever that recorded change in pressure on a rotating smoked drum. The system had a high inertia and a low elasticity, giving it a narrow range of usefulness.

Sensitivity. The sensitivity of such a measurement system may be defined as the ratio of the amplitude of the recorded signal to the amplitude of the input signal. With the Hürthle manometer, the more rigid the sensing membrane, the lower the sensitivity; conversely, the more flaccid the membrane, the higher the sensitivity. This general principle applies to manometers currently employed.

Frequency Response. A second crucial property of any pressure measurement system is its frequency response. The frequency response of a pressure measurement system may be defined as the ratio of output amplitude to input amplitude over a range of frequencies of

the input pressure wave. To accurately measure pressures, the frequency response (amplitude ratio) must be constant over a sufficient range of frequency variation. Otherwise, the amplitude of major frequency components of the pressure wave form may be attenuated while minor components are amplified, so that the recorded wave form becomes a distorted caricature of the physiologic event. Referring again to the Hürthle manometer, the range of good frequency response may be improved by stiffening the membrane, or it may be narrowed by making the membrane more flaccid, because the flaccid membrane cannot respond well to higher frequencies. Thus, it should be apparent that frequency response and sensitivity are related reciprocally, and one can be obtained only by sacrificing the other.

Natural Frequency and Damping. A third important concept is the natural frequency of a sensing membrane and the way it determines

Table 9–1. *Definitions of Terms Relevant to the Theory and Practice of Pressure Measurement*

Term	Definition
Pressure wave	Complex periodic fluctuation in force per unit area. Units: *dynes/cm²*: 1 dyne/cm² = 1 microbar = 10^{-1} N/M² = 7.5×10^{-4} mmHg *mmHg:* 1 mmHg = 1 Torr = 1/760 atmospheric pressure
Fundamental frequency	Number of times the pressure wave cycles in 1 second
Harmonic	Multiple of the fundamental frequency
Fourier analysis	Resolution of any complex periodic wave into a series of single sine waves of differing frequency and amplitude
Sensitivity of pressure measurement system	Ratio of the amplitude of the recorded signal to the amplitude of the input signal
Frequency response of pressure measurement system	Ratio of output amplitude to input amplitude over a range of frequencies of the input pressure wave
Natural frequency	The frequency at which the pressure measurement system oscillates or responds when shock-excited; also, the frequency of an input pressure wave at which the ratio of output/input amplitude of an undamaged system is maximal. Units: cycles/sec, Hz
Damping	Dissipation of the energy of oscillation of a pressure measurement system, due to friction. Units: Damping coefficient, D (see text)
Optimal damping	Damping that progressively blunts the increase in output/input ratio that occurs with increasing frequency of pressure wave input. Optimal damping can maintain frequency response "flat" (output/input ratio = 1) to 88% of the natural frequency of the system
Strain gauge	Variable resistance transducer in which the strain ($\Delta L/L$) on a series of wires is determined by the pressure on the transducer's diaphragm. Over a wide range, electrical resistance (R) of the wire is directly proportional to $\Delta L/L$
Wheatstone bridge	Arrangement of electrical connections in a strain gauge such that pressure-induced changes in resistance result in proportional changes in voltage across the bridge
Balancing a transducer	Interpolating a variable resistance across the output of a Wheatstone bridge/strain gauge transducer so that atmospheric pressure at the "zero level" (e.g., midchest) induces an arbitrary voltage output on the monitor/recording device (i.e., a voltage that positions the transducer output on the oscilloscopic pressure "baseline")

the degree of damping required for optimal recording. If the sensing membrane were shock-excited (like a gong), in the absence of friction it would oscillate for an indefinite period of time in simple harmonic motion. The frequency of this motion would be the natural frequency of the system. Any means of dissipating the energy of this system, such as friction, is called *damping*. The dynamic response characteristics of such a system are largely determined by the natural frequency and the degree of damping that the system possesses.[4]

The significance of the natural frequency and importance of proper damping are illustrated in Figure 9–3. Note that the amplitude of an output signal tends to be augmented as the frequency of the input signal approaches the natural frequency of the sensing membrane.

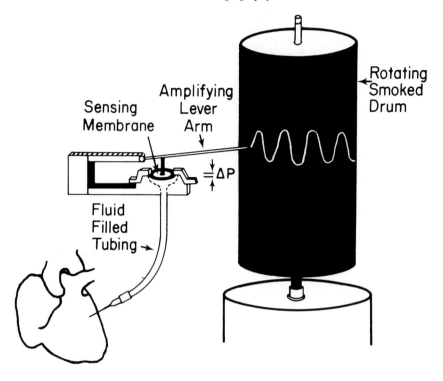

Fig. 9–2. Schematic illustration of the Hürthle manometer. A rubber tambour serves as the sensing membrane and is coupled with an amplifying lever arm that records changes in pressure (ΔP) on a rotating smoked drum. Pressure is transmitted from the heart (lower left hand corner) to the sensing membrane by fluid-filled tubing.

The physical counterpart of this augmentation of output amplitude as input frequency approaches the natural frequency is that the sensing membrane of the pressure transducer vibrates with increasing energy and violence. The same mechanism underlies the fracture of a crystal glass when an opera singer vocalizes the appropriate "input" frequency. *Damping* dissipates the energy of the oscillating sensing membrane, and optimal damping dissipates the energy gradually and thereby maintains the frequency response curve nearly flat (constant output/input ratio) as it approaches the region of the pressure measurement system's natural frequency.

As an analogy to further help the reader understand the significance of damping, consider the simple case of a weight suspended from a spring. If the weight is displaced and then released, the stretched spring will recoil so that the weight will move past its original position and then oscillate up and down. In the absence of frictional forces *(damping)*, the oscillation would continue indefinitely at a frequency determined by the stiffness of the spring and an amplitude determined by the mass of the weight. In practice there is always some damping, and this has two effects: (1) the *amplitude* of the oscillations gradually dies away, and (2) the *frequency* of oscillation is reduced. This second important consequence of damping—to reduce the natural frequency of a system—is not widely appreciated. If we continue with our analogy, imagine that the spring and its weight are suspended in a jar of syrup or honey; it will clearly vibrate with lesser amplitude of vibration *and* lesser frequency. The effect of the viscous medium is to further damp the oscillations, and if its viscosity is high enough, it will prevent any overshoot or oscillation: the weight will return to its original position regardless of its initial displacement. Further damping at this point simply slows the return of the weight to its equi-

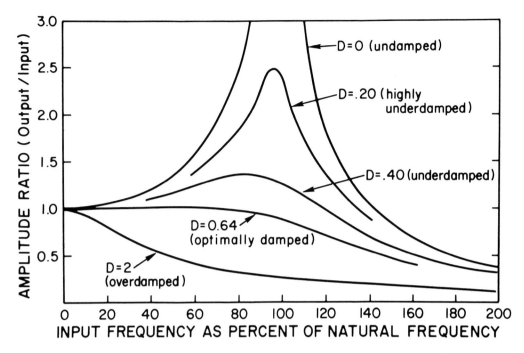

Fig. 9–3. Frequency response curves of a pressure measurement system, illustrating the importance of optimal damping. The amplitude of an input signal tends to be augmented as the frequency of that signal approaches the natural frequency of the sensing membrane. Optimal damping dissipates the energy of the oscillating sensing membrane gradually and thereby maintains a nearly flat natural frequency curve (constant output/input ratio) as it approaches the region of the pressure measurement system's natural frequency. D = damping coefficient. (See text.)

librium position, thereby depressing the frequency response characteristics of the system. Thus, damping helps to prevent overshoot artifacts resulting from resonance of the system, but at the cost of frequency response.

WHAT FREQUENCY RESPONSE IS DESIRABLE?

Wiggers suggested[2] that the shortest "significant" vibrations contained within physiologic pressure waves have one tenth the period of the entire pressure curve; that is, the essential physiologic information is contained within the first 10 harmonics of the pressure wave's Fourier series. At a heart rate of 120 beats/minute, the fundamental frequency is 2 cycles per second and the tenth harmonic is 20 cycles per second. Thus, a pressure measurement system with a frequency response range that is flat to 20 cycles per second should be adequate in such a circumstance, and sup-

port for this has come from experimental work comparing high frequency response systems with conventional catheter systems.[5]

The useful frequency response range of commonly used pressure measurement systems is generally less than 20 cycles per second unless special care is taken. Wood et al[6] and Gleason and Braunwald[7] found that frequency response was flat to less than 10 cycles per second with small-bore (6 Fr) catheters attached to standard strain gauge manometers.

To ensure a high-frequency response range, the pressure measurement system must be set up in such a way that it has the highest possible *natural frequency* as well as *optimal damping*. The natural frequency is directly proportional to the lumen radius of the catheter system. It is inversely proportional to the length of the catheter and associated tubing and to the square root of the catheter and tubing compliance and the density of fluid filling the system. The highest natural frequency will thus be obtained by using a short, wide-bore, stiff catheter connected to its transducer without intervening tubing or stopcocks and filled with a low density liquid from which small air bubbles, which increase compliance, have been excluded (e.g., boiled saline solution). Such a system may well be impractical for routine use, but it is important to bear in mind that deviation from such a system occurs only at a significant sacrifice.

If such a system is constructed, it will be found to be grossly underdamped (see Fig. 9–3). Accordingly, it will be important to introduce damping into the system to keep the frequency response flat as the frequency of the input signal approaches the natural frequency of the pressure measurement system. With optimal damping, the frequency response can be maintained flat ($\pm 5\%$) to within 88% of the natural frequency according to Fry,[4] although it is unusual to achieve more than 50% in most laboratories. Damping may be introduced by interposing a "damping needle" between the catheter and manometer[6] and gradually shortening it until optimal damping is obtained, by filling the manometer or tubing with a viscous medium, such as Renografin (a radiographic contrast agent); or by any of several other methods.

EVALUATION OF FREQUENCY RESPONSE CHARACTERISTICS

Ideally, the frequency response characteristics of a pressure measurement system should be evaluated using a sine wave pressure generator to construct curves similar to those seen in Figure 9–3. By altering the characteristics of the system discussed just previously, a reasonable compromise between frequency response, damping, and practicality can be achieved for each laboratory. Such a sine wave pressure generator has become commercially available.* An example of the use of this device in estimating frequency response of a pressure measurement system is seen in Figure 9–4.

*Millar instruments, Houston, TX.

Another method, which does not require the use of such a pressure waveform generator, is described here. This technique may be used for measuring the dynamic response characteristics of a pressure measurement system.

The catheter to be studied is connected by means of a three-way stopcock with or without intervening tubing to one arm of a strain gauge transducer (Fig. 9–5). The transducer used should be of the low-volume-displacement type (small chamber capacity) to enhance frequency response. The tip of the catheter is snugly projected through a hole in a No. 6 rubber stopper, which is tightly inserted into the cut-off barrel of a 60-ml plastic syringe.† The syringe plunger has been removed, and the barrel is fixed in a vertical position, pointing downward, so that the catheter enters from below. The manometer and catheter are filled with saline solution, care being taken to avoid even small air bubbles, and the catheter is flushed until the catheter tip and holes are submerged in approximately 30 ml of saline solution. The plunger is slowly inserted into the syringe, producing an upward deflection of the pressure trace on the recording apparatus oscilloscope. When the trace comes to rest at the top of the oscilloscope, the recorder is turned on at rapid paper speed and the plunger is suddenly withdrawn. This method, modified from Hansen,[8] produces shock excitation vibrations of the type seen in Figure 9–6. The mathematical foundation for analysis of such a shock excitation has been described by Wiggers[2] and Fry,[4] and may be summarized as follows:

The frequency of the after-vibrations produced by shock excitation is the damped natural frequency of the system. This is obtained by measuring the time, t, between two successive vibrations and obtaining the damped natural frequency, N_D as $1/t$. In the example in Figure 9–6, $N_D = 1/0.04 = 25$ cycles/sec. Next, the damping coefficient D is calculated as a function of the ratio by which successive single vibrations decrease. In Figure 9–6, this may be calculated from the ratio

†60-ml disposable plastic syringe, Monoject. Sherwood Medical Industries, Inc., DeLand, FL.

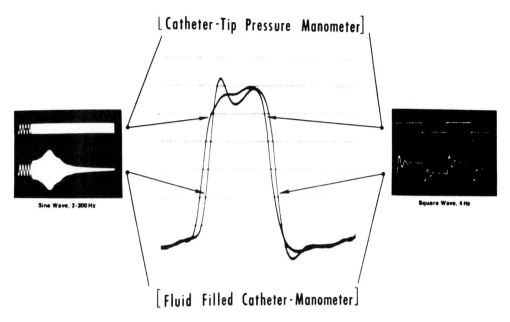

⌊Catheter-Tip Pressure Manometer⌋

⌊Fluid Filled Catheter-Manometer⌋

Sine Wave, 2-200 Hz

Square Wave, 4 Hz

Fig. 9–4. Left ventricular pressure (center panel) measured using fluid-filled standard catheter and micromanometer (catheter-tip pressure manometer) in a patient undergoing cardiac catheterization. Left- and right-hand panels show in-vitro comparisons of frequency response for micromanometer (upper) and fluid-filled (lower) systems. The left-hand panel recordings were obtained by continuously increasing the input frequency of a sine-wave pressure waveform from 2 to 200 Hz. The fluid-filled system resonates (natural frequency) at 37 Hz, but was "flat" (±5%) only to 12 Hz. Therefore its useful range is only to ~12 Hz. The right-hand panel shows the response of each system to a square wave pressure-input signal. (From Nichols et al.: Percutaneous left ventricular catheterization with an ultraminiature catheter-tip pressure transducer. Cardiovasc. Res. 12:566, 1978, with permission.)

of x_2 to x_1, the percent overshoot, as $D = \sqrt{\ln^2(x_2/x_1)/\{\pi^2 + \ln^2(x_2/x_1)\}}$, where $\ln(x_2/x_1)$ is the natural logarithm of the percent overshoot. In our example, $x_2/x_1 = 0.093$, $\ln(x_2/x_1) = -2.379$, and $D = 0.603$. From the damping coefficient D and the damped natural frequency N_D we may determine the undamped natural frequency N as $N = N_D/\sqrt{1 - D^2}$. A simple practical goal is to try to regulate the damping of an actual pressure measurement system so that its damping coefficient is as close to 0.64 (so-called "optimal" damping) as possible. At this value, the pressure measurement system shows uniform frequency response (±5%) to about 88% of its natural frequency according to Fry.[2] If such optimal damping is achieved for the system illustrated in Figure 9–6, its frequency response could be considered flat to 0.88N = 27.5 cycles per second. Improperly damped systems with a low natural frequency (because of small air bubbles, excessively compliant

tubing) may achieve uniform frequency response to less than 10 cycles per second.

TRANSFORMING PRESSURE WAVES INTO ELECTRICAL SIGNALS: THE ELECTRICAL STRAIN GAUGE

Pressure measurement systems in use today are essentially all electrical strain gauges and employ the principle of the Wheatstone bridge. The strain gauge is a variable resistance transducer whose operation depends on a simple phenomenon: when a wire is stretched, its electrical resistance increases. As long as the strain remains well below the elastic limit of the wire, there is a wide range within which the increase in resistance is accurately proportional to the increase in length.

Figure 9–7 illustrates how the Wheatstone bridge employs this principle in converting a pressure signal into an electrical signal. In this

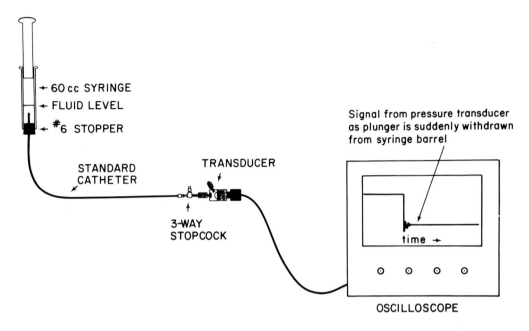

Fig. 9–5. Practical evaluation of dynamic response characteristics of catheter-transducer system. The catheter hub is connected by means of a three-way stopcock to one arm of a low-volume-displacement pressure transducer. The tip of the catheter is snugly projected through a hole in a No. 6 rubber stopper, which is tightly inserted into the cut-off barrel of a 60-ml plastic syringe. The manometer and catheter are filled with saline solution, care being taken to avoid even small air bubbles, and the catheter is flushed until the catheter tip and holes are submerged in approximately 30 ml of saline solution. Next, the plunger is slowly inserted into the syringe, producing an upward deflection of the pressure trace on the recording apparatus oscilloscope. When the pressure trace comes to rest at the top of the oscilloscope screen, the recorder is turned on and the plunger suddenly withdrawn from the syringe barrel. Dynamic response characteristics are then calculated as shown in Figure 9–6.

schematic representation of a pressure transducer, pressure is transmitted through port P and acts on diaphragm D, which is vented to atmospheric pressure on its opposite side. The manner of attachment is such that increased pressure on the diaphragm stretches and therefore increases the electrical resistance of G_1 and G_2, while having the opposite effect on G_3 and G_4. In the Wheatstone bridge, G_1, G_2, G_3, and G_4 are electrically connected, as in Figure 9–8, and are attached to a voltage source, B. If all four resistances are equal, then exactly half the voltage of battery B will exist at the junction of G_1 and G_4, and also at the junction of G_2 and G_3, and therefore no current will flow between the output terminals. However, when pressure is applied to the diaphragm in Figure 9–7, the resistances are unbalanced, so that the junction of G_1 and G_4 becomes negative, and a current will flow across the output terminals.

Since movement of the diaphragm D in Figure 9–7 is necessary to produce current flow in the Wheatstone bridge, a certain volume of fluid must actually move through the catheter and connecting tubing to produce a recorded pressure. Therefore, the use of low-volume-displacement transducers with a small chamber volume will improve frequency response characteristics of the system.

Balancing a transducer is simply a process whereby a variable resistance (the R balance of most amplifiers) is interpolated into the circuit of Figure 9–8, so that at an arbitrary baseline pressure the voltage across the output terminal can be reduced to zero. Some currently employed amplifiers use an alternating current (A-C) signal in place of the DC current source in Figure 9–8. When these "carrier current" amplifiers are employed, it becomes necessary to utilize a variable capacitor (the C balance) as well as a variable resistor in balancing the bridge.

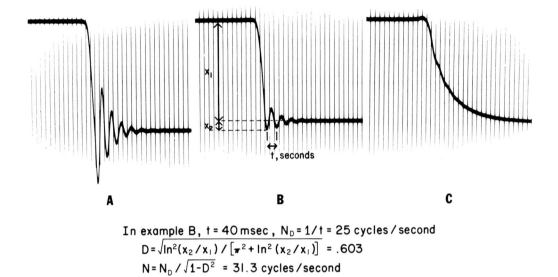

A   B   C

In example B, $t = 40$ msec, $N_D = 1/t = 25$ cycles/second

$$D = \sqrt{\ln^2(x_2/x_1) / [\pi^2 + \ln^2(x_2/x_1)]} = .603$$

$$N = N_D / \sqrt{1-D^2} = 31.3 \text{ cycles/second}$$

Fig. 9–6. Records of dynamic frequency response characteristics obtained using the system illustrated in Figure 9–5. Panels A, B, and C represent progressive increases in damping produced by introducing increasing amounts of a viscous radiographic contrast agent (Renografin-76) into the catheter-transducer system. The catheter was 80 cm long and its diameter was 8 Fr. Panel A is underdamped, Panel C overdamped, and Panel B nearly optimally damped. The percent overshoot x_2/x_1 is used in the calculation of the damping coefficient, D. The undamped natural frequency, *N,* is calculated from D and the damped natural frequency, N_D. Time lines are 20 msec. Using the curves illustrated in Figure 9–3 for various values of D, the frequency response of the system in Panel B can probably be considered flat ($\pm 5\%$) to 0.88N = 27.5 cycles per second.

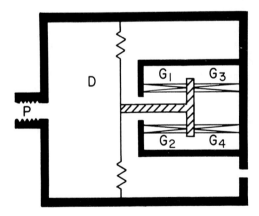

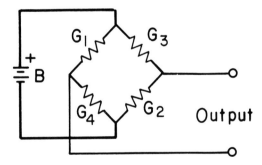

Fig. 9–7. Schematic representation of a strain-gauge pressure transducer. Pressure is transmitted through port P and acts on diaphragm D, which is vented to atmospheric pressure on its opposite side. Pressure on the diaphragm stretches and therefore increases the resistance of wires G_1 and G_2, while having the opposite effect on G_3 and G_4. The wires are electrically connected as shown in Figure 9–8.

Fig. 9–8. Strain-gauge connection of the Wheatstone bridge. In this arrangement, if all resistances are equal, then exactly half the voltage of battery B will exist at the junction of G_1 and G_4 and also at the junction of G_2 and G_3, and therefore no current will flow between the output terminals. However, when pressure is applied to the diaphragm in Figure 9–7, the resistances are unbalanced, so that the junction of G_1 and G_4 becomes negative, and a current will flow across the output terminals.

PRACTICAL PRESSURE TRANSDUCER SYSTEM FOR THE CATHETERIZATION LABORATORY

Trying to incorporate all of the principles discussed so far in this chapter, we have settled on a practical system in which a fluid-filled catheter is attached by means of a manifold to a small-volume-displacement strain-gauge type pressure transducer (Fig. 9–9).

The system illustrated is the simplest one employed in our laboratory, and is used for pressure measurement from the right heart and for arterial monitor lines. The system used for left heart pressure measurement is more complex, because it also incorporates ports for radiographic contrast and blood discard, as well as a syringe for coronary angiography (the left heart system is illustrated in Fig. 13–2, Chap. 13). We are currently using an inexpensive sterile disposable pressure transducer (Spectramed DTX Disposable Transducer), in which a tiny integrated circuit on a thin silicon diaphragm serves as the sensing element. Fluid pressure is transmitted to this element through a gel medium, bending the circuit, and altering the resistance of resistors in the silicon diaphragm. The circuit delivers an electrical output proportional to the pressure being applied, as discussed previously.

To the first sidearm of the manifold (Fig. 9–9), a fluid-filled connecting tube is attached, the distal end of which is adjusted to midchest level (zero reference). The second sidearm is connected by a fluid-filled tube to a pressurized flush bag containing heparinized saline solution. The cardiac catheter is connected directly to the front of the manifold through a built-in rotating adapter. By turning the stopcock attached to the flush solution, the catheter may be intermittently flushed clear of blood (e.g., every 3 minutes). Turning this stopcock the other way permits filling and flushing of the zero line or the pressure transducer. With this system, a frequency response flat ±5% to >20 Hz can be achieved routinely. The transducers may be sterilized with gas or Cidex between uses.

The establishment of a zero reference is an important practical undertaking that must be accomplished as a part of each catheterization procedure. As mentioned, we use midchest level as our zero reference, because fluoroscopic visualization in a lateral projection confirms that the left ventricle and aorta are generally located midway between the sternum and the table top with the patient supine. Establishment of zero reference level in our laboratory begins with measurement of the patient's antero-posterior (AP) thoracic diameter at the level of the angle of Louis. This is done using a large square chest caliper (Picker Instruments) as illustrated in Figure 9–10. The

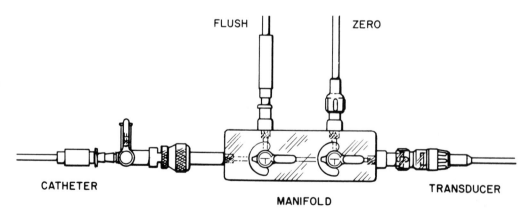

Fig. 9–9. A practical system for pressure measurement with excellent frequency response. The catheter is connected by a stopcock to a manifold, which is connected at its other end to a small volume fluid-filled pressure transducer. The manifold's two sidearms are connected by fluid-filled tubing to zero pressure level and to pressurized flush solution.

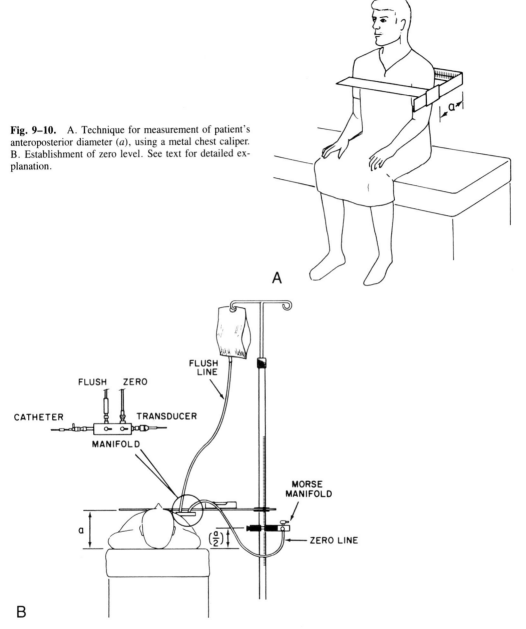

Fig. 9–10. A. Technique for measurement of patient's anteroposterior diameter (*a*), using a metal chest caliper. B. Establishment of zero level. See text for detailed explanation.

patient then lies supine on the catheterization table and is draped and otherwise prepared for catheterization (12 lead ECG is taken, skin sites are shaved and cleansed), and the zero level is established on an adjustable pole attached to the side of the table. This is accomplished using a yardstick to which a carpenter's level has been taped, placing one end of the yardstick on the patient's sternum at the angle of Louis and the other end of the yardstick against the adjustable metal pole. As illustrated in Figure 9–10, the metal pole has a centimeter-ruled tape attached to it, allowing identification of the level of midchest (one half of the patient's AP diameter below the angle of Louis). Using this technique, we set a Morse manifold (NAMIC, Medical Products Division, Hudson Falls, NY) that can be moved up and down the metal pole, at the midchest level and attach one end of the zero line (clear polyethylene tubing) to it, and the other end to the pressure measurement manifold (Fig. 9–9). The zero line, manifold, and pressure transducer are next filled with saline from the flush line, so that the pressure transducer can be connected directly with the zero line by the turn of a stopcock on the pressure manifold. The pressure transducers are calibrated by using a mercury manometer attached to a free port on the Morse manifold, with 100 mm Hg pressure transmitted through the fluid-filled zero line to all pressure transducers being used in a particular case (e.g., left heart, right heart, and arterial monitor). Otherwise, the free port of the Morse manifold is left open to air, in communication with the individual zero lines of the various left and right heart manifold systems by way of the series of stopcocks of which the Morse manifold is comprised, so referencing all of the transducer systems to a common "zero level."

PHYSIOLOGIC CHARACTERISTICS OF PRESSURE WAVEFORMS

Reflected Waves

Recognizing the normal appearance of pressure waveforms is a prerequisite to identifying abnormalities that characterize certain cardiovascular disorders. As shown in Figure 9–11, *forward* pressure and flow waves as seen in the central aorta are intrinsically identical in shape and timing. The pressure wave, however, is modified by summation with a *reflected* pressure wave ($P_{backward}$), and the resultant *measured* central aortic pressure wave shows a steady increase throughout ejection.[9,10] The flow wave is also modified by summation with a reflected flow wave ($F_{backward}$), but because flow is directional, $F_{backward}$ reduces the magnitude of flow in late ejection, giving the characteristic $F_{measured}$ as is seen with aortic flow meters or Doppler signals.

The reflections for pressure occur from many sites within the arterial tree, but the major effective reflection site in man appears to be the region of the terminal abdominal aorta.[10] As seen in Figure 9–12, ascending aortic pressure is substantially increased within 1 beat following bilateral occlusion of the femoral arteries by external manual compression (arrow, left). High-speed recordings (right panel) show that the major part of the increase in pressure occurs late in systole, consistent with an increase in the magnitude of the reflected pressure.

A variety of factors influence the magnitude of reflected waves, as listed in Table 9–2. Pressure reflections are diminished during the strain phase of the Valsalva maneuver,[9] with the result that pressure and flow waveforms become similar in appearance (Fig. 9–13). Following release of the Valsalva strain, reflected waves return and are exaggerated. Thus the commonly noted late-peaking appearance of central aortic and left ventricular pressure tracings in man (Fig. 9–14), referred to as the type A waveform pattern,[9] is a result of strong pressure reflections in late systole. In addition to the Valsalva maneuver, pressure reflections are diminished during hypovolemia, hypotension, and in response to a variety of vasodilator agents (Table 9–2). In these circumstances the left ventricular and central aortic pressure waves will exhibit a type C pattern (Fig. 9–14). On the other hand, vasoconstriction and hypertension may be expected to accentuate the normal type A waveform. Because the contribution of reflections to the arterial pressure waveform should move earlier in systole, it is not surprising that the closer one gets to the source of the reflections, the earlier the pressure peaks as the catheter is withdrawn from the central aorta to the periphery (Fig. 9–15).

Reflected waves can be of substantial magnitude, and are increased in the patient with heart failure.[11] Laskey and Kussmaul[11] showed that reflected pressure waves were increased in amplitude in 17 patients with heart failure secondary to idiopathic dilated cardiomyopathy, often producing an exaggerated dicrotic wave. The magnitude of these reflections did not decrease consistently during ex-

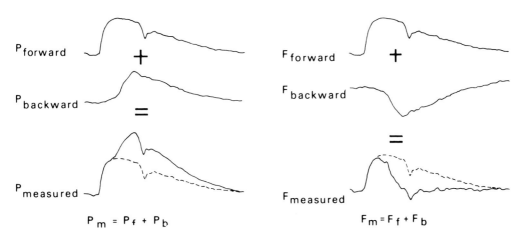

Fig. 9–11. Central aortic pressure (P) and flow (F) measured in a patient during cardiac catheterization. Computer-derived forward and backward pressure and flow components are shown individually: their sum results in the measured waves. See text for discussion. (From Murgo JP, et al., Circulation 63:122, 1981, with permission.)

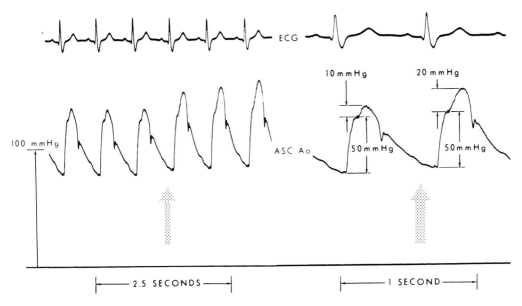

Fig. 9–12. Ascending aortic (ASC Ao) pressure waveform in a patient before and after bilateral occlusion of the femoral arteries by external manual compression (left, arrow). On the right, high speed recordings show that the major portion of the increase in pressure results from augmentation of the late (reflected) wave. (From Murgo JP, et al.: Circulation 62:105, 1980, with permission.)

ercise, as is characteristic of the normal circulation. Infusion of sodium nitroprusside intravenously markedly reduced the magnitude of the reflected pressure waves and delayed their timing; both of these changes were deemed beneficial with regard to left ventricular systolic load.[11]

Wedge Pressures. A physiologic aspect of pressure measurement that has been of interest for many years is the concept of the "wedge pressure." Broadly stated, a wedge pressure is obtained when an end-hole catheter is positioned in a "designated" blood vessel with its open end-hole facing a capillary bed, with no connecting vessel(s) conducting flow into or away from the designated blood vessel be-

Table 9–2.   *Factors That Influence the Magnitude of Reflected Waves*

1. Augment Pressure Wave Reflections:
   Vasoconstriction
   Heart failure
   Hypertension
   Aortic or iliofemoral obstruction
   Post-Valsalva release
2. Diminish Pressure Wave Reflections:
   Vasodilation
       physiologic (e.g., fever)
       pharmacologic (e.g., nitroglycerin,
       nitroprusside)
   Hypovolemia
   Hypotension
   Valsalva maneuver–strain phase

tween the catheter's tip and the capillary bed. *A true wedge pressure can be measured only in the absence of flow.* In the absence of flow, pressure equilibrates across the capillary bed so that the catheter tip pressure is equal to that on the other side of the capillary bed. If there is minimal damping between the catheter tip and the opposite side of the capillary bed (i.e., if there is a large, relatively dilated capillary bed, if the precapillary arterioles and postcapillary venules are not constricted, and if there is no other source of obstruction such as the presence of microthrombi), phasic as well as mean pressure may be transmitted to the wedged catheter. Thus, an end-hole catheter wedged in a hepatic vein may be used to measure portal venous pressure; a catheter wedged in a distal pulmonary artery will measure pulmonary venous pressure, and if it is wedged in a pulmonary vein it will measure pulmonary artery pressure. The details involved in measurement of pulmonary artery wedge pressure, commonly termed pulmonary capillary wedge pressure, are discussed in Chapter 4. Properly performed, pulmonary artery ("capillary") wedge pressure accurately measures pulmonary venous pressure. In the absence of cor triatriatum or obstruction to pulmonary venous outflow, the pulmonary venous and left atrial pressures are equal, so that pulmonary artery wedge pressure may be used as a substitute for left atrial pressure. Issues of damping and time delay need to be considered when using this pressure to assess a transmitral gradient in pa-

tients with mitral stenosis or prosthetic valve obstruction, and these issues have been addressed by Lange and co-workers.[12]

SOURCES OF ERROR AND ARTIFACT

Even when every effort has been made to design a pressure measurement system with high sensitivity, uniform frequency response, and optimal damping, distortions and inaccuracies in the pressure waveform may occur. Some of the common sources of error and artifact in clinical pressure measurement include deterioration in frequency response, catheter whip artifact, end-pressure artifact, catheter impact artifact, systolic pressure amplification in the periphery, and errors in zero level, balancing, and calibration.

Deterioration in Frequency Response. Although frequency response may be high and damping optimal during setup of the transducers, substantial deterioration in the characteristics may develop in the course of a catheterization study. Air bubbles may be introduced into the catheters, stopcocks, or tubing during the catheterization procedure, or dissolved air may come out of the saline solution used to fill the transducer (just as dissolved air may come out of solution in a glass of water allowed to stand unperturbed for a few hours). Even the smallest air bubbles have a drastic effect on pressure measurement as a result of lowering the natural frequency (by serving as an added compliance) as well as excessive damping. When the natural frequency of the pressure measurement system falls, high frequency components of the pressure waveform (such as those that occur with intraventricular pressure rise and fall) may set the system in oscillation producing the ventricular pressure "overshoot" commonly seen in early systole and diastole (Figs. 9–4 and 9–16).

Catheter Whip Artifact. Motion of the tip of the catheter within the heart and great vessels accelerates the fluid contained within the catheter, and such catheter whip artifacts may produce superimposed waves of ± 10 mmHg.

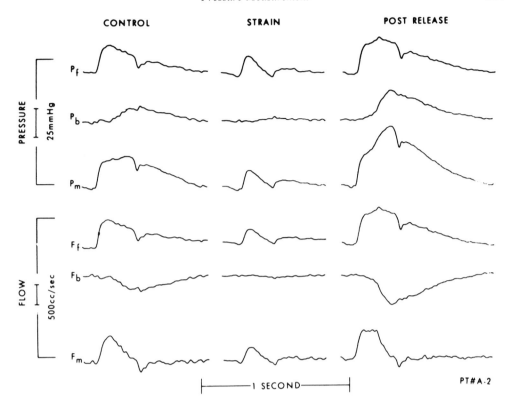

Fig. 9–13. Measurements of central aortic pressure (P_m) and flow (F_m) in a patient performing Valsalva maneuver during cardiac catheterization. Control, Valsalva strain, and post-Valsalva release tracings are shown. P_m is the sum of forward (P_f) and backward or reflected (P_b) pressure waves, and F_m is the sum of F_f and F_b. See text for discussion. (Reproduced from Murgo JP, et al.: Circulation 63:122, 1981, with permission.)

Catheter whip artifacts are particularly common in tracings from the pulmonary arteries, and are difficult to avoid.

End-Pressure Artifact. Flowing blood has a kinetic energy by virtue of its motion, and when this flow suddenly comes to a halt the kinetic energy is converted in part into pressure. Therefore, if an end-hole catheter is pointing upstream (e.g., radial or femoral arterial pressure monitoring line), it will record a pressure artifactually elevated by the converted kinetic energy. This added pressure may range from 2 to 10 mmHg.

Catheter Impact Artifact. This is similar but not identical to catheter whip artifact. When a fluid-filled catheter is ''hit'' (e.g., by valves in the act of opening or closing, or by the walls of the ventricular chambers), a pressure transient is created. Any frequency component of this transient that coincides with the natural

frequency of the catheter-manometer system will cause a superimposed oscillation on the recorded pressure wave. Catheter impact artifacts are common with pigtail catheters in the left ventricular chamber, where the terminal ''pigtail'' is often hit by the mitral valve leaflets as they open in early diastole.

Systolic Pressure Amplification in the Periphery. When radial, brachial, or femoral arterial pressures are measured and used to represent aortic pressure, it is important to recall that peak systolic pressure in these arteries may be considerably higher (e.g., by 20 to 50 mmHg) than peak systolic pressure in the central aorta (Fig. 9–17), although mean arterial pressure will be the same or slightly lower. There has been debate concerning the mechanism of this amplification of systolic pressure. McDonald[5] and Murgo[9,10] present convincing evidence that the change in waveform

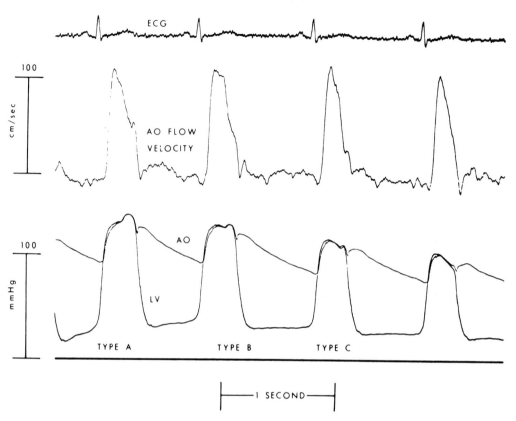

Fig. 9–14.　Left ventricular (LV) and central aortic (AO) pressure and aortic flow velocity tracings in a patient at the initiation of the strain phase of a Valsalva maneuver. See text for details. (From Murgo JP et al: Circulation 63:122, 1981, with permission.)

of arterial pressure as it travels away from the heart is largely a consequence of reflected waves. These waves, presumably reflected from the aortic bifurcation, arterial branch points, and small peripheral vessels, reinforce the peak and trough of the antegrade pressure waveform, causing amplification of the peak systolic and pulse pressures (Fig. 9–15). This phenomenon may tend to mask and distort pressure gradients across the aortic valve or left ventricular outflow tract. The transseptal technique with a second catheter in the central aorta offers one way of avoiding this problem (see Chapter 5). Giving special attention to performing careful pull-back tracings may also help the operator to avoid this particular error.

We routinely record central aortic pressure together with peripheral arterial pressure immediately before entering the left ventricle during retrograde left heart catheterization. If

this tracing shows a ''reverse gradient'' (peak systolic pressure in periphery higher than in central aorta), the amount of this pressure difference must be considered when subsequently comparing left ventricular and ''systemic arterial'' pressure for the detection of aortic or subaortic stenosis. The peripheral arterial systolic pressure may commonly appear to be 20 mmHg higher than left ventricular systolic pressure as a result of this phenomenon. This pressure amplification in the periphery is particularly marked in the radial artery (Fig. 9–17), especially if there is also some end-pressure artifact, and may mask the presence of aortic stenosis because of failure to appreciate a systolic gradient. If any doubt exists concerning the presence of a true pressure gradient, a full length catheter should be exchanged for the arterial pressure monitor and advanced to central aorta.

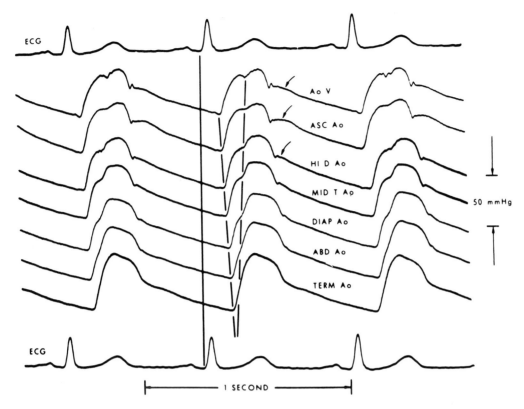

ECG

Ao V

ASC Ao

HI D Ao

MID T Ao

50 mmHg

DIAP Ao

ABD Ao

TERM Ao

ECG

├─────── 1 SECOND ───────┤

Fig. 9–15. Pressure waveforms in a patient undergoing cardiac catheterization as a function of distance from the aortic (Ao) valve (V). ASC, ascending; Hi D, high descending; MID T, midthoracic; DIAP, diaphragmatic; ABD, abdominal; TERM, just above aortic bifurcation. First vertical line marks onset of primary (forward) pressure wave, which occurs progressively later after the QRS complex with increasing distance from the aortic valve. Second vertical line marks onset of secondary pressure rise associated with the backward or reflected pressure wave. See text for discussion. (From Murgo, JP et al.: Circulation 62:105, 1980, with permission.)

Errors in Zero Level, Balancing, or Calibration. Error in the quantitation of pressures because of improper zero reference is common. As mentioned earlier, in our laboratory, the zero reference point is taken at the midchest with the patient supine, although some laboratories use 10 cm vertically up from the back or 5 cm vertically down from the sternal angle. All manometers must be zeroed at the same point (see Fig. 9–10), and the zero reference point must be changed if the patient's position is changed during the course of the study (e.g., if pillows are placed to prop him up). Transducers should be calibrated frequently against a standard mercury reference, preferably before each period of use. Electrical calibration signals and "calibration factors" should not be relied upon as a substitute for mercury calibration. Linearity of response should be checked by using mercury inputs of 25, 50, and 100 mmHg. If possible, all transducers should be exposed to the calibrating system simultaneously to avoid false "gradients" caused by unequal amplification of the same pressure signal. In our system, a bubble in the zero-reference line can give a false zero level; therefore, in tracking down an unexpected pressure gradient, flushing of the zero line is an important initial step. If the unexpected gradient persists, it is useful to switch catheter attachments between the two involved manifolds. An artifactual gradient reverses direction, whereas a real gradient persists after this maneuver.

MICROMANOMETERS

To reduce the mass and inertia of the pressure measurement system, improve the fre-

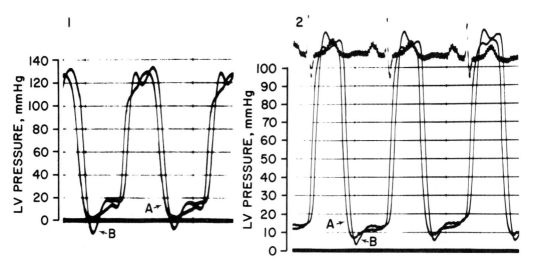

Fig. 9–16. Left ventricular (LV) pressure signals as recorded with micromanometer and a system employing long fluid-filled tubing and several interposed stopcocks between the pressure transducer and the 7F NIH catheter. The micromanometer tracing is labeled A and the fluid-filled catheter tracing is labeled B. Note both the early diastolic and early ejection phase overshoot seen with the fluid-filled catheter, indicating a poor frequency response, especially in panel 1.

quency response characteristics, and decrease artifacts associated with overdamping and catheter whip, miniaturized transducers have been developed that fit on the end of standard catheters and thus may be used as intracardiac manometers (Figs. 9–4, 9–16). Several models are commercially available, but many still have major technical shortcomings, such as fragility, electrical drift problems, temperature sensitivity, and inability to withstand the usual catheter sterilization techniques. After trying many varieties, we have settled on the Mikrotip,* which has met all the foregoing objections in our experience. Commercially available modifications of this catheter have multiple side holes and thus permit angiography and high-fidelity pressure measurement through the same catheter. A modification of this catheter has a pigtail tip. The catheter may be subjected to gas sterilization (ethylene oxide) along with other catheters and instruments, and it may be calibrated externally at room temperature because its response characteristics are not appreciably affected by temperature changes over a wide range. In our experience, it has proven remarkably stable and resistant to breakage over multiple periods

*Millar Instruments, Houston, TX.

of use. In addition, modifications are available with electromagnetic flow velocity sensors and other special capabilities for research applications. Some laboratories have used a *disposable* high-fidelity transducer catheter, and have shown that the pressures measured with these catheters are superior in waveform and accuracy to those measured with standard techniques.[13]

For accurate measurement of the rate of ventricular pressure rise (dP/dt) and other parameters of myocardial performance occurring during the first 40 to 50 msec of ventricular systole, high frequency response characteristics are necessary. Although there is some debate on this subject,[14] micromanometer-tipped catheters are generally required in patient studies when myocardial mechanics are being examined. In this regard, Gersh and co-workers have published a careful study on the physical criteria for measurement of left ventricular pressure and its first derivative.[15] They showed that pressure measurement flat to ±5% of the first 20 harmonics of the left ventricular pressure curve is required for accurate reproduction of the amplitude of maximal dP/dt. In their study, accuracy to six harmonics led to only a 20% underestimation of peak dP/dt. At a heart rate of 80 beats/min, the fundamental

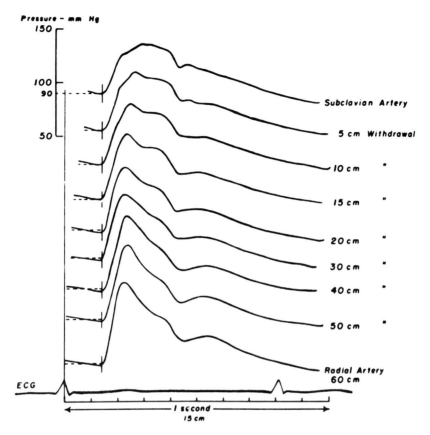

Fig. 9–17. Transformation of arterial pressure waveform with transmission to the periphery in a healthy 30-year-old man. Onset of pressures are aligned for purposes of comparison. As pulse wave moves peripherally, the upstroke steepens and increases in magnitude, giving the pressure a "spiky" appearance. Horizontal line intersecting onset of each pulse contour is calibration reference of 90 mmHg. (From Marshall, HW, et al.: Physiologic consequences of congenital heart disease. *In* Hamilton, WF, and Dow, P (eds.): Handbook of Physiology. Sect. 2. Circulation, Vol. 1. Washington, DC, American Physiological Society, 1962, p. 417.)

frequency is $80/60 = 1.33$ sec^{-1}, and the twentieth harmonic is 26.7 cycles/sec. As seen in Figure 9–6, this may be possible to achieve with a short, wide-bore catheter attached directly to the pressure transducer, with optimal damping. If the heart rate increases to 100 beats/min, however, the twentieth harmonic will now be $(100 \div 60) \times 20 = 33.3$ sec^{-1}, which exceeds the capacity for even this optimal fluid-filled system. Thus, to minimize the chance of error, we use micromanometer catheters exclusively when dP/dt is being measured. Examples of pressure recordings taken with and without micromanometer-tipped catheters may be seen in Figures 9–4 and 9–16.

REFERENCES

1. Hales S: *In* Willius FA, Keys TE (ed): Classics in Cardiology. New York, Dover Publications, 1961. pp 131–155.
2. Wiggers CJ: The Pressure Pulses in the Cardiovascular System. London, Longmans, Green and Co., 1928. pp 1–14.
3. Hürthle K: Beiträge zur Hämodynamik. Arch Ges Physiol 72:566, 1898.
4. Fry DL: Physiologic recording by modern instruments with particular reference to pressure recording. Physiol Rev 40:753, 1960.
5. McDonald DA: Blood Flow in Arteries, ed. 2. Baltimore, Williams & Wilkins, 1974.
6. Wood EH, Leusen IR, Warner HR, Wright JL: Measurement of pressures in man by cardiac catheters. Circ Res 2:294, 1954.
7. Gleason WL, Braunwald E: Studies on the first derivative of the ventricular pressure pulse in man. J Clin Invest 41:80, 1962.

8. Hansen AT: Pressure measurement in the human organism. Acta Physiol Scand 19(Suppl. 68):87, 1949–50.
9. Murgo JP, Westerhof N, Giolma JP, Altobelli SA: Manipulation of ascending aortic pressure and flow wave reflections with Valsalva maneuver: relationship to input impedance. Circulation 63:122, 1981.
10. Murgo JP, Westerhof N, Giolma JP, Altobelli SA: Aortic input impedance in normal man: relationship to pressure wave forms. Circulation 62:105, 1980.
11. Laskey WK, Kussmaul WG: Arterial wave reflection in heart failure. Circulation 75:711, 1987.
12. Lange RA, Moore DM, Jr., Cigarroa RG, Hillis LD: Use of pulmonary capillary wedge pressure to assess severity of mitral stenosis: Is true left atrial pressure needed in this condition? J Am Coll Cardiol 13:825, 1989.
13. Cha SD, Roman CF, Maranhao V: Clinical trial of the disposable transducer catheter. Cathet Cardiovasc Diagn 14:63, 1988.
14. Falsetti HL, Mates RE, Greene DG, Bunnell IL: V_{max} as an index of contractile state in man. Circulation 43:467, 1971.
15. Gersh BJ, Hahn CEW, Prys-Roberts C: Physical criteria for measurement of left ventricular pressure and its first derivative. Cardiovasc Res 5:32, 1971.

10

Clinical Measurement of Vascular Resistance and Assessment of Vasodilator Drugs

WILLIAM GROSSMAN

POISEUILLE'S LAW

In 1842, a French physician, Jean Léonard Marie Poiseuille, empirically derived a series of equations describing the flow of fluids through cylindrical tubes. Although Poiseuille was interested in blood flow, he substituted simpler liquids in his measurements of flow through rigid glass tubes.

Poiseuille's law may be stated as:

$$Q = \frac{\pi(Pi - Po)r^4}{8\eta l}$$

where:

$$
\begin{aligned}
Q &= \text{volume flow} \\
Pi - Po &= \text{inflow pressure} - \text{outflow} \\
&\quad \text{pressure} \\
r &= \text{the radius of the tube} \\
l &= \text{the length of the tube} \\
\eta &= \text{viscosity of the fluid}
\end{aligned}
$$

This relationship is applicable in the specific circumstance of steady state laminar flow of a homogeneous fluid through a rigid tube. Under these conditions, flow, Q, varies directly as

Note: Some material in this chapter has been retained from the first and second editions, to which Dr. L. P. McLaurin had contributed.

the pressure difference, Pi − Po, and the *fourth power* of the tube's radius, r. It varies inversely as the length, l, of the tube and the viscosity, η, of the fluid.

Hydraulic resistance, R, is defined by analogy to Ohm's law as the ratio of mean pressure drop, ΔP, to flow, Q, across the vascular circuit. The various factors contributing to vascular resistance can be illustrated by rearranging Poiseuille's law as follows:

$$R = \frac{Pi - Po}{Q} = \frac{8\eta l}{\pi r^4}$$

It is apparent from this equation that, in the condition of steady laminar flow of a homogeneous fluid through a rigid cylindrical tube, resistance to flow depends only on the dimensions of the tube and the viscosity of the fluid. In particular, the resistance is remarkably sensitive to changes in the radius of the tube, varying inversely with its fourth power.

VASCULAR RESISTANCE AND PRESSURE-FLOW RELATIONSHIPS

The applicability of laws derived from steady-state fluid mechanics in assessing vas-

143

cular resistance is somewhat ambiguous because blood flow is pulsatile, blood is a non-homogeneous fluid, and the vascular bed is a nonlinear, elastic, frequency-dependent system. In such a system, resistance varies continuously with pressure and flow and is influenced by many factors, such as inertia, reflected waves, and the phase angle between pulse and flow wave velocities.[1,2]

To assess both vessel caliber and elasticity, the resistive and compliant characteristics of the vascular system, the concept of *vascular impedance* has been used.[2] Vascular impedance has been defined as the instantaneous ratio of pulsatile pressure to pulsatile flow.[3,4] Because impedance may not be the same for all frequencies, its calculation requires resolution of the harmonic components of both pressure and flow pulsations. The *impedance modulus* so calculated is then expressed as a spectrum of impedance versus frequency.

As a consequence of the foregoing considerations and the many active and passive factors that influence pressure and flow in blood vessels, the concept of vascular resistance in its pure physical sense is limited in application. In the context of the clinical and physiologic setting, however, vascular resistance derived from hemodynamic measurements made during cardiac catheterization has acquired empiric pathophysiologic meaning and is often an important factor in clinical decision-making.

ESTIMATION OF VASCULAR RESISTANCE

Calculations of *vascular resistance* are usually applied to both the pulmonary and systemic circulations. Although many authors refer to systemic or pulmonary *arteriolar* resistances, I prefer the term *vascular* resistance because it is less committal concerning the anatomic site of the resistance. As will be discussed, arteriolar tone is only one determinant of vascular resistance to blood flow. To estimate pulmonary and systemic vascular resistances quantitatively, knowledge of both the pressure differential across the pulmonary and systemic circuits and the respective blood flow through them is required.

The formulae generally used are:

1. **Systemic Vascular Resistance** $= \dfrac{\overline{Ao} - \overline{RA}}{Q_s}$

2. **Total Pulmonary Resistance** $= \dfrac{\overline{PA}}{Q_p}$

3. **Pulmonary Vascular Resistance**

$$= \dfrac{\overline{PA} - \overline{LA}}{Q_p}$$

where: $\overline{Ao}$ = mean systemic arterial pressure, $\overline{RA}$ = mean right atrial pressure, $\overline{PA}$ = mean pulmonary arterial pressure, $\overline{LA}$ = mean left atrial pressure, Q_s = systemic blood flow, Q_p = pulmonary blood flow.

In many laboratories, the mean pulmonary capillary wedge pressure is used as an approximation of mean left atrial pressure. This should cause no problem because there is ample evidence that pulmonary capillary wedge pressure, properly obtained, closely approximates the level of left atrial pressure.[5–7] The flows are *volume* flows (as opposed to velocity flows), and are expressed in liters/minute, and pressures are in millimeters of mercury (mmHg). These equations yield resistance in arbitrary resistance units (R units) expressed in mmHg/(L/min), also called "hybrid units." These units are sometimes referred to as Wood units, since they were first introduced by Dr. Paul Wood. They may be converted to metric resistance units expressed in dynes-seconds-cm^{-5} by use of the conversion factor 80. In this system resistance is expressed as:

Resistance:

$$= \dfrac{\Delta P(\text{mmHg}) \times 1332 \text{ dynes/cm}^2/\text{mmHg}}{Q_s \text{ or } Q_p \text{ (L/min)} \times 1000 \text{ ml/L} \div 60 \text{ sec/min}}$$

$$= \dfrac{\Delta P}{Q_s \text{ or } Q_p} \times 80$$

$$= \text{dynes-sec-cm}^{-5}$$

There is no particular advantage to either system, since both express precisely the same ratio. Most pediatric cardiologists use hybrid units, whereas cardiologists with adult practices generally use metric units.

In pediatric practice it is conventional to normalize vascular resistances for body surface area (BSA), thus giving a resistance index. Although this is not commonly done in adult cardiac catheterization laboratories, the practice makes sense because normal cardiac output and therefore vascular resistance may be substantially different in a 260-pound man as compared to a 110-pound woman. The normalized resistance, however, is *not* obtained by dividing resistance as calculated in equations 1 to 3 by body surface area. Rather, normalized resistance is calculated by substituting blood flow index for blood flow in the resistance formula. Thus systemic vascular resistance index (SVRI) is calculated as

$$SVRI = (\overline{Ao} - \overline{RA})80/CI$$

where CI is the cardiac (or systemic blood flow) index. Therefore, *SVRI equals SVR multiplied by BSA.*

Cardiac output, usually measured by either the Fick or the thermal dilution method, is used as mean blood flow. It is important to realize that in conditions of intracardiac shunts or shunts between the pulmonary and systemic circulations, *pulmonary blood flow and systemic flow may not be equal,* and the respective flow through each circuit must be measured and used in the appropriate resistance calculation.

Normal values for vascular resistance in adults are given in Table 10–1.

CLINICAL USE OF VASCULAR RESISTANCE

As can be deduced from the Poiseuille equation, changes in systemic or pulmonary vascular resistance theoretically may result from one of three mechanisms. Because changes in *length* of the vascular beds are uncommon after growth has been completed, changes in vascular resistance reflect either altered *viscosity* of blood or a change in cross-sectional area *(radius)* of the vascular bed.

There is ample evidence that changes in blood viscosity alter measured vascular resistances. Nihill[8] has shown an approximate doubling of pulmonary vascular resistance with increases in hematocrit from 43% to 64%. Similarly, low values for measured vascular resistance are commonly seen in patients with severe chronic anemia, although the low vascular resistance in such cases probably represents more than a viscosity effect alone.

With regard to changes in cross-sectional area of the pulmonary or systemic vascular bed, such changes *do not invariably imply altered arteriolar tone.* In the normal systemic circulation, mean aortic pressure may be 100 mmHg, whereas right atrial pressure is only 5 mmHg. Although the greatest part of this pressure drop occurs at the arteriolar level (approximately 60%), about 15% occurs in the capillaries, 15% in small veins, and 10% in the arterial system proximal to the arterioles.[2] Thus, although systemic vascular resistance is dominated by the caliber of the arterioles, the other components of the systemic vascular bed are by no means negligible. For example, Read and co-workers[9] studied systemic vascular resistance in dogs with constant (pump-con-

Table 10–1. *Normal Values for Vascular Resistance*

Systemic Vascular Resistance	1170 ± 270 dynes-sec-cm^{-5}
Systemic Vascular Resistance Index	2130 ± 450 dynes-sec-cm$^{-5} \cdot M^2$
Pulmonary Vascular Resistance	67 ± 30 dynes-sec-cm^{-5}
Pulmonary Vascular Resistance Index	123 ± 54 dynes-sec-cm$^{-5} \cdot M^2$

Values are expressed as mean ± standard deviation, and are derived from 37 subjects without demonstrable cardiovascular disease (17 males, 20 females age 47 ± 9 years) who underwent diagnostic cardiac catheterization at the Peter Bent Brigham Hospital between July 1, 1975, and June 30, 1978.

trolled) cardiac output, and found that a rise in venous pressure consistently caused a fall in resistance. The magnitude of the fall was proportional to the increment in venous pressure rise and was about 20% for an increase in venous pressure of 20 mmHg. Other studies show no change in resistance when arterial pressure is so manipulated (in the absence of baroreceptor control). These findings have been interpreted by McDonald[2] to suggest that the decline in systemic vascular resistance with increased venous pressure results from dilation of small venous channels, whereas systemic arterioles do not distend passively with increased pressure. Therefore, measurement of vascular resistance is not a precise tool for assessing the dynamics of individual sections of the vascular bed.

The minute-to-minute control of vascular resistance, at least in the systemic bed, is an amalgam of autonomic nervous system influences and local metabolic factors. Hypotension or reduced cardiac output generally triggers increased systemic resistance by means of the baroreceptors, alpha-adrenergic neural pathways, and the release of humoral vasoconstrictor hormones, but these influences may be opposed by metabolic factors if the hypotension or low cardiac output results in decreased tissue perfusion with local hypoxia and acidosis. This latter circumstance is commonly seen in congestive heart failure or shock.

Knowledge of changes in systemic vascular resistance is also important in evaluating the hemodynamic response to stress tests, such as dynamic or isometric exercise.[10] In this regard, there is ample evidence that systemic vascular resistance normally falls in response to dynamic exercise, but pulmonary vascular resistance is unchanged (at least with supine bicycle exercise). Transient elevations in systemic vascular resistance have been provoked by infusions of vasopressor drugs in an effort to evaluate the left ventricular response to a sudden increase in afterload.[11] Such tests often provide useful information regarding left ventricular performance and reserve.

Low systemic vascular resistance may be seen in conditions in which blood flow is in-appropriately increased, such as arteriovenous fistula, severe anemia, and other high-output states. It is important to realize that in these circumstances there may well be regional differences in vascular resistance, and calculations based on mean pressure and flow in the entire systemic circulation may lead to inaccurate conclusions.

Total Pulmonary Resistance. Calculated as the ratio of mean pulmonary artery pressure to pulmonary blood flow, total pulmonary resistance expresses the resistance to flow in transporting a volume of blood from the pulmonary artery to the left ventricle in diastole, neglecting left ventricular diastolic pressure. This relationship is obviously influenced by alterations in left atrial pressure and will not consistently provide useful information about the condition of the pulmonary vasculature. Although widely used 25 years ago, it is rarely used today.

Pulmonary Vascular Resistance. Sometimes called pulmonary arteriolar resistance, pulmonary vascular resistance expresses the pressure drop across the major pulmonary vessels, the precapillary arterioles, and the pulmonary capillary bed, and is more precise in assessing the presence and degree of pulmonary vascular disease than is total pulmonary resistance. Simple calculation of pulmonary vascular resistance provides general information about the pulmonary circulation, but this must be interpreted in the context of the clinical situation and other hemodynamic data obtained during cardiac catheterization. The pulmonary vasculature is a dynamic system and is subject to many mechanical, neural, and biochemical influences. Some of these factors are listed in Table 10–2.

Several investigators have taken advantage of this responsiveness of the pulmonary circulation to various manipulations in the hope of assessing the reversibility of pulmonary hypertension. Oxygen inhalation,[12] infusions of acetylcholine,[13] and infusions of tolazoline[14] have all been used in attempts to relieve whatever reflex pulmonary vasoconstriction may be present.

The tolazoline test is generally performed

Table 10–2. *Factors That May be Related to Rapid, Transient Changes in Pulmonary Vascular Resistance*

I. Mechanical
  A. Changes in pulmonary venous pressure
  B. Changes in pulmonary blood flow
  C. Changes in pulmonary blood volume
  D. Changes in alveolar pressures
  E. Changes in intrathoracic pressure
  F. Pericapillary edema
  G. Changes in size of pulmonary vascular bed
II. Neural
  A. Autonomic nervous system
  B. Intravascular chemoreceptors
  C. Intravascular mechanoreceptors
  D. Changes in neuroregulation of ventilation
III. Biochemical and Hormonal
  A. Changes in oxygen tension
  B. Acute hypercapnia
  C. Acute acidosis
  D. Catecholamines (esp. isoproterenol)
  E. Acetylcholine
  F. Tolazoline
  G. Serotonin
  H. Histamine
  I. Prostaglandins

in the following manner.[14,15] After a complete set of baseline data including pulmonary blood flow, pulmonary artery and pulmonary artery wedge pressures are measured, 1.0 mg/kg of tolazoline is infused over a one-minute period into the pulmonary artery. Patients frequently experience a sense of warmth accompanied by cutaneous flushing soon after injection. This rapidly passes and the pulmonary arterial and systemic arterial pressures are monitored at 1-minute intervals. After 10 minutes, pulmonary blood flow and pulmonary artery and pulmonary artery wedge pressures are again determined.

Using this test, Brammel and his associates identified a small number of patients with the Eisenmenger syndrome and high pulmonary resistance who had a drop in total pulmonary resistance to less than 450 dynes-sec-cm^{-5} m^2 in response to tolazoline.[15] Postoperative cardiac catheterization confirmed a substantial drop in pulmonary resistance and pulmonary artery pressure. These patients were considered to be "pulmonary vascular hyperreac-

tors" who respond to increased pulmonary blood flow with pulmonary vasoconstriction. When pulmonary hypertension has been present for many years, permanent obliterative changes in the pulmonary vasculature occur, and reactive vasoconstriction is less significant. For this reason, the tolazoline test has its widest application in young children, and has less value in assessing adults with pulmonary hypertension.

The value of oxygen inhalation in assessing pulmonary vascular reactivity is substantial. Any patient with high pulmonary vascular resistance (i.e., ≥ 600 dynes-sec-cm^{-5}) in association with a central shunt (e.g., ventricular septal defect) should be given 100% oxygen by face mask before concluding that the changes are fixed. Older patients with a combination of left heart failure and chronic obstructive lung disease may have considerable pulmonary vasoconstriction due to alveolar hypoventilation and its resultant hypoxia. Inhalation of 100% oxygen in such cases may result in a dramatic fall in pulmonary arterial pressure and vascular resistance.

Pulmonary Vascular Disease in Patients with Congenital Central Shunts. The decision as to whether or not a patient with congenital heart disease would profit from corrective surgery often hinges on the pulmonary vascular resistance. Although each case must be evaluated on its own characteristics, many criteria for operability have been proposed.[16,17] It has been suggested that the ratio between pulmonary vascular resistance and systemic vascular resistance (resistance ratio PVR/SVR) be used as a criteria for operability in dealing with congenital heart disease.[16] Normally this ratio is ≤ 0.25. Values of 0.25 to 0.50 indicate moderate pulmonary vascular disease, and values greater than 0.75 indicate severe pulmonary vascular disease. When the PVR/SVR resistance ratio equals 1.0 or more, surgical correction of the congenital defect is considered contraindicated because of the severity of the pulmonary vascular disease.

We have been impressed with the clinical value of the resistance ratio. It has the value of factoring in miscellaneous neural, hormonal and blood viscosity influences that may be affecting *both* pulmonary and systemic vascular beds, and which may be primarily related to the patient's immediate clinical status rather than to intrinsic pulmonary vascular changes. Many patients with left ventricular failure and low systemic output (from any cause) have associated high systemic and pulmonary vascular resistance, but the resistance ratio will be normal in the absence of intrinsic vascular pathology.

We have reported[16] three patients with congenital heart disease (two with atrial septal defect and one with patent ductus arteriosus) having cyanosis and pulmonary arterial hypertension at nearly systemic levels. Each patient had progressive improvement in pulmonary vascular resistance toward normal following operative closure of the shunts. These cases illustrate the importance of increased blood viscosity associated with the polycythemia of cyanosis (hematocrits in the 56 to 66% range), which may contribute substantially to the measured increase in pulmonary and systemic vascular resistances. This influence, as well as the generalized vasoconstriction often seen in patients with advanced cardiac disease, will be factored out by the ratio of PVR/SVR. Each of our patients[16] had PVR/SVR ratios of less than 0.50 and net left-to-right shunts despite severe pulmonary hypertension (e.g., pulmonary artery pressure 110/55 mmHg).

In his classic description of the Eisenmenger syndrome, Wood pointed out that attempted surgical repair of the shunt defect was a major source of death in these patients.[17] He stated that in patients with pulmonary blood flow less than 1.75 times systemic flow or with total pulmonary vascular resistance greater than 12 Wood or "hybrid" units (960 dynes-sec-cm^{-5}), ordinary surgical repair of the defect should not be attempted. Others have suggested similar criteria for special instances or conditions. Briefly summarized, it can be stated that surgical repair should be limited to patients in whom the net shunt is left to right and the total pulmonary vascular resistance is less than systemic vascular resistance, preferably with a resistance ratio of less than 0.50.

Pulmonary Vascular Disease in Patients with Mitral Stenosis. Marked elevations in pulmonary vascular resistance may also be seen in acquired heart disease, notably in mitral stenosis. The effect of mitral valve replacement in patients with mitral stenosis and/or regurgitation associated with pulmonary hypertension has been evaluated.[18,19] Most patients experience significant reduction in pulmonary vascular resistance following successful repair of the mitral valve lesion. Although some degree of pulmonary hypertension may persist postoperatively, significant palliative benefit usually occurs, and the decision regarding surgery must be made in light of information regarding left and right ventricular function as well as the degree of pulmonary hypertension.

Recently, percutaneous balloon mitral valvuloplasty has been used as an alternative to surgery for treating patients with advanced mitral stenosis.[20–24] The procedure results in an immediate improvement in mitral valve area and in pulmonary hypertension.[25] Its effects on pulmonary vascular resistance have been studied by our group in a cohort of 14 patients with critical mitral stenosis and severe pulmonary hypertension. Balloon mitral valvuloplasty resulted in an immediate improvement in mitral valve area (0.7 ± 0.2 cm^2 to 1.6 ± 0.7 cm^2, $p < 0.01$), mean left atrial pressure (26 ± 6 mmHg to 15 ± 5 mmHg, $p < 0.01$), mean pulmonary artery pressure (51 ± 17 mmHg to 40 ± 14 mmHg), and pulmonary vascular resistance (630 ± 570 dynes-sec-cm^{-5} to 447 ± 324 dynes-sec-cm^{-5}, $p < 0.01$). At an average of 7 months followup (Fig. 10–1), repeat catheterization showed that pulmonary vascular resistance had declined further and now averaged 280 ± 183 dynes-sec-cm^{-5}. Of note, two patients who showed substantial restenosis to mitral valve areas of less than 1.0 cm^2 exhibited a return of pulmonary vascular resistance to pre-valvuloplasty values.[25] The decline in pulmonary vascular resistance after balloon valvuloplasty is not offset by the bronchopulmonary stresses

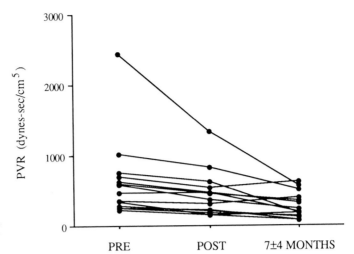

Fig. 10–1. Pulmonary vascular resistance before (PRE), immediately after (POST), and at an average of 7 months follow-up in 14 patients with mitral stenosis and severe pulmonary hypertension undergoing balloon valvuloplasty. See text for details. Data adapted from Levine et al (Circulation 79:1061, 1989) with permission.

associated with thoracotomy and general anesthesia, making mitral balloon valvuloplasty appealing as either an alternative to surgery or as a preparatory procedure before surgery in patients with mitral stenosis and advanced pulmonary hypertension.

ASSESSMENT OF VASODILATOR DRUGS

Cardiac catheterization provides an ideal opportunity for assessing the potential response of a patient to a change in medical regimen, particularly with regard to vasodilator drugs. In recent years, vasodilator drugs have assumed a major role in the treatment of patients with congestive heart failure. There is, however, great variability among currently used vasodilator agents and the relative effects of a particular drug on resistance and capacitance vessels is of major importance in predicting its hemodynamic effects.[26] This problem may become complex in the circumstance in which a particular drug may have different effects depending on the level of resting tone in resistance and capacitance beds. For example, nitrate preparations are well known to influence venous capacitance; this is presumably responsible (at least in part) for the fact that ventricular filling pressures and pulmonary congestion are consistently improved when nitrate therapy is given to patients with congestive heart failure. Despite this consistent effect

on preload, the effect of nitrates on forward cardiac output has been variable,[27–29] and studies have reported decreases, increases, or mixed effects on cardiac output in normal subjects and in patients with heart failure. Goldberg et al.[30] studied 15 patients with chronic congestive heart failure who were given an oral nitrate (erithrityl tetranitrate) at the time of cardiac catheterization to identify predictors of nitrate effect on cardiac output. There were significant reductions in right atrial, pulmonary capillary wedge, and mean arterial pressure in nearly all patients. Augmentation in cardiac output by $\geq 10\%$ occurred in 8 patients (thereby defined as "responders"), but no change or decline occurred in 7 patients ("nonresponders"). The level of peripheral vasoconstriction, as reflected by resting systemic vascular resistance, was significantly higher for the "responders" than for the "nonresponders" (2602 ± 251 versus 1744 ± 193 dynes-sec-cm^{-5}, $p < .02$). Furthermore, a significant reduction in systemic vascular resistance occurred only in "responders," and the decline was a linear function of resting resistance (Fig. 10–2).

Thus, although reductions in arterial pressure and left and right ventricular filling pressures are a constant result of nitrate therapy, significant augmentation in forward cardiac output is likely only in patients with the most intense resting peripheral vasoconstriction. The design of a catheterization protocol in a

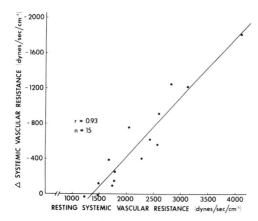

Fig. 10–2. The change (Δ) in systemic vascular resistance following administration of erythrityl tetranitrate plotted as a function of resting systemic vascular resistance in 15 patients with congestive heart failure. Patients with the greatest degree of vasoconstriction at rest demonstrated the greatest fall in resistance in response to the nitrate. (From Goldberg et al: Nitrate therapy of heart failure in valvular heart disease. Am J Med 65:161, 1978.)

sures and systemic vascular resistance are normal, vasodilator drugs will probably do more harm than good, and a therapeutic trial of preload elevation (administration of colloid) with or without an inotropic agent could be tested during the catheterization.

These examples are presented merely to illustrate the principle of using cardiac catheterization parameters (i.e., resistances, flows, and filling pressures) to design a therapeutic regimen and then, while the catheters are still in place, put it to the test. We have found this most useful with regard to the patient with heart failure, and we feel strongly that cardiac catheterization in such patients must include full right and left heart catheterization with measurement of cardiac output, left and right heart pressures, and systemic and pulmonary vascular resistances.

patient with congestive heart failure can include assessment of vasodilator therapy based on these principles. For example, if the resting cardiac output is low and if right and left ventricular filling pressures as well as systemic vascular resistance are high, a long-acting nitrate or a balanced agent (e.g., an angiotensin-converting-enzyme inhibitor) might be expected to be particularly beneficial, and can be tested while the catheters are still in place. Alternatively, if the output is low, resistance is high, but filling pressures are near normal, a nitrate might not help because the lowered resistance may be offset by the fall of the already normal preload, with the result being no increase in output. In such a patient, a selective lowering of resistance would be desirable, and hydralazine could be tested before removing the catheters. If the cardiac output is low but resistance is normal, nitrate or converting-enzyme inhibitor most likely will not increase output, and should be tested only if filling pressures are high and symptoms of congestion are a prominent part of the clinical picture. In such patients, the combination of an inotropic agent and a nitrate may be particularly helpful and could be tested at the time of catheterization. Finally, if the output is low, but filling pres-

REFERENCES

1. O'Rourke MF: Arterial Function in Health and Disease. Edinburgh, Churchill Livingstone, 1982.
2. McDonald DA: Blood Flow in Arteries, 2nd ed. Baltimore, Williams & Wilkins, 1974.
3. Milnor WR: Hemodynamics, 2nd ed. Baltimore, Williams & Wilkins, 1989.
4. Murgo JP, Westerhof N, Giolma JP, Altobelli SA: Aortic input impedance in normal man: Relationship to pressure wave forms. Circulation 62:105, 1980.
5. Connolly DC, Kirklin JW, Wood CH: The relationship between pulmonary artery pressure and left atrial pressure in man. Circ Res 2:434, 1954.
6. Rapaport E, Dexter L: Pulmonary "capillary" pressure. Meth Med Res 7:85, 1958.
7. Lange RA, Moore DM Jr, Cigarroa RG, Hillis LD: Use of pulmonary capillary wedge pressure to assess severity of mitral stenosis: Is true left atrial pressure needed in this condition? J Am Coll Cardiol 13:825, 1989.
8. Nihill MR, McNamara DG, Vick RL: The effects of increased blood viscosity on pulmonary vascular resistance. Am Heart J 92:65, 1976.
9. Read RC, Kuida H, Johnson JA: Venous pressure and total peripheral resistance in the dog. Am J Physiol 192:609, 1958.
10. Grossman W, et al: Changes in inotropic state of the left ventricle during isometric exercise. Br Heart J 35:697, 1973.
11. Ross J Jr, Braunwald E: The study of left ventricular function in man by increasing resistance to ventricular ejection with angiotensin. Circulation 29:739, 1964.
12. Fishman AP: Respiratory gases in the regulation of the pulmonary circulation. Physiol Rev 41:214, 1961.
13. Wood P, Besterman EM, Towers MK, McIlroy MB: The effect of acetylcholine on pulmonary vascular

resistance and left atrial pressure in mitral stenosis. Br Heart J 19:279, 1957.

14. Grover RF, Reeves JT, and Blount SG Jr: Tolazoline hydrochloride (Priscoline): An effective pulmonary vasodilator. Am Heart J 61:5, 1961.

15. Brammel HL, Vogel JHK, Pryor R, Blount SG Jr: The Eisenmenger syndrome. Am J Cardiol 28:679, 1971.

16. DiSesa VJ, Cohn LH, Grossman W: Management of adults with congenital bidirectional shunts, cyanosis, and pulmonary vascular obstruction: successful operative repair in 3 patients. Am J Cardiol 51:1495, 1983.

17. Wood P: The Eisenmenger syndrome or pulmonary hypertension with reversal central shunt. Br Med J 2:701, 1958.

18. Braunwald E, Braunwald NS, Ross J Jr, Morrow AG: Effects of mitral-valve replacement on the pulmonary vascular dynamics of patients with pulmonary hypertension. N Engl J Med 273:509, 1965.

19. Dalen JE et al: Early reduction of pulmonary vascular resistance after mitral valve replacement. N Engl J Med 277:387, 1967.

20. McKay RG, Lock JE, Keane JF, Safian RP, Aroesty JM, Grossman W: Percutaneous mitral valvuloplasty in an adult patient with calcific rheumatic mitral stenosis. J Am Coll Cardiol 7:1410, 1986.

21. McKay RG, Lock JE, Safian RD, Come PC, Diver DJ, Baim DS, Berman AD, Warren SE, Mandell VE, Royal AD, Grossman W: Balloon dilatation of mitral stenosis in adult patients: postmortem and percutaneous mitral valvuloplasty studies. J Am Coll Cardiol 9:723, 1987.

22. Lock JE, Khalilullah M, Shrivasta S, Bahl V, Keane JF: Percutaneous catheter commissurotomy in rheumatic mitral stenosis. N Engl J Med 313:1515, 1985.

23. Palacios IF, Lock JE, Keane JF, Block PC: Percutaneous transvenous balloon valvotomy in a patient with severe calcific mitral stenosis. J Am Coll Cardiol 7:1416, 1986.

24. Al Zaibag M, Ribeiro PA, Kasab S, Al Fagih MR: Percutaneous double balloon mitral valvotomy for rheumatic mitral valve stenosis. Lancet 1:757, 1986.

25. Levine MJ, Weinstein JS, Diver DJ, Berman AD, Wyman RM, Cunningham MJ, Safian RD, Grossman W, McKay RG: Progressive improvement in pulmonary vascular resistance following percutaneous mitral valvuloplasty. Circulation 79:1061, 1989.

26. Braunwald E, Colucci WS: Vasodilator therapy of heart failure. Has the promissory note been paid? N Engl J Med 310:459, 1984.

27. Ferrer MI et al: Some effects of nitroglycerin upon the splanchnic, pulmonary and systemic circulations. Circulation 33:357, 1966.

28. Williams JF, Glick G, Braunwald E: Studies on cardiac dimensions in intact unanesthetized man V. Effects of nitroglycerin. Circulation 32:767, 1965.

29. Gold HK, Leinbach RC, Sanders CA: Use of sublingual nitroglycerin in congestive failure following acute myocardial infarction. Circulation 46:389, 1972.

30. Goldberg S, Mann T, Grossman W: Nitrate therapy of heart failure in valvular heart disease: importance of resting level of peripheral vascular resistance in determining cardiac output response. Am J Med 65:161, 1978.

11

Calculation of Stenotic Valve Orifice Area

BLASE A. CARABELLO and WILLIAM GROSSMAN

T he normal cardiac valve offers little resistance to the flow of blood, even when blood flow velocity across it is high. As valvular stenosis develops, the valve orifice produces progressively greater resistance to flow, resulting in a fall in pressure *(pressure gradient)* across the valve. At any stenotic orifice size, greater flow across the orifice yields a greater pressure gradient. Using this principle together with two fundamental hydraulic formulas, Dr. Richard Gorlin and his father developed a formula for the calculation of cardiac valvular orifices from flow and pressure-gradient data.[1]

GORLIN FORMULA

The first hydraulic formula that the Gorlins used was Torricelli's law, which describes flow across a round orifice:

$$F = AVC_c \qquad (1)$$

where F = flow rate, A = orifice area, V = velocity of flow, and C_c = coefficient of orifice contraction. The constant C_c compensates for the physical phenomenon that, except for a perfect orifice, the area of a stream flowing through an orifice will be less than the true area of the orifice.

Rearranging the terms:

$$A = \frac{F}{VC_c} \qquad (2)$$

The second hydraulic principle used in the derivation of Gorlin's formula relates pressure gradient and velocity of flow:

$$V^2 = (C_v)^2 \cdot 2gh \text{ or } V = (C_v) \sqrt{2gh} \qquad (3)$$

where V = velocity of flow, C_v = coefficient of velocity, correcting for energy loss as pressure energy is converted to kinetic or velocity energy, g = acceleration due to gravity (980 cm/sec/sec) and h = pressure gradient in cm H_2O.

Combining the two equations:

$$A = \frac{F}{C_v \sqrt{2gh} \cdot C_c} = \frac{F}{C_v C_c \sqrt{2 \cdot 980 \cdot h}} \qquad (4)$$

$$A = \frac{F}{(C)(44.3) \sqrt{h}}$$

where C is an empiric constant accounting for C_v nd C_c, the expression of h in mm Hg, and correcting calculated valve area to actual measured valve area at surgery or autopsy.

It is obvious that antegrade flow across the mitral and triscuspid valves occurs only in diastole, whereas that across the aortic and pulmonic valves occurs only in systole. Accordingly, the flow (F) for equation 4 is the total cardiac output expressed in terms of the seconds per minute during which there is actually forward flow across the valve. For the mitral and tricuspid valves this is calculated by multiplying the diastolic filling period (sec/beat) times the heart rate (beats/min), yielding the number of seconds/minute during which there is diastolic flow. The cardiac output in ml/min (or cm³/min) is then divided by the seconds per minute during which there is flow, yielding diastolic flow in cm³/second. For the aortic and pulmonic valves the systolic ejection period is substituted for diastolic filling period. The manner in which the diastolic filling period and systolic ejection period are measured is shown in Figure 11–1. The diastolic filling period begins at mitral valve opening and continues until end diastole. The systolic ejection period begins with aortic valve opening and proceeds to the dicrotic notch or other evidence of aortic valve closure.

Thus, the final equation for the calculation of valve orifice area (A, in cm²) is

$$A = \frac{CO/(DFP \text{ or } SEP)(HR)}{44.3 \ C \ \sqrt{\Delta P}} \qquad (5)$$

where CO = cardiac output (cm³/min), DFP = diastolic filling period (sec/beat), SEP = systolic ejection period (sec/beat), HR = heart rate (beats/min), C = empiric constant, and P = pressure gradient. The empiric constant for the tricuspid, pulmonic, and aortic valves, as well as for a patent ductus arteriosus or ventricular septal defect, is assumed to be 1.0. The empiric constant for the mitral valve was originally reported by Gorlin and Gorlin to be 0.7, but in their early studies DFP was derived from an arterial pressure tracing by subtracting the systolic ejection period from the RR interval.[1] This method overestimates DFP, because it neglects the isovolumic contraction and relaxation periods. When the DFP is measured directly from left ventricular versus pulmonary capillary wedge or left atrial pressure tracings, as in Figure 11–1, an empiric con-

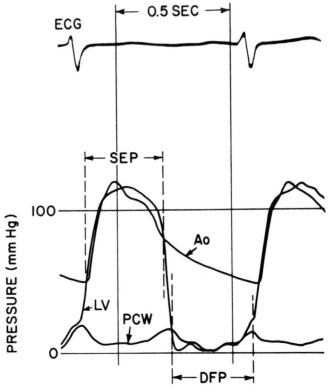

Fig. 11–1. Left ventricular (LV), aortic (Ao), and pulmonary capillary wedge (PCW) pressure tracings from a patient without valvular heart disease, illustrating the definition and measurement of diastolic filling period (DFP) and systolic ejection period (SEP). See text for discussion.

stant for the mitral valve of 0.85 should be used.[2]

In their initial correlations, Gorlin and Gorlin compared the calculated mitral valve area to actual measured area from autopsy or surgical specimens in 11 patients.[1] The maximum deviation of calculated valve area from measured valve area was 0.2 cm[2]. To date there has been remarkably little validation of the empiric constant for the aortic, pulmonic, and tricuspid valves. Nonetheless, the Gorlin formula remains the "gold standard" for assessing the severity of stenotic cardiac valves.

MITRAL VALVE AREA

By rearranging the terms of equation 5, one sees that for the mitral valve:

$$\Delta P = \left[\frac{CO/(HR)(DFP)}{(MVA)(44.3)(0.85)} \right]^2 \qquad (6)$$

where ΔP = mean transmitral pressure gradient, and MVA = mitral valve area. Thus, by doubling cardiac output, one will quadruple the gradient across the valve, if heart rate and diastolic filling period remain constant. The normal mitral orifice in an adult has a cross-sectional area of 4.0–5.0 cm[2] when the mitral valve is completely open in diastole. Considerable reduction in this orifice area can occur without symptomatic limitation, but when the area is ≤1.0 cm[2], a substantial resting gradient will be present across the mitral valve, and any demand for increased cardiac output will be met by increases in left atrial and pulmonary capillary pressure that lead to pulmonary congestion and edema.

As can be seen in Figure 11–2, a cardiac output of 5 liters/min can be maintained with only a minimal mitral diastolic gradient as the mitral orifice area contracts from its normal 4.0–5.0 cm[2] to a moderately stenotic area of 2.0 cm[2]. After that, the gradient rises so that at an orifice area of 1.0 cm[2] a resting gradient of 8 to 10 mm Hg is required to maintain cardiac output at 5 liters/minute, with a normal resting heart rate of 72 beats/min (Fig. 11–2A). Note that even at this level of cardiac output, substantial increases in gradient may

occur in response to tachycardia (Fig. 11–2, B and C), which reduces the total time per minute available for diastolic filling. Thus 1.0 cm[2] is generally viewed as the "critical" mitral valve area, because only small increases in cardiac output lead to pulmonary congestion and severe dyspnea. Some allowance, however, needs to be made for the patient's size in assessing critical valve area. Larger patients need greater flows to maintain tissue perfusion than smaller patients and have higher gradients because of higher cardiac output for any given valvular area. Thus, 1.2 cm[2] could be a critical mitral valve area for a larger patient. Currently, no uniform agreement exists on indexing critical valve area to body size.

Example of Valve Area Calculation in Mitral Stenosis. Figure 11–3 shows pulmonary capillary wedge (PCW) and left ventricular (LV) pressure tracings in a 40-year-old woman with rheumatic heart disease and severe mitral stenosis. This woman also had hypertension and significant elevation of her left ventricular diastolic pressure. The valve area is calculated with the aid of a form reproduced as Table 11–1. In this patient, five beats were chosen from the recordings taken closest in time to the Fick cardiac output determination. Planimetry of the area between PCW and LV pressure tracings (Fig. 11–3) was done for these five beats, and these areas were divided by the length of the diastolic filling periods for each beat, giving an average gradient deflection in millimeters (mm). The mean gradient in mm Hg (Table 11–1, B) was calculated as the average gradient deflection in millimeters (mm) multiplied by the scale factor (mm Hg/mm deflection). In this case, the mean gradient was 30 mm Hg. Next, the average diastolic filling period is calculated (Table 11–1, C) using the average measured length between initial PCW-LV crossover in early diastole and end diastole (peak of the R wave by ECG). This average length in mm is divided by the paper speed (mm/sec) to give the average diastolic filling period, which in this case was 0.40 seconds. Heart rate and cardiac output (Table 11–1 D and E) are recorded, ideally from data collected simultaneously with the recording of the

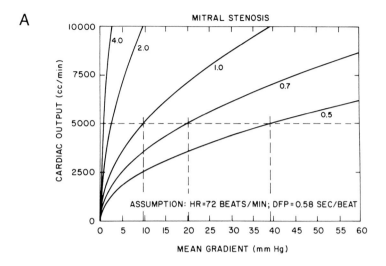

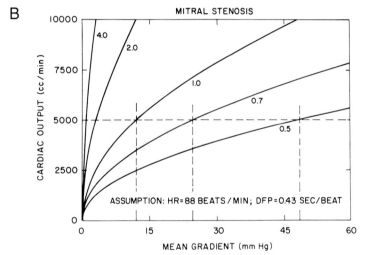

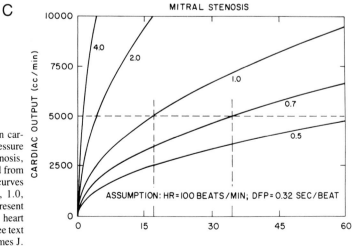

Fig. 11–2. Relationships between cardiac output and mean diastolic pressure gradient in patients with mitral stenosis, calculated using Equation 6 derived from the Gorlin formula. Individual curves represent orifice areas of 4.0, 2.0, 1.0, 0.7, and 0.5 cm². A, B, and C represent flow-gradient relations at differing heart rates and diastolic filling periods. See text for discussion. (Courtesy of Dr. James J. Ferguson, III.)

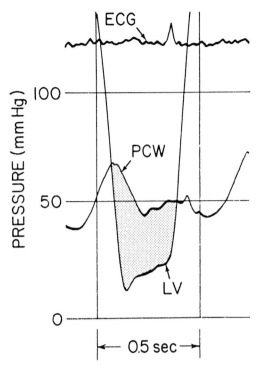

Fig. 11–3. Pulmonary capillary wedge (PCW) and left ventricular (LV) pressure tracings in a 40-year-old woman with mitral stenosis. This woman also had hypertension and significant elevation of her LV diastolic pressure. See text for discussion.

PCW-LV pressure gradient. Heart rate was 80 beats/min and cardiac output was 4680 cm³/minute in the case illustrated in Figure 11–3. Note that cardiac output must be expressed in cm³/min if valve area is expressed in cm² cross-sectional area.

Entering these values in the formula given in Table 11–1 F, and using a constant of 0.85(44.3) = 37.7 for the mitral valve, we get:

Mitral Orifice Area =

$$\frac{(4680 \text{ cm}^3/\text{min})/(80 \text{ beats/min})(0.40 \text{ sec/beat})}{37.7 \sqrt{30 \text{ mm Hg}}}$$

Mitral Orifice Area = 0.71 cm²

Because the accuracy of the method to hundredths of a cm² has not been demonstrated, the resultant valve area is rounded off and expressed as 0.7 cm².

Pitfalls

Pulmonary Capillary Wedge Tracing. In most cases, pulmonary capillary wedge pressure is substituted for left atrial pressure under the assumption that a *properly confirmed wedge pressure* accurately reflects left atrial pressure. Schoenfeld et al. have suggested that in prosthetic valve mitral stenosis, pulmonary capillary wedge pressure obtained from a flexible Swan-Ganz catheter overestimated the transvalvular gradient when compared to the actual gradient measured using direct left atrial pressure obtained by transseptal technique.[3] The authors noted, however, that oximetric confirmation of the pulmonary capillary wedge pressure was not performed. More recently, Lange and colleagues examined directly measured (transseptal) left atrial pressure versus oximetrically confirmed wedge pressure obtained using a stiff woven Dacron catheter.[4] In this study, overestimation of true left atrial pressure was only 1.7 ± 0.6 mm Hg. Thus, we and others believe that the weight of evidence[5] and our own experience support the use of the pulmonary capillary wedge pressure as a satisfactory substitution for left atrial pressure, except in some patients with pulmonary veno-occlusive disease or cor triatriatum. Failure to wedge the catheter properly may, however, cause one to compare a damped pulmonary artery pressure to the left ventricular pressure, yielding a falsely high gradient. To ensure that the right heart catheter is properly wedged, one should verify that:

1. The mean wedge pressure is lower than the mean pulmonary artery pressure.
2. Blood withdrawn from the wedged catheter is 95% or more saturated with oxygen, or at least equal in saturation to arterial blood.

Alignment Mismatch. Alignment of the pulmonary capillary wedge and left ventricular pressure tracings does not match alignment of simultaneous left atrial and left ventricular tracings because there is a time delay in the transmission of the left atrial pressure signal back through the pulmonary venous and capillary beds. The resulting pressure mismatch is small when pulmonary capillary wedge pres-

Table 11–1. *Valve Orifice Area Determination*

Patient _____ Age _____ Unit Number _____ Date _____

A. Complex No.	Area of Gradient (mm²)	/	Length of Diastolic or Systolic Period (mm)	=	Average Gradient (deflection, mm)
1.	_____	/	_____	=	_____
2.	_____	/	_____	=	_____
3.	_____	/	_____	=	_____
4.	_____	/	_____	=	_____
5.	_____	/	_____	=	_____

B. Mean Gradient = Average Gradient (mm deflection) × Scale Factor (mm Hg/mm deflection)

= _____ × _____ = _____ mm Hg

C. Average Diastolic or Systolic Period = Average Length (mm)/Paper Speed (mm/sec)

= _____ / _____ = _____ sec/beat

D. Heart Rate = _____ beat/min

E. Cardiac Output (Fick or Indicator dilution) = _____ cc/min

F. Valve Area = $\dfrac{\text{Cardiac Output/(Heart Rate} \times \text{Avg. Diastolic or Systolic Period)}}{\text{Valve Constant* } \times \sqrt{\text{Mean Gradient}}}$

= $\dfrac{\underline{\quad\quad} / (\underline{\quad\quad} \times \underline{\quad\quad})}{\underline{\quad\quad} \times \sqrt{\underline{\quad\quad}}}$ = _____ cm²

G. Valve Area Index = Valve Area/Body Surface Area = _____ cm²/m²

*Valve Constants: for mitral valve use 37.7; for aortic, tricuspid, and pulmonic valves use 44.3.

sure is measured in the distal pulmonary arteries using a 7F or 8F Cournand or Goodale-Lubin catheter but may be larger when wedge pressure is measured more proximally in the pulmonary arterial tree, using a balloon-tipped flow-directed catheter. As illustrated in Chapter 4, Figure 4–8, the ''a'' and ''v'' waves in an optimally damped pulmonary capillary wedge tracing are delayed typically by 50 to 70 msec compared to a simultaneous left atrial pressure tracing. Thus, ideally, the wedge pressure should be realigned with the left ventricular pressure (using tracing paper) by shifting it leftward by 50 to 70 msec.

The V wave, which is normally present in the left atrium (where it represents pulmonary venous return), peaks immediately before the downstroke of the left ventricular pressure tracing. With a wedge pressure measured distally using a 7F Goodale-Lubin catheter (Fig. 11–3), the peak of the V wave is bisected by the rapid downstroke of left ventricular pressure decline. Realignment of a wedge tracing so that the V wave peak is bisected by (or slightly to the left of) the downstroke of left

ventricular pressure is a practical method for achieving more physiologic realignment.

Calibration Errors. Failure to calibrate pressure transducers properly and adjust them to the same zero reference point may yield an erroneous gradient. A quick way to check the validity of an unsuspected mitral gradient is to switch left and right heart catheters to opposite transducers, which if calibrated equally yields the same gradient.

Cardiac Output Determination. Cardiac output must be determined accurately, as described in Chapter 8. The cardiac output used in valve area calculation should be the value measured simultaneously with the gradient determination. The measurement used in the valve area formula is usually the *forward* cardiac output determined by Fick or indicator dilution methods. If mitral valvular regurgitation exists, the gradient across the valve will reflect not only net forward flow but forward plus regurgitant or total transmitral diastolic flow. Thus, using only net forward flow to calculate the valve area will underestimate the actual anatomic valve area in cases where regurgitation coexists with stenosis.

Early Diastasis. Even when left atrial and left ventricular pressures equalize (diastasis) before the end of diastole, there will generally still be flow through the mitral valve after diastasis. The *diastolic filling period thus includes all of nonisovolumic diastole,* not just the period during which the gradient is present.

AORTIC VALVE AREA

An aortic valve area of 0.7 cm² or less is generally considered severe enough to account for the symptoms of angina, syncope, or heart failure in a patient with aortic stenosis.

Figure 11–4 illustrates the relationship between cardiac output and aortic pressure gradient over a range of values for aortic valve area at three values for heart rate and systolic ejection period. For the aortic valve, equation 4 can be rearranged as:

$$\Delta P = \left[\frac{CO/(HR)(SEP)}{44.3 \; AVA} \right]^2 \qquad (7)$$

As can be seen in Figure 11–4A, at a normal resting cardiac output of 5.0 liters/min, an aortic orifice area of 0.7 cm² will result in a gradient of approximately 33 mm Hg across the aortic valve. Doubling of the cardiac output, as might occur with exercise, would increase the gradient by a factor of 4 to 132 mm Hg if the systolic time/minute did not change. This increase in gradient would require a peak left ventricular pressure in excess of 250 mm Hg to maintain a central aortic pressure of 120 mm Hg. Such a major increase in left ventricular pressure obviously increases myocardial oxygen demand and also limits ejection performance; these factors contribute to the symptoms of angina and congestive heart failure, respectively.[6,7] The limitations in cardiac output imposed by high afterload may contribute to hypotension when peripheral vasodilation occurs during muscular exercise. Actually, the systolic time per minute *does not* remain constant during the increase in cardiac output associated with exercise. As heart rate increases during exercise, the systolic ejection period tends to become shorter, but the tendency is counteracted by both increased venous return and systemic arteriolar vasodilation, factors that normally help to maintain left ventricular stroke volume constant (or even increased) during exercise. Thus, heart rate is increasing, but systolic ejection period is diminishing only slightly, so that their product (systolic ejection time per minute) increases. This is the counterpart of the decreased diastolic filling time per minute during exercise, discussed above. Examining equation (7), it can be seen that the increase in cardiac output will be partially offset by the increase in (HR)(SEP), so that the gradient will not quadruple with a doubling of cardiac output during exercise.

Figure 11–4 B and C show that with *decreasing* heart rate, the gradient increases in aortic stenosis for any value of cardiac output. This is opposite to the effect of heart rate in mitral stenosis and reflects the opposite effects of heart rate on systolic and diastolic time per minute. Viewed another way, as the heart rate slows in aortic stenosis, the stroke volume increases if cardiac output remains constant. Thus, the flow/beat across the aortic valve increases, and so does the pressure gradient.

As with mitral stenosis, some allowance must be made for body size in deciding what is a critical valve area in aortic stenosis: larger patients who require higher output may become symptomatic at somewhat larger valve areas. Thus, a very large man with a body surface area of 2.4 m² and a cardiac index of 3.0 L/min/m² would have a cardiac output of 7200 ml/min. At a heart rate of 68 beats/min (Fig. 11-4 C), this man might have a 50 mm Hg aortic valve gradient with an orifice area of 0.9–1.0 cm². Thus, for him, this might be a critical valve area.

Example. Figure 11–5 demonstrates simultaneous pressure tracings from the left ventricle (LV) and right femoral artery (RFA) in a patient with exertional syncope. Since the pulse wave takes a finite period of time to travel from the left ventricle to the femoral artery, the femoral artery tracing is somewhat delayed (Fig. 11–5A). Figure 11–5B shows the LV and RFA tracings realigned to correct for the delay in transmission time. This is ac-

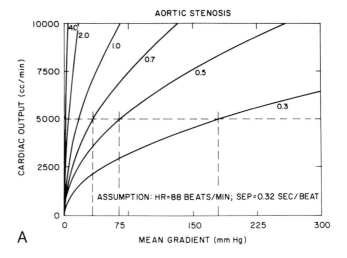

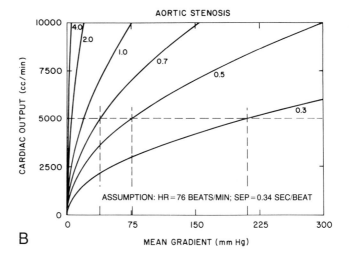

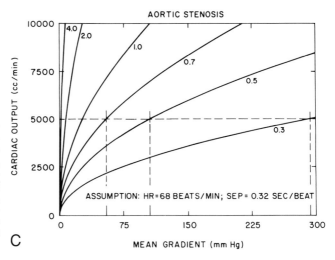

Fig. 11–4. Relationships between cardiac output and mean aortic systolic pressure gradient in patients with aortic stenosis, calculated using equation 7, derived from the Gorlin equation. Individual curves represent orifice areas of 4.0, 2.0, 1.0, 0.7, 0.5, and 0.3 cm². A, B, and C represent flow-gradient relations at differing heart rates and systolic ejection periods. (Courtesy of Dr. James J. Ferguson, III.)

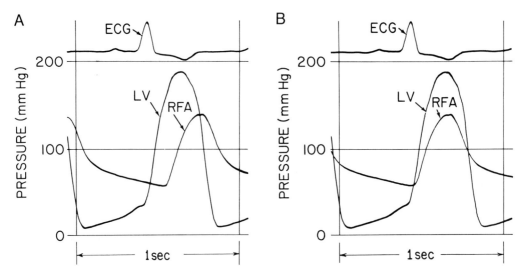

Fig. 11–5. Left ventricular (LV) and right femoral artery (RFA) pressure tracings in a patient who presented with exertional syncope due to aortic stenosis. A shows the tracings actually recorded, and demonstrates the significant time delay for the pressure waveform to reach the RFA. B shows realignment using tracing paper. See text for discussion.

complished using tracing paper and aligning the arterial upstroke to coincide with the LV upstroke. After such alignment, the mean pressure gradient can now be obtained by planimetry, and the orifice area can be calculated using the form given in Table 11–1. For this example, the average aortic pressure gradient was 40 mm Hg, the systolic ejection period 0.33 sec, the heart 74 beats/min, and the cardiac output 5000 cm³/min. Using these values together with an aortic valve constant of (1)(44.3) = 44.3 in the equation in Table 11–1 gives:

Aortic valve area =

$$\frac{(5000 \text{ cm}^3/\text{min})/(74 \text{ beats/min})\cdot(0.33 \text{ sec/beat})}{44.3 \sqrt{40 \text{ mm Hg}}}$$

Aortic valve area = 0.7 cm²

As discussed in Chapter 9, peripheral arterial pressure waveforms are distorted in ways other than time delay. These distortions include systolic amplification and spreading out (widening) of the pressure waveform. To assess possible errors introduced by the use of peripheral arterial pressure as a substitute for ascending aortic pressure, Folland and co-workers compared the left ventricular-ascending aortic (LV-Ao) mean gradient in 26

patients with aortic stenosis with the left ventricular femoral artery (LV-FA) systolic gradient, with and without realignment (Fig. 11–6).[8] Without realignment, the LV-FA gradient *overestimated* the LV-Ao gradient by about 9 mm Hg. In contrast, aligned LV-FA gradients *underestimated* the LV-Ao gradient by about 10 mm Hg, possibly representing the fact that peak systolic arterial pressure is higher in peripheral arterial pressure tracings than in central aortic tracings, so that the planimetered gradient will be smaller when using LV-FA. Without realignment, this effect is offset by the fact that much of the arterial systolic waveform is outside and to the right of the left ventricular pressure tracing (Fig. 11–6). When the transvalvular gradient is large (more than 50 mm Hg), these differences are of little clinical importance. When a small transvalvular gradient is present in conjunction wth a low cardiac output, however, the differences between aligned and unaligned tracings may affect the decision whether or not to replace the valve. In such instances, we recommend that the problem be obviated by placing a second catheter in the proximal ascending aorta without need for alignment (Fig. 11–6A).[8] As an alternative, the difference between peak central aortic and peripheral arterial pressure is

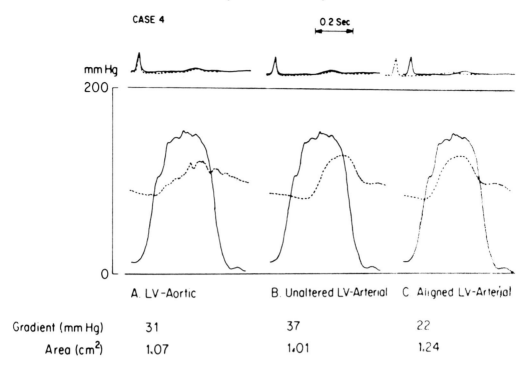

CASE 4   0 2 Sec

	A. LV–Aortic	B. Unaltered LV-Arterial	C Aligned LV-Arterial
Gradient (mm Hg)	31	37	22
Area (cm^2)	1.07	1.01	1.24

Fig. 11–6. Pressure gradients in aortic stenosis. (A) the left ventricular (LV)-central aortic gradient; (B) LV-femoral artery gradient without alignment; and (C) LV-femoral artery gradient with alignment obtained by moving the femoral artery tracing leftward so that its upstroke coincides with the LV pressure upstroke. (Reproduced with permission from Folland ED, Parisi AF, Carbone C: Is peripheral arterial pressure a satisfactory substitute for ascending aortic pressure when measuring aortic valve gradients? J Am Coll Cardiol 4:1207, 1984.)

added to the planimetered gradient measured during the Fick output determination. This compensates for the fact that the planimetered gradient with realignment (Fig. 11–6C) underestimates the true gradient (Fig. 11–6A). The most accurate approach, however, involves the use of a second catheter positioned in the ascending aorta, as discussed above.

Another approach to increasing the accuracy of transaortic valve gradient measurement using simultaneous left ventricular and femoral artery pressures has been introduced by Krueger and co-workers at the University of Utah.[9] As seen in Figure 11–7, the mean LV systolic pressure during interval "A" and the mean FA systolic pressure during interval "B" are determined by planimetry. Their difference was nearly identical to the gradient measured by planimetry of simultaneous LV and central aortic pressures, and was more accurate than other techniques commonly used.[9]

If a second catheter is not used to obtain simultaneous left ventricular and peripheral pressure, the gradient may be obtained by recording left ventricular pressure and superimposing it upon the aortic pressure obtained immediately after the left ventricular catheter is pulled back into the aorta.

Pitfalls

Transducer Calibration. As with calculation of mitral valve area, attention to cardiac output determination and transducer calibration is critical. Assurance that proper transducer calibration has been accomplished can be obtained by comparing the left heart catheter pressure to the peripheral arterial catheter pressure prior to insertion of the left heart catheter into the left ventricle. Since in the absence of peripheral stenosis mean arterial pressure will be the same throughout the arterial tree,

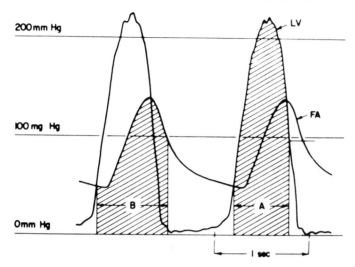

Fig. 11–7. Simultaneous recordings of left ventricular (LV) and femoral artery (FA) pressures in a patient with aortic stenosis. The mean LV systolic pressure during interval "A" and the mean FA systolic pressure during interval "B" are determined by planimetry, and the systolic LV-aortic gradient is estimated as the difference between these mean pressures. (Reproduced with permission from Krueger SK, Orme EC, King CS, and Barry WH: Accurate determination of the transaortic valve gradient using simultaneous left ventricular and femoral artery pressures. Cathet Cardiovasc Diagn 16:202, 1989.)

the mean pressure recorded by both catheters should be identical, confirming identical transducer calibration. Further gradient verification is made by comparing the left ventricular pressure to aortic pressure obtained by the left heart catheter during catheter pullback. In this case, both left ventricular and aortic pressures are recorded by the same catheter and transducer, eliminating the second transducer as a source of error.

Low Flow States. In low cardiac output states, only a small gradient may be present across a critically narrowed aortic valve. For instance, at a cardiac output of 3 liters/minute, a pressure gradient of 20 mm Hg will yield an aortic valve area of 0.7 cm^2. In such cases, small errors in gradient or cardiac output measurement may substantially alter the hemodynamic assessment of stenosis severity and may lead to an incorrect conclusion concerning the need to replace the aortic valve. Furthermore, at low flows a valve that is sclerotic, but not truly stenotic, may fail to open fully. This results in a reduced effective valve area.[10–12] In such cases, the use of exercise or infusion of a positive inotropic agent allows for calculation of gradient and valve area at a higher and more reliable cardiac output.

Pullback Hemodynamics. When the aortic valve area is diminished to 0.6 cm^2 or less, a 7F or 8F catheter placed retrograde across the valve takes up a significant amount of the residual orifice area, and the catheter may ac-

tually increase the severity of stenosis. Conversely, removal of the catheter reduces the amount of stenosis. We have observed that a peripheral pressure rise occurs in severe aortic stenosis when the left ventricular catheter is removed from the aortic valve orifice.[13] In our experience, an augmentation in peripheral systolic pressure of over 5 mm Hg at the time of left ventricular catheter pullback indicates that significant aortic stenosis is present. This sign is present in more than 80% of patients with an aortic valve area of 0.5 cm^2 or less, a point that is discussed further in Chapter 31.

AREA OF TRICUSPID AND PULMONIC VALVES

Because of the rarity of tricuspid and pulmonic stenosis in adults, no general agreement exists as to what constitutes a critical orifice area for these valves. In general, a mean gradient of 5 mm Hg across the tricuspid valve is sufficient to cause symptoms of systemic venous hypertension. Gradients across the pulmonic valve of less than 50 mm Hg are usually well tolerated, but gradients of greater than 100 mm Hg indicate a need for surgical correction. Between 50 mm Hg and 100 mm Hg, decisions regarding surgical correction depend on the clinical features in each individual case.

ALTERNATIVES TO THE GORLIN FORMULA

A simplified valve formula for the calculation of stenotic cardiac valve areas has been proposed by Hakki et al. and tested in 100 consecutive patients with either aortic or mitral stenosis.[14] The simplified formula is simply:

$$\text{Valve area} = \frac{\text{Cardiac output (L/min)}}{\sqrt{\text{Pressure gradient}}}$$

and is based on their observation that the product of heart rate, SEP or DFP, and the Gorlin equation constant was nearly the same for all patients whose hemodynamics were measured in the resting state, and the value of this product was close to 1.0. For the examples given earlier in this chapter, the simplified formula works reasonably well. Thus, for the patient with mitral stenosis (Fig. 11–3) with a cardiac output of 4680 ml/min and a mitral diastolic gradient of 30 mm Hg, mitral valve area = $4.68 \div \sqrt{30} = 0.85$ cm^2 using the simplified formula, as opposed to the value of 0.71 cm^2 calculated using the Gorlin formula. For the patient with aortic stenosis whose tracings are shown in Figure 11–5 (cardiac output 5 L/min, aortic gradient 40 mm Hg), the aortic valve area by the simplified formula is $5 \div \sqrt{40} = 0.79$ cm^2, as opposed to 0.73 cm^2 by the Gorlin formula. Because the percentage of time per minute spent in diastole or systole changes substantially at higher heart rates, the simplified formula may be less useful in the presence of substantial tachycardia. This point, however, has not been tested adequately.

Angel et al.[15] have introduced a modification of Hakki's simplified formula for calculation of valve areas. They added a correction for heart rate, dividing Hakki's equation by 1.35 when heart rate was below 75 beats/min for patients with mitral stenosis and above 90 beats/min for patients with aortic stenosis.[15] This empiric correction improved the predictive accuracy of Hakki's formula.

FLOW DEPENDENCE OF VALVE AREA CALCULATIONS

Previous studies have demonstrated that valve area calculated using the Gorlin formula varies directly with flow; valve area increases as flow increases. This is particularly true of the aortic valve. Although this fact has been known for some time,[16,17] recent need to assess the results of balloon valvuloplasty have refocused attention on the hemodynamic assessment of stenotic valves.[18,19] Two potential mechanisms exist by which the calculated area increases with cardiac output: (1) increased flow through the stenotic aortic valve in conjunction with increased left ventricular pressure physically opens the valve to a greater orifice area and thus the valve orifice really is wider during increased flow; or (2) inaccuracies in the Gorlin formula cause the calculated area (but not necessarily the actual orifice area) to be flow-dependent. The Gorlins themselves noted that they had no data from which to calculate an empiric constant for the aortic valve;[1] thus, one was never calculated but assumed to be 1.0, not by the Gorlins but by the rest of the cardiologic community.

Existing data suggest that both of the above proposed mechanisms play a role in the flow dependence of calculated valve areas. Richards and co-workers inserted a balloon catheter into the orifice of stenotic aortic valves at the time of aortic valve replacement.[11] By inflating the balloon to varying pressures achievable by the normal left ventricle, they were able to effect a significantly larger orifice area at higher pressures than at lower pressures. This study demonstrated that even in severe calcific aortic valve stenosis, the orifice is not "fixed" but can vary with differing pressures. On the other hand, Cannon et al.[20] using a flow chamber and valves of known *fixed* orifice area found that increasing cardiac output increased calculated but not actual valve area. They also found that the Gorlin "constant" was not a constant at all, but varied with the square root of the mean pressure gradient (Fig. 11–8).[20] If the constant in the Gorlin formula is proportional to the square root of the mean pres-

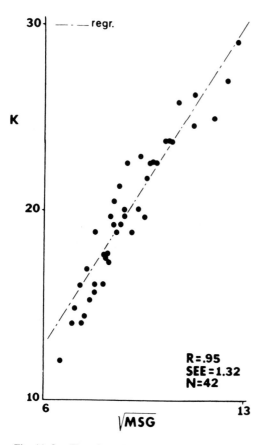

Fig. 11–8. The valve area constant (K) is demonstrated to vary linearly with the square root of the mean systolic gradient (MSG) across the valve. Thus, K is not fixed but varies with the valve gradient. Regr. = regression line. (Reproduced by permission of the American Heart Association, Inc. from Cannon SR et al., Hydraulic estimation of stenotic orifice area: A correction of the Gorlin Formula, Circulation 71:1170, 1985).

sure gradient, it is necessary to multiply the square root of the mean pressure gradient in the Gorlin formula by the square root of the mean pressure gradient:

$$A = \frac{F}{44.3 \cdot (C \cdot \sqrt{MPG}) \cdot \sqrt{MPG}}$$

where A = valve area, F = cardiac output, C = empiric constant, and MPG = mean pressure gradient. Because multiplication of square root by square root removes the square root sign, a modification to the original Gorlin formula was proposed by Cannon et al. in

which the square root sign disappears.[20] The general form of this equation is:

$$A = \frac{F}{C' \cdot MPG}$$

where C' is a new constant. This modification greatly reduced the tendency for calculated valve area to be flow-dependent. This formula reliably predicted actual valve areas in a group of patients with normally functioning porcine aortic valves. An interesting prediction of Cannon's formula is that for any given value of A, F is a linear function of ΔP. Thus, Figures 11–2 and 11–4 would consist of a series of straight lines, if constructed by Cannon's formula.

The original concept of the Gorlin formula, which assesses valve area by relating flow to pressure gradient, is valid and has endured for 40 years. Recent data, however, indicate that modifications of this concept need to be made to account for real or calculated flow-dependent changes in valve area.

ACKNOWLEDGMENT

The authors express their appreciation to Dr. James J. Ferguson, III, who supplied Figures 11–2 and 11–4, constructed by him from computer simulation.

REFERENCES

1. Gorlin R, Gorlin G: Hydraulic formula for calculation of area of stenotic mitral valve, other cardiac values and central circulatory shunts. Am Heart J 41:1, 1951.
2. Cohen MV, Gorlin R: Modified orifice equation for the calculation of mitral valve area. Am Heart J 84:839, 1972.
3. Schoenfeld MH, Palacios IF, Hutter AM Jr, et al: Underestimation of prosthetic mitral valve areas: Role of catheterization in avoiding unnecessary repeat mitral valve surgery. J Am Coll Cardiol 5:1387, 1985.
4. Lange RA, Moore DM, Cigarroa RG, Hillis LD: Use of pulmonary capillary wedge pressure to assess severity of mitral stenosis: Is true left atrial pressure needed in this condition? J Am Coll Cardiol 13:825, 1989.
5. Alpert JS: The lessons of history as reflected in the pulmonary capillary wedge pressure. J Am Coll Cardiol 13:830, 1989.
6. Strauer BE, Burger SB: Systolic stress, coronary

hemodynamics and metabolic reserve in experimental and clinical cardiac hypertrophy. Basic Res Cardiol 75:234, 1980.

7. Carabello BA, et al: Hemodynamic determinants of prognosis of aortic valve replacement in critical aortic stenosis and advanced congestive heart failure. Circulation 62:42, 1980.

8. Folland ED, Parisi AF, Carbone C: Is peripheral arterial pressure a satisfactory substitute for ascending aortic pressure when measuring aortic valve gradients? J Am Coll Cardiol 4:1207, 1984.

9. Krueger SK, Orme EC, King CS, Barry WH: Accurate determination of the transaortic valve gradient using simultaneous left ventricular and femoral artery pressures. Cathet Cardiovasc Diagn 16:202, 1989.

10. Gasper J, et al: Overestimation of aortic stenosis with the Gorlin equation in low flow states. J Am Coll Cardiol 1:639, 1983.

11. Richards KL, Hart TT, Cannon SR, et al: Confirmation of variable orifice native valves in adults with severe aortic stenosis (abstract). Circulation 74 (suppl II):II–314, 1986.

12. Wyman RM, Diver DJ, Lorell BH: The effects of increasing inotropy and transvalvular flow on Gorlin formula aortic valve area calculations in aortic stenosis (abstract). Circulation 78 (suppl II):II–124, 1988.

13. Carabello BA, Barry WH, Grossman W: Changes in arterial pressure during left heart pullback in patients with aortic stenosis: A sign of severe aortic stenosis. Am J Cardiol 44:424, 1979.

14. Hakki AH, et al: A simplified valve formula for the calculation of stenotic cardiac valve areas. Circulation 63:1050, 1981.

15. Angel J, Soler-Soler J, Anivarro I, Domingo E: Hemodynamic evaluation of stenotic cardiac valves: II. Modification of the simplified formula for mitral and aortic valve area calculation. Cathet Cardiovasc Diagn 11:127, 1985.

16. Richter HS: Mitral valve area: Measurement soon after catheterization. Circulation 28:451, 1963.

17. Bache RJ, Wang Y, Jorgensen CR: Hemodynamic effects of exercise in isolated valvular aortic stenosis. Circulation 44:1003, 1971.

18. Carabello BA: Advances in the hemodynamic assessment of stenotic cardiac valves. J Am Coll Cardiol 10:912, 1987.

19. Gorlin R: Calculations of cardiac valve stenosis: Restoring an old concept for advanced applications. J Am Coll Cardiol 10:920, 1987.

20. Cannon SR, Richards KL, Crawford M: Hydraulic estimation of stenotic orifice area: A correction of the Gorlin formula. Circulation 71:1170, 1985.

12

Shunt Detection and Measurement

WILLIAM GROSSMAN

etection, localization, and quantification of intracardiac shunts are an
integral part of the hemodynamic
evaluation of patients with congenital heart
disease. In most cases, an intracardiac shunt
is suspected on the basis of the clinical evaluation of the patient before catheterization.
There are several circumstances, however, in
which data obtained at catheterization should
alert the cardiologist to look for a shunt that
had not been suspected previously:

1. Unexplained arterial desaturation should
immediately raise the suspicion of a right-to-
left intracardiac shunt, which may then be assessed by the methods to be discussed. Most
commonly, arterial desaturation (i.e., arterial
blood oxygen saturation under 95%) detected
at the time of cardiac catheterization represents
alveolar hypoventilation. The causes for this
alveolar hypoventilation and its associated
"physiologic" right-to-left shunt include (a)
excessive sedation from the premedication,
(b) chronic obstructive lung disease or other
pulmonary parenchymal disease, and (c) pulmonary congestion/edema secondary to the
patient's cardiac disease. Alveolar hypoventilation associated with each of these problems
is exacerbated by the supine position of the
patient during the catheterization procedure.

Helping the patient to assume a more upright
posture (head-up tilt, or propping the patient
up with a large wedge if tilt mechanism is not
available), and encouraging the patient to take
deep breaths and to cough will correct or substantially ameliorate arterial hypoxemia in
most cases. If arterial desaturation persists,
oxygen should be administered by face mask
for both therapeutic and diagnostic purposes.
If full arterial blood oxygen saturation cannot
be achieved by face-mask administration of
oxygen (it is best in this regard to use a re-
breathing mask that fits snugly), a right-to-left
shunt must be presumed to be present, and its
anatomic site and magnitude determined using
the methods described later in this chapter.

2. Conversely, when the oxygen content of
blood in the pulmonary artery is unexpectedly
high, that is, if the pulmonary artery (PA)
blood oxygen saturation is above 80%, the
possibility of a left-to-right intracardiac shunt
should be considered. It is for these two reasons that arterial and pulmonary artery saturation should be measured routinely *during* the
catheterization.

3. When the data obtained at catheterization
do not confirm the presence of the suspected
lesion, one should consider the presence of an
intracardiac shunt. For example, if left ventricular cineangiography fails to reveal mitral
regurgitation in a patient in whom this was
judged to be the cause of a systolic murmur,
it is prudent to look for evidence of a ventric-

Some material in this chapter has been retained from
the first and second editions, to which Dr. James E. Dalen
had contributed.

ular septal defect (VSD) with left-to-right shunting.

DETECTION OF LEFT-TO-RIGHT INTRACARDIAC SHUNTS

Many different techniques are available for the detection, localization, and quantification of left-to-right intracardiac shunts. They vary in their sensitivity, in the type of indicator they use, and in the equipment needed to sense and read out the presence of the indicator.

Measurement of Blood Oxygen Saturation and Content in the Right Heart (Oximetry Run)

In this basic technique for detecting and quantifying left-to-right shunts, the oxygen content or percent saturation is measured in blood samples drawn sequentially from the pulmonary artery, right ventricle (RV), right atrium (RA), superior vena cava (SVC), and inferior vena cava (IVC). A left-to-right shunt may be detected and localized if a significant "step-up" in blood oxygen saturation or content is found in one of the right heart chambers. A significant step up is defined as an increase in blood oxygen content or saturation that exceeds the normal variability that might be observed if multiple samples were drawn from that cardiac chamber.

The technique of the oximetry run is based on the fundamental studies of Dexter and his associates in 1947.[1] They found that multiple samples drawn from the right atrium could vary in oxygen content by as much as 2 volumes percent (vol%).* This variability has been attributed to the fact that the right atrium receives its blood from three sources of varying oxygen content: the superior vena cava, the inferior vena cava, and the coronary sinus. The maximal normal variation within the right ventricle was found to be 1 vol%. Because of more adequate mixing, a maximal variation within the pulmonary artery of only $\frac{1}{2}$ vol% was found by Dexter. Thus, using the Dexter

*1 volume percent = 1 ml O_2/100 ml blood or 10 ml O_2/liter of blood.

criteria, a significant step-up is present at the atrial level when the highest oxygen content in blood samples drawn from the right atrium exceeds the highest content in the venae cavae by ≥ 2 vol%. Similarly, a significant step-up at the ventricular level is present if the highest right ventricular sample is ≥ 1 vol% higher than the highest right atrial sample, and a significant step-up at the level of the pulmonary artery is present if the pulmonary artery oxygen content is more than $\frac{1}{2}$ vol% greater than the highest right ventricular sample.

Dexter's classic study described normal variability and gave criteria for a significant oxygen step-up only for measurement of blood oxygen content. This, in part, reflects the methodology available to him because reflectance oximetry was not widely used at that time. In recent years, most cardiac catheterization laboratories (especially those primarily involved in pediatric catheterization) have moved toward the measurement of percent saturation by reflectance oximetry as the routine method for oximetric analysis of blood samples. Oxygen content may then be calculated from knowledge of percent saturation, the patient's blood hemoglobin concentration, and an assumed constant relationship for oxygen carrying capacity of hemoglobin, as discussed in Chapter 8 (1.36 ml O_2/gm hemoglobin). When oxygen content is derived in this manner, rather than by measurement by the Van Slyke or other direct oximetric technique, it is no more accurate (and probably less so because of the potential presence of carboxyhemoglobin or hemoglobin variants with O_2 capacity other than 1.36) than the percent oxygen saturation values from which it is calculated.

To clarify this situation, Antman and coworkers studied prospectively the normal variation of both oxygen content and oxygen saturation of blood in the right heart chambers.[2] The study population consisted of patients without intracardiac shunts who were undergoing diagnostic cardiac catheterization for evaluation of coronary artery disease, valvular heart disease, cardiomyopathy, or possible pulmonary embolism. Each patient had a complete right heart oximetry run (see below) with sampling of multiple sites in each chamber. Oxygen content was measured directly by an electrochemical fuel-cell method (Lex-02-Con*), a method that had been validated previously against the Van Slyke method. Oxygen saturation was calculated as blood oxygen content divided by oxygen-carrying capacity. It is obvious that the relationship between oxygen content and oxygen saturation depends on the hemoglobin concentration of the patient's blood; e.g., 75% oxygen saturation of pulmonary artery blood will be associated with a substantially lower oxygen content in an anemic patient than in one with normal hemoglobin concentration. Also, systemic blood flow may be an important determinant of oxygen variability in the right heart chambers because high systemic flow tends to equalize the differences across various tissue beds.

In the context of these considerations, I have listed in Table 12–1 criteria for a significant step-up in right heart oxygen content and percent oxygen saturation associated with various types of left-to-right shunt, based on the study of Antman and co-workers[2] and other investigators.[1,3,4] As can be seen from the bottom line (ANY LEVEL) of Table 12–1, the simplest way to screen for a left-to-right shunt is to sample SVC and PA blood and measure the difference, if any, in percent O_2 saturation. As stated in Chapters 4 and 5, we routinely obtain blood samples from SVC and PA at the time of right heart catheterization and determine their O_2 saturation by reflectance oximetry. If the ΔO_2 saturation between these samples is $\geq 8\%$, a left-to-right shunt may be present at atrial, ventricular, or great vessel level, and a full oximetry run should be done.

Oximetry Run. The blood samples needed to localize a step-up in the right heart are obtained by performing what is called an oximetry run. The samples needed, and the order in which we recommend they be obtained, follow.

Obtain a 2-ml sample from each of the following locations:

1. Left and/or right pulmonary artery

*Lexington Instruments, Lexington, MA.

*2. Main pulmonary artery
*3. Right ventricle, outflow tract
†4. Right ventricle, mid
*†5. Right ventricle, tricuspid valve or apex
*6. Right atrium, low or near tricuspid valve
7. Right atrium, mid
8. Right atrium, high
9. Superior vena cava, low (near junction with right atrium)
10. Superior vena cava, high (near junction with innominate vein)
11. Inferior vena cava, high (just below diaphragm)
12. Inferior vena cava, low (at L4–L5)
13. Left ventricle
14. Aorta (distal to insertion of ductus)

In performing the oximetry run, an end-hole catheter or one with side holes close to its tip (e.g., a Goodale-Lubin catheter‡) is positioned in the right or left pulmonary artery. Cardiac output is measured by the Fick method. As soon as the determination of oxygen consumption is completed, the operator begins to obtain 2-ml blood samples from each of the locations indicated. This is done under fluoroscopic control, with catheter tip position further confirmed by pressure measurement at the sites noted. The entire procedure should take less than seven minutes. If a sample cannot be obtained from a specific site because of ventricular premature beats, that site should be skipped until the rest of the run has been completed.

Oxygen saturation and/or content in each of the samples is determined as discussed previously, and the presence and localization of a significant step-up are determined by applying the criteria listed in Table 12–1.

An alternative method for performing the oximetry run is to withdraw a fiberoptic catheter from the pulmonary artery through the right heart chambers and the inferior and superior venae cavae. This permits a continuous

*Confirm location by pressure measurement.
†If frequent extrasystoles occur, do not persist. Obtain samples from three different locations in right ventricle and right atrium.
‡United States Catheter and Instrument Corp., Billerica, MA.

Table 12–1. *Detection of Left-to-Right Shunt by Oximetry*

Level of Shunt	Criteria For Significant Step-Up				Approximate Minimal Q_p/Q_s Required for Detection (Assuming SBFI = $3L/min/M^2$)	Possible Causes of Step-Up
	Mean of Distal Chamber Samples – Mean of Proximal Chamber Samples		Highest Value in Distal Chamber – Highest Value in Proximal Chamber			
	O_2% Sat	O_2 Vol%	O_2% Sat	O_2 Vol%		
Atrial (SVC/IVC to RA)	≥7	≥1.3	≥11	≥2.0	1.5–1.9	Atrial septal defect; partial anomalous pulmonary venous drainage; ruptured sinus of Valsalva; VSD with TR; coronary fistula to RA
Ventricular (RA to RV)	≥5	≥1.0	≥10	≥1.7	1.3–1.5	VSD; PDA with PR; primum ASD; coronary fistula to RV
Great Vessel (RV to PA)	≥5	≥1.0	≥5	≥1.0	1.3	PDA; aorta-pulmonic window; aberrant coronary artery origin
ANY LEVEL (SVC to PA)	≥7	≥1.3	≥8	≥1.5	1.5	All of the above

Abbreviations: SVC and IVC, superior and inferior vena cavae; RA, right atrium; RV, right ventricle; PA, pulmonary artery; VSD, ventricular septal defect; TR, tricuspid regurgitation; PDA, patent ductus arteriosus; PR, pulmonic regurgitation; ASD, atrial septal defect, SBFI, systemic blood flow index; Q_p/Q_s, pulmonary to systemic flow ratio.

readout of oxygen saturation that allows detection of a step-up in oxygen content.

If the oximetry run reveals that a significant step-up is present, the pulmonary blood flow, systemic blood flow, and the magnitude of left-to-right and right-to-left shunts may be calculated according to the following formulae.

Calculation of Pulmonary Blood Flow **(Q_P).** Pulmonary blood flow is calculated by the same formula used in the standard Fick equation:

$$\underset{\text{(L/min)}}{Q_P} = \frac{O_2 \text{ consumption (ml/min)}}{\left[\begin{array}{c} PV\ O_2 \\ \text{content} \\ \text{(ml/L)} \end{array}\right] - \left[\begin{array}{c} PA\ O_2 \\ \text{content} \\ \text{(ml/L)} \end{array}\right]}$$

If a pulmonary vein (PV) has not been entered, systemic arterial oxygen content may be used in the preceding formula, if systemic oxygen saturation is 95% or more. If systemic oxygen saturation is <95%, one must determine whether a right-to-left intracardiac shunt is present. If there is an intracardiac right-to-left shunt, an assumed value for pulmonary venous oxygen content of 98% × oxygen capacity should be used in calculating pulmonary blood flow. If arterial desaturation is present and is not due to a right-to-left intracardiac shunt, the observed systemic oxygen saturation should be used to calculate pulmonary blood flow.

Example. Let us suppose that a patient is found to have an atrial septal defect with a left-to-right shunt clearly detected by oximetry run. Furthermore, the catheter crosses the defect and a pulmonary vein is entered, from which a blood sample shows O_2 saturation of 98%. Let us further suppose, however, that systemic arterial blood saturation is 90% and that this is due to chronic pulmonary disease. After ruling out a right-to-left shunt (e.g., inhalation of 100% oxygen, indocyanine green dye injection in inferior vena cava, echocardiogram-bubble study), should we use 98% or 90% for pulmonary venous blood O_2 saturation in the calculation of Q_p? As indicated above, because arterial desaturation is not caused by a right-to-left intracardiac shunt, the observed systemic arterial O_2 saturation (90%) should

be used because this summates all the pulmonary veins draining both lungs, not just the one with 98% O_2 saturation.

Calculation of Systemic Blood Flow (Q_s).

$$\underset{\text{(L/min)}}{Q_s} = \frac{O_2 \text{ consumption (ml/min)}}{\left[\begin{array}{c} SA\ O_2 \\ \text{content} \\ \text{ml/L} \end{array}\right] - \left[\begin{array}{c} MV\ O_2 \\ \text{content} \\ \text{ml/L} \end{array}\right]}$$

The key to the measurement of systemic blood flow in the presence of an intracardiac shunt is that the mixed venous oxygen content must be measured in the chamber immediately proximal to the shunt, as shown in Table 12–2.

The formula to be used for the calculation of venous content in the presence of an atrial septal defect (ASD) was derived by Flamm et al.[5] They found that systemic blood flow calculated from mixed venous oxygen content as determined from the formula listed in Table 12–2 most closely approximates systemic blood flow as measured by left ventricular to brachial artery (BA) dye curves in patients with atrial septal defect studied at rest. It should be noted that Flamm's formula "weights" blood returning from the superior vena cava more heavily than might be expected on the basis of relative flows in the superior and inferor cavae. The success of this empirical weighting of the relatively desaturated superior vena cava blood (O_2 saturation is almost always less in blood from the superior as opposed to the inferior vena cava) probably reflects the fact that the third contributor to mixed venous blood—desaturated coronary sinus blood—is not sampled during the oximetry run and therefore cannot be included directly in the formula. It must also be pointed out that the formula (3 SVC O_2 + 1 IVC O_2)/ 4 was validated by Flamm and associates for mixed venous oxygen content at rest.[5] Thus, in 18 patients without shunt, this value agreed closely with pulmonary artery blood oxygen content at rest. During supine bicycle exercise, however, a different relationship was found to apply, in which mixed venous (pulmonary artery) oxygen content in patients without shunts was best approximated as (1 SVC O_2 + 2 IVC

Table 12–2. *Calculation of Systemic Blood Flow in the Presence of Left-to-Right Shunt*

Location of Shunt as Determined by Site of O_2 Step-up	Mixed Venous Sample to Use in Calculating Systemic Blood Flow
1. Pulmonary artery (e.g., patent ductus arteriosus)	Right ventricle, average of samples obtained during oximetry run
2. Right ventricle (e.g., ventricular septal defect)	Right atrium, average of all samples during oximetry run
3. Right atrium (e.g., atrial septal defect)	$\dfrac{3(\text{SVC } O_2 \text{ content}) + 1(\text{IVC } O_2 \text{ content})}{4}$

O_2)/3. This formula was then used for patients with atrial septal defect *during exercise,* and it reliably predicted systemic blood flow measured by left ventricular to brachial artery dye-dilution curve. Therefore, for patients with left-to-right shunt at the atrial level, the formula in Table 12–2 should be used only for calculation of *resting* mixed venous O_2 content.

Obviously, calculations from the formula in Table 12–2 would be little changed in many cases by ignoring inferior vena cava blood altogether, and this is done in some laboratories (especially those involved in pediatric catheterization). Flamm and associates, however, examined the effects of assuming that superior vena cava O_2 content equaled mixed venous O_2 content, and concluded that this was somewhat less accurate (in both the 18 subjects without shunt and the 9 patients with atrial septal defect and left-to-right shunt) than the formula given in Table 12–2.[5]

Calculation of Left-to-Right Shunt. If there is no evidence of an associated right-to-left shunt, the left-to-right shunt is calculated by:

$$\text{L} \rightarrow \text{R Shunt} = Q_p - Q_s$$
$$(\text{L/min})$$

Examples of Left-to-Right Shunt Detection and Quantification

Some examples of oximetry runs are presented to illustrate interpretation.

Atrial Septal Defect. In the example seen in Figure 12–1, there is a step-up in oxygen saturation in the mid-right atrium. The average or mean value for the vena caval samples in this patient is calculated as [3(SVC) + 1(IVC)] ÷ 4. SVC is the average of SVC samples (i.e., 67.5% in this example), and IVC is the value for the IVC sample taken at the level of the diaphragm only (i.e., 73%). Thus, the vena caval mean O_2 saturation for

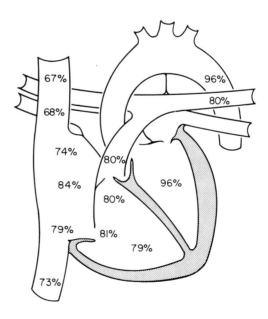

Fig. 12–1. Schematic representation of the results of an oximetry run in a patient with a small to moderate size atrial septal defect. Values represent % O_2 saturation of blood at multiple locations. See text for details.

the patient in Figure 12–1 is $[3(67.5) + 1(73)] \div 4 = 69\%$. The right atrial mean O_2 saturation for this patient is $(74 + 84 + 79) \div 3 = 79\%$. The 10% step-up in mean O_2 saturation from vena cava to right atrium is higher than the 7% value listed in Table 12–1 as a criterion for a significant step-up at the atrial level. Note that for this example, the highest-to-highest approach (highest right atrial O_2 saturation − highest vena caval O_2 saturation) would barely meet criteria for a significant step-up, because of the high value for IVC saturation (73%) compared to SVC saturation. Thus, for the detection of a significant step-up at the atrial level using the highest-to-highest approach, it is best to use the highest SVC sample and compare it to the highest RA sample. In this case, the result would be $(84\% − 68\%) = 16\%$, which is clearly above the 11% value listed in Table 12–1 for detection of a significant step-up. Also, the *"screening samples"* that we recommend for all right heart catheterizations (single sample from SVC and PA) would have strongly indicated a shunt at some level in the right heart, since ΔO_2 saturation from SVC to PA is 12 to 13%, well above the 8% value for a significant step-up.

To calculate pulmonary and systemic blood flows for the example given in Figure 12–1, we need to know O_2 consumption and blood O_2 capacity. If the patient's O_2 consumption determined by the methods described in Chapter 8 is 240 ml O_2/min and the blood hemoglobin concentration is 14 gm%, pulmonary and systemic blood flows may be calculated as follows:

$$Q_p = \frac{O_2 \text{ consumption (ml/min)}}{\begin{bmatrix} PV\ O_2 \\ \text{content} \\ \text{(ml/L)} \end{bmatrix} - \begin{bmatrix} PA\ O_2 \\ \text{content} \\ \text{(ml/L)} \end{bmatrix}}$$

PV O_2 content was not measured, but LV and arterial blood O_2 saturation was 96% (effectively ruling out a right-to-left shunt) and therefore it may be assumed that PV blood O_2 saturation was 96%. As described in Chapter

8, oxygen content for PV blood is calculated as:

$$0.96\left(\frac{14 \text{ gm Hgb}}{100 \text{ ml blood}}\right) \times \left(\frac{1.36 \text{ ml } O_2}{\text{gm Hgb}}\right)$$

$$= 18.3 \text{ ml } O_2/100 \text{ ml blood}$$

$$= 183 \text{ ml } O_2/L$$

Similarly, PA O_2 content is calculated as:

$$0.80(14)1.36 \times 10 = 152 \text{ ml } O_2/L$$

Therefore,

$$Q_p = \frac{240 \text{ ml } O_2/\text{min}}{[183 − 152] \text{ ml } O_2/L} = 7.74 \text{ L/min}$$

Systemic blood flow for the patient in Figure 12–1 is calculated as

$$Q_s = \frac{240 \text{ ml } O_2/\text{min}}{\begin{bmatrix} \text{systemic} \\ \text{arterial} \\ O_2 \text{ content} \end{bmatrix} - \begin{bmatrix} \text{mixed} \\ \text{venous} \\ O_2 \text{ content} \end{bmatrix}}$$

$$= \frac{240}{(0.96 − 0.69)14(1.36)10}$$

$$= 4.6 \text{ Liters/min}$$

For this calculation, mixed venous O_2 saturation was derived from the formula given in Table 12–2, as 69%. Thus, the ratio of Q_p/Q_s in this example is $7.74/4.6 = 1.68$, and the magnitude of the left-to-right shunt is $7.7 − 4.7 = 3$ liters/min. This patient has a small to moderate sized atrial septal defect.

Ventricular Septal Defect. Figure 12–2 shows another example of findings in an oximetry run. In this case, the patient has a large O_2 step-up in the right ventricle, indicating the presence of a ventricular septal defect. If O_2 consumption is 260 ml/min and hemoglobin is 15 gm%,

$$Q_p = \frac{260}{(0.97 − 0.885)15(1.36)10} = 15 \text{ L/min}$$

$$Q_s = \frac{260}{(0.97 − 0.66)15(1.36)10} = 4.1 \text{ L/min}$$

$$Q_p/Q_s = 15/4.1 = 3.7$$

$$L \rightarrow \text{shunt} = 15 − 4.1 = 10.9 \text{ L/min}$$

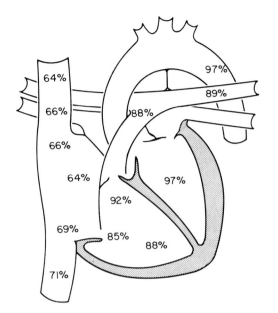

Fig. 12–2. Findings from an oximetry run performed in a patient with a large ventricular septal defect. See text for details.

In this case, the O_2 saturation of mixed venous blood is calculated by averaging the right atrial O_2 saturations because the right atrium is the chamber immediately proximal to the O_2 step-up.

Flow Ratio. The ratio Q_p/Q_s gives important physiologic information about the magnitude of a left-to-right shunt. In addition, because it factors out other variables (e.g., O_2 consumption), it can be calculated from knowledge of blood O_2 saturation alone. A Q_p/Q_s ratio of <1.5 signifies a small left-to-right shunt and is often felt to argue against operative correction, particularly if the patient has an otherwise uncomplicated atrial or ventricular septal defect. A ratio of ≥2.0 indicates a large left-to-right shunt and is generally considered suffi-

cient evidence to recommend surgical repair of the defect, in order to prevent late pulmonary vascular disease as well as other complications of prolonged circulatory overload. Flow ratios between 1.5 and 2.0 are obviously intermediate in magnitude: surgical correction is generally recommended if operative risk is low.

A flow ratio of less than 1.0 indicates a net right-to-left shunt, and is often a sign of the presence of irreversible pulmonary vascular disease.

A *simplified formula* for calculation of flow ratio can be derived by combining the equations for systemic and pulmonary blood flow to obtain:

$$\frac{Q_p}{Q_s} = \frac{(SA\ O_2 - MV\ O_2)}{(PV\ O_2 - PA\ O_2)}$$

where $SA\ O_2$, $MV\ O_2$, $PV\ O_2$, and $PA\ O_2$ are systemic arterial, mixed venous, pulmonary venous, and pulmonary arterial blood oxygen saturations, respectively. For the patient illustrated in Figure 12–1, $Q_p/Q_s = (96\% - 69\%)/(96\% - 80\%) = 1.68$.

Calculation of Bidirectional Shunts. If there is evidence of a right-to-left shunt, as well as a left-to-right shunt, the formulae at the bottom of this page[6] are used.

This formula for calculation of bidirectional shunts tends to be too complex for easy use during the procedure. A quick approximation can be obtained by using a hypothetic quantity known as the *effective blood flow,* the flow that would exist in the absence of any left-to-right or right-to-left shunting:

$$Q_{eff} = \frac{O_2\ consumption\ (ml/min)}{\left[\begin{array}{c}PV\ O_2 \\ content \\ (ml/L)\end{array}\right] - \left[\begin{array}{c}MV\ O_2 \\ content \\ (ml/L)\end{array}\right]}$$

$$L \rightarrow R = \frac{Q_p\ (MV\ O_2\ content - PA\ O_2\ content)}{(MV\ O_2\ content - PV^*\ O_2\ content)}$$

$$R \rightarrow L = \frac{Q_p\ (PV^*\ O_2\ content - SA\ O_2\ content)(PA\ O_2\ content - PV^*\ O_2\ content)}{(SA\ O_2\ content - MV\ O_2\ content) \times (MV\ O_2\ content - PV^*\ O_2\ content)}$$

*If pulmonary vein is not entered, use 98% × O_2 capacity.

The approximate left-to-right shunt then equals $Q_p - Q_{eff}$, while the approximate left-to-right shunt equals $Q_s - Q_{eff}$.

Limitations of Oximetry Method. There are several limitations and potential sources of error in the calculations of blood flow using the data obtained from an oximetry run. A primary source of error may be the absence of a steady state during the collection of blood samples. That is, if the oximetry run is prolonged because of technical difficulties, if the patient is agitated, or if arrhythmias occur during the oximetry run, the data may not be consistent.

An important limitation of the oxygen step-up method for detecting intracardiac shunts is that it lacks sensitivity. Most shunts of a magnitude that would lead to a recommendation for surgical closure of a ventricular septal defect or patent ductus arteriosus are detected by this method. Small shunts, however, are not consistently detected by this technique.

As pointed out by Antman and co-workers,[2] the normal variability of blood oxygen saturation in the right heart chambers is strongly influenced by the magnitude of systemic blood flow. High levels of systemic flow tend to equalize the arterial and venous oxygen values across a given vascular bed. Therefore, elevated systemic blood flow will cause the mixed venous oxygen saturation to be higher than normal, and interchamber variability due to streaming will be blunted. Even a small increase in right heart oxygen saturation under such conditions might indicate the presence of a significant left-to-right shunt; larger increases would indicate voluminous left-to-right shunting of blood. For a patient with a systemic blood flow index of ≤ 3.0 L/min/M[2], minimum shunt sizes that could be detected reliably by oximetry are listed in Table 12–1.

Fundamental to the oximetric method of shunt detection is the fact that left-to-right shunting across an intracardiac defect will cause an increase in *blood O_2 saturation* in the chamber receiving the shunt proportional to the magnitude of the shunt. The increase in *blood O_2 content* in the chamber receiving the shunt, however, depends not only on the magnitude of the shunt, but on the O_2 carrying capacity of the blood (i.e., the hemoglobin concentration). As reported by Antman et al.,[2] the influence of blood hemoglobin concentration may be important when blood O_2 content (rather than O_2 saturation) is used to detect a shunt (Table 12–3).

Thus, the same shunt giving the same blood O_2 saturation step-up would give markedly different blood O_2 content step-ups if the blood hemoglobin concentration varied significantly. Accordingly, when evaluating oximetric data for shunt detection, it is more precise to exclude the potential influence of blood oxygen carrying capacity and use only O_2 saturation data. This is especially true in pediatric cases[4] where the normal blood O_2 carrying capacity may vary from 20 to 28 volumes percent in the neonate to 12 to 16 volumes percent in infancy.

To minimize errors and maximize the physiologic strengths of the oximetry method for shunt detection and quantification, the guidelines listed in Table 12–4 should be followed.

Many more sensitive techniques are avail-

Table 12–3. *Expected Value of O_2 Content (Volumes Percent) for Various Levels of O_2 Step-up and Blood Hemoglobin Concentration†*

Increase in O_2 Saturation	Hemoglobin Concentration (gm/100 ml)		
	10	12	15
5%	0.68 vol%	0.82 vol%	1.02 vol%
10%	1.36 vol%	1.63 vol%	2.04 vol%
15%	2.04 vol%	2.45 vol%	3.06 vol%
20%	2.72 vol%	3.26 vol%	4.08 vol%

†Modified from Antman et al[2] with permission.

able to detect smaller left-to-right shunts, and these are discussed in the following sections.

Early Recirculation of an Indicator

In the presence of a left-to-right shunt, standard indicator dilution curves performed by injection of indocyanine green into the pulmonary artery with sampling in a systemic artery will demonstrate early recirculation on the downslope of the dye curve[7] (Fig. 12–3).

This technique is easily performed and can detect left-to-right shunts too small to be de-

tected by the oxygen step-up method.[8] Thus, if there is no evidence of a left-to-right shunt by this method, there is no need to perform an oximetry run. The studies of Castillo et al[9] suggest that left-to-right shunts as small as 25% of the systemic output can be detected by standard pulmonary artery to systemic artery dye curves.

Although a simple pulmonary to systemic artery dye curve may detect the presence of a shunt, it does not localize it. That is, a pulmonary artery to systemic artery dye curve will show evidence of early recirculation in the presence of a left-to-right shunt due to an atrial septal defect, ventricular septal defect, or patent ductus arteriosus.

Intracardiac defects with left-to-right shunts too small to cause detectable early recirculation on a standard pulmonary to systemic artery dye curve would rarely require surgical closure. When it is pertinent to detect shunts even smaller than those detected by this technique, however, a variety of more sensitive techniques are available.

Early Appearance of an Indicator in the Right Heart

In this technique, an indicator such as indocyanine green[10] is injected into the left heart at the level of, or proximal to, the origin of a left-to-right shunt. Early appearance of the indicator is sought by measuring the appearance of the indicator in right heart blood.

If indocyanine green is used, blood is withdrawn from a standard catheter whose tip is positioned in the pulmonary artery; the blood is passed through a densitometer to determine the appearance time of the indocyanine green in the pulmonary artery. In the presence of a left-to-right shunt, the appearance time will be nearly instantaneous: less than 1 to 2 seconds. In the absence of a left-to-right shunt, the appearance time will be more than 4 to 6 seconds.

The site of the shunt may be localized by varying the injection site (e.g., left atrium, left ventricle, or aorta), or by varying the sampling site until early appearance is no longer present.

Figure 12–4 illustrates the use of this tech-

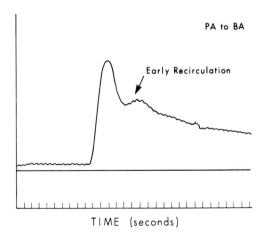

PA to BA

Early Recirculation

TIME (seconds)

Fig. 12–3. Left-to-right shunt. This indicator dilution curve, performed by injecting indocyanine green into the pulmonary artery with sampling in the brachial artery, demonstrates early recirculation on the downslope, indicating a left-to-right shunt. Injection was at time zero. This technique does not localize the site of the left-to-right shunt.

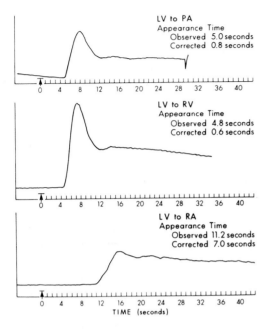

LV to PA
Appearance Time
    Observed 5.0 seconds
    Corrected 0.8 seconds

LV to RV
Appearance Time
    Observed 4.8 seconds
    Corrected 0.6 seconds

LV to RA
Appearance Time
    Observed 11.2 seconds
    Corrected 7.0 seconds

TIME (seconds)

Fig. 12–4. Left-to-right shunt, localization by left-sided injection of indocyanine green dye into the left ventricular (LV) chamber with sampling in the pulmonary artery (PA), right ventricle (RV), and right atrium (RA), demonstrating a ventricular septal defect. See text for details.

nique to detect and localize a left-to-right shunt. The top panel is a dye curve obtained by injecting 1 ml of indocyanine green into the left ventricle with sampling in the pulmonary artery. The appearance time of the dye, when corrected for the time necessary to withdraw blood from the pulmonary artery catheter to the densitometer (4.2 seconds), is less than one second. This early appearance of dye is consistent with a left-to-right shunt at the level of the ventricle (ventricular septal defect) or the aorta (e.g., patent ductus arteriosus), or it could be due to an ostium primum defect with shunting from the left ventricle to the right atrium. The site of the shunt is further localized in the middle panel by sampling from the right ventricle. The appearance remains less than a second; thus the shunt is from the left heart to the right ventricle or to the right atrium. The lower panel shows that the appearance time from the left ventricle to the right atrium is normal. Thus, the shunt is from the left ventricle or aorta to the right ventricle. A subsequent injection into the ascending aorta with

sampling in the right ventricle demonstrated a normal appearance time. This series of dye curves demonstrated that the left-to-right shunt was due to a ventricular septal defect.

This method is very sensitive in detecting small left-to-right shunts across a ventricular septal defect or a patent ductus arteriosus. It is not as well adapted to detecting atrial septal defects because they require entry into the left atrium.

A variety of specialized indicators (e.g., hydrogen gas, krypton-85, nitrous oxide, ascorbic acid, freon, ether) have been used in shunt detection in the past and are still used by some laboratories. The interested reader is referred to the 2nd edition of this textbook, and to the literature.[11–18]

Angiography

Selective angiography is effective in visualizing and localizing the site of left-to-right shunts. In fact, because angiographic demonstration of anatomy has become a routine part of the preoperative evaluation of patients with congenital or acquired shunts, the role of the indicator-dilution techniques just described in localizing the anatomic site of the shunt has been largely superseded. Actually, the use of angiography in this fashion should be considered an indicator-dilution method, with the radiographic contrast agent being the indicator and the cinefluoroscopy unit serving as the "densitometer."

In our laboratory, assessment of the patient with a left-to-right shunt virtually always includes a left ventriculogram. If this is performed in the left anterior oblique projection with cranial angulation (or done as a biplane study with both left and right anterior oblique views), excellent visualization of the interventricular septum, sinuses of Valsalva, and ascending and descending thoracic aorta will allow diagnosis and localization of essentially all the causes of left-to-right shunt other than atrial septal defect and anomalous pulmonary venous return.

Complicated lesions (e.g., endocardial cushion defects, coronary artery-right heart fistulae, ruptured aneurysms at the sinus of Valsalva) commonly require angiographic delineation before surgical intervention can be undertaken. Angiography also helps to assess the "routine" cases more completely. For instance, does the patient with secundum atrial septal defect have associated left ventricular dysfunction or mitral valve prolapse? Does the patient with ventricular septal defect have associated aortic regurgitation (caused by prolapse of the medial aortic leaflet) or infundibular pulmonic stenosis?

Angiography, however, cannot replace the important physiologic measurements that allow quantitation of flow and vascular resistance. Without quantitative evaluation of pulmonary and systemic flows (Q_p and Q_s) and their associated resistances (PVR and SVR), decisions regarding patient management cannot be made, nor can prognosis be assessed.

Radionuclide Techniques

Radionuclide techniques have been developed that have proven to be of substantial value in the detection and quantitation of intracardiac shunts. Because these are not methods that involve cardiac catheterization and angiography, they are discussed only briefly here, and the reader is referred elsewhere for details.[19] The radionuclide techniques rely on the indicator dilution theory. In one method, after oral administration of potassium perchlorate (to block uptake of radionuclide by the thyroid and speed its excretion), technetium 99m as sodium pertechnetate is injected intravenously as a bolus. The adequacy of the bolus should always be checked on a time-activity curve obtained over the superior vena cava. The duration of the bolus should be 2 sec or less. A pattern similar to a left-to-right shunt can be created artificially by a double-peaked injection.

Calculation of the magnitude of a left-to-right shunt by this method assumes that there are no complicating conditions, such as valvular incompetence, large bronchial collaterals, congestive heart failure, or a right-to-left shunt. The technique uses quantitation of radioactivity from various regions of interest within the central circulation. The time activity curves closely resemble indicator dilution curves obtained with indocyanine green. In a patient with a left-to-right shunt, there will be a delay in the disappearance of radionuclide due to early pulmonary recirculation of the left-to-right shunt. Using computer techniques, the area (A) under the first pass curve is extrapolated, as is the area (B) under the early pulmonary recirculation component of the curve. Assuming that the areas are proportional to flows, the following equation is used:

$$\frac{\text{area A}}{\text{area A} - \text{area B}} = \frac{Q_p}{Q_s}$$

where Q_p and Q_s are the pulmonary and systemic flows. Thus, this technique yields a flow ratio but does not give values for the actual flows. The use of collimator techniques and angulated views has greatly increased the ability of this technique to distinguish radioactivity from different cardiac chambers and blood pools. Using such techniques, the *level* of the left-to-right shunt can be detected as the first chamber in which early recirculation is identified.

DETECTION OF RIGHT-TO-LEFT INTRACARDIAC SHUNTS

The primary indication for the use of techniques to detect and localize right-to-left intracardiac shunts is the presence of cyanosis or, more commonly, hypoxemia. The presence of hypoxemia raises two specific questions: First, is the observed hypoxemia due to an intracardiac shunt, or is it due to a ventilation/perfusion imbalance secondary to a variety of forms of intrinsic pulmonary disease? This problem is particularly important in patients with coexistent congenital heart disease and pulmonary disease. Second, if hypoxemia is caused by an intracardiac shunt, what is its site and what is its magnitude?

Attempts to measure right-to-left shunts in patients with cyanotic heart disease date back at least to 1941. Prinzmetal,[20] in a series of ingenious experiments, expanded the earlier observation of Benenson and Hitzig that ether injected intravenously in patients with cyanotic heart disease will cause a prickly, burning sensation of the face.[18] This sensation is caused by the entrance of ether into the systemic circulation of patients with right-to-left shunts. In normal subjects without right-to-left shunts, the ether is eliminated by the lungs and thus does not reach the systemic circulation. Prinzmetal then measured the time necessary for an intravenous injection of a dilute solution of saccharin to be tasted. This time is equal to the transit time from a peripheral vein through the lungs, through the left heart, and then to the systemic circulation. By increasing the concentration of the saccharin he found that a second, much shorter appearance time occurred in patients with cyanotic heart disease because of the presence of a right-to-left shunt bypassing the pulmonary circulation. He then estimated the percent right-to-left shunt by the following formula:

$$\% \, R \rightarrow L \text{ Shunt} = \frac{A}{A + C}$$

where A is the smallest concentration of saccharin to be tasted by way of the long circuit, and C is the smallest concentration of saccharin to be tasted by the short circuit. Our current methods of documenting and quantitating right-to-left shunts may not be as ingenious and certainly are not as sweet, but they are nonetheless effective.

Angiography

With appropriate techniques, angiography may be used to demonstrate right-to-left intracardiac shunts. This method is particularly important in detecting right-to-left shunting due to a pulmonary arteriovenous fistula. In this circumstance, the shunt cannot be detected by indicator dilution curves on the basis of a shortened appearance time. That is, the difference in transit time when the pulmonary capillaries are bypassed is not perceptible by standard indicator dilution techniques. Although angiography may localize right-to-left shunts, it does not permit quantification.

Oximetry

The site of right-to-left shunts may be localized if blood samples can be obtained from a pulmonary vein, the left atrium, left ventricle, and aorta. The pulmonary venous blood of patients with hypoxemia caused by an intracardiac right-to-left shunt is fully saturated. Therefore, the site of a right-to-left shunt may be localized by noting which left heart chamber is the first to show desaturation; i.e., a step-down in oxygen concentration. That is, if left atrial saturation is normal, but desaturation is present in the left ventricle and in the systemic circulation, the right-to-left shunt is across a ventricular septal defect. The only disadvantage of this technique is that a pulmonary vein and the left atrium must be entered. This is not feasible in adults as often as it is in infants, in whom the left atrium may be entered by way of the foramen ovale.

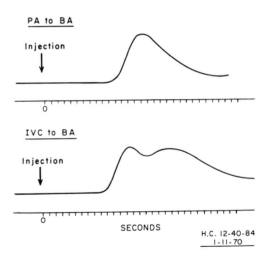

Fig. 12–5. Demonstration of a right-to-left shunt by indicator dilution curves. The top panel illustrated injection of indocyanine green into the pulmonary artery (PA) with sampling at the brachial artery (BA). There is a normal upstroke, with no early appearance of indicator in the systemic circulation. The lower panel shows a "double hump" contour, indicating early appearance of indicator in the systemic circulation when it is injected into the inferior vena cava (IVC). These two curves suggest the presence of a right-to-left shunt at either the atrial or ventricular level.

Early Appearance of an Indicator in the Systemic Circulation

A variety of techniques are based on the fact that, if an indicator is injected proximal to the site of a right-to-left shunt, its appearance time in the systemic circulation will be perceptibly shortened.

Swan and co-workers[21] demonstrated that injection of Evans blue proximal to the site of a right-to-left shunt with sampling in a systemic artery produces a distinctive indicator dilution curve. There is an early hump in the dye curve before the primary peak (Fig. 12–5). This technique, using *indocyanine green,* can detect right-to-left shunts as small as 2.5% of the systemic output.[9] This method is simple and sensitive. Injection of indocyanine green into the inferior vena cava will detect right-to-left shunts at the level of the atrium, ventricle, and pulmonary artery. The site of the shunt is then localized by injecting

more distally until the early appearance hump is no longer noted in the dye curve. For example, if the right-to-left shunt is an atrial septal defect, early appearance of the dye will be noted with injection into the inferior vena cava, but not with injection into the right ventricle. It should be noted that right-to-left shunting across an atrial septal defect or patent foramen ovale is best detected by injection into the inferior vena cava, because of preferential streaming of blood from the inferior vena cava toward the region of the fossa ovalis.[22]

In the case of small right-to-left shunts at the atrial level, the magnitude of the shunt can be increased and thus more easily detected if dye is injected into the IVC while the patient performs a Valsalva maneuver (Fig. 12–6). This maneuver transiently increases right atrial pressure more than left atrial pressure, and thus increases the volume of the right-to-left shunt.[23]

The prime advantage of the indocyanine green method for detecting right-to-left shunts is that it is on-line and requires equipment that is available in most cardiac catheterization laboratories.

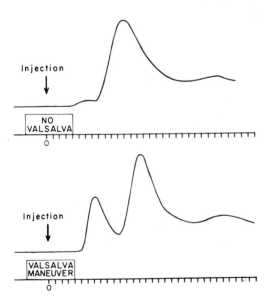

Fig. 12–6. Detection of right-to-left shunt by inferior vena cava (IVC) dye curves with and without Valsalva maneuver. A small right-to-left shunt is suggested by the early appearance in the upstroke of an IVC to brachial artery dye curve in the top panel. The early appearance becomes much more obvious when the dye curve is recorded during a Valsalva maneuver (bottom panel). The Valsalva maneuver transiently increases right atrial pressure with respect to left atrial pressure and thereby increases the magnitude of right-to-left shunts at the atrial level.

Echocardiographic Methods

Finally, echocardiographic methods have proven sensitive for the detection and localization of left-to-right and right-to-left shunts. The so-called echocardiographic contrast or "bubble study" using agitated saline solution with microbubbles can detect small shunts, and the use of two-dimensional echocardiographic techniques can often localize the site of the shunt to the atrial or ventricular septum. Combined echocardiographic and cardiac catheterization studies allow injection of the echo contrast agent into the right or left heart chambers sequentially, thus permitting localization of the shunt and determination as to whether it is unidirectional or bidirectional. Echo-Doppler techniques can also be used to detect and localize intracardiac shunts. In this regard, color Doppler echocardiography is particularly useful in detecting and localizing small intracardiac shunts without the need for

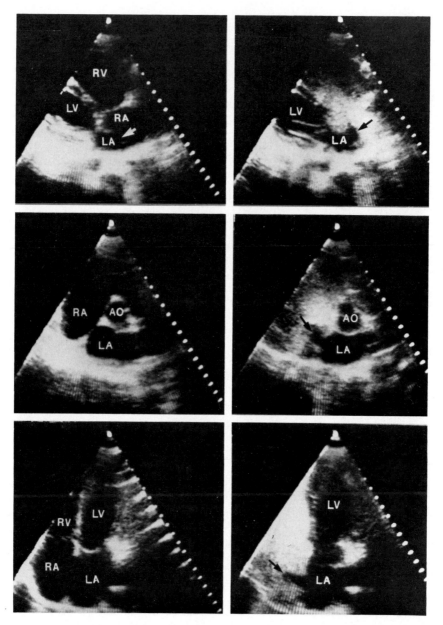

Fig. 12–7. Two-dimensional echo showing right ventricular (RV) inflow tract (upper panels), short axis views at the base (middle panels) and four chamber apical view (bottom panels) in a patient with an atrial septal defect (ASD) shown at cardiac catheterization to be associated with a Q_p/Q_s of 3.0. The left side of each panel shows the anatomy before echo contrast injection. Following an intravenous injection of agitated saline solution (right side of each panel), a negative contrast effect (black arrows) is seen within the right atrium (RA), compatible with entry of unopacified blood from the left atrium (LA) across the ASD into the RA. The ASD is visualized (white arrow) as an area of septal dropout. (Reproduced from Come PC, Riley M: Contrast echocardiography. *In* Come PC (ed.): Diagnostic Cardiology: Noninvasive Imaging Techniques. Philadelphia: JB Lippincott Co, 1984, p. 294, with permission.)

injection of an echo contrast agent. An example of the use of echo-contrast technique for the detection of an atrial septal defect with left-to-right shunting is shown in Figure 12–7. A full description of the use of echo-Doppler techniques in the detection of shunts is given in Dr. Patricia Come's textbook.[24]

REFERENCES

1. Dexter L et al: Studies of congenital heart disease. II. The pressure and oxygen content of blood in the right auricle, right ventricle, and pulmonary artery in control patients, with observations on the oxygen saturation and source of pulmonary capillary blood. J Clin Invest 26:554, 1947.
2. Antman EM, Marsh JD, Green LH, Grossman W: Blood oxygen measurements in the assessment of intracardiac left to right shunts: a critical appraisal of methodology. Am J Cardiol 46:265, 1980.
3. Barratt-Boyes BF, Wood EH: The oxygen saturation of blood in the vena cavae, right heart chambers, and pulmonary vessels of healthy subjects. J Lab Clin Med 50:93, 1957.
4. Freed MD, Miettinen OS, Nadas AS: Oximetric determination of intracardiac left to right shunts. Br Heart J 42:690, 1979.
5. Flamm MD, Cohn KE, Hancock EW: Measurement of systemic cardiac output at rest and exercise in patients with atrial septal defect. Am J Cardiol 23:258, 1969.
6. Dexter L et al: Studies of congenital heart disease. I. Technique of venous catheterization as a diagnostic procedure. J Clin Invest 26:547, 1947.
7. Swan HJC, Wood EH: Localization of cardiac defects by dye-dilution curves recorded after injection of T-1824 at multiple sites in the heart and great vessels during cardiac catheterization. Proc Staff Meet Mayo Clin 28:95, 1953.
8. Hyman AL et al: A comparative study of the detection of cardiovascular shunts by oxygen analysis and indicator dilution methods. Ann Intern Med 56:535, 1962.
9. Castillo CA, Kyle JC, Gilson WE, Rowe GG: Simulated shunt curves. Am J Cardiol 17:691, 1966.
10. Braunwald E, Tannenbaum HL, Morrow AG: Localization of left-to-right cardiac shunts by dye-dilution curves following injection into the left side of the heart and into the aorta. Am J Med 24:203, 1958.
11. Long RTL, Braunwald E, Morrow AG: Intracardiac injection of radioactive krypton: clinical applications of new methods for characterization of circulatory shunts. Circulation 21:1126, 1960.
12. Levy AM, Monroe RG, Hugenholtz PG, Nadas AS: Clinical use of ascorbic acid as an indicator of right-to-left shunt. Br Heart J 29:22, 1967.
13. Hugenholtz PG et al: The clinical usefulness of hydrogen gas as an indicator of left-to-right shunts. Circulation 28:542, 1963.
14. Amplatz K et al: The Freon test: a new sensitive technic for the detection of small cardiac shunts. Circulation 39:551, 1969.
15. Singleton RT, Dembo DH, Scherlis L: Krypton-85 in the detection of intracardiac left-to-right shunts. Circulation 32:134, 1965.
16. Morrow AG, Sanders RJ, Braunwald E: The nitrous oxide test: An improved method for the detection of left-to-right shunts. Circulation 17:284, 1958.
17. Long RT, Waldhausen JA, Cornell WP, Sanders RJ: Detection of right-to-left circulatory shunts: A new method utilizing injections of krypton-85. Proc Soc Exp Biol Med 102:456, 1959.
18. Benenson W, Hitzig LWM: Diagnosis of venous arterial shunt by ether circulation time method. Proc Soc Exp Biol Med 38:256, 1938.
19. Parker JA, Treves S: Radionuclide detection, localization, and quantitation of intracardiac shunts and shunts between the great arteries. Prog Cardiovasc Dis 20 (No. 1–4):189, 1977–1978.
20. Prinzmetal M: Calculation of the venous arterial shunt in congenital heart disease. J Clin Invest 20:705, 1941.
21. Swan HJC, Zapata-Diaz J, Wood EH: Dye dilution curves in cyanotic congenital heart disease. Circulation 8:70, 1953.
22. Swan HJC, Burchell HB, Wood EH: The presence of venoarterial shunts in patients with interatrial communications. Circulation 10:705–713, 1954.
23. Banas JS et al: A simple technique for detecting small defects of the atrial septum. Am J Cardiol 28:467, 1971.
24. Come P (ed.): Diagnostic Cardiology: Non-Invasive Imaging Techniques. Philadelphia, JB Lippincott Co., 1984, p 294.

Part IV

Angiographic Techniques

13

Coronary Angiography

DONALD S. BAIM and WILLIAM GROSSMAN

B ecause of progressive evolution in catheter design, radiographic imaging, contrast media, and options for the treatment of coronary artery disease (bypass surgery and angioplasty), diagnostic coronary angiography has become a safe and widely practiced component of cardiac catheterization. It is estimated that more than 600,000 coronary angiographic procedures (roughly 300/100,000 population) are performed each year in the United States, with a procedure-related mortality of 0.1%.[1,2] In each procedure, the objective is to examine the entire coronary tree, recording details of coronary anatomy, including individual variations in arterial distribution, anatomic or functional pathology (atherosclerosis, thrombosis, congenital anomalies, or focal coronary spasm), and the presence of inter- and intracoronary collateral connections. With repeat intracoronary contrast injections in a series of angulated views, a high-resolution image intensifier, and 35 mm cineangiographic film or other recording media, it is possible to define all portions of the coronary arterial circulation down to vessels as small as 0.2 mm, and to eliminate artifacts caused by vessel overlap or foreshortening.

CURRENT INDICATIONS

There are a variety of current indications for coronary angiography, based on the principle stated by F. Mason Sones that coronary arteriography is indicated when a problem is encountered that may be resolved by the objective demonstration of the coronary tree, provided competent personnel and adequate facilities are available and the potential risks are acceptable to the patient and his physician. The most frequent such indication is the further evaluation of patients in whom the diagnosis of coronary atherosclerosis is almost certain.[3] This includes patients with angina pectoris refractory to medical therapy, in whom anatomic correction by means of coronary bypass surgery or transluminal coronary angioplasty is contemplated. In such patients, angiographic evaluation of coronary anatomy provides a crucial anatomic guide to the revascularization procedure. In patients with less severe anginal symptoms, coronary angiography may still be indicated if the clinical setting or noninvasive testing suggest a higher-than-usual probability of severe multivessel disease or left main coronary stenosis.[3,4] Some cardiologists also favor angiographic evaluation of patients with new onset, unstable, or postinfarction angina, as well as younger patients recovering from an uncomplicated myocardial infarction.[4] Moreover, while patients with acute myocardial infarction were formerly subjected to coronary angiography only when ongoing ischemic events or the presence of a mechanical defect (papillary muscle rupture, ventricular septal defect, or large left ventricular aneurysm with

185

shock) compelled early surgical intervention, the advent of thrombolytic therapy and coronary angioplasty has demonstrated the relative safety of coronary angiography in this setting. Controlled trials, however, have failed to demonstrate a clear benefit for routine catheterization or angioplasty in acute infarction patients treated with intravenous tissue plasminogen activator within 4 hours of symptom onset.[5]

A second group of indications for coronary angiography concerns patients in whom the presence or absence of coronary artery disease is unclear. This includes patients with troublesome chest pain syndromes but ambiguous noninvasive test results, patients with unexplained heart failure or ventricular arrhythmias, and patients with suspected or proven variant angina.[4] Finally, coronary angiography is widely used in the preoperative evaluation of patients scheduled for the correction of congenital or valvular pathology. Patients with congenital defects such as tetralogy of Fallot frequently have anomalies of coronary distribution that may lead to surgical complications if unrecognized,[6] and other patients with valvular disease may have advanced coronary atherosclerosis. Although younger patients with valvular disease are commonly operated on without prior coronary angiograms, most surgical centers believe it critical to recognize and correct significant coronary lesions to provide the best and safest outcome during concurrent valve replacement.[7]

TECHNIQUE

The initial attempts to perform coronary angiography used nonselective injections of contrast medium into the aortic root with simultaneous opacification of both the left and right coronary arteries and recording of the angiographic images on conventional sheet film.[8] To improve contrast delivery into the coronary ostia, some early investigators employed transient circulatory arrest induced by the administration of acetylcholine or by elevation of intrabronchial pressure, followed by occlusion of the ascending aorta by gas-filled balloon and

injection of the contrast bolus. Although nonselective aortic root injection is still used today to evaluate ostial lesions, anomalous coronary ostia, or coronary bypass grafts, intentional circulatory arrest is no longer practiced, and the nonselective technique has largely been replaced by selective coronary injection using specially designed catheters advanced from either the brachial or the femoral approach.

In most patients, successful coronary angiography can be performed by either the brachial or the femoral approach, leaving the choice up to physician and patient. The brachial approach may offer a selective advantage in patients with severe peripheral vascular disease or known abdominal aortic aneurysm, whereas small elderly women are frequently more easily studied by the femoral approach. In either case, it is important for the catheterization team to meet the patient before the actual procedure to evaluate the best approach to catheterization, to gain an appreciation of the clinical questions that need to be answered by coronary angiography, to uncover any history of adverse reaction to medications or organic iodine compounds, and to explain the procedure in detail. Although coronary angiography has been widely performed as an inpatient procedure, many centers have adopted outpatient protocols for selected low-risk patients,[9,10] usually using either the brachial or the femoral approach. In either case, preparation for catheterization should include proscription of oral intake except for medications and limited quantities of clear liquids over the 6 to 8 hours before catheterization, a baseline 12-lead electrocardiogram, and a suitable sedative premedication (usually diazepam, 5 to 10 mg p.o., and diphenhydramine, 50 mg p.o.) administered on call to the catheterization laboratory. We do not routinely premedicate patients with either atropine or nitroglycerine, although both are immediately on hand if needed.

The Femoral Approach

As described in Chapter 5, the femoral approach to left heart catheterization involves insertion of the catheter either directly over a guide wire or through an introducing sheath. Systemic anticoagulation (heparin, 5000 units) is used by most laboratories utilizing this approach.[8] A series of preformed catheters are employed, usually a pigtail catheter for left ventriculography and separate catheters (either Judkins or Amplatz shapes) for cannulation of the left and right coronary arteries. Coronary catheters are available in either 7 or 8 Fr endhole design, with a shaft that tapers to 5 Fr near the tip. They may be constructed of either polyethylene (Cook Inc, Bloomington, IN) or polyurethane (Cordis, Miami, FL, and USCI, Billerica, MA) and contain either steel braid or nylon within the catheter wall to provide the excellent torque control needed for coronary cannulation. Although the 8 Fr catheters have traditionally permitted more rapid contrast delivery, recent improvements in the design of 7 Fr catheters (Cordis High Flow, USCI Nycore or Proflow) allow a lumen comparable in diameter to that of a standard 8 Fr catheter. Smaller (6 and even 5 Fr) coronary angiographic catheters have been designed and promoted for outpatient examinations, but we still prefer the large lumen 7 Fr catheters for their superior maneuverability and contrast injection characteristics.[11] On occasion, we even resort to 8 Fr catheters for better catheter control in the face of a widened aortic root or marked iliac tortuosity. Coronary catheters used for either the femoral or brachial approach are shown in Figure 13–1.

The desired catheter is advanced to the level of the left mainstem bronchus with the guide wire in place. The guide wire is then removed, and the catheter is attached to a specially designed manifold system which permits the maintenance of a "closed system" during pressure monitoring, catheter flushing, and contrast agent administration (Fig. 13–2). The catheter is immediately double-flushed: blood is withdrawn and discarded, and heparinized saline flush is injected through the catheter lumen. Difficulty in blood withdrawal suggests apposition of the catheter tip to the aortic wall, which can be rectified by slight advancement or rotation of the catheter until free blood withdrawal is possible. If an introducing sheath is used, its lumen should also be flushed immediately during each catheter insertion, after each catheter removal, and every 5 minutes thereafter to prevent the encroachment of blood into the sheath. Once the catheter has been flushed with saline solution, tip pressure should be monitored at all times except during actual contrast injections. Next, the catheter lumen should be gently filled with contrast agent under fluoroscopic visualization, avoiding selective contrast administration into small arterial vessels. Filling with contrast results in a slight reduction in high frequency components of the aortic pressure waveform, which should be noted carefully and compared continuously to the femoral sidearm pressure. Any change in waveform during coronary angiography (see damping and ventricularization, below) may signify an ostial coronary stenosis or an unfavorable catheter position within the coronary artery. The coronary angiographic catheter is then advanced around the arch into the ascending aorta under continuous pressure monitoring and fluoroscopic imaging in the left anterior oblique projection.

Cannulation of the left coronary ostium with the Judkins technique is usually easy to accomplish. As Judkins himself has stated, "No points are earned for coronary catheterization—the catheters know where to go if not thwarted by the operator."[12] If a left Judkins catheter with a 4 cm curve (commonly referred to as a JL4) is simply allowed to remain en face as it is advanced down into the aortic root, it will engage the left coronary ostium without further manipulation in 80 to 90% of patients (Fig. 13–3). Engagement should take place with the arm of the catheter traversing the ascending aorta at an angle of approximately 45 degrees, the tip of the catheter in a more or less horizontal orientation, and with no change in the pressure waveform recorded from the catheter tip.

Damping and Ventricularization. A fall in overall catheter tip pressure (damping) or a fall in diastolic pressure only (ventricularization) (Fig. 13–4) indicates restriction of coronary inflow because of insertion of the catheter tip

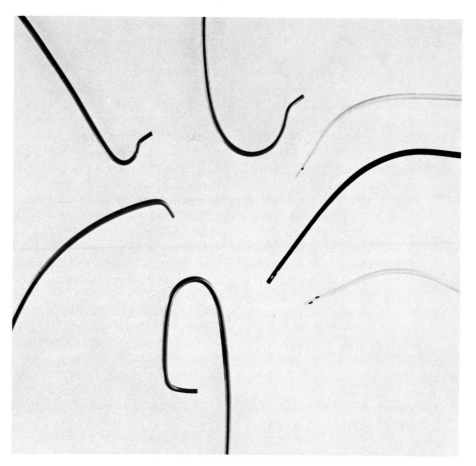

Fig. 13–1.   Different types of catheters currently in wide use for selective coronary angiography. At the bottom, center, is the left coronary Judkins catheter. Proceeding clockwise from this catheter are the right coronary Judkins catheter, the right (R2) and left (L3) Amplatz catheters, the Schoonmaker multipurpose catheter, the Standard Sones catheter (woven Dacron, USCI), the polyurethrane, Sones-type catheter (Cordis). (See text for discussion.)

into a proximal coronary stenosis or to an adverse catheter lie against the coronary wall. If either of these phenomena is observed, the catheter should be withdrawn into the aortic root immediately until the operator can analyze the situation further using nonselective injections into the sinus of Valsalva or cautious small injections into the coronary artery followed immediately by catheter withdrawal. *Vigorous injection despite a damped or ventricularized pressure waveform predisposes to dissection of the proximal coronary artery, and may lead to major ischemic complications.*

In patients with a widened aortic root due to aortic valve disease or long-standing hy-pertension, the 4 cm left Judkins curve may be too short to allow successful engagement: the catheter arm may lie nearly horizontally across the aortic root with the tip pointing vertically against the roof of the left main artery, or the catheter may even refold into its packaged shape during advancement into the aortic root. In this case, a left Judkins catheter with a larger (5 cm or even 6 cm) curve should be selected, rather than persevering in an effort to make an unsuitable catheter work. On the other hand, even the 4 cm Judkins curve may be too long for the occasional patient with a short or narrow aortic root: the catheter arm may lie nearly vertically with the tip pointing inferiorly. Despite this somewhat unfavorable

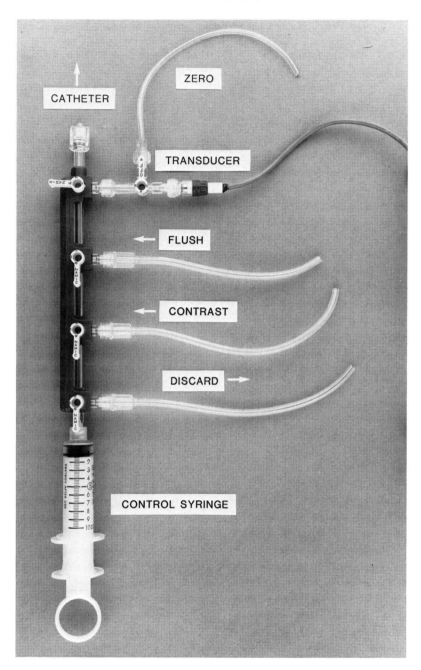

Fig. 13–2. Four-port coronary manifold (Namic). This manifold provides a closed system with which blood can be withdrawn from the catheter and discarded, the catheter can be filled with either flush solution or contrast medium, and catheter pressure can be observed, all under the control of a series of stopcocks. The fourth port is connected to an empty plastic bag and is used as a discard port (for blood from the double flush, air bubbles) so that the syringe need not be disconnected from the manifold at any time during the procedure. Attachment of the transducer directly to the manifold allows optimum pressure waveform fidelity (see Chapter 9), and the fluid-filled reference line allows zeroing of the transducer to midchest level.

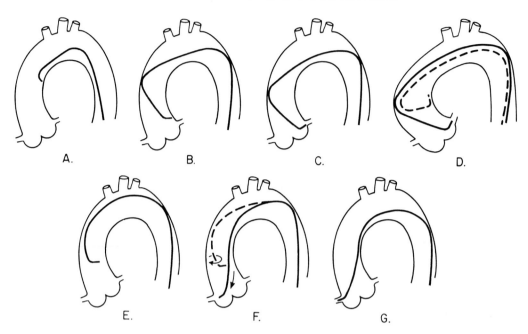

Fig. 13–3. Judkins technique for catheterization of the left and right coronary arteries as viewed in the LAO projection. In a patient with a normal sized aortic arch, simple advancement of the JL4 catheter leads to intubation of the left coronary ostium (A, B, and C). In a patient with an enlarged aortic root (D) the arm of the JL4 may be too short, causing the catheter tip to point upward or even flip back into its packaged shape (dotted catheter). A catheter with an appropriately longer arm (a JL5 or JL6) is required. To catheterize the right coronary ostium, the right Judkins catheter is advanced around the aortic arch with its tip directed leftward, as viewed in the LAO projection, until it reaches a position 2 to 3 cm above the level of the left coronary ostium (E). Clockwise rotation causes the catheter tip to drop into the aortic root and point anteriorly (F). Slight further rotation causes the catheter tip to enter the right coronary ostium (G).

situation, the left ostium may still be engaged by pushing the catheter down into the left sinus of Valsalva for approximately 10 seconds to tighten the angle on the catheter tip, and then withdrawing the catheter slowly. Having the patient take a deep breath during this maneuver pulls the heart into a more vertical position and may also assist in engagement of the left ostium. The most satisfactory approach, however, is exchanging for a catheter with a 3.5 cm curve.

Occasionally, the operator may choose a left Amplatz catheter (Fig. 13–1) (available in progressively larger curves—1, 2, 3, 4) rather than a left Judkins catheter. The Amplatz family of catheters is more tolerant of rotational maneuvering during engagement of left coronary ostia which are positioned out of the conventional Judkins plane, and allows easy subselective engagement of the left anterior descending and circumflex coronary arteries in

patients with short left main coronary segments or separate left coronary ostia.[13] The left Amplatz is advanced around the arch oriented toward the left coronary ostium (Fig. 13–5). The tip of the catheter usually comes to rest in the sinus of Valsalva below the coronary ostium. As the catheter is advanced further, however, the Amplatz shape causes the tip of the catheter to ride up the wall of the sinus until it engages the ostium. At that point, slight withdrawal of the catheter causes deeper engagement of the coronary ostium, whereas further slight advancement causes paradoxical retraction of the catheter tip.

Cannulation of the right coronary ostium by the Judkins technique requires slightly more catheter manipulation than cannulation of the left coronary ostium.[8,12] After being flushed and filled with contrast in the descending aorta (with the catheter tip directed anteriorly to avoid injection into the intercostal arteries),

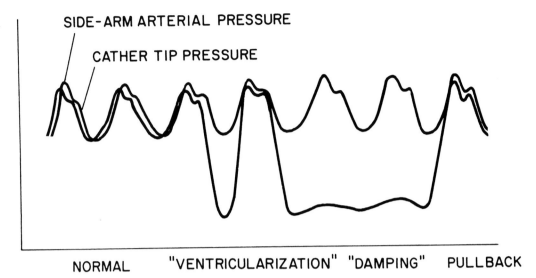

SIDE-ARM ARTERIAL PRESSURE

CATHER TIP PRESSURE

NORMAL   "VENTRICULARIZATION" "DAMPING"   PULLBACK

Fig. 13–4.   Pressure tracings as recorded during coronary angiography. Except for its earlier phase and slightly lower systolic pressure, catheter tip pressure should resemble the pressure waveform simultaneously monitored by way of the femoral sidearm sheath or other arterial monitor (e.g., radial artery). In the presence of an ostial stenosis or an unfavorable catheter position against the vessel wall, the waveform shows either ''ventricularization'' (in which systolic pressure is preserved but diastolic pressure is reduced) or frank ''damping'' (in which both systolic and diastolic pressures are reduced). In either case, the best approach is to withdraw the catheter immediately until the waveform returns to normal and to attempt to define the cause of the problem by nonselective injections in the sinus of Valsalva.

the right Judkins catheter with a 4 cm curve (JR4) is brought around the aortic arch with the tip facing inward until it comes to lie against the right side of the aortic root with its tip aimed toward the left coronary ostium (Fig. 13–3). In a left anterior oblique projection, the operator slowly and carefully rotates the catheter clockwise by nearly 180 degrees to engage the right coronary artery. Because of its tertiary

curve, the tip of the right Judkins catheter tends to drop more deeply into the aortic root as the catheter is rotated toward the right ostium. To compensate for this effect, the operator must either begin the rotational maneuver with the tip 2 to 3 cm above the coronary ostium, or withdraw the catheter slowly during rotation. Care must be taken to avoid ''over-rotation'' of the catheter, which may lead to undesirably

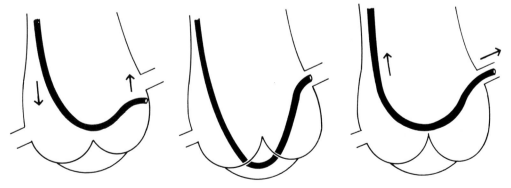

Fig. 13–5.   Catheterization of the left coronary with an Amplatz catheter. The catheter should be advanced into the ascendng aorta with its tip pointing downward, so that the terminal catheter configuration resembles a diving duck. As the Amplatz catheter is advanced into the left sinus of Valsalva, its tip initially lies below the left coronary ostium (left). Further advancement causes the tip to ride up the aortic wall and enter the ostium (center). Slight withdrawal of the catheter causes the tip to seat more deeply in the ostium (right).

deep engagement of the right coronary artery. To avoid this common technical error, it is wise to apply a small amount of counterclockwise torque as soon as the catheter has entered the ostium. Catheters with smaller (3.5 cm) or larger (5 or 6 cm) Judkins curves or right Amplatz catheters (AR 1 or AR 2) may be of value if aortic root configuration and proximal right coronary anatomy make engagement difficult. Damping and ventricularization are far more common in the right coronary artery than in the left, and may be caused by: (1) the generally smaller caliber of the vessel, (2) ostial spasm around the catheter tip, (3) subselective engagement of the conus branch, or (4) true ostial stenosis. These problems in right coronary engagement can usually be elucidated by nonselective injections into the right sinus of Valsalva or cautious injections in a damped position with immediate postinjection withdrawal of the catheter.

Bypass Graft Catheterization. As increasing numbers of patients develop recurrent angina after prior bypass surgery, roughly 10% of our diagnostic procedures now involve cannulating one or more bypass grafts. The most common graft conduit remains the saphenous vein graft, originating from the right or left anterior aortic surface several centimeters above the sinuses of Valsalva. Because many surgeons resist the practice of placing radioopaque markers on the proximal graft anastomosis, the catheterizer must generally rely on the operative report or diagram, and his knowledge of surgical practice in his own institution.

Most commonly, grafts to the left coronary arise from left anterior surface of the aorta, with grafts to the left anterior descending, originating somewhat lower than grafts to the circumflex system. Grafts to the right coronary (or the distal portions of a dominant circumflex) usually originate from the right anterior surface of the aorta, somewhat behind the plane of the native right coronary ostium. To engage these grafts, the catheter tip should be oriented against the appropriate aortic wall, and slowly advanced and withdrawn until it "catches" in a graft ostium, a process that is

repeated until all graft sites have been identified. The right Judkins and Amplatz catheters can be used for this purpose, but their tips do not always remain in contact with the wall of the ascending aorta and frequently do not align well with the proximal portion of the vein graft (particularly grafts to the right coronary that originate somewhat posteriorly, and then course anteriorly). Although some operators rely on multipurpose (i.e., Schoonmaker[14]) or special preformed vein graft catheters, we prefer using a soft catheter with a pronounced secondary curve and no primary curve (Wexler catheter, Cook or Angiomedics). It remains in contact with the aortic wall, and can be rotated or flexed into alignment with the proximal graft once the ostium has been selected.

Based on a demonstrated superior 10-year patency compared to saphenous venous grafts, the left (and now the right) internal mammary arteries have become increasingly more common graft conduits[15] (Fig. 13–6). In our center, nearly 90% of current elective bypass procedures involve at least one such graft. Despite excellent long-term results, these grafts may develop stenoses (particularly at the distal mammary-coronary anastomosis), and must be evaluated during a catheterization performed for post-bypass angina.

Although mammary grafts can be studied easily from the ipsilateral brachial approach, we prefer the femoral approach using a soft-tip preformed internal mammary catheter (Angiomedics), which resembles a right Judkins catheter except for a tighter primary curve. This catheter is advanced with 1 to 2 cm or J guide wire protruding from its tip, until it lies just inside the left (or right) edge of the wedge-like shadow formed by the upper mediastinum against the lung fields. Counterclockwise rotation sweeps the wire into the subclavian artery origin, from whence it can be advanced well out into the axillary artery (Fig. 13–6B). The mammary catheter is then advanced over the wire, after which the guide wire is removed and the catheter is flushed and filled with contrast. A nonionic or dimeric (Hexabrix) contrast agent should be used to avoid potential CNS toxicity by reflux of hyperosmolar ionic

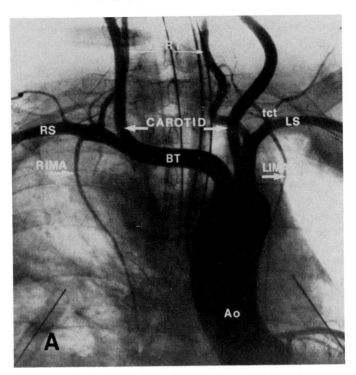

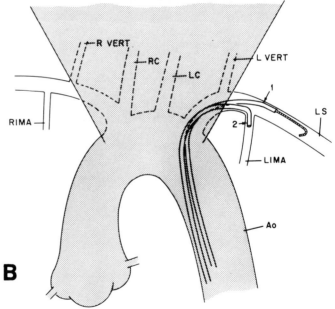

Fig. 13–6. Internal mammary angiography. A. Aortic arch injection shows the left internal mammary artery (LIMA) originating from the left subclavian (LS), just opposite the thyrocervical trunk (tct) and distal to the right vertebral (VERT). The right internal mammary artery (RIMA) originates from the right subclavian (RS), just distal to the bifurcation of the right carotid from the brachiocephalic trunk (BT). B. Schematic diagram shows the corresponding arch vessel origins. Note that the left subclavian originates just inside the patient's leftmost edge of the wedge-shaped shadow cast by the upper-mediastinal structures in the left anterior oblique projection. Catheter manipulation in this projection facilitates advancement of a guide wire into the LS (step 1), facilitating selective cannulation of the LIMA during catheter withdrawal and slight counterclockwise rotation (step 2, see text).

contrast up the verterbral arteries. The catheter is rotated somewhat anteriorly, using intermittent gentle contrast puffs as it is withdrawn slowly in the straight AP projection until the internal mammary is engaged. Great care should be taken to avoid catheter tip trauma/ dissection of the relatively delicate mammary vessel. If selective cannulation is difficult because of tortuosity or anatomic variations, a variety of super-selective or non-selective techniques can be used to permit internal mammary angiographic evaluation.[15]

Taken together, the left and right internal mammary arteries can be used to revascularize most lesions in the left anterior descending, proximal circumflex, and proximal right coronary arteries, but most revascularization procedures still suffer the limitations associated with the use of saphenous veins. More recently, several groups have begun exploring the use of the right gastroepiploic artery as a graft to the posterior descending or other vessels on the inferior surface of the heart.[16] The right gastroepiploic artery originates from the gastroduodenal branch of the celiac artery, and normally supplies the majority of the greater curvature of the stomach. Angiography of this vessel is possible using standard visceral angiographic catheters,[17] but remains uncommon enough that few laboratories have accumulated significant experience.

The Brachial Approach

The technique of brachial artery cutdown has been described previously in Chapter 4. The catheter designed by Dr. F. Mason Sones, Jr., is a thin-walled radiopaque woven Dacron catheter with a 2.67 mm (8 French) external diameter to its shaft.[18]* The tip is open, and in current models two side holes are arranged in opposed pairs within 7 mm of its distal end. The shaft tapers abruptly to 5 Fr external diameter at a point 5 cm from its tip. As Sones has stated, this provides a "flexible finger" that may be curved upward into the coronary orifices by pressure of the more rigid shaft against the aortic valve cusps. This standard catheter is available in lengths of 80, 100, and 125 cm and in 7 and 8 Fr sizes.

Some operators use a Sones type of coronary catheter constructed of polyurethane and made by Cordis Corporation.† This catheter has the same shape and taper as the woven Dacron catheter and has an end hole with four side holes within 7 mm of its tip. This catheter traverses a tortuous subclavian system with

*United States Catheter and Instrument Co., Billerica, MA.

†80 cm Cordis brachial coronary A, Sones technique, type II.

much greater facility and smoothness than does the woven Dacron catheter, and its enhanced torque control and reduced friction coefficient permit greater ease in engaging the coronary ostia. It is the first choice for coronary angiography of one of us (WG). It will pass an 0.035-inch guide wire, and is an excellent catheter for crossing a stenotic aortic valve. Figure 13–1 shows a variety of coronary catheters effective with the brachial approach.

When the Sones method is used, once the catheter enters the brachial artery, pressure should be monitored, and further passage of the catheter into the subclavian and innominate arteries should be accomplished with pressure monitoring and fluoroscopic visualization. Occasionally, it will be difficult to pass the catheter from the subclavian artery to the aortic arch, but a simple maneuver by the patient, such as a deep inspiration, shrugging the shoulders, or turning his head to the left, often facilitates passage of the catheter into the ascending aorta. If passage of the catheter from the subclavian artery to the ascending aorta is not accomplished immediately and with complete ease, the operator should stop catheter manipulation and use a soft J-tipped 0.035-inch guide wire. Once the catheter is in the ascending aorta, the guide wire is removed and the catheter is aspirated, flushed, and reconnected to the rotating adaptor of the manifold, either directly or by a short length of large-bore flexible connecting tubing.

With the Sones technique, selective engagement of the *left coronary artery* is accomplished as follows. In a left anterior oblique projection, the sinus of Valsalva containing the ostium of the left coronary artery lies to the left, and the sinus containing the ostium of the right coronary artery lies to the right. The noncoronary sinus lies posteriorly. The operator advances the catheter to the aortic valve and then continues to advance the catheter until its tip bends cephalad and points toward the left coronary ostium. When the catheter is properly positioned with its tip bent cephalad, slightly advancing or rotating the catheter usually results in selective engagement of the left coronary ostium, which is verified by a small injection of radiographic contrast agent. Occasionally, a deep breath taken by the patient will facilitate this selective engagement. Once the catheter tip is engaged, it commonly (but not always) appears to be fixed by the coronary orifice. There is more than one way to successfully engage the left coronary artery with the Sones catheter. Our usual approach, illustrated in the upper left panel of Figure 13–7, involves forming a smooth shallow loop and gradually "inching up" to the ostium from below. If the distal 2 to 3 mm of the catheter tip bends downward during this "inching up" process, the tip may enter the left coronary

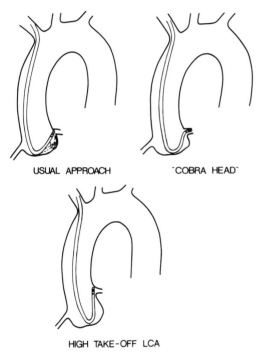

USUAL APPROACH   **"COBRA HEAD"**

HIGH TAKE-OFF LCA

Fig. 13–7. Selective catheterization of the left coronary artery using the Sones catheter. The standard approach involves forming a smooth shallow loop and gradually "inching up" to the ostium from below. If the distal 2 to 3 mm of the catheter tip bends downward during this inching-up process, the tip may enter the left coronary artery, giving a "cobra-head" appearance (upper right). When the left coronary ostium originates high in the left sinus of Valsalva ("high take-off" left coronary artery), the catheter may have the appearance seen in the bottom panel, where the tip is lying across the ostium, at right angles to the course of the left main coronary artery. During coronary injection in this instance, coronary blood flow generally carries the contrast medium down the vessel, giving good opacification of the entire left coronary artery.

artery, giving a "cobra head" appearance (Fig. 13–7, upper right panel) similar to that achieved with the left Amplatz catheter (Fig. 13–5). This is a stable position that allows rotation of the patient in a cradle-type table top without disengaging the catheter. For the high take-off left coronary ostium, the catheter may have the appearance as in Figure 13–7, bottom, in which the catheter tip is lying across the ostium, at right angles to the course of the left main coronary artery. During contrast injection in this instance, coronary blood flow generally carries the contrast agent down the vessel, giving good opacification of the entire left coronary artery.

When the catheter tip has engaged the coronary ostium and no damping of pressure from the catheter tip is observed, cineangiography may be performed with selective injection of radiopaque material in a variety of views, as described below.

Selective engagement of the right coronary orifice may be accomplished as illustrated in steps 1 to 3 of Figure 13–8. In the shallow LAO projection, the catheter is curved up toward the left coronary artery (step 1) and clockwise torque is applied. While the operator is gradually applying clockwise torque, a gentle to-and-fro motion of the catheter (the to-and-fro excursions are not more than 5 to 10 mm in length) helps to translate the applied torque to the catheter tip. When the tip starts moving in its clockwise sweep of the anterior wall of the aorta, the operator maintains (but does not increase) a clockwise torque tension on the catheter and simultaneously pulls the catheter back slightly (step 2, Fig. 13–8) because the right coronary ostium is lower than that of the left coronary artery. At this point, the catheter usually makes an abrupt turn into the right coronary ostium, at which time the operator must release all torque to prevent the catheter tip from continuing its sweep past the ostium. On occasion, the Sones catheter literally leaps into the right coronary artery and will be 4 to 5 cm down its lumen. If this occurs, the catheter should be gently withdrawn until its tip is stable just within the ostium. Another technique for catheterizing the right coronary

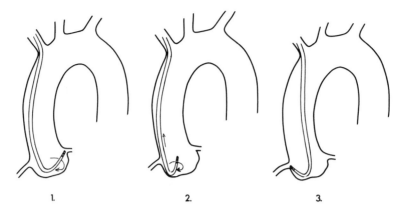

Fig. 13–8.   Selective catheterization of the right coronary artery using the Sones catheter. In the shallow LAO projection, the catheter is curved upward and to the left (1) and clockwise torque is applied. While the operator is gradually applying clockwise torque, a gentle to-and-fro motion of the catheter helps to translate the applied torque to the catheter tip. When the tip starts moving in its clockwise sweep of the anterior wall of the aorta, the operator maintains (but does not increase) a clockwise torque tension on the catheter and simultaneously pulls the catheter back slightly (2), because the right coronary ostium is lower than that of the left coronary artery. At this point the catheter usually makes an abrupt leap into the right coronary ostium (3), at which time the operator must release all torque to prevent the catheter tip from continuing its sweep and passing by the ostium. See text for details and alternative methods.

artery involves a more direct approach by way of the right coronary cusp. With the catheter in the right sinus, the operator should make a small curve on the tip, directed rightward. A small dose of contrast material in the right sinus of Valsalva will allow visualization of the right coronary orifice and thus facilitate selective engagement. Occasionally, a deep inspiration by the patient accompanied by gentle advancement of the catheter to the right of the aortic root results in selective engagement of the right coronary artery.

In addition to the Sones catheter, many other catheters may be used for coronary arteriography from the brachial approach, including the Amplatz, Schoonmaker, Bourassa, Judkins, and other specially designed catheters. Some of these catheters are illustrated in Figure 13–1. The Amplatz catheters* come in different shapes for the right and left coronary artery and basically incorporate a preformed Sones curvature. The left Amplatz comes in sizes L1, L2, L3, and L4; we have found the L2 adequate for most patients with normal aortic roots, whereas the L3 may be necessary for a dilated ascending aorta or in large men. Occasionally an L4 is needed for pronounced aortic dilatation or for a left coronary artery whose

ostium originates very high in the left sinus of Valsalva ("high take-off" left coronary artery). The Amplatz right coronary catheter comes in R1 and R2 sizes; the R1 is usually adequate for patients with a normal aortic root. Although the Amplatz catheters were originally devised for use by the percutaneous femoral approach, we have found these catheters highly useful from the brachial approach in cases in which there was difficulty in seating the Sones catheter. The Amplatz catheter traverses the subclavian artery easily over a guide wire and is effective for bypass graft angiography. It cannot be used safely for ventriculography, however, as can the Sones catheter. We have also used the Judkins catheters, particulary from the *left* brachial artery approach, with success. We have not had experience with the Bourassa or Schoonmaker catheters from the brachial approach, but large published series attest to the effectiveness of these catheters from the femoral artery approach, and they should be effective from the brachial approach as well.

ADVERSE EFFECTS OF CORONARY ANGIOGRAPHY

Once the coronary vessels have been engaged, selective angiography requires tran-

---

*Cook, Inc., Bloomington, Ind.

sient but nearly complete replacement of blood flow with a radiopaque contrast agent. A wide variety of iodine-containing agents are currently used for coronary angiography, and are discussed in greater detail in Chapter 2.

To a greater or lesser degree, coronary injection of any of these agents has potentially deleterious effects including: (1) transient (10 to 20 second) hemodynamic depression marked by arterial hypotension and elevation of the left ventricular end diastolic pressure, (2) electrocardiographic effects with T-wave inversion or peaking in the inferior leads (during right and left coronary injection, respectively), sinus slowing or arrest, and prolongation of the PR, QRS, and QT intervals,[19–21] (3) significant arrhythmia (asystole or ventricular tachycardia/fibrillation),[22] (4) myocardial ischemia due to interruption of oxygen delivery or inappropriate arteriolar vasodilatation (coronary "steal"), (5) allergic reaction, and (6) cumulative renal toxicity.

To recognize, treat, and hopefully prevent these adverse effects, patients undergoing coronary angiography should be monitored continuously in terms of clinical status, surface electrocardiogram, and arterial pressure from the catheter tip (and the sheath side-arm or arterial monitor line, if one is used). In patients with baseline left ventricular dysfunction or marked ischemic instability, we also like to monitor pulmonary artery pressure continuously (using the right heart catheter and displaying pulmonary arterial pressure on the same scale as the arterial pressure to avoid visual confusion). Pulmonary artery pressure monitoring frequently provides the earliest indication of procedural problems or decompensation; a significant rise in pulmonary artery mean or diastolic pressure should prompt temporary suspension of angiography and initiation of treatment (e.g., intravenous furosemide, nitroglycerin, nitroprusside) before frank pulmonary edema develops. The venous sheath provides a ready route for the rapid administration of fluid or medications through its sidearm, and also allows rapid insertion of a temporary pacing electrode if needed.

We do not, however, endorse the routine prophylactic placement of temporary pacing electrodes in patients undergoing coronary angiography. Most episodes of bradycardia or asystole are brief and are resolved promptly by having the patient give a forceful cough, which elevates central aortic pressure and probably helps wash residual contrast out of the myocardial capillary bed. True life-threatening bradycardia is very uncommon[23,24] and can be managed successfully by having the patient cough at 1 to 2 second intervals while a temporary pacing lead is inserted through the indwelling venous sheath and attached to a generator kept at standby at the foot of the catheterization table. Similarly, prophylactic drugs are not given routinely to prevent ventricular tachyarrhythmias, although drugs (lidocaine, procainamide, atropine, epinephrine, etc.), a defibrillator, and airway management equipment are always kept at the ready, and can be brought into play within seconds.

One of the most common adverse effects seen during coronary angiography is the provocation of myocardial ischemia, particularly in patients with unstable angina. In such patients, we commonly do not interrupt any precatheterization heparin infusion (in fact, additional heparin is required during the catheterization itself), do not reverse heparin at the completion of the procedure, and do not follow our usual practice of performing the left ventriculogram before coronary angiography (lest an adverse reaction to the ventriculogram compromise the more important coronary study). When myocardial ischemia does occur during coronary angiography, the best course of action is to remove the catheter from the coronary ostium and temporarily suspend injections until angina resolves. If this takes more than 30 seconds, we typically administer nitroglycerine (200 μg bolus, repeated at 30-second intervals up to a total of 1000 μg) into either the involved coronary artery or the pulmonary artery catheter. If marked arterial hypertension is present and fails to respond to nitroglycerine, we administer sublingual nifedipine, 10 mg every 5 minutes. In patients with inappropriate tachycardia in the setting of angina and reasonable systolic left ventricular function, intravenous propranolol (1 mg every minute to a total dose of 0.1 to 0.15 mg/ kg), or an infusion of a short-acting beta-blocking agent (esmolol) is frequently beneficial. Only rarely (in patients with severe three-vessel and/or left main coronary disease and those whose ischemia is associated with hypotension) is myocardial ischemia severe and refractory to the above management program, prompting placement of an intra-aortic counterpulsation balloon in the contralateral femoral artery before completion of coronary angiography. In any patient with prolonged or refractory ischemia, it is also worthwhile to perform limited re-examination of the coronary vessels to determine whether the angiographic procedure has caused a problem (spasm, dissection, thrombosis) that might require immediate treatment with additional vasodilators, balloon angioplasty, thrombolysis, or emergency bypass surgery.

Severe allergic reactions are uncommon during coronary angiography, and are best prevented by 18 to 24 hours of premedication (prednisone 20 to 40 mg and cimetidine 300 mg every 6 hours) and/or use of a nonionic contrast agent in patients with a history of prior allergic reaction to radiographic contrast.[25] When a severe unexpected reaction does occur, it usually responds promptly to the intravenous administration of epinephrine (0.1 mg = 1 ml of the 1:10,000 solution available on most emergency carts, repeated every 2 minutes until the blood pressure and/or wheezing improves). Larger bolus doses of epinephrine are to be avoided because they may provoke marked tachycardia, hypertension, and arrhythmia.

Renal insufficiency may develop after coronary angiography, particularly in patients who are hypovolemic, who receive large volumes of contrast (more than 3 ml/kg), or who have had prior renal insufficiency, diabetes, or multiple myeloma.[26–27] In these patients, every effort should be made to give adequate hydration pre- and post-procedure (see also Chaps. 2 and 3).

INJECTION TECHNIQUE

As mentioned previously, high-quality coronary angiography requires selective injection of radiographic contrast at an adequate rate and volume to essentially replace the blood contained in the involved vessel and cause slight but continuous reflux into the aortic root. Too timid an injection allows intermittent entry of nonopaque blood into the coronary artery (producing streaming, which makes interpretation of lesions difficult), and fails to visualize the coronary ostium and proximal coronary branches. On the other hand, too vigorous an injection may cause coronary dissection or excessive myocardial blushing, and too prolonged an injection may contribute to increased myocardial depression or bradycardia.

We train our fellows to adjust the rate and duration of manual contrast injection to match the filling pattern observed during the run. Injection velocity should be built up gradually during the first second until it is adequate to completely replace antegrade blood flow into the coronary ostium (Fig. 13–9). This injection rate should be maintained until the entire vessel is opacified, and then terminated while cine filming of distal vessels or late-filling branches continues. If there is any question about whether the body of the injection has provided adequate reflux to visualize the coronary ostium, an additional burst of contrast (extra reflux) should be given before the injection is terminated. To avoid problems, each injection should begin with a completely full (and bubble-free) injection syringe, held with the tip slightly depressed so that any microbubbles drift up toward the plunger. Recent changes in contrast labeling also suggest that the injection syringe be managed in such a way as to avoid mixtures of blood and contrast because such mixtures may promote formation of thrombi (particularly when nonionic contrast agents are used).

While manual contrast injection is the standard technique in coronary angiography, some operators favor use of a power injector (as used in left ventriculography or aortography) to perform coronary injections.[28] The injector is preset for a rate to match the involved vessel (2 to 3 ml/sec for the right and 3 to 4 ml/sec for the left coronary), and activated by a foot switch for a sufficient period of time to fill the coronary with contrast (generally 2 to 3 sec-

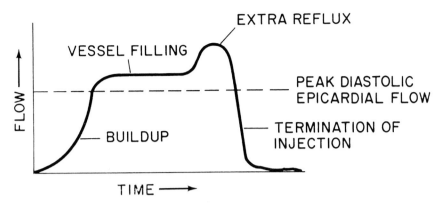

Fig. 13–9. Suggested injection pattern for coronary angiography. To appropriately replace antegrade coronary blood flow with contrast medium throughout the cardiac cycle, the operator should build up the velocity of injection over 1 to 2 seconds until no unopacified blood is seen to enter the ostium and there is reflux of contrast medium into the aorta during systole and diastole. This injection is maintained until the entire coronary artery is filled with contrast medium. If the ostium has not been well seen, a brief extra push should be given to cause adequate reflux into the aortic root, and the injection should be terminated. Prolonged held inspiration with some degree of Valsalva maneuver reduces coronary flow considerably and makes it much easier to replace blood flow by manual injection.

onds). This approach allows a single operator to perform injections and move the table, and has proven safe in thousands of procedures; however, we still prefer the greater flexibility and control afforded by manual injection.

ANGIOGRAPHIC VIEWS AND QUANTITATION OF STENOSIS

Coronary Anatomy. The coronary angiographer must develop a detailed familiarity with normal coronary arterial anatomy and its common variations. The main coronary trunks can be considered to lie in one of two orthogonal planes (Fig. 13–10). The anterior descending and posterior descending coronary arteries lie in the plane of the interventricular septum, and the right and circumflex coronary trunks lie in the plane of the atrioventricular valves. In the 60-degree left anterior oblique (LAO) projection, one is looking down the plane of the interventricular septum, with the plane of the AV valves seen en face; in the 30-degree right anterior oblique (RAO) projection, one is looking down the plane of the AV valves, with the plane of the interventricular septum seen en face.

Right-Dominant Circulation. In 85% of patients, the coronary circulation is "right-dominant"; that is, the right coronary artery sup-

plies the inferior aspect of the interventricular septum by giving rise to the posterior descending artery and also supplies one or more posterior left ventricular branches after the origin of the posterior descending artery (Fig. 13–10). The left anterior descending artery has septal branches that curve down into the interventricular septum and diagonal branches that wrap over the anterolateral free wall of the left ventricle. In the right-dominant coronary circulation, the circumflex artery has one or more obtuse marginal branches that supply the lateral free wall of the left ventricle, as well as one or more left atrial branches. In some patients, a large intermedius or ramus medianus branch (neither a diagonal nor a marginal) may originate directly from the left main trunk, bisecting the angle between the left anterior descending and circumflex arteries, so that there is a trifurcation of the left main coronary artery. The right coronary artery gives rise to the AV nodal artery in right-dominant circulations and also supplies the right ventricular outflow tract (conus branch), the sinus node (in 60% of patients), and the free wall of the right ventricle (acute marginal branches) whether the circulation is right-dominant or not.

Left-Dominant Circulation. In 8% of patients, the coronary circulation is "left-dom-

CORONARY ANGIOGRAPHIC ANATOMY: REPRESENTATION IN STANDARD PROJECTIONS

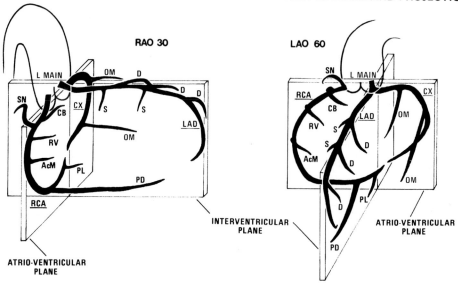

Fig. 13–10. Representation of coronary anatomy relative to the interventricular and atrioventricular valve planes. Coronary branches are as indicated—L Main (left main), LAD (left anterior descending), D (diagonal), S (septal), CX (circumflex), OM (obtuse marginal), RCA (right coronary), CB (conus branch), SN (sinus node), AcM (acute marginal), PD (posterior descending), PL (posterolateral left ventricular).

inant''; that is, the posterolateral ventricular, posterior descending, and AV nodal arteries are supplied by the terminal portion of the left circumflex coronary artery, and the right coronary artery supplies only the right atrium and right ventricle.

Finally, about 7% of hearts exhibit a codominant or balanced system, with the right coronary artery giving rise to the posterior descending artery and then terminating, while the circumflex artery gives rise to all the posterior left ventricular branches and perhaps also a parallel posterior descending branch to the interventricular septum. Within this general description, it should be noted that there is considerable patient-to-patient variability in the size and position of different branches.

Moreover, 1 to 2% of patients may have more divergent coronary anatomic features, such as anomalous origin of the circumflex from the right coronary artery, separate ostia of the left anterior descending and left circumflex arteries, or separate ostia of the right coronary and its conus branch (Fig. 13–11).[29] The operator must be thoroughly familiar with these anatomic anomalies, and continually vigilant for their occurrence, lest failure to recognize an anomaly result in an incomplete and therefore inadequate examination. Anomalous vessels that originate unusually high or out of the normal coronary plane are generally easier to cannulate using left Amplatz rather than Judkins catheters.

Angiographic Views. To quantitate a coronary stenosis accurately, it must be seen in profile, free from artifact related to foreshortening or obfuscation by a crossing vessel. Multiple views are important, particularly in the evaluation of eccentric or slitlike stenoses, whose true severity may be underestimated if viewed only in a single projection. These severely eccentric stenoses can often be recognized by their marked lucency in the major axis projection caused by thinning of the contrast column. It is important to confirm the presence of significant stenosis in an orthogonal projection, however, because similar lucency may be seen adjacent to areas of denser contrast caused by tortuosity or overlapping vessels, as the result of a perceptual artifact

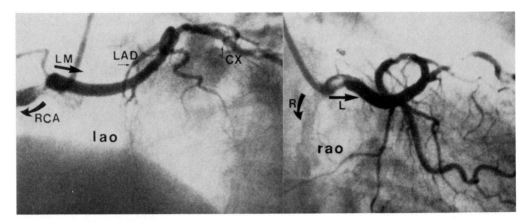

Fig. 13–11. Anomalous origin of the left coronary artery. Left panel: Left anterior oblique (lao) projection shows normal origin of the right coronary artery (RCA), but anomalous origin of the left coronary artery (LM) from the anterior portion of the right sinus of Valsalva. It then passes anterior to the pulmonary artery before dividing into the LAD and Cx. Right panel: Right anterior oblique (rao) projection shows engagement of the anomalous ostium with a left Amplatz catheter.

(Mach effect) in the absence of any true abnormality at the site.[30]

The degree of stenosis (Fig. 13–12) is usually quantitated from the moving cineangiogram by visual evaluation of the percentage of diameter reduction relative to the caliber of the adjacent normal segments.[31] This is fairly accurate in very mild or very severe stenoses, although overestimation of stenosis severity is common. There is also substantial interobserver variability (frequently ±20%) in the visual quantitation of moderate stenoses between 40 and 80%.[32] This range of stenosis is particularly important because a 50% diameter (75% cross-sectional area) stenosis is barely "hemodynamically significant" at peak coronary flows, but a 70% diameter (90% cross-sectional area) stenosis is restrictive at these same peak flows.[33,34] Direct measurement using a digital caliper[35] or optical reticule, video processing with visual[36] or automated edge detection,[37] or densitometric analysis[38] offers the possibility of more consistent stenosis quantitation, but these techniques are not currently in wide clinical use. In addition to noting the degree of stenosis, it is increasingly important

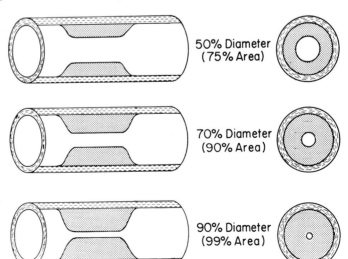

Fig. 13–12. Coronary stenoses of 50, 70, and 90% diameter reduction are shown in longitudinal and cross section. The corresponding reductions in cross-sectional area are indicated in parentheses.

50% Diameter (75% Area)

70% Diameter (90% Area)

90% Diameter (99% Area)

to evaluate lesion *morphology* for the features (eccentricity, ulceration, thrombus) associated with unstable clinical patterns,[39] as well as features that determine suitability for balloon angioplasty (calcification, bend, involvement of bifurcation, etc.).

Accurate coronary diagnosis requires coronary injections in multiple views. When earlier cradle systems were used, these views were usually limited to different degrees of left or right anterior obliquity in the transverse plane, including the 60-degree LAO and 30-degree RAO projections (Fig. 13–13). Cradle systems have subsequently been modified to allow concurrent cranial angulation of the x-ray beam by propping the patient's shoulders up on a foam wedge—hence the name "sit-

up" view for the LAO-cranial projection. By mounting the x-ray tube and image intensifier on a parallelogram or a rigid U-arm supported by a rotating pedestal, however, modern gantries now allow combination of any conventional transverse angulation with cranial or caudal angulation up to 45 degrees. While these views increase the demand on the generator and the scattered radiation (due to greater x-ray tube-intensifier separation and soft tissue depth), there is no doubt that they have improved our ability to define coronary anatomy.[40–42] It is important to point out that all potential views are not necessary in a given patient to constitute an adequate study. Rather, a series of "screening views" should be used as the foundation of the study, supplemented

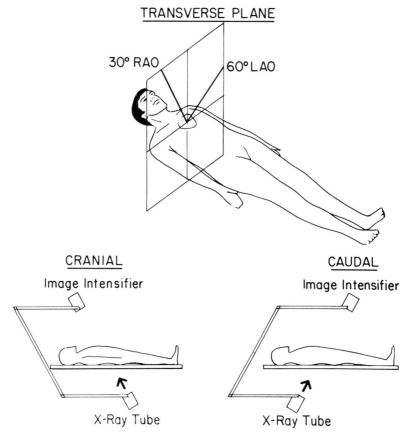

Fig. 13–13. Geometry of angulated views. Conventional coronary angiography was performed previously using angulation only in the transverse plane (top), as demonstrated by the 60-degree left anterior oblique (LAO) and 30-degree right anterior oblique (RAO) views. Currently, improved x-ray equipment permits simultaneous cranial or caudal angulation in the sagittal plane. Each view is named based on the location of the image intensifier, rather than the older nomenclature specifying the location of both the x-ray tube and intensifier (i.e., cranial = caudocranial).

by one or more "special" views selected to define more completely suspicious areas observed on live fluoroscopy or on review of the videotape images that are recorded concurrently with cine film exposure. This requires the operator to interpret the coronary anatomy as each injection is made (rather than simply shooting a series of routine views and hoping that the study will prove adequate when the cine film is developed) and to understand the influence of angulation on the projected coronary anatomy. In respect to the latter issue, a coronary anatomic model is a valuable training tool (Fig. 13–14).[43]

RAO Projection. For historic reasons, the screening views used in many laboratories are the conventional LAO-RAO angulations. In our laboratory, however, we have found that certain cranial and caudal angulated views may be preferable. The conventional 30-degree RAO projection suffers from overlap and foreshortening in both the left anterior descending and circumflex territories (Fig. 13–14). The shallow RAO-cranial projection (0 to 10 degrees RAO and 25 to 40 degrees cranial) pro-

vides a superior view of the mid and distal left anterior descending artery, with clear visualization of the origins of the septal and diagonal branches. The shallow RAO cranial view is also quite good for examination of the distal right coronary artery because it "unstacks" the posterior descending and posterolateral branches and projects them without foreshortening. Because of foreshortening and overlap, however, this view seldom provides useful information about the left main or circumflex coronary artery. In contrast, the shallow RAO-caudal projection (0 to 10 degrees RAO and 15 to 20 degrees caudal) provides an excellent view of the left main bifurcation, the proximal left anterior descending artery, and the proximal to mid circumflex artery and is our initial view of choice in studying unstable patients.

LAO Projection. The conventional 60-degree LAO projection of the left coronary artery is limited by overlap and foreshortening, but is useful in the evaluation of the proximal and mid-right coronary artery. The addition of 15 to 30 degrees of cranial angulation has the effect of elongating the left main and proximal

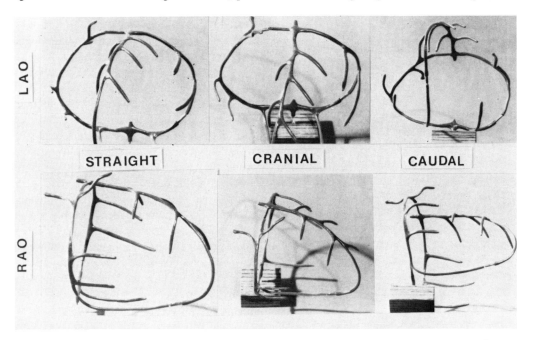

Fig. 13–14. Demonstration of angiographic projections using the author's coronary model. LAO and RAO projections are photographed straight (i.e., with no cranial or caudal angulation), as well as with moderate cranial and moderate caudal angulation (see text for details).

left anterior descending arteries while projecting the intermedius or first diagonal branch downward off the proximal circumflex. If radiographic penetration in this view is difficult, reducing the LAO angulation to 30 to 40 degrees will usually allow the left anterior descending artery to fall into the lucent wedge between the right hemidiaphragm and the spine. The LAO-caudal view (40 to 60 degrees LAO and 10 to 20 degrees caudal) projects the left coronary artery in the appearance of a spider and offers improved visualization of the left main, proximal LAD, and proximal circumflex arteries. This view is particularly valuable in patients whose heart has a horizontal lie, i.e., the origin of the left main artery projects at or below the proximal left anterior descending artery in the standard LAO projection, but stresses the radiographic capacity of most older installations. This "spider view" (LAO-caudal) can often be enhanced by filming during forced maximal expiration, which accentuates a horizontal cardiac position and allows a better look from below.

AP and Left Lateral Projections. Two underused views are the AP and left lateral projections. Because the left main coronary artery curves from a more leftward to an almost anterior direction along its length, the AP projection frequently provides the best view of the left main ostium, whereas the shallow RAO caudal view frequently provides a better look at the more distal left main artery. The left lateral projection is particularly useful in examining the proximal circumflex and the proximal and distal left anterior descending arteries, particularly if combined with slight (10 to 15 degrees) cranial angulation. It also provides an excellent look at the midportion of the right coronary artery and has the advantage of allowing easy radiographic penetration in most patients when performed with both of the patient's hands positioned behind his or her head.

Over the past several years, operators in our laboratory have adopted a uniform sequence of "screening views," the exact angles of which are modified slightly as dictated by test

puffs of contrast. Beginning with the left coronary artery, these vews include:

1. RAO-CAUDAL to visualize the left main, proximal LAD and proximal Cx
2. RAO-CRANIAL to visualize the mid and distal LAD without overlap of septal or diagonal branches
3. LAO-CRANIAL to visualize the mid and distal LAD in an orthogonal projection
4. LAO-CAUDAL to visualize the left main and proximal Cx.

One or more supplemental views (AP, LATERAL-CRANIAL, LATERAL-CAUDAL) may then be taken to clarify any areas of uncertainty. The right coronary catheter is then placed, after which three screening views are obtained:

1. LAO to visualize the proximal RCA
2. RAO-CRANIAL to visualize the posterior descending and posterolateral branches
3. LATERAL to visualize the mid-RCA.

Coronary Collaterals. In reviewing the coronary angiogram, one basic principle is that there should be evident blood supply to all portions of the left ventricle. Previously occluded vessel branches are usually manifest as truncated stumps, but no stump may be evident if there has been a "flush-occlusion" at the origin of the involved vessel. These occluded or severely stenotic vessels will be seen frequently to fill late in the injection by antegrade (so-called bridging) collaterals or collaterals that originate from the same ("intracoronary") or an adjacent ("intercoronary") vessel, which are reviewed in an excellent paper by Levin[44] and illustrated in Figures 13–15 through 13–17. Finally, coronary occlusion may present in some patients simply as an "angiographically arid" area to which there is no evidence of either antegrade or collateral flow and no evident vascular stump. If such an area fails to show regional hypokinesis on the left ventriculogram, however, the operator should search carefully for blood supply by way of anomalous vessels or unopacified collaterals (i.e., a separate origin conus branch that was not opacified during the main right coronary injections), because the myocardium

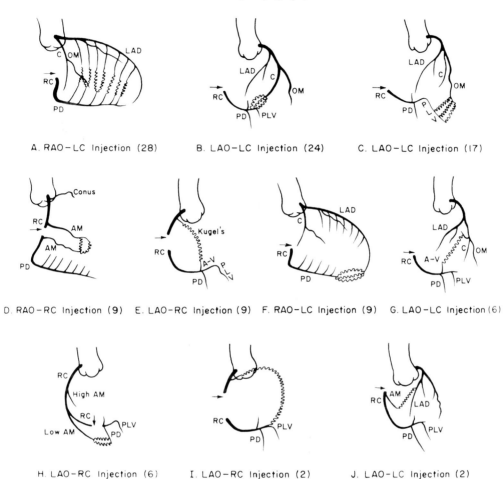

A. RAO-LC Injection (28)   B. LAO-LC Injection (24)   C. LAO-LC Injection (17)

D. RAO-RC Injection (9)   E. LAO-RC Injection (9)   F. RAO-LC Injection (9)   G. LAO-LC Injection (6)

H. LAO-RC Injection (6)   I. LAO-RC Injection (2)   J. LAO-LC Injection (2)

Fig. 13–15. Ten collateral pathways observed in patients with right coronary (RC) obstruction (total occlusion or >90% stenosis). Abbreviations for arteries: LAD, left anterior descending; C, circumflex; OM, obtuse marginal; PD, posterior descending; PLV, posterior left ventricular branch; AM, acute marginal branch of right coronary artery; A-V, atrioventricular nodal; LC, left coronary. Numbers in parentheses represent numbers of cases in this series. (From Levin DC: Pathways and functional significance of the coronary collateral circulation. Circulation 50:831, 1974. By permission of the American Heart Association, Inc.).

cannot continue to function normally with no visible means of support.

NONATHEROSCLEROTIC CORONARY ARTERY DISEASE

Although atherosclerotic stenosis is far and away the most common pathologic process identified on the coronary angiogram, the angiographer must be aware of a variety of other potential findings.[45] These include congenital anomalies of coronary origin,[29] coronary fistulae (Fig. 13–18), and muscle bridges (Fig.

13–19).[5,45–48] The latter are sections of a coronary artery (almost always the left anterior descending) which run under a strip of left ventricular muscle and are compressed during ventricular systole but appear normal during diastole. These congenital anomalies are important to recognize because they can be associated with ischemic symptoms in some patients in whom catheterization fails to demonstrate the expected finding of coronary atherosclerosis and can be surgically repaired if necessary. With regard to muscle bridges, there is evidence that they prevent a normal increase in coronary blood flow during tach-

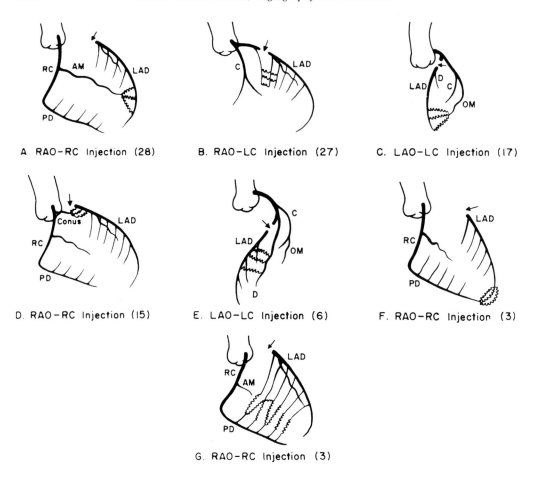

A. RAO-RC Injection (28) B. RAO-LC Injection (27) C. LAO-LC Injection (17)

D. RAO-RC Injection (15) E. LAO-LC Injection (6) F. RAO-RC Injection (3)

G. RAO-RC Injection (3)

Fig. 13–16. Seven collateral pathways observed in patients with left coronary artery obstruction. Abbreviations and format are the same as in Figure 13–15. (From Levin DC: Pathways and functional significance of the coronary collateral circulation. Circulation 50:831, 1973. By permission of the American Heart Association, Inc.).

ycardia, when both systolic and diastolic coronary flow may be important. Surgical relief of such bridges has led to subjective and objective improvement in selected patients.

Finally, some patients who come to catheterization have *no* demonstrable coronary abnormality to account for their clinically suspected ischemic heart disease. Although angina-like pain can be seen in patients with noncoronary cardiac abnormality (mitral valve prolapse, hypertrophic cardiomyopathy, aortic stenosis, myocarditis) or extracardiac conditions (esophageal dysmotility,[49,50] cholecystitis), one must also consider the possibility of coronary vasospastic disease.[51] Vasospasm of an epicardial coronary artery is likely when a patient has episodes of rest pain despite well-preserved effort tolerance. An electrocardiogram recorded during an episode of spontaneous pain usually shows ST elevation in the territory supplied by the vasospastic artery, confirming the diagnosis of variant angina (Fig. 13–20). In these patients, the main purpose of coronary angiography is to look at the extent of underlying atherosclerosis,[52] we generally do not attempt to provoke spasm in patients with documented variant angina. In patients with no prior documented spontaneous ST elevation and insufficient coronary stenosis to explain chest pain, however, provocational testing for coronary spasm is frequently helpful.

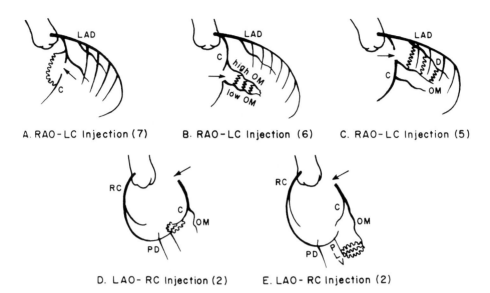

A. RAO-LC Injection (7)   B. RAO-LC Injection (6)   C. RAO-LC Injection (5)

D. LAO- RC Injection (2)   E. LAO- RC Injection (2)

Fig. 13–17. Five collateral pathways observed in patients with circumflex coronary artery obstruction. Abbreviations and format are the same as in Figure 13–15. (From Levin DC: Pathways and functional significance of the coronary collateral circulation. Circulation 50:831, 1974. By permission of the American Heart Association, Inc.).

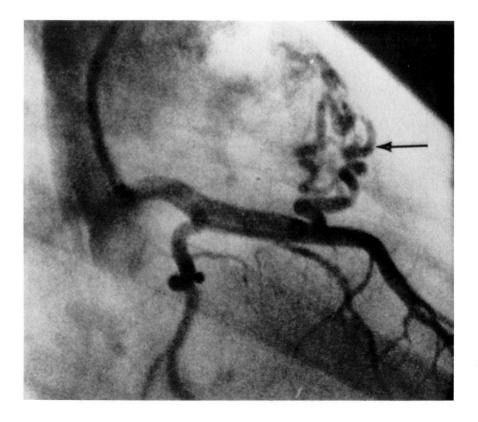

Fig. 13–18. Coronary artery fistula (arrow) between the mid-left anterior descending coronary artery and the pulmonary artery, shown in the right anterior oblique view.

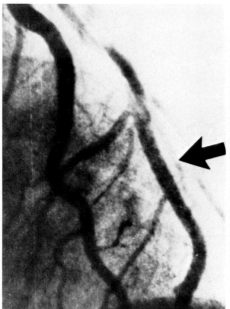 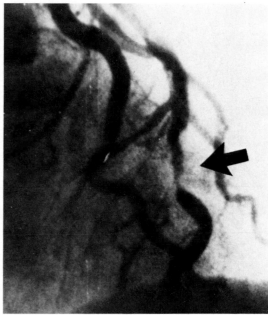

Fig. 13–19. Muscle bridge. Moderately severe muscle bridge of the left anterior descending coronary artery (arrow) as seen in diastole (left) and systole (right).

DETECTION OF CORONARY VASOSPASM

If provocational testing for coronary spasm is contemplated, the patient should be withdrawn from calcium-channel blockers for at least 24 hours and long-acting nitrates for at least 12 hours before study and not be premedicated with either atropine or sublingual nitroglycerin. Ongoing therapy with any of these agents may render provocational tests falsely negative.[53] Although a variety of provocational tests have been used (methacholine, epinephrine and propranolol, hyperventilation and tris-buffer, cold pressor), the most commonly used provocational agent is ergonovine maleate,[54–57] a stimulant of the alpha-adrenergic and serotonin receptors in coronary vascular smooth muscle.

Testing for coronary spasm should be performed only after baseline angiographic evaluation of both the left and right coronary arteries. According to our protocol, a total of 0.4 mg (400 μg = 2 ampules) of ergonovine maleate is diluted to a total volume of 8 ml in a 10-ml syringe that is appropriately labeled.

The provocational test consists of intravenous administration of 1 ml (0.05 mg), 2 ml (0.10 mg), and 5 ml (0.25 mg) of this mixture at 3 to 5 minute intervals. *Parenteral nitroglycerin (100 to 200 μg/ml) must be premixed and loaded in a labeled syringe before the testing is begun.* At 1 minute before each ergonovine dose, the patient is interrogated about symptoms similar to those of his clinical complaint and a 12-lead electrocardiogram is recorded. After each electrocardiogram, coronary angiography is performed, looking either at both arteries or only at the artery of highest clinical suspicion for vasospasm. In the absence of clinical symptoms, electrocardiographic changes, or focal coronary vasospasm exceeding 70% diameter reduction, the next ergonovine dose is administered and the cycle is repeated until the total dose of 0.4 mg has been given.

Clinical symptoms in the absence of electrocardiographic or angiographic evidence of vasospasm in either coronary artery suggest an alternative diagnosis such as esophageal dysmotility.[49,50] Even if there are no symptoms or electrocardiographic changes, both coronary

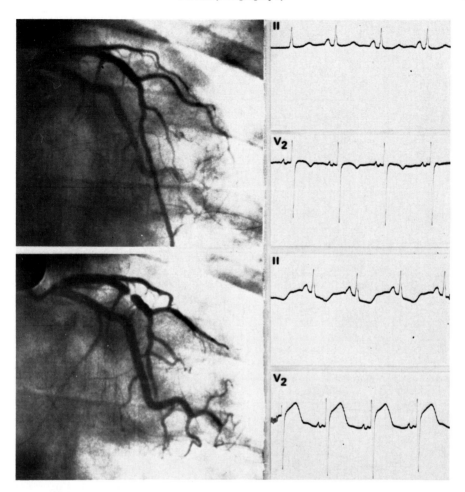

Fig. 13–20. True coronary spasm. Intense focal vasospasm of the left anterior descending coronary artery is shown in RAO projection in a patient with variant angina. Note the absence of a significant underlying atherosclerotic stenosis in the top panel, the absence of vasoconstriction of other vessel segments, and the marked ST elevation in the anterior leads during the spontaneous vasospastic episode. (From Baim DS, Harrison DC: Nonatherosclerotic coronary heart disease. *In* Hurst JW (ed): The Heart, 5th ed. New York, McGraw-Hill Book Company, 1985, with permission.)

arteries should be opacified at the end of the ergonovine test, and the generalized ergonovine vasoconstrictor effect should be terminated by administration of nitroglycerin. Coronary artery spasm may occur in two vessels simultaneously (Fig. 13–21), and visualization of only one vessel may fail to adequately assess the response to ergonovine. The provocational test should be considered positive only if focal spasm occurs and is associated with clinical symptoms and/or electrocardiographic changes. The patient is then treated immediately with parenteral nitroglycerin in the dose of 200 μg administered either by vein or, preferably, directly into the spastic coronary artery. The involved artery should then be reopacified 1 minute after nitroglycerin administration, to document the resolution of spasm and the extent of underlying atherosclerotic stenosis. The operator should be prepared to use additional doses of parenteral nitroglycerin, sublingual nifedipine, or sodium nitroprusside to treat refractory spasm or the occasional severe hypertensive reaction that can occur following ergonovine administration. Low doses of intracoronary verapamil (0.1 mg) have also proven useful in refractory spasm, although care must be taken to avoid

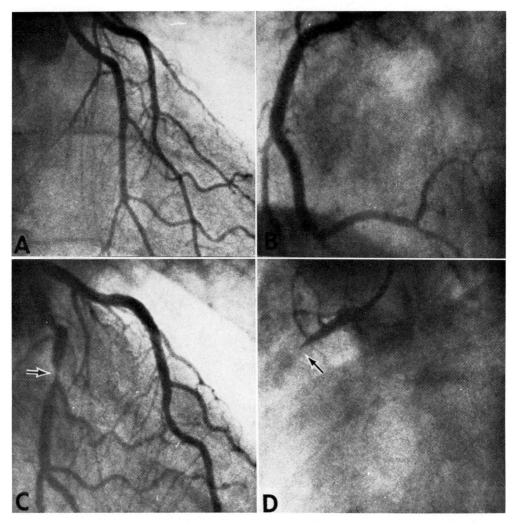

Fig. 13–21.   Coronary angiograms before (A and B) and after (C and D) coronary artery spasm induced by ergonovine maleate in a patient with Prinzmetal's variant angina. Severe spasm occurred in both the circumflex and right coronary arteries. Catheterization was by Sones technique. (From Heupler FA, et al: Ergonovine maleate provocative test for coronary arterial spasm. Am J Cardiol 41:631, 1978.)

excessive bradycardia or myocardial depression. Temporary pacing and defibrillatory equipment should also be available to treat the brady- or tachyarrhythmias that sometimes accompany coronary spasm.

Several additional comments about ergonovine are in order. Our group does not perform ergonovine testing in patients with severe atherosclerotic stenosis (80% or greater) in whom spasm is not required to explain the clinical symptoms. In these patients, however,

we frequently *do* repeat coronary angiography of the stenosed vessel after the intracoronary administration of 200 μg of nitroglycerin, to exclude the possibility that spontaneous focal vasospasm is contributing to the appearance of severe atherosclerotic stenosis. Secondly, it is important to distinguish the intense focal spasm seen in patients with variant angina from the normal mild (15 to 20%) diffuse coronary narrowing seen as a pharmacologic response to ergonovine in normal patients[58,59] or from "catheter tip" spasm (Fig. 13–22).[60] The latter is most common in the right coronary artery, is not associated with clinical symptoms or electrocardiographic changes, and does not indicate variant angina. It should be recognized as such, however, and treated by withdrawal of the catheter, administration of nitroglycerin, and nonselective or cautious repeat selective opacification of the involved vessel, to avoid mistaking catheter-tip spasm for an atherosclerotic lesion. Finally, the operator should be aware that the positivity rate of ergonovine testing depends strongly on the patients studied; the test is almost always positive in patients with known variant angina (if their disorder is active and medications have been withheld), is positive in approximately one third of patients with clinically suspected variant angina, but is positive in fewer than 5% of patients whose symptoms do not suggest variant angina.[57,61]

Abnormal Coronary Vasodilator Reserve

Evidence has been accumulating that the patient group with angina and angiographically normal coronary arteries may contain a subgroup of patients who have myocardial ischemia on the basis of abnormal vasodilator reserve.[62–64] In these patients, coronary sinus blood flow measured by thermodilution technique (as described in Chapter 21) fails to rise normally with pacing tachycardia or ergonovine, and the coronary vascular resistance is increased abnormally. Also, many of these patients show an abnormal rise in left ventricular end diastolic pressure following pacing tachycardia, and show less lactate consumption than normal subjects in response to pacing tachycardia. A failure of small vessel coronary vasodilation, inappropriate vasoconstriction[62,63] at the arteriolar level, or histologic abnormalities of capillary endothelial cells[64]

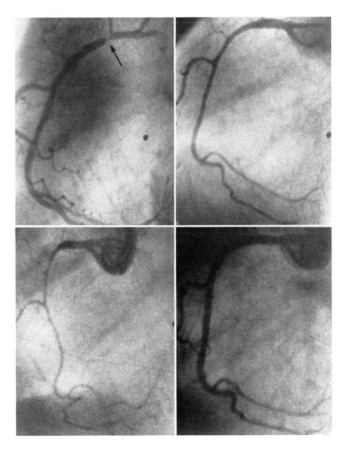

Fig. 13–22. Vasomotor changes *not* representing true coronary spasm. During right coronary catheterization with a Judkins catheter (upper left), this patient developed severe catheter-tip spasm. Recatheterization 24 hours later with an Amplatz catheter (upper right) showed neither catheter-tip spasm nor an atherosclerotic stenosis. Following ergonovine 0.4 mg, marked diffuse coronary narrowing was observed (lower left), without angina or electrocardiographic changes. After the intracoronary administration of nitroglycerin 200 μg (lower right), there is marked diffuse vasodilation.

have been postulated to account for these findings, and a beneficial response to calcium antagonist therapy has been described. Coronary angiography in these patients is entirely normal.

MISTAKES IN INTERPRETATION

An inexperienced operator often produces an incomplete, uninterpretable, or misinterpreted study, especially if he is using poor equipment. The following discussion summarizes some of the more common pitfalls mentioned earlier that may lead the inexperienced coronary angiographer to mistaken conclusions.

Inadequate Number of Projections. There is no standard number of projections that will always provide complete information. Each major vessel must be viewed in an isolated fashion as it stands apart from other vessels. Usually, the angulated views discussed earlier in this chapter are necessary to visualize clearly the anatomy of the proximal left anterior descending and circumflex arteries.

Inadequate Injection of Contrast Material. The inexperienced operator or assistant has a tendency to hold back on the volume and force of injection into the coronary circulation. This results in inadequate opacification of the coronary arterial tree and pulsatile filling because the contrast flow may exceed coronary flow only during systole. Because there is inadequate mixing of contrast agent and blood, pockets of nonradiopaque blood may give the appearance of arterial narrowing.

Superselective Injection. It is not uncommon to catheterize the left anterior descending or circumflex coronary artery superselectively, especially when the left main coronary artery is short and its bifurcation is early. To the inexperienced operator, this may give the impression of total occlusion of the nonvisualized vessel (e.g., if only the circumflex artery is opacified, the operator may conclude that the left anterior descending artery is occluded). If adequate filling of the noncannulated vessel cannot be achieved by reflux, selective cannulation of the LAD may be obtained by *coun-*

terclockwise rotation or use of the next-smaller-size Judkins catheter (e.g., JL 3.5), whereas selection cannulation of the Cx may be obtained by *clockwise* rotation or use of the next-larger-size Judkins catheter (e.g., JL 5). With the right coronary artery, superselective injection may occur if the catheter tip is too far down the vessel, leading to failure to visualize the conus and sinus node arteries. Because these are important sources of collateralization of the left coronary system, important information may be missed. Adequate injection to give a continuous (nonpulsatile) reflux of contrast agent back into the sinus of Valsalva will help the operator to recognize vessels that originate proximally to the catheter tip and thus avoid the interpretation error of superselective injection.

Catheter-Induced Coronary Spasm. Coronary artery spasm may be related to the catheter itself, possibly caused by mechanical irritation and a myogenic reflex (Fig. 13–22). It is seen most commonly when the right coronary artery is engaged selectively, but it may occur in the left anterior descending artery as well. Although it can occur with either the brachial or femoral approach, it is probably more common with the right Judkins catheter, especially if the catheter tip enters the right coronary ostium at an angle and produces tenting of the proximal vessel. If coronary narrowing suggests the occurrence of spasm to the operator, sublingual, intravenous, or intracoronary nitroglycerin should be given and the injection repeated.

Congenital Variants of Coronary Origin and Distribution. This topic has been discussed earlier in this chapter, but it bears reemphasis. Variation in origin and distribution of the coronary artery branches may confuse the operator and cause him to mistakenly diagnose coronary occlusion. For example, a small right coronary artery that terminates in the AV groove well before the crux may be interpreted as an abnormal or occluded artery, whereas it is a normal finding in 7 to 10% of human hearts. Double ostia of the right coronary artery or origin of the circumflex artery from the right coronary artery may be similarly confusing and lead to misdiagnosis.

Myocardial Bridges. As discussed earlier, coronary arteries occasionally dip below the epicardial surface under small areas of myocardium. During systole the segment of the artery surrounded by myocardium is narrowed and appears as a localized stenosis. These "myocardial bridges" occur most commonly in the distribution of the left anterior descending artery and its diagonal branches. The key to the recognition of these bridges is that the apparent localized stenosis returns to normal during diastole. Although it is likely that these bridges can cause true myocardial ischemia under certain circumstances, they may be seen in patients with normal hearts and no evidence of ischemia.

Total Occlusion. If a coronary artery or branch is totally occluded at its origin, it may not be visualized and the occlusion may be missed. If the occlusion is "flush" with the parent vessel, no stump will be seen. Such occlusions are primarily recognized by visualization of the distal segment of the occluded vessel by means of collateral channels or by noting the absence of the usual vascularity seen in a particular portion of the heart.

REFERENCES

1. Kennedy RH, et al: Cardiac-catheterization and cardiac-surgical facilities. Use, trends and future requirements. N Engl J Med 307:986, 1982.
2. Johnson LW, et al: Coronary arteriography 1984–1987: a report of the registry of the Society for Cardiac Angiography and Interventions. I. Results and complications. Cathet Cardiovasc Diagn 17:5, 1989.
3. Silverman K, Grossman W: Angina pectoris: Natural history and strategies for evaluation and management. N Engl J Med 310:1712, 1984.
4. Ross J, et al: Guidelines for coronary angiography: A report of the American College of Cardiology/American Heart Association Task Force on assessment of diagnostic and therapeutic cardiovascular procedures. Circulation 76:963A, 1987.
5. The TIMI Study Group: Comparison of invasive and conservative strategies after treatment with intravenous tissue plasminogen activator in acute myocardial infarction. N Engl J Med 320:618, 1989.
6. Neufeld NH, Blieden LC: Coronary artery disease in children. Prog Cardiol 4:119, 1975.
7. Roberts WC: No cardiac catheterization before cardiac valve replacement—a mistake. Am Heart J 103:930, 1982.
8. Conti CR: Coronary arteriography. Circulation 55:227, 1977.
9. Maher PR, Young C, Magnusson PT: Efficacy and safety of outpatient cardiac catheterization. Cathet Cardiovasc Diagn 13:304, 1987.
10. Fierens E: Outpatient coronary arteriography. Cathet Cardiovasc Diagn 10:27, 1984.
11. Kohli RS, Vetrovec GW, Lewis SA, Cole S: Study of the performance of 5 French and 7 French catheters in coronary angiography: A functional comparison. Cathet Cardiovasc Diagn 18:131, 1989.
12. Judkins MP: Selective coronary arteriography, a percutaneous transfemoral technic. Radiology 89:815, 1967.
13. Amplatz K, Formanek G, Stanger P, Wilson W: Mechanics of selective coronary artery catheterization via femoral approach. Radiology 89:1040, 1967.
14. Schoonmaker FW, King SB: Coronary arteriography by the single catheter percutaneous femoral technique, experience in 6,800 cases. Circulation 50:735, 1974.
15. Kuntz RE, Baim DS: Internal mammary angiography: a review of technical issues and newer methods. Cathet Cardiovasc Diagn 20:10–16, 1990.
16. Mills NL, Everson CT: Right gastroepiploic artery: a third arterial conduit for coronary artery bypass. Ann Thorac Surg 47:706, 1989.
17. Tanimoto Y, et al: Angiography of right gastroepiploic artery for coronary artery bypass graft. Cathet Cardiovasc Diagn 16:35, 1989.
18. Sones FM, Shirey EK: Cine coronary arteriography. Mod Concepts Cardiovasc Dis 31:735, 1962.
19. Ovitt T, et al: Electrocardiographic changes in selective coronary arteriography: the importance of ions. Radiology 102:705, 1972.
20. Tragardh B, Bove AA, Lynch PR: Mechanism of production of cardiac conduction abnormalities due to coronary arteriography in dogs. Invest Radiol 11:563, 1976.
21. Higgins CB: Effect of contrast media on the conduction system of the heart: Mechanism of action and identification of toxic component. Radiology 124:599, 1977.
22. Paulin S, Adams DF: Increased ventricular fibrillation during coronary arteriography with a new contrast medium preparation. Radiology 101:45, 1971.
23. Gilchrist IC, Cameron A: Temporary pacemaker during coronary arteriography. Am J Cardiol 60:1051, 1987.
24. Harvey JR, et al: Use of balloon flotation pacing catheters for prophylactic temporary pacing during diagnostic and therapeutic catheterization procedures. Am J Cardiol 62:941, 1988.
25. Lasser EC, et al: Pretreatment with corticosteroids to alleviate reactions to intravenous contrast material. N Engl J Med 317:845, 1987.
26. Parfrey PS, et al: Contrast material-induced renal failure in patients with diabetes mellitus, renal insufficiency, or both. N Engl J Med 329:143, 1989.
27. Schwab SJ, et al: Contrast nephrotoxicity: A randomized controlled trial of a nonionic and an ionic radiographic contrast agent. N Engl J Med 320:149, 1989.

28. Ireland MA et al: Safety and convenience of a mechanical injector pump for coronary angiography. Cathet Cardiovasc Diagn 16:199, 1989.

29. Click RL, et al: Anomalous coronary arteries: Location, degree of atherosclerosis and effect on survival—a report from the Coronary Artery Surgery Study. J Am Coll Cardiol 13:531, 1989.

30. Randall PA: Mach bands in cine coronary arteriography. Radiology 129:65, 1978.

31. Arnett EN, et al: Coronary artery narrowing in coronary heart disease: comparison of cineangiographic and necropsy findings. Ann Intern Med 91:350, 1979.

32. Zir LM, et al: Interobserver variability in coronary angiography. Circulation 54:627, 1976.

33. Wilson RF, Marcus ML, White CW: Prediction of physiologic significance of coronary arterial lesions by quantitative lesion geometry in patients with limited coronary artery disease. Circulation 75:723, 1987.

34. Kirkeeide RL, Gould KL: Cardiovascular imaging: coronary artery stenosis. Hosp Pract 1984 (April) 160.

35. Rafflenbeul W, et al: Quantitative coronary arteriography—coronary anatomy of patients with unstable angina pectoris reexamined 1 year after optimal medical therapy. Am J Cardiol 43:699, 1979.

36. Brown BG, Bolson E, Frimer M, Dodge HT: Quantitative coronary arteriography—estimation of dimensions, hemodynamic resistance, and atheroma mass of coronary artery lesions using the arteriogram and digital computation. Circulation 55:329, 1977.

37. Spears JR, et al: Computerized image analysis for quantitative measurement of vessel diameter from cineangiograms. Circulation 68:453, 1983.

38. Crawford DW, Brooks SH, Barndt R, Blankenhorn DH: Measurement of atherosclerotic luminal irregularity by radiographic densitometry. Invest Radiol 12:307, 1977.

39. Ambrose JA, Hjemdahl-Monsen CE: Angiographic anatomy and mechanisms of myocardial ischemia in unstable angina. J Am Coll Cardiol 9:1397, 1987.

40. Aldridge HE: A decade or more of cranial and caudal angled projections in coronary arteriography—another look. Cathet Cardiovasc Diagn 10:539, 1984.

41. Elliott LP, et al: Advantage of the cranial-right anterior oblique view in diagnosing mid left anterior descending and distal right coronary artery disease. Am J Cardiol 48:754, 1981.

42. Grover M, Slutsky R, Higgins C, Atwood JE: Terminology and anatomy of angulated coronary arteriography. Clin Cardiol 7:37, 1984.

43. Taylor CR, Wilde P: An easily constructed model of the coronary arteries. Am J Radiol 142:389, 1984.

44. Levin DC: Pathways and functional significance of the coronary collateral circulation. Circulation 50:831, 1974.

45. Baim DS, Harrison DC: Nonatherosclerotic coronary heart disease. *In* Hurst JW (ed): The Heart. 6th ed. New York, McGraw-Hill Book Company, 1986.

46. Razavi M: Unusual forms of coronary artery disease. Cardiovasc Clin 7:25, 1975.

47. Engel HJ, Torres C, Page HL: Major variations in anatomical origin of the coronary arteries: Angiographic observations in 4,250 patients without associated congenital heart disease. Cathet Cardiovasc Diagn 1:157, 1975.

48. Levin DC, Fellows KE, Abrams HL: Hemodynamically significant primary anomalies of the coronary arteries, angiographic aspects. Circulation 58:25, 1978.

49. Cohen S: Motor disorders of the esophagus. N Engl J Med 301:183, 1979.

50. Kaye MD: Recognizing and managing esophageal spasm. Drug Therapy 1982 (March) 137.

51. Maseri A, Chierchia S: Coronary artery spasm: demonstration, definition, diagnosis, and consequences. Prog Cardiovasc Dis 25:169, 1982.

52. Mark DB, et al: Clinical characteristics and long-term survival of patients with variant angina. Circulation 69:880, 1984.

53. Waters DD, Theroux P, Szlachcic J, Dauwe F: Provocative testing with ergonovine to assess the efficacy of treatment with nifedipine, diltiazem and verapamil in variant angina. Am J Cardiol 48:123, 1981.

54. Schroeder JS, et al: Provocation of coronary spasm with ergonovine maleate. Am J Cardiol 40:487, 1977.

55. Heupler FA, et al: Ergonovine maleate provocative test for coronary arterial spasm. Am J Cardiol 41:631, 1978.

56. Raizner AE, et al: Provocation of coronary artery spasm by the cold pressor test. Circulation 62:925, 1980.

57. Meyers DG: Ergonovine provocation of coronary artery spasm. Cardiovasc Rev Reports 3:855, 1982.

58. Cipriano PR, et al: The effects of ergonovine maleate on coronary arterial size. Circulation 59:82, 1979.

59. Curry RC, et al: Effects of ergonovine in patients with and without coronary artery disease. Circulation 56:803, 1979.

60. Friedman AC, Spindola-Franco H, Nivatpumin T: Coronary spasm: Prinzmetal's variant angina vs. catheter-induced spasm; refractory spasm vs. fixed stenosis. Am J Radiol 132:897, 1979.

61. Bertrand ME, et al: Frequency of provoked coronary arterial spasm in 1089 consecutive patients undergoing coronary arteriography. Circulation 65:1299, 1982.

62. Cannon RO III, Watson RM, Rosing DR, Epstein SE: Angina caused by reduced vasodilator reserve of the small coronary arteries. J Am Coll Cardiol 1:1359–1373, 1983.

63. Cannon RO III, et al: Left ventricular dysfunction in patients with angina pectoris, normal epicardial coronary arteries, and abnormal vasodilator reserve. Circulation 72:218–226, 1985.

64. Mosseri M, et al: Histologic evidence for small-vessel coronary artery disease in patients with angina pectoris and patent large coronary arteries. Circulation 74:964, 1986.

14

Cardiac Ventriculography

L. DAVID HILLIS and WILLIAM GROSSMAN

Cardiac ventriculography has been used extensively to define the anatomy of the ventricles and related structures in patients with congenital, valvular, coronary, and cardiomyopathic heart disease.[1-5] Specifically, *left ventriculography* may provide valuable information about global and segmental left ventricular function, mitral valvular incompetence, and the presence, location, and severity of a number of other abnormalities, including ventricular septal defect and hypertrophic cardiomyopathy. As a result, it should be a routine part of catheterization in patients being evaluated for coronary artery disease, aortic or mitral valvular disease, unexplained left ventricular failure, or congenital heart disease. Similarly, *right ventriculography* may provide information about global and segmental right ventricular function and can be especially helpful in patients with congenital heart disease.

INJECTION CATHETERS

To achieve adequate opacification of the left or right ventricles it is necessary to deliver a relatively large amount of contrast material in a relatively short time. In adults, a 7 or 8 Fr catheter with multiple side-holes is usually required, keeping in mind that the ease of de-

Some of the material in this chapter has been obtained from the first and second editions, to which Drs. Charles E. Rackley and William P. Hood, Jr. contributed.

livery of contrast material is related to catheter lumen size. For left and right ventriculography at Parkland Memorial Hospital, every attempt is made to use a catheter in which the lumen is equivalent to that of a standard 8 Fr catheter, unless, of course, the size of the artery through which it is advanced mandates that it be smaller. For adult ventriculography, a 6 Fr (or smaller) catheter is often unsatisfactory.

The ideal catheter for ventriculography should offer minimal resistance to the rapid delivery of contrast material, so that it remains in a stable position during injection and, therefore, produces no disturbance of cardiac rhythm. A catheter with only an end-hole, such as the *Cournand* or *multipurpose,* is unsatisfactory for ventriculography because it often recoils during contrast delivery, causing ventricular ectopic beats and inadequate ventricular opacification, and may produce myocardial penetration (so-called endocardial staining) or even perforation.

Pigtail Catheter. The pigtail catheter has several advantages for left and right ventriculography (Fig. 14–1). First, its end-hole permits its insertion and manipulation with a J-tipped guide wire, so that it can be advanced safely to the left ventricle from the arm or leg even in the patient with brachiocephalic or iliac arterial tortuosity. Second, the design of the catheter virtually eliminates the possibility of endocardial staining, because the end-hole usually is not positioned adjacent to ventricular

215

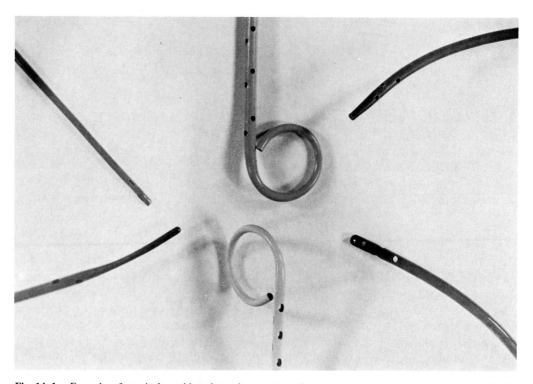

Fig. 14–1. Examples of ventriculographic catheters in current use. Beginning at the top and moving clockwise: pigtail, 8.2 Fr (Cook); Gensini, 7 Fr; NIH, 8 Fr, pigtail, 8 Fr (Cordis); Lehman ventriculographic, 8 Fr; Sones, 7.5 Fr, tapering to a 5.5 Fr tip. The advantages and disadvantages of each catheter are discussed in the text. The Gensini and Sones catheters may cause endocardial staining because of the high pressure jet of contrast material exiting the end-hole; therefore, ventriculography with them should be performed with special attention to catheter position and rate of contrast injection.

trabeculae. Third, the catheter's shape substantially reduces the occurrence of ventricular ectopic beats. As noted, the pigtail can be used with the femoral or brachial approach. Its introduction through a brachial arteriotomy is made easier if a guide wire is used to straighten the curved end of the catheter. In many catheterization laboratories, including the one at Parkland Memorial Hospital, the pigtail is the preferred catheter for left ventriculography by the brachial as well as the femoral approach. In our experience, the pigtail catheter can easily be passed across a porcine aortic valve bioprosthesis—more easily, in fact, than straight catheters—such as the NIH or Eppendorf. In such a situation, the pigtail configuration seems to prevent the catheter from glancing off the large valve cusps and sliding down into the lateral sinuses.

Recently, several catheter manufacturers

have made available pigtail catheters of a "thinwall" variety. These polyurethane catheters are produced with little or no metal reinforcement in the wall. As a result, the wall is distinctly thinner, yielding a larger lumen for a given outer Fr size. Thus, a thin-wall pigtail 7 Fr in outer size has a lumen similar in diameter to a conventional 8 Fr catheter. Because of the larger lumen, these thinwall catheters allow a greater delivery of contrast material without recoil or catheter movement. At the same time, the removal of metal reinforcement from the wall renders these catheters less stiff and, therefore, somewhat more likely to cause ventricular ectopy by moving within the ventricle during systole. We have found the thinwall pigtail catheter to be of particular advantage in patients in whom, for some reason, an unusually large amount of contrast material must be given quickly (i.e., a patient with a very high cardiac output or an individual whose left ventricle is greatly enlarged).

For right ventriculography, the NIH and Eppendorf catheters are practical and effective, but the standard pigtail catheter is preferred at Parkland Memorial Hospital. In addition, the Grollman catheter (which has a pigtail tip and an angulated shaft) is used occasionally for right ventriculography and pulmonary angiography.

Sones Catheter. The Sones catheter is used widely for left ventriculography when catheterization is from the brachial approach. It is the preferred catheter for left ventriculography by the brachial approach at the Beth Israel Hospital in Boston. The polyurethane Sones catheter* is particularly suitable for left ventriculography because it has four side-holes in addition to its end-hole. The catheter comes in 7 and 8 Fr sizes, and tapers to a 5 Fr external diameter near its tip. It will accept an 0.035-inch guide wire, which can be useful in crossing a severely stenotic aortic valve. Techniques for traversing a tortuous subclavian artery system and entering the left ventricle with the Sones catheter are discussed in Chapter 4. For left ventriculography, the Sones catheter should be positioned in an axial orientation (parallel to the ventricular long axis), with its tip midway between the aortic valve and left ventricular apex. Low injection rates (see following paragraphs) usually minimize the extent and forcefulness of catheter recoil. Catheter recoil may still occur, however, with induction of multiple ventricular extrasystoles and potential danger of endocardial staining. Accordingly, the operator should hold the catheter during injection and be prepared to withdraw it if significant recoil develops.

NIH and Eppendorf Catheters. The NIH and Eppendorf catheters have multiple side-holes and no end-hole (Fig. 14–1). They are easily inserted through an arteriotomy (by the brachial approach) or a percutaneously introduced femoral arterial sheath. The 7 Fr and 8 Fr NIH catheters prepared by USCI are made

of woven Dacron with nylon reinforcement and are especially stiff. The Cordis NIH catheter (polyurethane) and Cook NIH torcon blue catheter (polyethylene) are much softer and less likely to cause dissection or perforation. The Eppendorf catheter (USCI, woven Dacron construction) is less stiff as well, and the tips of both the Cordis NIH and the USCI Eppendorf catheters are sufficiently soft that they can be gently prolapsed across the aortic valve. In our catheterization laboratories, the Eppendorf catheter (USCI) and polyurethane or polyethylene NIH catheters (Cordis, Cook Inc.) are sometimes used for left ventriculography by the brachial approach. In some patients, especially those whose left ventricles are small, left ventriculography with an NIH or Eppendorf catheter induces frequent ventricular premature beats. Despite the absence of an end-hole, endocardial staining occasionally occurs with these catheters, usually in patients in whom the end of the catheter is wedged within the ventricular trabeculae.

Lehman Catheter. The Lehman ventriculographic catheter has a tapered closed tip which extends beyond multiple side-holes (Fig. 14–1). The tapered tip may assist the operator in manipulating the catheter through tortuous arteries and across a stenotic aortic valve. Once in the left ventricle, the tip lessens the likelihood of endocardial staining, but, in our experience, it increases the chance of ventricular ectopy during the injection of contrast material.

INJECTION SITE

The adequate opacification of either ventricle is accomplished only if a large amount of contrast material is delivered to it. Satisfactory opacification of the left ventricle can usually be achieved by the injection of contrast material into the left atrium, with cineangiographic acquisition as the left ventricle is filled. Such a left atrial injection is advantageous because it seldom causes atrial or ventricular ectopic activity. It introduces the hazard of transseptal catheterization, however; does not allow an evaluation of mitral valvular

---

*80 cm Cordis SON-II, Sones Technique, Cordis Corporation, Miami, FL

incompetence; and may obscure the basal portion of the left ventricle and the aortic valve. If the patient has aortic regurgitation, the left ventricle may be opacified by aortography, but adequate opacification is usually accomplished only in patients whose regurgitation is severe. Similarly, the right ventricle may be opacified satisfactorily by injecting contrast material into the venae cavae or right atrium. These peripheral injections, however, do not allow an assessment of tricuspid valvular incompetence, and it is often difficult to film the injection in an obliquity that eliminates overlap of the venae cavae, right atrium, and right ventricle.

Ventriculography in the adult is best accomplished by injecting contrast material directly into the ventricular chamber. In the left ventricle, the optimal catheter position is the midcavity, provided that ventricular ectopy is not a problem (Fig. 14–2). Such a midcavitary position ensures (1) that adequate contrast material is delivered to the chamber's body and apex; (2) that the catheter does not interfere with mitral valvular function, thereby producing factitious mitral regurgitation; and (3) that the holes through which the contrast material is injected are not wedged within the ventricular trabeculae (possibly causing endocardial staining). In some patients, a midcavitary position induces repetitive ventricular ectopy, especially with an NIH or Eppendorf catheter. In these individuals, the tip of the catheter is best positioned in the left ventricular *inflow tract,* immediately in front of the posterior leaflet of the mitral valve (Figs. 14–3 and 14–4). This position usually does not cause ventricular ectopy, but mitral regurgitation may be produced if the catheter is too close to the mitral valve.

In the right ventricle, the optimal catheter position is the midcavity, provided, of course, that repetitive ventricular ectopy does not occur. If ectopy is uncontrollable, the catheter may be positioned in the outflow tract, below the pulmonic valve. Even here, however, repetitive ventricular ectopy may present a difficult problem. In our experience, right ventriculography is often accompanied by frequent ventricular premature beats irrespective of catheter position.

INJECTION RATE AND VOLUME

The rapid delivery of an adequate amount of contrast material requires the use of a power injector. There are two types of power injectors. The *pressure injector* allows one to select the volume of contrast material and its delivery pressure, but the rate of delivery is determined by the lumen size and length of the catheter, the viscosity of the contrast material, and the size of the injector syringe. The rapid delivery of contrast material is facilitated by a large-bore and short catheter, prewarmed contrast material, and an injector syringe of small diameter. The pressure injector is now outmoded and does not have the versatility of the flow injector.

The *flow injector* allows one to select both the volume and rate of delivery of contrast material. These injectors develop automatically a pressure sufficient to deliver a selected volume of injectate in a selected time. They are designed to shut down immediately if the pressure required exceeds a preset maximum, however. In most catheterization laboratories, the maximal pressure cutoff is set at 1000 psi. This high pressure is not actually delivered to the catheter tip; instead, most of it is dissipated by frictional losses in the shaft of the catheter.

Some injectors permit synchronization of the injection of contrast material with the R-wave of the electrocardiogram, so that a set flow rate is delivered in each of several successive diastolic intervals.[6,7] Although this technique has been said to lessen the incidence of ventricular ectopic beats and to minimize the volume of contrast material required for adequate ventricular opacification, our impression is that it offers no clear advantage over nonsynchronized methods.

Cine left ventriculography is accomplished using an injection rate and volume that depend on (1) the type and size of catheter, (2) the size of the ventricular chamber to be opacified, (3) the approximate ventricular stroke volume, and (4) the preventriculography hemody-

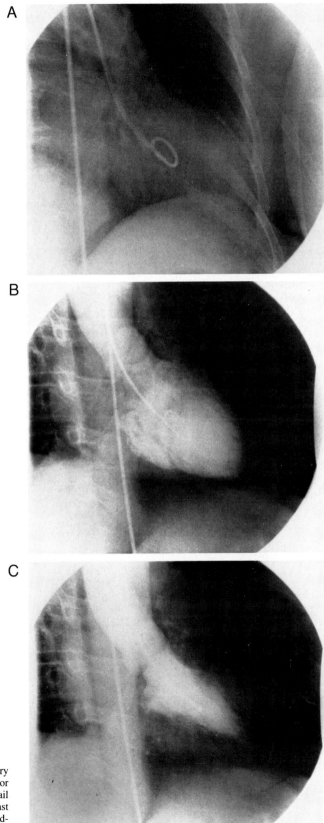

Fig. 14–2. An example of midcavitary catheter position for 30-degree right anterior oblique left ventriculography using a pigtail catheter: (A) before the injection of contrast material. (B) at end-diastole; and (C) end-systole.

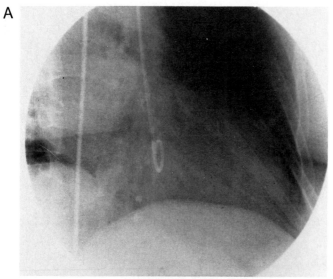

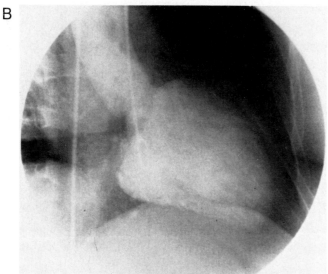

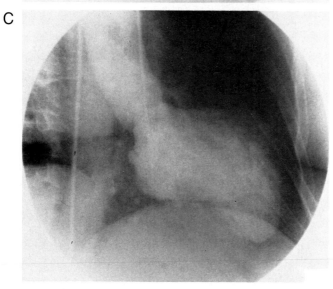

Fig. 14–3. An example of left ventricular inflow tract catheter position for 30-degree right anterior oblique left ventriculography using a pigtail catheter: (A) before the introduction of contrast material; (B) at end-diastole; and (C) end-systole. Note that this patient has a large anteroapical aneurysm.

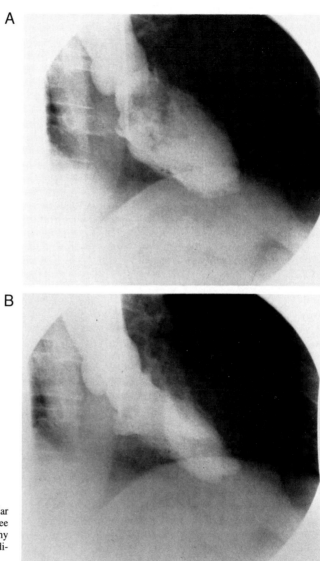

Fig. 14–4. An example of left ventricular inflow tract catheter position for 30-degree right anterior oblique left ventriculography using an Eppendorf catheter: (A) at end-diastole; and (B) end-systole.

namics. We have asked our colleagues in several laboratories to tell us their usual parameters for left ventricular injection using various catheters and either femoral or brachial techniques, and these parameters are listed in Table 14–1. As can be seen, there is a fairly wide spectrum of injection rates and volumes for the pigtail catheter for either femoral or brachial approach. For the pigtail, Eppendorf, and NIH catheters, an injection rate of from 10 to 16 ml/sec (higher for high cardiac output and large ventricular chamber) and a total volume of 30 to 55 ml (depending on ventricular size)

represent average values from Table 14–1. If a Sones catheter is used for left ventriculography, the rate of injection of contrast material should not exceed 7 to 12 ml/sec, thus lessening the chance of recoil and staining.

In the patient with hemodynamic evidence of severe left ventricular dysfunction (mean pulmonary capillary wedge pressure > 25 mm Hg), left ventriculography should be performed using a non-ionic contrast agent. Nonionic contrast agents, discussed in Chapter 2, have substantially improved the safety of left ventriculography in patients with depressed

Table 14-1. *Catheter Type, Injection Rate, and Volume of Contrast Material Used for Left Ventriculography*

Institution & City	Femoral Approach			Brachial Approach		
	Catheter Used	Injection Rate (ml/sec)	Volume (ml)	Catheter Used	Injection Rate (ml/sec)	Volume (ml)
Parkland Hospital Dallas, TX	pigtail	12–16	40–55	pigtail	12–16	40–55
Beth Israel Hospital Boston, MA	pigtail	12–15	36–45	Sones	7–10	30–45
U of Pennsylvania Philadelphia, PA	pigtail	10–14	40–50	pigtail, Sones	10–14 / 8–10	40–50 / 40–45
Barnes Hospital St. Louis, MO	pigtail	10–14	30–40	NIH	10–14	30–40
Nat'l Inst. Health Bethesda, MD	pigtail	10–15	30–45	NIH	10–15	30–45
U of Washington Seattle, WA	pigtail	15–20	40–50	few catheterizations by this approach		
Baylor University Houston, TX	pigtail	12–15	36–45	Sones	8–10	32–40
Brown University Providence, RI	pigtail	15–20	35–50	pigtail, NIH	15–20	35–50
Yale University New Haven, CT	pigtail	12–16	36–48	pigtail, NIH	12	36
Mayo Clinic Rochester, MN	pigtail	12–18	40–55	NIH, Rodriguez	12–18	40–55
U of Florida Gainesville, FL	pigtail	8–12	25–36	Sones	8–12	25–36
New York Hospital New York, NY	pigtail	8–12	30–45	Sones	8–12	30–45
U of Iowa Hospital Iowa City, IA	pigtail	12–15	45–60	pigtail	12–15	45–60
U of N Carolina Chapel Hill, NC	pigtail	10–14	30–42	pigtail	10–14	30–42

myocardial function, severe coronary artery disease, and/or aortic stenosis. Compared to so-called ionic agents (e.g., sodium meglumine diatrizoate), the non-ionic agents (e.g., iohexol) produce only minor decreases in ionized calcium in the coronary circulation, and thus have a minimal myocardial depressant effect.[8,11] One drawback preventing even more widespread use of the newer non-ionic contrast agents is their cost, which is currently 5 to 10 times that of ionic agents. As an alternative to use of non-ionic contrast, left ventriculography should be limited, if possible (i.e., 12 to 16 ml/sec for only 2 seconds, giving a total volume of 24 to 32 ml), and the ventriculogram should be performed during the administration of an acutely imposed "protective regimen." In the patient whose abnormal filling pressures are attributable to coronary artery disease, cardiomyopathy, or severe aortic or mitral regurgitation, left ventriculography is best performed after the administration of sublingual nitroglycerin or during the intravenous infusion of nitroglycerin or sodium nitroprusside. If the pulmonary capillary wedge pressure is greatly elevated because of mitral stenosis, left ventriculography should be preceded by the intravenous administration of morphine sulfate and furosemide. *Failure to take a highly elevated preventriculography pulmonary capillary wedge pressure seriously can lead to disastrous consequences, such as intractable pulmonary edema and even death.* In our experience, the left ventricular end-diastolic pressure is not as reliable a predictor of impending pulmonary edema as the wedge pressure because (as discussed elsewhere) the left ventricular end-diastolic and mean pulmonary capillary wedge pressures may be widely disparate.

As another approach to improved safety, left ventriculography may be performed with a small amount of contrast material (12 to 20 ml given in 3 seconds) using radiographic equipment with digital subtraction capability.[12]

Before the power injection of contrast material, one should (1) do a test injection of 3 to 5 ml to confirm proper catheter and patient position and (2) take appropriate precautions

in filling and firing the power injector to prevent air embolism. In our catheterization laboratories, a Medrad Mark IV power injector with a 130 ml translucent syringe is used. These syringes are made of siliconized plastic so that the contrast medium and any air may be easily seen. The injector is loaded with contrast material through roentgenography tubing 30 inches long while the syringe barrel is pointed upward. With the injector in the vertical position, air is expelled from the syringe and tubing by holding the load switch in the forward position as the operator taps the syringe and its Luer-Lok connector to discharge all air bubbles. Subsequently, the injector is inverted, and a "running connection" is made between the roentgenography tubing and the catheter. Specifically, the connection is accomplished while blood is spurting from the hub of the catheter as the operator of the injector depresses the forward position of the load switch. After the connection is made, the injector operator presses the reverse position of the load switch, withdrawing gradually until the "interface" between contrast material and blood in the roentgenography tubing is easily visible and is noted to be free of air bubbles. A test injection of contrast material can then be done under fluoroscopic visualization, enabling the physician to assess catheter and patient position.

The physician performing the catheterization should look closely at the injector syringe to be sure that it is filled with contrast medium and free of air. This physician should also plan to hold the catheter at the point of its insertion into the body during the power injection of contrast, so that he may pull the catheter back instantaneously if ventricular extrasystoles, myocardial staining, or other untoward events develop during injection. Thus, the physician operator must have good visualization of the fluoroscopic screen during ventriculography. The technician or other individual firing the injector should be prepared to abort the injection upon command from the physician operator in the event of an untoward occurrence. In many laboratories the physician performing the catheterization holds the connection between catheter and roentgenography tubing tightly in one hand during the power injection to prevent a leak of contrast material at this point.

Proper catheter positioning is important to avoid extrasystoles during ventriculography, as discussed earlier in this chapter. If extrasystoles develop, it is our policy to withdraw the ventriculographic catheter immediately after the first extrasystole a distance of approximately 2 to 3 cm. This usually results in a quiet position for the remainder of the 3 to 4 second contrast injection, and is particularly effective when the Sones catheter is being used for left ventriculography: this technique has not resulted in ventricular staining in a very large experience.

Instructions to the patient regarding respiration during contrast ventriculography vary from laboratory to laboratory. Previously, imaging systems were often inadequate to give good definition of the left ventricular silhouette unless ventriculography was performed during deep inspiration to move the diaphragm out of the radiographic field. With modern imaging systems, excellent definition of the ventricular silhouette can be achieved without performing ventriculography during held deep inspiration. Left ventriculography done during normal quiet breathing allows physiologic interpretation of left ventricular volumes, angiographic stroke volume, and calculated left ventricular regurgitant fraction in cases of valvular regurgitation. In the catheterization laboratory at Parkland Memorial Hospital, most left ventriculograms are performed after the patient simply has stopped breathing (without first inspiring deeply).

FILMING PROJECTION AND TECHNIQUE

As a general rule, *biplane* ventriculography is preferable to *single plane* ventriculography because it allows one to obtain more information at essentially no additional risk to the patient. For example, in the patient with coronary artery disease, biplane left ventriculography is superior to single plane left ventric-

ulography in providing information on the location and severity of segmental wall motion abnormalities. In the patient with congenital heart disease, biplane right ventriculography allows one to assess accurately the anatomy of the right ventricular outflow tract, the pulmonic valve, and the proximal portions of the pulmonary artery. Biplane ventriculography, however, has several disadvantages, including (1) the increased expense of biplane cineangiographic equipment; (2) the reduced quality of cineangiographic imaging in each plane that results from the radiation scatter caused by the opposite plane; (3) the additional time required to position the biplane equipment appropriately, especially when the brachial approach is used; and (4) the additional radiation exposure to personnel in the room.

Whether doing biplane or single plane ventriculography, one should use the projection(s) that provide(s) maximal delineation of the structure(s) of interest and minmal overlapping of other structures. Most laboratories doing biplane left ventriculography prefer a 30° right anterior oblique (RAO) and a 60° left anterior oblique (LAO) view. The 30° RAO projection eliminates overlap of the left ventricle and the vertebral column, allows one to assess anterior, apical, and inferior segmental wall motion, and places the mitral valve in profile, thus providing a reliable assessment of the presence and angiographic severity of mitral regurgitation. As seen in Figure 14–5, the 30-degree RAO projection allows excellent visualization of the extent of an anterior wall aneurysm of the left ventricle in a patient with isolated proximal occlusion of the left anterior descending artery. The 60-degree LAO view allows one to assess ventricular septal integrity and motion, posterior segmental function, and aortic valvular anatomy. *Cranial angulation* of the 60-degree LAO view may prevent the foreshortening of the left ventricle that commonly occurs with LAO views and places the entire length of the interventricular septum in profile.

If biplane cineangiographic equipment is not available, the single-plane projection that provides the best delineation of structures of interest should be used. For example, the 30-

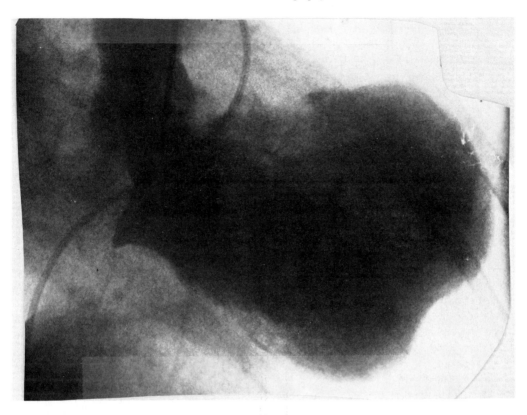

Fig. 14–5. Left ventriculogram in a 30-degree RAO projection (end systolic frame) showing a large anterior wall aneurysm. The patient was a 65-year-old man who had a massive myocardial infarction (peak CK 4460 units) and showed subsequently a progressively enlarged cardiac silhouette on a roentgenogram. Catheterization 4 weeks following infarction demonstrated a large anterior wall LV aneurysm, with LV pressure 95/40 mmHg, PCW pressure 34 mmHg, and occlusion of the left anterior descending artery proximal to the first septal perforator. Ejection fraction was 18%, and the other coronary arteries were normal.

degree RAO projection allows a reliable assessment of mitral regurgitation, whereas a 45-degree to 60-degree LAO view (with cranial angulation of 15 degrees if possible) provides the opportunity to visualize a ventricular septal defect and the associated left-to-right shunting.

Almost all cineangiographic systems in use today employ a 35-mm camera. For routine left or right ventriculography, we perform cineangiography at 60 frames/second and use a 9-inch image intensifier, which allows us to visualize the entire ventricle within the field. In many patients, ventriculography performed with a greater degree of magnification (e.g., 6-inch intensifier) is not adequate for assessment of the entire ventricular silhouette together with the left atrium and ascending aorta.

INTERVENTION VENTRICULOGRAPHY

Segmental dysfunction of the left ventricular wall can be caused by ischemia or infarction. Over the past 10 to 15 years, several techniques have been described that allow one to determine during left ventriculography if an asynergic segment of the left ventricle is ischemic or infarcted. With each of these techniques, segments whose abnormal wall motion is caused by *ischemia* show improvement in systolic motion, whereas segments whose abnormal wall motion is due to *infarction* fail to improve.

First, left ventricular segmental wall motion can be improved substantially by the administration of catecholamines.[13] Two left ventriculograms are performed—the first in the resting (baseline) state, the second during a steady-state infusion of epinephrine (1 to 4 μg/min). Segments that are ischemic and, as a result, hypokinetic or akinetic on baseline ventriculography improve their contractile pattern during epinephrine infusion; in contrast, segments that are asynergic due to infarction show no alteration in contractility when stimulated by epinephrine.

Second, left ventricular segmental wall motion can be influenced by nitroglycerin.[14] Here, also, two left ventriculograms are performed, one before and the other after sublingual administration of nitroglycerin, when there is evidence of a nitroglycerin-induced fall in systemic arterial pressure. Segments of the left ventricle in which contraction is abnormal on the baseline ventriculogram but which improve after nitroglycerin are reversibly injured (that is, ischemic), whereas those in which asynergy is present before nitroglycerin and is not altered by it are most likely irreversibly damaged (that is, infarcted). Segments in which motion improves with nitroglycerin generally maintain this level of improvement after successful surgical revascularization; in contrast, segments in which contractile function is not influenced by nitroglycerin are not improved by revascularization.

Third, left ventricular segmental wall motion can be influenced by postextrasystolic potentiation.[15] A single ventricular premature beat is introduced during left ventriculography and is followed by a compensatory pause and then a potentiated beat. Segmental wall motion during one of the preceding sinus beats is compared to that of the post-extrasystolic beat. Left ventricles with asynergic wall motion during a preceding sinus beat which improves on the potentiated beat are ischemic, whereas those in which asynergy is similar on the preceding sinus beat and on the postextrasystolic beat are infarcted. Augmentation ventriculography by this technique offers the advantage that both baseline and potentiated left ventricular wall motion can be characterized on a single ventriculogram. Postextrasystolic potentiation

may be provided by introducing a timed stimulus (delivered through a right ventricular pacing catheter) or by pullback of a right ventricular catheter during left ventriculography. It is probably unwise to attempt to induce the ventricular extrasystole by manipulating the left ventriculographic catheter during the injection of contrast material, since such manipulation may cause endocardial staining.

Other types of intervention ventriculography may be of use in the patient with chronic left ventricular volume overload caused by aortic or mitral regurgitation. In the patient with aortic regurgitation and well-preserved left ventricular function, angiotensin in a dose sufficient to increase left ventricular systolic pressure by 20 to 50 mmHg causes no change in left ventricular ejection fraction.[16] In the patient whose aortic regurgitation has caused a loss of left ventricular contractile reserve, a similar amount of angiotensin caused a fall in left ventricular ejection fraction of more than 0.10. Thus, left ventriculography during "afterload stress" may provide additional information about left ventricular functional capability. Alternatively, intervention ventriculography using sodium nitroprusside may be used in patients with mitral regurgitation, aortic regurgitation, or dilated cardiomyopathy to assess the potential benefit of chronic vasodilator therapy.

COMPLICATIONS AND HAZARDS

Although complications of cardiac catheterization and angiography are discussed in detail in Chapter 3, certain specific points relevant to ventriculography are presented here.

Complications of Injection

Arrhythmias. Ventricular extrasystoles occur frequently during ventriculography and are usually caused by mechanical stimulation of the ventricular endocardium by the catheter or a jet of contrast agent. Such extrasystoles can usually be eliminated or at least minimized by repositioning the catheter. Although short runs of ventricular tachycardia occur during an occasional ventriculogram, they almost always cease promptly when the catheter is removed from the ventricle. Rarely, the ventricular tachycardia caused by ventriculography is sustained even after catheter removal. It should be treated quickly with a bolus of intravenous lidocaine and, if necessary, direct current countershock. Ventricular fibrillation has been reported to be induced by an improperly grounded power injector.[17]

Intramyocardial Injection (So-called Endocardial Staining). The deposition of contrast material within the endocardium and myocardium is usually caused by improper positioning of the ventriculographic catheter. Although a small endocardial stain usually causes no problem, a large stain may lead to medically refractory ventricular tachyarrhythmias, including ventricular tachycardia or fibrillation. In the catheterization laboratory at Parkland Memorial Hospital, about 3500 left ventriculograms have been performed with a pigtail catheter. A very small endocardial stain occurred in only one and was not accompanied by ventricular tachyarrhythmias. Rarely, the power injection of contrast material causes myocardial perforation, with the resultant leakage of blood and contrast material into the pericardial space and the development of cardiac tamponade. This must be treated by emergency pericardiocentesis, and immediate consultation obtained from a cardiothoracic surgeon.

Embolism. The inadvertent injection of air or thrombus probably poses the greatest risk associated with ventriculography. The presence of thrombi on the ventriculographic catheter is minimized by (1) frequent flushing of the catheter with a solution containing heparin and (2) systemic heparinization of the patient when the ventriculographic catheter is first introduced. For all adult patients, we administer 5000 units of heparin intravenously when the first arterial catheter (brachial or femoral) is introduced into the aorta.

An occasional patient is referred for catheterization in whom there is suspicion (from noninvasive testing) of a thrombus in the left ventricular apex. If left ventriculography is required in such a patient, great care should be taken to position the ventriculographic catheter in the left ventricular inflow tract avoiding the apical portion completely. Partially organized thrombi may be dislodged from the left ventricular cavity by the catheter tip or the force of a power injection. Accordingly, the ventricular angiographic catheter should not be advanced to the left ventricular apex except under exceptional circumstances (e.g., suspicion of IHSS).

Complications of Contrast Material

For 20 to 30 seconds after ventriculography, the patient has a "hot flash," due to the powerful vasodilation caused by the contrast material. Transient nausea and vomiting used to occur in 20 to 30% of patients, but with current formulations of contrast agent, this is uncommon. The immediate but short-lived hemodynamic effects of ventriculography with ionic contrast agents include a modest fall in systemic arterial pressure, a reflex increase in heart rate, and a transient depression of left ventricular contractility. Within 1 to 2 minutes, these effects usually resolve.

REFERENCES

1. Hildner FJ, et al: New principles for optimum left ventriculography. Cathet Cardiovasc Diagn 12:266, 1986.
2. Grossman W: Assessment of regional myocardial function. J Am Coll Cardiol 7:327, 1986.
3. Herman MV, Gorlin R: Implication of left ventricular asynergy. Am J Cardiol 23:538, 1969.
4. Bruschke AVG, Proudfit WL, Sones FM Jr: Progress study of 590 consecutive nonsurgical cases of coronary disease followed 5–9 years. II. Ventriculographic and other correlations Circulation 47:1154, 1973.
5. Rackley CE, Hood WP Jr: Quantitative angiographic evaluation and pathophysiologic mechanisms in valvular heart disease. Prog Cardiovasc Dis 15:427, 1973.
6. Schad N, et al: The intermittent phased injection of contrast material into the heart. Am J Roentgenol 104:464, 1968.
7. Viamonte M Jr: Innovations in angiography. Radiol Clin North Am 9:361, 1971.
8. Bourdillon PD, et al: Effects of a new nonionic and a conventional ionic contrast agent on coronary sinus ionized calcium and left ventricular hemodynamics. J Am Coll Cardiol 6:845, 1985.

9. Salem DN, Konstam MA, Isner JM, Bonin JD: Comparison of the electrocardiographic and hemodynamic response to ionic and nonionic radiocontrast media during left ventriculography: a randomized double-blind study. Am Heart J 111:533, 1986.

10. Benotti JR: The comparative effects of ionic versus nonionic agents in cardiac catheterization. Invest Radiol 23 (Suppl 2):5366, 1988.

11. Wisneski JA, Gertz EW, Dahlgren M, Muslin A: Comparison of low osmolality ionic (ioxaglate) versus nonionic (iopamidol) contrast media in cardiac angiography. Am J Cardiol 63:489, 1989.

12. Mancini GB, et al: Quantitative assessment of global and regional left ventricular function with low-contrast dose digital subtraction ventriculography. Chest 87:598, 1985.

13. Horn HR, et al: Augmentation of left ventricular contraction pattern in coronary artery disease by an inotropic catecholamine. The epinephrine ventriculogram. Circulation 49:1063, 1974.

14. Helfant RH, et al: Nitroglycerin to unmask reversible asynergy. Correlation with post coronary bypass ventriculography. Circulation 50:108, 1974.

15. Dyke SH, Cohn PF, Gorlin R, Sonnenblick EH: Detection of residual myocardial function in coronary artery disease using postextrasystolic potentiation. Circulation 50:694, 1974.

16. Bolen JL, et al: Evaluation of left ventricular function in patients with aortic regurgitation using afterload stress. Circulation 53:132, 1976.

17. Rowe GG, Zarnstorff WC: Ventricular fibrillation during selective angiography. JAMA 192:947, 1965.

15

Pulmonary Angiography

JOSEPH R. BENOTTI and WILLIAM GROSSMAN

INDICATIONS

Pulmonary angiography is most frequently required to confirm or exclude the diagnosis of pulmonary embolism.[1,2] Other cardiovascular conditions in which pulmonary angiography is indicated for diagnosis in anticipation of corrective surgery include branch pulmonary artery stenosis (Fig. 15–1) and pulmonary arteriovenous malformation (Fig. 15–2).[2,3] The effect of occluding the arteriovenous malformation (by inflating the balloon on the tip of a flotation catheter) on the magnitude of right-to-left shunt can be determined. Pulmonary arteriovenous malformations have been closed successfully by embolizing the communication with thrombogenic material or placement of occlusion coils. This is particularly advantageous in a patient with multiple pulmonary arteriovenous malformations that, by the diffuse nature of the process, preclude successful surgical management with segmental pulmonary resection. Pulmonary angiography is also sometimes indicated in the evaluation of bullous lung disease in which resection of one or more blebs is being considered. Selective pulmonary angiography may be important in the evaluation of patients with suspected primary pulmonary hypertension to exclude large unresolved pulmonary embolism,[4] particularly when there are segmental or lobar perfusion abnormalities detected by the lung scan.[5] Pulmonary angi-ography is required to evaluate sarcomatous tumors.[6] These arise from the component tissues of the pulmonary vasculature, present as compressive central or peripheral lung masses, and may cause symptoms from compression of adjacent structures. In the evaluation of these rare tumors, pulmonary angiography (in addition to computerized axial tomography of the thorax) is often needed to characterize the extent of the malignancy, its vascular origin and resectability, and to guide technical aspects of the operative approach. Wedge or balloon occlusion pulmonary angiography has been used in evaluating the severity of hypertrophic changes in the small pulmonary arteries. This information may be useful in assessing the morphology and reversibility of reactive pulmonary vascular changes in congenital heart disease, particularly when there is a long-standing left-to-right shunt that has become bidirectional as a result of reactive pulmonary hypertension. Levo-phase pulmonary angiography may be useful in confirming or excluding a left atrial myxoma when echocardiographic findings are equivocal.

Pulmonary angiography is also occasionally used to identify the insertion site(s) of anomalous pulmonary veins(s). Because of high pulmonary blood flow from the left-to-right shunt, however, a large volume of contrast medium must be injected rapidly to opacify an anomalous vein with sufficient resolution. Hand-powered contrast injection through the

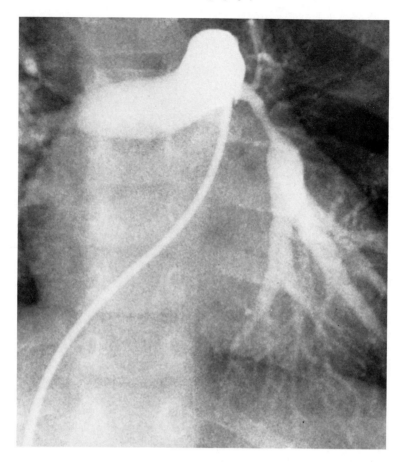

Fig. 15–1. Pulmonary angiogram of branch pulmonary stenosis in an adolescent male. The catheter tip is positioned 1 to 2 cm beyond the origin of the right pulmonary artery so that with the power injection of contrast agent the catheter tip recoils into the main pulmonary trunk to optimally opacify the left pulmonary artery and its ramifications.

distal lumen of a balloon-tipped catheter with the balloon inflated may be a useful technique for such a study. The inflated balloon stops antegrade pulmonary flow into the lobar artery from which the anomalous vein originates. Filming as contrast medium is injected and again later as the balloon is deflated allows the contrast medium to enter and satisfactorily opacify the anomalous vein. This technique may facilitate identification of anomalous pulmonary veins with much greater resolution and with a much lower cumulative contrast load.

Role of the Lung Scan. Pulmonary arteriography is certainly not indicated in every patient whenever pulmonary embolism is suspected; rather, its performance is predicated on logical interpretation of all relevant clinical data including the ventilation-perfusion lung scan. Except in the patient with cardiogenic shock and cor pulmonale, where emergency pulmonary angiography is required for diagnostic confirmation before embolectomy, it is advisable to obtain a ventilation perfusion lung scan in all patients with suspected pulmonary embolism. A normal perfusion lung scan reliably excludes pulmonary embolism, sparing the patient the needless morbidity and expense of pulmonary angiography. Similarly, in a patient in shock a small unilateral regional perfusion abnormality on the lung scan would make it highly unlikely that massive pulmonary embolism could account for this hemodynamic derangement. Recognizing that pulmonary embolism of such a small magnitude could not account for the clinical signs, the clinician should look for other causes of cir-

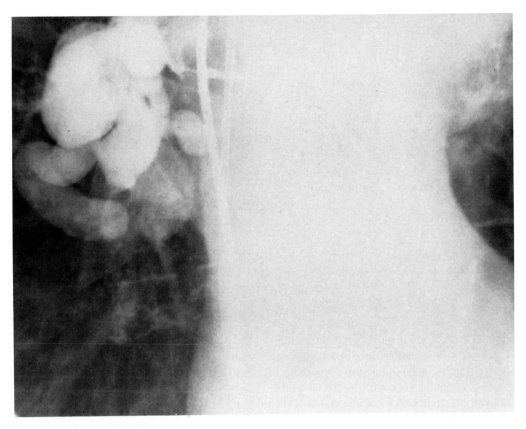

Fig. 15–2. Pulmonary angiogram of pulmonary arteriovenous malformation involving the right upper lobe pulmonary artery and vein in a 48-year-old woman. Contrast agent is injected by hand through a balloon-tipped pulmonary artery catheter with the tip positioned at the origin of the right upper lobe vessel. The balloon is inflated so that the fistula is occluded, and it is adequately opacified with less than 10 ml of contrast agent.

culatory inadequacy (e.g., hemorrhage, sepsis, myocardial infarction).

Pulmonary angiography is most commonly indicated when there is a strong clinical suspicion of pulmonary embolism, but the ventilation-perfusion lung scan reveals one or more "matched" defects where perfusion and ventilation abnormalities coincide. Though the chest roentgenogram may be helpful in identifying localized pulmonary parenchymal findings (pneumonia, atelectasis, bullous disease) that satisfactorily account for the perfusion lung scan abnormalities in the absence of pulmonary embolism, angiography is usually required to confirm or exclude pulmonary embolism if, in the appropriate clinical setting, such findings cannot be explained otherwise. Even when the lung scan findings would not obviate the need for pulmonary angiography, it is often helpful to have obtained a lung scan before pulmonary angiography because location of the perfusion defect(s) directs the angiographer in his choice of lung regions for selective study. A strategy for deciding when to perform pulmonary angiography based on the combined findings of lung scan and chest roentgenogram is presented in Table 15–1.

CONTRAINDICATIONS

A relative contraindication to pulmonary arteriography is a history of allergic reaction to contrast material. However, with proper premedication with corticosteroids and antihistaminic agents (see Chapter 2) angiographic procedures can almost always be performed safely in such patients.

Pulmonary angiography is remarkably safe

Table 15–1. *Clinically Suspicious Pulmonary Embolism: Role of Pulmonary Angiography*

	Lung Scan	Chest Roentgenogram	Fraction of Patients with Documented Embolism
Angiography not ordinarily required	Normal		1/8*
	Low probability	No signs of embolism†	0/18
	High probability	2 or more signs	17/17
Angiography may be required	High probability	No signs of embolism	4/8
	High probability	Only one sign	16/21
	Low probability	At least one sign	7/32
Angiography normally required	Any abnormality	Cardiomegaly or left heart failure	7/15

*Single small embolus in affected patient.

†Signs include infiltrate, effusion, atelectasis, elevated hemidiaphragm, and segmental oligemia (Westermark's sign).

(Adapted from Moses DC, et al: The complementary roles of chest radiography, lung scanning, and selective pulmonary angiography in the diagnosis of pulmonary embolism. Circulation 49:179, 1974.)

even in critically ill patients when performed by an experienced physician. Certainly, a carefully performed pulmonary angiogram that establishes the diagnosis and aids in selection of therapy carries less risk than treating a patient with anticoagulants empirically when there really is no pulmonary embolism, or withholding anticoagulant therapy from a patient who has actually sustained pulmonary embolism.

COMPLICATIONS

Pulmonary angiography may be associated with complications related to right heart catheterization (cardiac perforation, arrhythmia) or to administration of radiographic contrast agent (allergic reactions, intimal injection, hypotension, pulmonary edema). Iodinated angiographic contrast medium causes an immediate acute depression in myocardial contractility and associated peripheral vasodilation. Minutes to hours later, it causes osmotic diuresis, thereby reducing afterload and preload. A clinical correlate in patients with normal underlying cardiovascular function is postural hypotension with warm, flushed, and well-perfused extremities one to several hours following the angiographic procedure. Pulmonary edema may develop in patients with severe myocardial depression within a few

minutes to 1 hour following angiography. This is usually a result of myocardial depression and acute volume expansion resulting from the osmotic load of contrast medium. To the extent that the pulmonary angiogram requires a rather large total contrast volume and is performed in patients with underlying heart disease, these problems can be anticipated and managed effectively.

Serious underlying cardiopulmonary disease increases the risk of pulmonary angiography, particularly when multiple contrast injections into the main and proximal pulmonary arteries subject the patient to a cumulative contrast dose exceeding 200 ml. Mainstream pulmonary angiography has been associated with acute myocardial depression and death in patients with primary pulmonary hypertension.[7] The risk is greatest when the pulmonary artery pressure approaches that in the systemic arterial circuit. Through preload augmentation and antecedent hypertrophy, the chronically pressure overloaded right ventricle may already be functioning at the limit of its preload reserve. The abrupt increase in right ventricular afterload and depression in contractility engendered by rapid contrast injection exceeding 25 to 30 ml into a major pulmonary artery acutely exceeds the limits of right ventricular compensation, sometimes with a fatal outcome. In reviewing 15 series involving over 400 pulmonary arteriograms, Goodman found a mortality rate of 0.2%, a cardiac perforation rate of 0.4% and a risk of cardiac arrhythmia of 0.7%.[8]

Although there have been no systematic studies examining the effect of substituting the *newer (low-osmolar) contrast agents* on the safety of pulmonary angiography, it seems likely that major hemodynamic complications should be sharply reduced. Thus, in patients with severe pulmonary hypertension, low-osmolar agents should be used preferentially for pulmonary angiography.

HEMODYNAMIC EVALUATION AS PART OF PULMONARY ANGIOGRAPHY

Although the most common reason for requesting pulmonary angiography is to confirm or exclude the presence of pulmonary embolism with the highest degree of certainty, a carefully performed angiographic study that includes complete hemodynamic evaluation provides much additional information of clinical value. Hemodynamic assessment preceding an angiographic evaluation that demonstrates pulmonary embolism allows rational selection of appropriate supportive, therapeutic, and prophylactic measures. For example, the patient with a depressed cardiac output and end-organ hypoperfusion in conjunction with massive pulmonary embolism and right ventricular failure requires supportive measures dictated by the hemodynamic findings. These might include colloid infusion to elevate right ventricular filling pressure and inotropic drugs to improve the force of right ventricular contraction, thereby overcoming the acute increase in right ventricular afterload imposed by the obstructing emboli. If prompt correction of the circulatory inadequacy cannot be achieved, definitive therapeutic measures to remove the obstructing emboli (e.g., administration of a thrombolytic agent, surgical pulmonary embolectomy, or catheter removal of pulmonary embolism) must be undertaken. Management of the patient with pulmonary embolism is predicated upon careful hemo-dynamic assessment, which can be accomplished at the time of pulmonary angiography. Conversely, hemodynamic assessment in conjunction with an angiogram that is negative or nondiagnostic for pulmonary embolism may enable the cardiologist to diagnose *other cardiopulmonary conditions* that may be responsible for the patient's clinical presentation and then to proceed with specific therapy. Careful hemodynamic evaluation may point to left ventricular failure, cardiac tamponade, occult constrictive pericardial disease, or cor pulmonale as a result of chronic obstructive lung disease as the underlying problem. In a patient with suspected pulmonary embolism referred for pulmonary angiography, one of us (JB) has observed cardiac tamponade resulting from right atrial perforation by the fine wire stylet of a central venous pressure catheter, hardly visible by image intensification fluoroscopy. This diagnosis was suggested initially by a continuously monitored femoral artery pressure demonstrating pulsus paradox of a magnitude insufficient to be detected by a sphygmomanometric pressure measurement, and by a right atrial pressure elevation not evident by visual inspection of the jugular meniscus because of the patient's obesity.

Hemodynamic evaluation before angiography also provides important information that facilitates technical performance of an optimal study at minimal risk to the patient. Pulmonary blood flow, measured by Fick or thermodilution technique or estimated from measurements of pulmonary artery and systemic arterial oxygen saturation, will influence, in part, selection of the injection parameters (contrast volume and flow rate) required for adequate vascular opacification. The pulmonary artery wedge pressure, if elevated, may restrict the total allowable contrast volume and directs the operator to treat the patient with diuretics or vasodilators. These interventions may permit administration of a sufficient total volume of contrast for performance of an adequate study. If *paradoxic embolism* is suspected, it is appropriate to perform indicator-dilution studies with injection of indocyanine green dye into the inferior vena cava to verify the potential for right-to-left shunting.

VASCULAR ACCESS

Pulmonary angiography has been performed traditionally using a catheter advanced by way of a brachial vein by exposed cutdown in the antecubital fossa. This approach facilitates catheter manipulation between right and left pulmonary arteries, so that more selective views can be obtained in either lung. The percutaneous subclavian, internal jugular, and femoral venous approaches carry the potential serious risk of delayed bleeding with anticoagulant and particularly with thrombolytic therapy. Also, there is always concern over the potential for dislodging loosely adherent iliofemoral or vena caval thrombi when a catheter is advanced from the femoral vein. If the thrombus has become organized in the iliofemoral venous system, it may not be possible to advance the catheter through this region. It is also usually more difficult to manipulate a catheter from the left to the right pulmonary artery or vice versa, when it has been introduced from the femoral vein. For these reasons we favor the brachial venous approach.

TECHNIQUES

The standard technique of pulmonary angiography involves power injection of radiographic contrast medium at a high flow rate (10 to 30 ml/sec) through a suitable 5 to 8 Fr angiographic catheter positioned in a first or second order pulmonary artery.[9] The 7 Fr or 8 Fr Eppendorf catheter,* a woven Dacron catheter, which has four side holes and lacks an end hole, is excellent for pulmonary angiography. The end-hole occluded design minimizes catheter tip recoil, which usually accompanies forceful contrast injection. A disadvantage of this catheter is that a soft-tipped guide wire cannot be extruded from the tip of the catheter for guiding purposes to facilitate safe catheter passage. End-hole catheters allow use of a guide wire to facilitate safe catheter passage through difficult-to-traverse right heart chambers. However, end-hole catheters have a much greater propensity to recoil proximally during angiography. The Grollman catheter† (a pigtail catheter with an acute angle on the terminal shaft, near the tip) has a natural shape that facilitates right heart catheterization and an end hole so that it can be advanced over a guide wire. It does not recoil because of its pigtail configuration and because contrast medium exits from side holes positioned opposite to one another. The result is that the forces responsible for catheter tip recoil cancel one another out. However, because of its preformed permanent shape and looped tip, the Grollman catheter usually cannot be advanced beyond the main right or left pulmonary artery into lobar vessels and is not ideal for more selective injections. The Berman angiographic catheter‡ is a balloon-flotation catheter with multiple side holes designed especially for pulmonary angiography and is the preferred catheter for this procedure in some laboratories.

In patients with *left bundle branch block,* one should have a pacing catheter prepared and ready to be advanced to the right ventricle in case right bundle branch block and asystole develop during placement of the angiographic catheter in the pulmonary artery.

For mainstream pulmonary angiography, the catheter is usually positioned in the right pulmonary artery with its tip 1 to 2 cm proximal to the takeoff of the upper lobe pulmonary artery branch and 1 to 2 cm distal to the origin of the right pulmonary artery. A wide or open loop is placed in the proximal catheter segment as it traverses the right ventricle to support the catheter to minimize recoil. Mainstream angiography usually requires 40 to 50 ml radiographic contrast medium injected at a rate of 20 to 30 ml/sec. Selective studies of lobar vessels usually require a total volume of 20 to 40 ml injected at a rate of 15 to 20 ml/sec. Subselective injections may be done at lower volumes and injection rates. Technical factors influencing selection of injection parameters

*USCI, Billerica, MA.

†Cook, Inc., Bloomington, IN.
‡Elecath, Rahway, NJ.

(total contrast dose and injection rate) include the quality of the imaging equipment, the size of the vascular region of interest, pulmonary blood flow, the Fr size of the angiographic catheter, and the strong suspicion of major proximal emboli as evidenced by the perfusion scan or by a previous test injection. Low pulmonary blood flow or major proximal emboli reduce the total contrast volume required for an adequate study, and smaller catheter sizes limit the maximal injection rate. Selective views require a slower delivery rate and lower-contrast dose relative to mainstream studies.

RADIOGRAPHIC FILMING

Filming is accomplished during a maximal inspiration either by the large film or the cineangiographic technique. Each method has advantages and disadvantages, and the laboratory performing pulmonary angiography should be equipped to use both methods.

Large Film Method. Before large film study, one or more scout films of the chest are obtained to select the kilovoltage that optimizes a gray-scale contrast between bone, vasculature, other soft-tissue structures, and the pulmonary parenchyma. Large film, either roll or cutfilm, is exposed serially by a programmed automatic film changer, activated at the start of the power contrast injection. Usually, peak opacification of the pulmonary arterial phase occurs 2 to 4 sec after injection, and when large film is used an exposure rate of 2 to 4 films/sec is utilized for this phase. The pulmonary venous-left heart phase occurs 5 to 7 sec after starting the injection and should be filmed at 1 to 2 films/sec. The systemic arterial phase peaks 7 to 10 sec after injection and may be recorded at 1 film/sec, so that for a complete run 14 to 20 films are obtained over 10 sec. If the cardiac output is reduced and the circulation time is prolonged, filming should continue for a total of 12 to 14 sec. Filming beyond the first 6 to 8 sec is usually performed at a frequency of 1 sec to minimize radiation and conserve film. As exemplified in Figure 15–3, the advantages of large film include quality of resolution, the clarity of vas-

cular detail, and versatility in field size (from the entire thorax to a single lobe depending upon how the tube is positioned and how the field is coned). Large film views enable the angiographer to study the entire thorax, a whole lung, or a single lobe with the excellent demonstration of the detailed anatomy of each and every vascular branch. Filming during the levophase of a mainstream injection gives reasonably detailed anatomic information about left heart structures and the thoracic aorta.

The mainstream pulmonary angiogram recorded on large film provides information from which *the percentage of pulmonary vascular obstruction* resulting from pulmonary embolism can be estimated. In patients with no underlying cardiopulmonary disease, this correlates directly with the severity of pulmonary hypertension and hypoxemia.[10]

An unequivocal angiographic diagnosis of pulmonary embolism requires demonstration of intralumenal filling defects and abrupt total or near-total cutoff of vessels resulting from embolic obstruction, as illustrated in Figure 15–3. Such findings are specific for pulmonary embolism. A disadvantage of the large film method is that vessels overlapping or crossing one another, viewed as consecutive static images, may mimic pulmonary embolism. Also, it is tedious and time-consuming to reposition the patient repetitively between the fluoroscopic image intensifier and the large film changer for catheter repositioning before selective studies. Indeed, if the patient is very ill, repositioning may not be possible and may limit the adequacy of the study. Even though the catheter is carefully positioned under fluoroscopic guidance, there is always concern that it may migrate during the interval required to position the patient between the x ray generator and large film changer. Proximal catheter dislodgement usually results in a subselective and less than adequate study. Migration of the catheter tip more distally may result in an injection at excessive pressure and flow that may damage or even disrupt a smaller pulmonary artery branch.

Cineangiographic Method. Pulmonary cineangiography, though not useful for main-

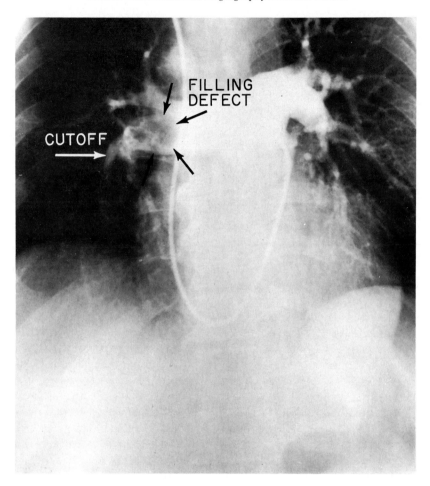

Fig. 15–3. Mainstream pulmonary angiogram of bilateral pulmonary embolism (PE) in a 48-year-old man. The tip of an Eppendorf catheter is positioned in the proximal right pulmonary artery 1 to 2 cm beyond its takeoff from the main pulmonary trunk. There are intralumenal filling defects and vessel cutoffs involving the right and left pulmonary arteries and their branches. Regional oligemia and asymmetry of flow are also evident. (From Benotti JR, Ockene IS, Alpert JL, Dalen JE: The clinical profile of unresolved pulmonary problems. Chest 84:670, 1984.)

stream studies because of the smaller field size, may confer advantages over the large film method for visualizing lobar arteries under certain circumstances.[11,12] In an acutely ill patient, the catheter can be positioned rapidly for selective study of the right and left pulmonary arteries. Figure 15–4 illustrates a frame from a right main pulmonary cineangiogram and depicts the technical advantages and limitations of this technique. The quality of current cineangiographic and videotape equipment is sufficiently good that large proximal emboli are usually evident immediately to the angiographer during the actual performance of the an-

giogram or on immediate replay of the study recorded on videotape. This advantage may shorten the procedure considerably and allow more rapid therapeutic intervention. Thrombi in second or third order vessels are sometimes diagnosed more readily as the interface between thrombus and flowing blood moves to and fro in the pulsatile stream. Indeed, what often appears on the static large film study as an oligemic area, suggestive but not diagnostic of pulmonary embolism, may be easily appreciated on the cineangiogram to represent a subtotally occluded vessel as some contrast agent flows slowly around the occluding thrombus.

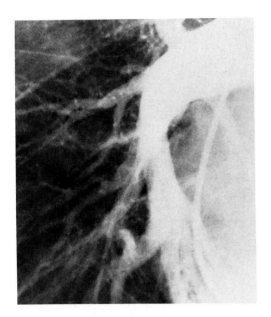

Fig. 15–4. Frame from a right main pulmonary cineangiogram where contrast agent was power injected through an Eppendorf catheter with its tip positioned in the midportion of the right main pulmonary artery. This technique allows prompt, unequivocal identification of emboli to the right or left pulmonary arteries and to the most proximal segments of the lobar branches. The obvious disadvantage is a small field, precluding adequate study of the entire pulmonary vasculature. (From Benotti JR, Ockene IS, Alpert JS, Dalen JE: Balloon occlusion pulmonary cineangiography to diagnosing pulmonary embolism. Cathet Cardiovasc Diagn 10:524, 1984.)

Recently, a relatively new and complimentary technique using a soft flexible balloon-tipped double-lumen catheter has been developed for pulmonary angiography.[13–15] In this method, either a standard 7 Fr Swan-Ganz double-lumen catheter with a balloon capacity of 1.8 ml or a specially designed catheter with a balloon capacity of 3 ml (Edwards Laboratories, Santa Ana, CA) may be used. Both balloons may be filled with room air, although carbon dioxide is a safer inflation medium.

The catheter is positioned proximally in the lobar vessel perfusing the area suspected of harboring pulmonary embolism, as identified by regional perfusion defects on the lung scan. The balloon is then slowly inflated with air to its maximum volume according to the manufacturer's specifications, or until it occludes the lobar vessel in its most proximal segment. Under fluoroscopic guidance, 5 to 10 ml of contrast agent is then delivered by a hand-powered injection into the distal lumen of the catheter, so that the pulmonary arterial segment downstream from the inflated balloon is opacified. Because the inflow of blood into the lobe has been temporarily arrested by the inflated balloon, this small volume of contrast delivered by hand injection opacifies the regional pulmonary vasculature completely and permits identification of pulmonary emboli in third- to fifth-order vessels with great specificity. Filming may be by either the cineangiographic or large film methods, but cine is usually quite adequate.

Figures 15–5 through 15–8 illustrate the technique, results, and advantages of balloon-occlusion pulmonary angiography in selected patients. A major advantage of the cineangiogram method is that it can be performed rapidly. The balloon occlusion guarantees prompt identification of pulmonary emboli as intraluminal filling defects that readily stand out as contrast agent slowly flows around them to fill out the regional pulmonary vasculature; usually the diagnosis is readily evident even on the test injection performed under fluoroscopy and filming is required only to generate a permanent record, rather than for critical diagnostic scrutiny. Small emboli to fifth-order vessels and beyond, which may be detected only as nonspecific multiple regions of oligemia on large film study, are particularly obvious on balloon-occlusion cineangiography. As depicted in Figure 15–6, when the balloon is deflated, unopacified blood enters the regional vessels and streams around the blood-thrombus interface. Radiographic contrast agent then hangs up selectively around the embolus and highlights its perimeter as it is washed out of the lobe. Balloon occlusion pulmonary angiography permits excellent regional opacification of more distal pulmonary arteries with a very small injection of contrast agent (5 to 10 ml) delivered by a hand-powered injection. This also minimizes the motion artifact that may result from the uncontrollable coughing often induced by standard angiographic technique that requires rapid injection of a large volume of contrast agent. With the

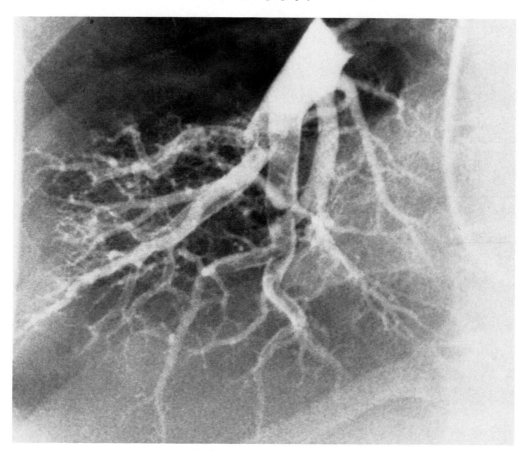

Fig. 15–5. Frame from a right lower lobe balloon-occlusion pulmonary cineangiogram in a 38-year-old woman who developed chest pain and dyspnea 1 week after an abdominal operation. The tip of the pulmonary artery catheter was positioned in the most proximal segment of the right lower lobe artery, the balloon was inflated with air to a volume of 1.5 ml (which occluded flow in this vessel), and the study was performed with a hand injection of 7 ml radiographic contrast medium. Intraluminal filling defects diagnostic of pulmonary embolism occupy almost the entire visualized segment of the artery to the right lower lobe. (From Benotti JR, Ockene IS, Alpert JS, Dalen JE: Balloon occlusion pulmonary cineangiography to diagnosing pulmonary embolism. Cathet Cardiovasc Diagn 10:525, 1984.)

aid of a guide wire the balloon-tipped catheter can usually be manipulated selectively into every lobar vessel implicated by the perfusion lung scan. All five pulmonary lobes can usually be studied selectively using a cumulative contrast dose rarely exceeding 75 ml. As illustrated in Figure 15–7, this may be particularly advantageous in patients with congestive heart failure or pulmonary hypertension, in whom administration of large cumulative contrast volume will aggravate heart failure. The occlusion technique prevents catheter recoil and retrograde reflux of contrast agent back out of the vessel of interest. This prevents simultaneous opacification of multiple vessels

and minimizes artifacts caused by vessel overlap and crossing changes. Thus, in addition to speed, advantages of balloon-occlusion pulmonary cineangiography include its resolving power and the minimal contrast requirement for identifying pulmonary embolism in lobar vessels and beyond. This latter point is particularly important if the perfusion abnormalities on the lung scan are less than segmental in distribution. If perfusion defects are lobar or involve an entire lung, this finding suggests large proximal pulmonary embolism to the right or left pulmonary arteries, as illustrated in Figure 15–3. In this case it is advisable to confirm or exclude their presence by the in-

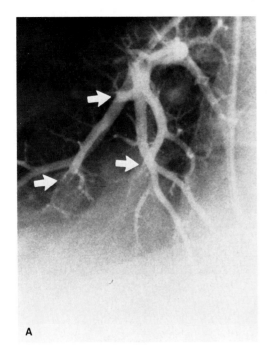
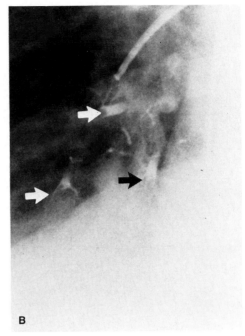

A

B

Fig. 15–6. Frame from a right lower lobe balloon-occlusion pulmonary cineangiogram filmed during contrast injection (A) and during contrast washout following balloon deflation (B). The tip of the catheter is positioned in the most proximal segment of the right lower lobe artery and the balloon is inflated to occlude arterial inflow. Occluded fifth-order vessels show sudden interruption of the contrast-filled vessel (vessel cutoff) during the injection phase (white arrows). These stand out clearly as intraluminal filling defects (pulmonary emboli) during the washout phase (black arrow) as contrast flows around the perimeter of the embolus.

jection of a large contrast volume at high pressure into the proximal vessel(s) in question through a standard angiographic catheter (e.g., Eppendorf catheter). If this study is negative, consideration should then be given to proceeding with balloon-occlusion pulmonary cineangiography of the lobar vessels.

Although we have not had any complications using the balloon-occlusion technique just described, a word of caution is in order. Previous investigators have reported on pulmonary angiography using temporary unilateral pulmonary artery occlusion.[16–19] Some authors have reported that prolonged exposure of the pulmonary vasculature to radiographic contrast may be harmful.[17,18] In addition, high injection pressures (injection pressures exceeding pulmonary capillary wedge pressure by $\leq$ 20 mm Hg) may cause extravasation of contrast into the pulmonary parenchyma with a resultant pulmonary infiltrate.[17] Accordingly, to reduce risks of pulmonary vascular damage, balloon-occlusion pulmonary angiography should be performed with small amounts of radiographic contrast injected under low pressures, with a minimal time of intravascular stasis.

Digital Subtraction Angiography. In recent years, several reports[20–23] have appeared in which digital subtraction angiography was used to visualize the pulmonary arterial tree in an attempt to assess the presence or absence of pulmonary embolism. The technique involves peripheral venous injection of radiographic contrast using high-resolution radiographic equipment and computer-assisted digital subtraction imaging. Patients must be able to hold their breath for 10 to 20 seconds, and the technique cannot be used in patients who are unable to suppress a cough, are very dyspneic, or have a low cardiac output. The technique has high sensitivity for pulmonary embolism[21,22] but rather low specificity,[21] and at least one group[23] found it substantially in-

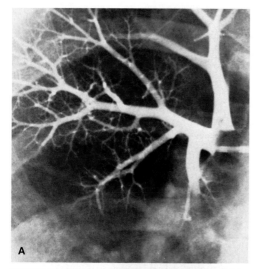

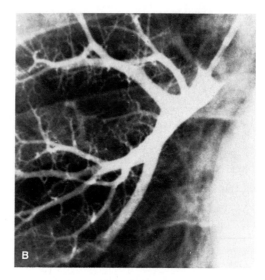

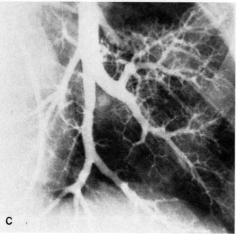

Fig. 15–7. Frames from balloon occlusion cineangio-grams of the right upper lobe (A), right lower lobe (B), and the left lower lobe (C) in a 52-year-old man with congestive heart failure in whom pulmonary embolism was considered as a cause for the patient's acute deteri-oration and a perfusion lung scan revealed multiple sub-segmental defects. There is attenuation of vascularity com-patible with lung disease, but no pulmonary emboli are identified. In each study the catheter tip is positioned in the most proximal segment of the artery in question and the balloon is inflated to occlude inflow of unopacified blood. Such a study, performed with less than 10 ml of contrast agent to opacify the vasculature of each lobe carries little increase in risk compared to bedside right heart catheterization, a procedure now frequently per-formed for hemodynamic monitoring in critically ill pa-tients.

ferior to standard technique using direct injec-tion of radiographic contrast into a pulmonary artery.

ANGIOGRAPHIC DIAGNOSIS OF PULMONARY EMBOLISM

A normal pulmonary arteriogram is rela-tively easy to recognize. Contrast flows sym-metrically from its site of proximal entry to uniformly fill second, third, and fourth order vessels that become progressively smaller in caliber. Similarly, as unopacified blood washes contrast from the pulmonary arterial to the pul-monary venous circulation, vascular definition is lost in a symmetric fashion.

As discussed earlier in this chapter, the an-giographic features specific for pulmonary em-bolism include *intraluminal filling defects* (Fig. 15–3, 15–5, 15–8) and *abrupt vessel cutoffs* (Fig. 15–6). Intraluminal filling defects result from flow of contrast around pulmonary emboli. Vessel cutoffs result from lobar or seg-mental vessels that have been totally occluded by embolic material. The pulmonary vascular anatomy is somewhat variable from patient to patient, and the angiographer frequently can-not be certain of the "normal" location and course of the smaller pulmonary arterial

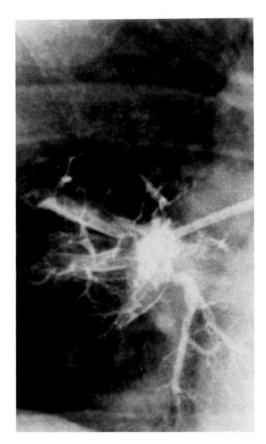

Fig. 15–8. Frame from a balloon-occlusion cineangiogram of the right lower lobe in a 72-year-old man with pulmonary embolism. The tip of the catheter is positioned proximally in the artery to the right lower lobe and the balloon is inflated to prevent contrast dilution and washout by inflow of unopacified blood during the injection of contrast agent. This study, performed with 8 ml of radiographic contrast agent injected through the distal lumen of the balloon-tipped catheter, demonstrates several "railroad track" signs, as contrast streams about partially occlusive thrombi. Intraluminal filling defects and abrupt vessel cutoffs, diagnostic of pulmonary embolism, are also evident.

branches in an individual patient. Therefore, it may be very difficult to identify cutoff of vessels when third-order (segmental) or smaller vessels are flush-occluded at their point of origin. In this circumstance, as demonstrated in Figure 15–8, when contrast flows slowly about the perimeter of a nearly totally occlusive embolus in a lobar or segmental artery giving rise to the so-called "railroad track" sign, the diagnosis of pulmonary embolism is unequivocal. When intraluminal filling defects, vessel cutoff, or "railroad tracking" are present, the diagnosis of pulmonary embolism can be made with a high degree of confidence.

Nonspecific angiographic findings in pulmonary embolism include localized asymmetry of flow and regional oligemia, defined as impaired local pulmonary artery flow. These findings are nonspecific because they can be due to conditions other than pulmonary embolism including pneumonia, asthma, bullous lung disease, atelectasis, or emphysema. When there is regional oligemia or asymmetry of flow without corresponding abnormality on the chest roentgenogram or ventilation lung scan, however, it is advisable to regard the patient as having probable pulmonary embolism so that he or she receives the potential benefit of anticoagulant therapy.

HEMODYNAMIC FINDINGS ASSOCIATED WITH PULMONARY EMBOLISM

The hemodynamic impact of pulmonary embolism is determined by the extent of pulmonary vascular cross-sectional compromise by embolic material and the patient's underlying cardiopulmonary status.[10,24,25] Acute pulmonary arterial obstruction augments the afterload opposing right ventricular ejection. This increases the wall tension the right ventricle must generate to eject its stroke volume. In the patient free of underlying cardiopulmonary disease, pulmonary artery hypertension (mean pressure above 25 mm Hg) develops as the magnitude of embolic obstruction exceeds 30 to 50% of the pulmonary arterial bed. As pulmonary arterial obstruction approaches 75%, mean pulmonary artery pressure approaches 35 to 45 mm Hg. At this point, the previously unstressed right ventricle can no longer generate sufficient systolic tension to eject its stroke volume against such an extreme elevation in impedance. The consequence is a reduction in stroke volume and cardiac output, an increase in end-systolic and end-diastolic volumes, acute right ventricular dilation, and an increase in right atrial pressure.[24,25] The reduction in cardiac output usually evokes reflex sympathetic nervous system activation with a resultant increase in systemic vascular resistance and heart rate, and these adjustments tend to preserve blood pressure and cardiac output. The reflex increase in venous tone reduces vascular capacitance and translocates blood from the peripheral systemic venous reservoir to the central circulation, resulting in an elevation in right atrial pressure. Thus, in the patient with no underlying cardiopulmonary disease, the presence of pulmonary hypertension indicates at least 30 to 50% obstruction of the pulmonary circulation, whereas acute cor pulmonale and right ventricular failure usually occur when at least 75% of the pulmonary arterial tree has been obstructed by embolism. If pulmonary vascular compliance has been reduced and pulmonary vascular resistance increased by preexisting heart or lung disease, the increase in pulmonary artery pressure in response to pulmonary embolism will be greater. A chronically pressure-overloaded right ventricle, however, having undergone hypertrophy, can often tolerate acute pulmonary hypertension of a

more severe degree as a result of embolic pulmonary artery obstruction before the ventricle fails and the right atrial pressure rises. Specific hemodynamic and clinical profiles in pulmonary embolism are discussed in Chapter 33.

REFERENCES

1. Robbins E: Overdiagnosis and overtreatment of pulmonary embolism: the emperor may have no clothes. Ann Int Med 87:775, 1977.
2. Menzioan JO, Williams JF: Is pulmonary angiography essential for the diagnosis of acute pulmonary embolism? Am Surg 137:543, 1979.
3. Dines DE, Arms RA, Bernatz PE, Gomes MR: Pulmonary arteriovenous fistulas. Mayo Clin Proc 49:460, 1974.
4. Benotti JR, Ockene IS, Alpert JS, Dalen JE: The clinical profile of unresolved pulmonary embolism. Chest 84:661, 1983.
5. Fishman AJ, Moser KM, Fedullo PF: Perfusion lung scans vs. pulmonary angiography in evaluation of suspected primary pulmonary hypertension. Chest 54:671, 1983.
6. Cook DJ, Tanser PH, Dobranowski J, Tuttle RJ: Primary pulmonary artery sarcoma mimicking pulmonary thromboembolism. Can J Cardiol 4:393, 1988.
7. Marsh JD, Glynn M, Torman HA: Pulmonary angiography. Application in a new spectrum of patients. Am J Med 75:763, 1983.
8. Goodman PG: Pulmonary angiography. *In* Symposium of Pulmonary Embolism and Hypertension: Clinics in Chest Medicine. Hyers TM (ed): Philadelphia, W.B. Saunders Co., 1984, pp. 465–477.
9. Bookstein JJ: Segmental arteriography in pulmonary embolism. Radiology 93:1007, 1969.
10. McIntyre KM, Sasahara AA: The hemodynamic response to pulmonary embolism in patients without prior cardiopulmonary disease. Am J Cardiol 78:288, 1971.
11. Meister SG, et al: Pulmonary cineangiography in acute pulmonary embolism. Am Heart J 84:33, 1972.
12. Meyerovitz MF, Levin DC, Harrington DP, et al: Evaluation of optimized biplane pulmonary cineangiography. Invest Radiol 20:945, 1985.
13. Bynum LJ, et al: Radiographic techniques for balloon-occlusion pulmonary angiography. Radiology 133:518, 1979.
14. Ferris EJ, et al: Angiography of pulmonary emboli: digital studies and balloon-occlusion cineangiography. Am J Radiol 142:369, 1984.
15. Benotti JR, Ockene IS, Alpert JS, Dalen JS: Balloon occlusion pulmonary cineangiography to diagnosing pulmonary embolism. Cathet Cardiovasc Diagn 10:519, 1984.
16. Nordenstrom B: Temporary unilateral occlusion of the pulmonary artery. Acta Radiol, Suppl 108:1–141, 1954.
17. Becu L, Paulin S, Varnauskas E: Pulmonary wedge angiography. Acta Radiol 57:209, 1962.
18. Bell ALV, et al: Wedge pulmonary arteriography. Ap-

plications in congenital and acquired heart disease. Radiology 73:566, 1959.

19. Dotter CT, Rosch J: Pulmonary arteriography: Technique. *In* Abrams Angiography, 3rd ed. Abrams HL (ed): Boston, Little Brown, 1983, pp. 707–708.

20. Pond GD, Chernin MM: Digital subtraction angiography of the pulmonary arteries. J Thorac Imaging 1:21, 1985.

21. Musset D, Rosso J, Petitpretz P, et al: Acute pulmonary embolism: Diagnostic value of digital subtraction angiography. Radiology 166:455, 1988.

22. Bjork L: Digital angiography in pulmonary embolism. Acta Radiol Diagn 27:179, 1986.

23. Gutierrez FR, Biello D, McKnight RC: Digital venous angiography in the diagnosis of pulmonary thromboembolism. Cathet Cardiovasc Diagn 10:343, 1984.

24. Dalen JS, et al: Resolution rate of acute pulmonary embolism in man. N Engl J Med 280:1194, 1969.

25. McIntyre KM, Sasahara AA: Pulmonary angiography, scanning and hemodynamics in pulmonary embolism: Critical review and correlations. Crit Rev Radiol Sci 3:489, 1972.

16

Aortography

SVEN PAULIN

A ortography, the radiographic demonstration of the contrast-filled central
large vessel from which all organ systems of the human body derive their arterial
blood supply, has a long history. In 1929, the
year when W. Forssmann[1] reported that he had
passed a catheter from an arm vein into his
own right atrium, dos Santos and his
colleagues[2] reported the successful performance of abdominal aortography after direct
puncture of this vessel with a needle. A more
daring approach to inject the ascending aorta
in similar fashion, resulting in angiographic
visualization of the thoracic aorta, was described by Nuvoli in 1936.[3] Since that time,
contrast angiography of the aorta has undergone many modifications aiming at greater patient safety, higher image quality, and optimal
diagnostic yield. Angiographic study of the
aorta may be performed to quantitate the degree of aortic valve incompetence, to delineate
the topography of abnormal vascular pathways
related to congenital malformations, or to
search for congenital or acquired vascular
lesions that might be the cause of systemic
hypertension. These procedures may be performed for reasons of different urgency, reaching from the emergency condition of a traumatic aortic perforation, dissection, or rupture
to the screening examination of an asymptomatic patient with an unexplained bruit. It
should not be surprising, therefore, that a great

variety of different technical and procedural
approaches to aortography are available.

TECHNICAL ASPECTS

The relatively large size of the aorta—the
thoracic portion alone under normal conditions
has a volume of several hundred milliliters
—poses special demands regarding technical
performance. These requirements differ substantially from those applicable to selective
arteriography of different organ systems. Unrelated to the mode by which the central aorta
has been filled with contrast medium, an unavoidable consequence is that all arterial com-
partments of the systemic circulation will be
exposed to a temporary flow of contrast agent
in proportion to their share of blood supply.
This fact opens on one hand the possibility of
extending the angiographic examination to include additional views by using special equipment, such as automatic stepwise table transport, so useful, for example, to follow the
"runoff" of contrast medium completely
through both lower extremities. On the other
hand, the fact that the contrast medium reaches
all organ systems has to be taken into consideration with regard to side effects and potential
complications.

Patient Preparation

Although the rapid injection of contrast medium in the amount necessary for an aortogram

244

may be recognized by the patient in the form of a profound ''heat wave'' through the entire body, the intensity of this phenomenon when using modern tri-iodinated water-soluble compounds is not excessive, and may be absent if low-osmolar agents are used. It is prudent practice for the operator to explain fully to the patient the purpose of the procedure, describe the side effects to be expected, and disclose the potential hazards. The latter may differ from one examination to the other and relate to a number of factors such as the technique chosen for the examination, the risk factor profile of the patient population under study, and the individual patient's condition at the time of the examination. The operator also must ask the patient if there is any previous history of adverse reaction to radiographic contrast media or of allergy to iodine-containing foods, which otherwise would call for special precautions such as premedication with steroids and/or cimetidine. Because aortography, particularly when including the proximal ascending aorta, may result in the contrast medium contacting the heart and the coronary circulation, precautions similar to those for coronary angiography are recommended (see Chapter 13). These should include ECG monitoring, review of cardiotropic medication, and pacemaker and defibrillator standby. Finally, the establishment of a good patient-operator relationship cannot be overemphasized.

Injection Techniques

Although injection of contrast medium in sufficient amount into the circulation at any site would eventually outline the aortic lumen, the general principle prevails that increased selectivity of delivery of contrast medium increases the quality of angiographic information. This strongly influences the choice of technique.

Catheter Aortography

Retrograde advancement of the arterial catheter to the central portion of the arterial circulation can be accomplished from different sites using puncture and/or surgical exposure of an artery.

Percutaneous Puncture of Femoral Artery.

By far the most popular is the percutaneous puncture of a femoral artery by Seldinger's technique for catheter replacement of a needle using a flexible guide wire.[4] This procedure is described in detail in Chapter 5. Because the length of the catheter determines to a high degree the resistance to injection, thoracic aortography requires a larger catheter (≥ 7 Fr) than abdominal aortography (5 or 6 Fr). Guide wire and catheter manipulations, as well as advancement, are performed under fluoroscopic control. J-shaped ends of the guide wires and similar catheter end configurations are helpful to avoid entry into small side branches, to negotiate arterial tortuosity and wall irregularities, and to prevent perforations or entrances into false channels, e.g., dissections. So-called pigtail catheters with a diameter approaching the expected caliber of the vessel stabilize the catheter position during the phase of rapid injection, decrease catheter whipping, and accomplish good mixing of radiographic contrast medium with blood because of the multiple jets of contrast agent emerging from the appropriately placed multiple side holes. These catheters are similar to those used for selective left ventricular angiography (Chapter 14). For aortography, however, we prefer thin-walled catheters, which allow higher injection rates.

Throughout the procedure, the catheter is flushed meticulously and frequently (every 3 to 5 minutes) with isotonic saline solution containing a small amount of heparin. Alternatively, a pressure-bag infusion set may be used for continuous catheter irrigation. Temporary total-body heparinization is not used widely for aortography alone, but should be considered when the procedure involves more time-consuming catheter manipulations in the thoracic aorta, potentially affecting the coronary and carotid circulation.

In spite of the known higher incidence of atherosclerotic changes in the arteries of the lower extremities and tortuosity of iliac vessels, particularly in the older population, the femoral approach has a high success rate when appropriate technique is used. Certain conditions, however, such as thoracic or abdominal coarctation, threatening abdominal aortic aneurysm, or complete occlusion may preclude this retrograde approach.

Percutaneous Puncture of Axillary Artery. An alternative approach is the percutaneous puncture of the axillary artery.[5–7] In general, catheter approach to the descending aorta is accomplished from the left and to the ascending aorta from the right axillary artery, but no great difficulty exists to advance the catheter to both aortic territories from either side. Because the axillary and higher brachial artery can be quite mobile, they need to be fixed by the operator's hand while the needle puncture is performed, similar to the approach to the femoral artery. The procedure is not more difficult, but reluctance to its more frequent use arises from a higher complication rate.[8,9] This seems to be related mostly to local formation of hematomas affecting the brachial nerve plexus; therefore, meticulous post-procedure compression and observation are mandatory. If delayed bleeding occurs, early surgical exploration and axillary sheath decompression are advisable. Catheter shape and side holes are similar to those used for the femoral approach, but in general a smaller catheter caliber (5 or 6 Fr) will permit a sufficient injection rate of contrast medium because the catheter can be kept shorter.

Surgical cutdown on the brachial artery, as in cardiac catheterization from the brachial approach (Chapter 4), can also be used when a percutaneous femoral approach cannot be employed.

Translumbar Aortography. Another percutaneous approach, rarely used today, is translumbar aortography, which was described as early as 1929 by dos Santos.[2] This procedure, performed with the patient in prone position, is done with a No. 18 gauge needle which is advanced through the skin below the inferior margin of the lowest left rib, some 10 cm to the left of the midline. This procedure can be performed with surprising ease and rapidity and finds its use mostly for delineation of the abdominal aorta and its branches to the lower extremities. More recently, this technique has been modified using catheter replacement and retrograde advancement into the thoracic aorta, and successful selective coronary arteriograms have even been reported when all other arterial approaches were blocked.[10]

Transseptal Angiocardiography. Percutaneous direct approaches to the thoracic aorta have historical importance only and are not practiced any more because of the obvious risk of uncontrollable hemorrhage. Transseptal angiocardiography offers a reasonable alternative for aortography in special cases.[11]

Antegrade Angiography and Venous Injections. Less selective approaches resulting in angiographic delineation of the aorta and its branches are the rapid bolus injection of contrast medium in the right side of the circulation, either selectively in the pulmonary artery—so-called antegrade angiography of the left heart—injections close to the right atrium by way of catheters, or even venous injections through one or two wide bore needles simultaneously. These approaches require, however, a larger total dose of contrast medium in order to compensate for the unavoidable dilution effect. These less selective approaches are frequently enhanced by using conventional subtraction radiography and have received more importance with the recent introduction of computerized *digital subtraction techniques.*

Contrast Agent

In the interest of obtaining a good aortographic result, the contrast medium injected into the thoracic aorta should have a relatively high concentration of iodine. Preparations containing 350 to 400 mg iodine per ml (76% contrast agent solution) seem to satisfy these requirements and are marketed by a number of companies: the solutions contain either diatrizoate, metrizoate, or iothalamate as anions. These compounds are all similar in chemical structure, contain three iodine atoms per molecule, and belong to the so-called ionic conventional contrast agents that over many years have proven to be well tolerated clinically in all forms of intravascular use. Higher concentrations, advocated by some, do not really improve the angiogram, and the increased viscosity may reduce the injection rate. Increased side effects and more intense sensation of heat by the patient are good arguments against their use. Lower concentration levels of 280 to 300 mg iodine per ml (60% contrast agent solution) can be used in the interest of lesser patient discomfort, particularly in situations of favorable radiographic conditions such as small object size and nondilated aorta. More important than the absolute concentration (which will undergo an unavoidable significant dilution in the aortic blood pool) is the mode of injection; i.e., a sufficiently high injection rate and delivery through multiple catheter holes to assure rapid and homogeneous mixing.

With regard to side effects, one has to pay attention to the cation concentration. In particular, the content of free sodium ion should be close to the normal serum level (approximately 140 meq/L), because both experimental and clinical studies have shown clearly that unphysiologic sodium content increases the risk of arrhythmias in selective coronary arteriography.[12,13] Mention must be made of the new *nonionic contrast* agents that offer equal radiographic density at lesser osmolarity. They have been associated with fewer side effects and better patient tolerance,[12,13] albeit at a considerably increased cost (8 to 10 times that of standard ionic agents).

The recommended contrast dose for a thoracic aortogram lies between 40 and 60 ml; slightly lesser amounts will suffice for an abdominal aortogram. More than one injection is frequently required and is usually well tolerated. Individual injections should be separated by a time interval of at least 5 to 10 minutes, and attention should be paid that the temporary hemodynamic reaction (such as increased heart rate and/or decreased blood pressure) has abated before delivery of another contrast injection. A general recommendation not to exceed 300 ml of contrast agent for the average adult patient during one examination is prudent, and lower limits may be set in particular patients such as those with heart failure or marginal renal function.

Radiographic Techniques

The most widely used radiographic technique is the direct large film series. Indirect methods are cinefluorography and spot-film fluorography, both using an image intensifier. Ongoing development in electronic image recording can be expected to benefit both methods, and it may be possible that in the future film recording will be replaced by video display in analog or digital form. Presently, it may be concluded that for the purpose of aortography direct film series are preferred when the indications for the examination require greatest anatomic detail, whereas cinematography is more suitable for the detection of abnormal dynamic events, i.e., valve motion and incompetence, abnormal contrast flow in shunts, AV fistulae, arterial bleeding sites, or extravasations.

Large-Film Series. Optimal radiographic detail important for precise anatomic definition is classically achieved with large-film series, and this is still the most widely used method. An important inherent advantage is the field size, covering up to 14 × 14 inches. This implies that in one projection the image may easily encompass the entire thoracic aorta, including the proximal portions of the large aortic arch branches, intercostal arteries, bronchial arteries, and internal mammary arteries. Modern large-film changers, less bulky than those of the past, allow varying film sequence up to a rate of 3 to 4 exposures per second, sufficient for the purpose of accurate sequential delineation of arterial filling and runoff. Powerful x-ray tubes with high speed rotating anodes (10,000 RPM) and optimal heat dissipation characteristics and small focal spot anode target (0.6 to 1.0 mm) fed by high output (80 to 100 kW) 12-pulse generators guarantee the production of high-contrast and high-resolution images on the films.

Biplane equipment, essentially an independent duplication of the equipment, increases the cost of the installation and may, therefore, not be available except in larger institutions. Two x-ray tubes placed slightly offset from each other and firing alternately on the same film changer are less expensive than a biplane system and provide stereoscopic pairs of images that enhance the information derived from one injection.[14] Similar to biplane examinations, these studies allow viewing of the same object in different projections. Single-plane technique more frequently require a second injection following appropriate repositioning of the patient. Film subtraction for enhancement of contrast medium and magnification techniques to depict greater detail can easily be applied.

Cinefluorography. In contrast to direct radiography, cinefluorography implies an indirect radiographic method. After having penetrated and being attenuated by the object, the x-ray photons activate the input phosphor of an image intensifier that by means of electron acceleration, generates an image of considerably increased brightness on the smaller output phosphor. (See Chapter 2 for a full discussion of radiographic principles.) By means of an appropriate optical lens system, this image is photographed by a movie camera, usually employing 35 mm film at a frame rate of 24 to 60 per second. Smaller 16-mm cameras allow even higher frame speed and may find use in imaging for physiologic research but are not recommended for practical clinical use. Technical improvements, in particular the introduction of cesium iodide screens, have led to near perfection of this cine technique, which is widely preferred in cardiac angiography. Its main advantage is the continuous imaging of the angiographic events, whereas the main disadvantage is the limited field size determined by the input aperture of the electron intensifier. Another disadvantage lies in the lesser resolution of details compared to direct radiography. This can be compensated for in part by electronic magnification, but as a general rule, it has to be recognized that the higher the definition the smaller the field size and vice versa. The high film rate of cinematography reduces the time available for exposure of each individual frame (3 to 10 msec); correspondingly, each individual pulse x-ray burst is of lesser intensity (25 to 35 microroentgen). Total patient dose per film run, however, is similar to that of a direct film series.

Spot-film Fluorography. This technique takes an intermediate position and delivers 100 mm cut film or 105 mm roll film images at a rate of 6 per second. Using also an image intensifier and a larger x-ray dose per frame at the input plane (150 microroentgen), a resolution of significantly greater detail can be achieved compared to cinematography. This technique is not as popular and widely available but has found advocates for certain indications such as examination of congenital abnormalities in children.

ANATOMY AND ANGIOGRAPHIC APPEARANCE OF THE NORMAL THORACIC AORTA

The thoracic portion of the aorta (Fig. 16–1) reaches from the aortic valve to its exit from the thoracic cavity into the abdomen at the level of the diaphragm. In frontal presentation the aortic root projects in the midline superimposed on the dense shadow of the spine. Because the aortic valve apparatus is directed cranially with a slight inclination to the right and posteriorly, the ascending aorta assumes a gentle curve with convexity to the right; however, it does not normally exceed the border of the right upper mediastinal shadow, which is usually represented by the superior vena cava. The ascending aorta has a rather constant caliber varying between 22 and 38 mm in adults and is related to individual body dimensions and probably also to general physical activity. A slight increase in dimensions occurs with age. Approximately at the origin of its first large branch, the brachiocephalic trunk, the thoracic aorta curves to the left and posteriorly in front of the trachea and gives off the left carotid and left subclavian arteries in sequence before it assumes a caudal direction at the site of the aortic isthmus to continue in the descending portion of the thoracic aorta slightly to the left and in front of the vertebral column.

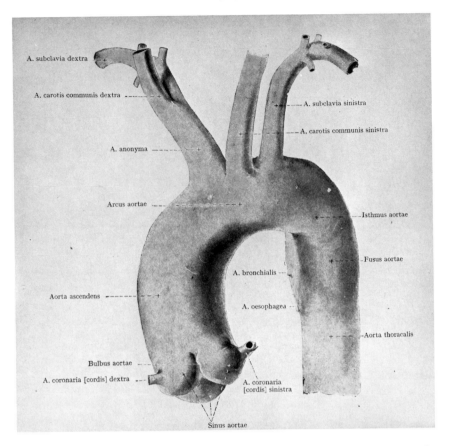

A. subclavia dextra

A. carotis communis dextra

A. anonyma

Arcus aortae

Aorta ascendens

Bulbus aortae

A. coronaria [cordis] dextra

A. subclavia sinistra

A. carotis communis sinistra

Isthmus aortae

Fusus aortae

A. bronchialis

A. oesophagea

Aorta thoracalis

A. coronaria [cordis] sinistra

Sinus aortae

Fig. 16–1. Thoracic aorta in LAO position according to Spalteholz. (From Paulin, S.: Coronary Angiography: A technical anatomic and clinical study. Acta Radiol., Suppl. 233, 1964, with permission.)

At the site of the isthmus and the fetal ductus arteriosus, a slight anteriorly directed bulge in the contour may be seen. Likewise, a slightly more distally located fusiform dilatation may occur, the so-called aortic spindle. Both findings are probably related to slight distortions affected by the ligamentum arteriosum and are more marked in the young, but can persist in adult life.

Important vessels deriving from the descending portion of the thoracic aorta are the anteriorly directed bronchial arteries and the intercostal arteries with corresponding ramifications. Commensurate with the branching of the large arch arteries, the descending aorta has a slightly smaller caliber than the ascending aorta.

Left Anterior Oblique (LAO) Projection. The left anterior oblique (or right posterior oblique) projection (Figs. 16–1 and 16–2) delineates the aortic arch optimally as it opens its curvature to the greatest extent. In most instances this projection also offers the tangential depiction of the large vessel orifices and may disclose variations in their relative position, which are frequent. This view also discloses most favorably the increased elongation and tortuosity of the aortic arch as it occurs in the elderly (Fig. 16–2).

Right Anterior Oblique (RAO) Projection. In the right anterior oblique (or left posterior oblique) projection, the ascending and descending aorta are more or less superimposed, and the aortic arch is markedly foreshortened.

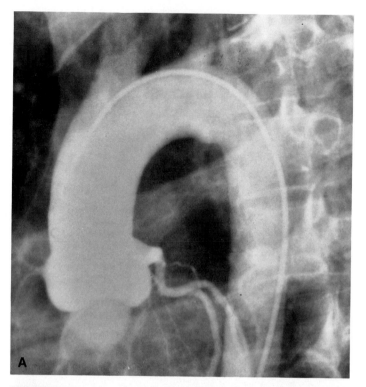

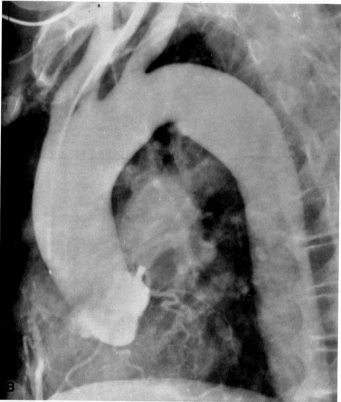

Fig. 16–2. Normal thoracic aortography in LAO projection: (A) young adult; (B) elderly person. Note the increased width of the aortic arch, resulting in a more proximal origin of the large vessels in the older individual. A small shallow bulge at the inner curvature of the arch just distally to the origin of the left subclavian artery corresponds to the obliterated ductus arteriosus, which is a common normal finding. The diameter of the descending aorta is slightly diminished compared to that of the ascending aorta.

Consequently, this view is less favorable to delineate the takeoff of the large branches of the arch, but both oblique views may be useful to illustrate the proximal portions of the corresponding intercostal arteries.

Cranial and Caudal Tilts. As in coronary angiography, cranial and caudal tilts may be added to achieve optimal visualization of specific anatomic details, e.g., an LAO projection with cranial tilt will result in a tangential depiction of the three aortic valve cusps (Fig. 16–3). A steep RAO projection with cranial tilt can demonstrate the aortic ostium en face.

COMMON INDICATIONS FOR AORTOGRAPHY

Indications for thoracic aortography vary widely. They may extend from the evaluation of congenital vascular abnormalities in asymp-

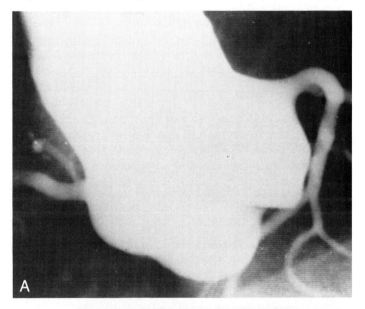

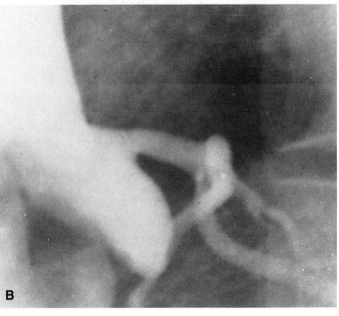

Fig. 16–3. Detail of aortic valve apparatus as seen in thoracic aortography. (A) Presentation of aortic bulb during diastole in LAO projection with cranial tilt. Both coronary cusps are identified by the orifices of the corresponding coronary arteries. The noncoronary cusp is located in the middle and slightly below. (B) Detail of left coronary cusp during systole. Note the straight border of the contrast-filled valve leaflet against the nonopacified blood ejected from the left ventricle.

tomatic patients to the preoperative study of tumor vessel supply to assess operability. Because aortography, when performed selectively, includes a certain risk, the question should always be asked whether the information gained is important for the patient's management or whether the situation can be sufficiently assessed by less invasive diagnostic procedures or examinations. The most common conditions in which aortography is likely to render important information are aortic valve disease, aortic valve incompetence, aortic aneurysms, aortic coarctation, patent ductus arteriosus, and coronary bypass grafts.

Aortic Valve Disease

Aortic Valve Stenosis. Although it is indisputable that the degree of functional impairment requires hemodynamic evaluation, angiographic examination contributes significantly to an optimal assessment of the condition. Anatomic delineation of the site and degree of abnormality is particularly important for the cardiovascular surgeon because it might influence the technical operative approach, including choice of vessel substitutes or valve prosthesis. Obviously, angiography is the optimal method to distinguish between supravalvular, valvular, and subvalvular position of the lesion. In most instances such lesions are studied selectively by injections into the left ventricle (Fig. 16–4), but the supravalvular aortogram may render important, albeit partially inferential, information. In the presence of a valvular lesion a cineangiographic study in conjunction with a supravalvular injection in the proximal portion of the ascending aorta is considered optimal. Catheter position close to the valve apparatus improves image quality; however, care has to be taken that catheter and contrast jets, particularly through an open end hole, does not interfere with valve function and thus generate artifactual findings. The optimal position to separate the aorta clearly from the left ventricle and allow assessment of the interpositional relationship of the aortic cusps is approximately 45 degrees LAO, which, when added to 10 to 15 degrees of cranial tilt,

results in a practically true tangential depiction of the valve plane.

Cineangiography permits study of the motion of the three aortic valve leaflets, which normally move upward rapidly during systole. The normal cusps are so thin that they are seen only if the projection demonstrates them on edge. In diastole the closed valve is represented by the three semilunar cusps in LAO projection, the right and left coronary cusp side by side with their free edges adapting against each other in the center, and the noncoronary cusp slightly below posteriorly and seen en face.

An important aortographic sign of valvular aortic stenosis is the presence of poststenotic dilatation, a finding that is readily made and quantified by comparing the width of the mid-ascending aorta and that of the aortic root. The cause of this finding is the flow turbulence that ensues immediately distally to the increased flow velocity through the significantly narrowed ostium and may assume asymmetric accentuation with a bulge to the right in cases of a narrow forceful blood jet.

The degree of poststenotic dilatation relates poorly to the tightness of the stenosis and to the existing systolic gradient between the left ventricle and the aorta. It has been shown, however, that it is consistently greater in patients with congenital aortic valve stenosis than in those with acquired types.

A characteristic finding for congenital aortic valve stenosis, at least in the early stages of life, is that the frequently fused but still pliable leaflets assume an *upward-directed dome* (Fig. 16–4). As congenital aortic stenosis frequently includes developmental abnormalities of the cusps, an asymmetric appearance of the closed valve with the point of leaflet coaptation in a markedly eccentric position should be looked for, as it is typical for a bicuspid aortic valve. The angiographic appearance of the valve apparatus in acquired aortic stenosis is characterized by decreased mobility of the leaflets, frequently associated with marked thickening and irregular contours. It is advisable to begin filming the area of interest one or two heartbeats before the start of the contrast injection,

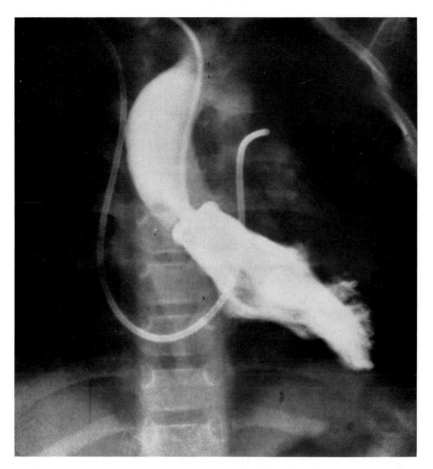

Fig. 16–4. Anteroposterior view of congenital aortic valve stenosis illustrates typical dome shape of pliable but fused aortic valve leaflets with centrally located narrowed opening. In this instance a selective left ventricular injection was performed. A supravalvular aortogram would show the findings with reversed contrast. The left heart catheter was passed retrograde from the right brachial artery. A right heart catheter is also seen, positioned in the pulmonary artery.

so that the presence of calcification can be assessed. This is also helpful in differentiating calcium located in the free aortic valve, the proximal coronary arteries, the atrioventricular ring, and the upper portion of the interventricular septum. In advanced stages of acquired aortic stenosis extensive calcification is often present, and a dense, rather fixed, irregularly contoured plate is the counterpart of the so-called fishmouth appearance of the valve as seen by the cardiac surgeon or pathologist.

Although the supravalvular aortogram contributes little in the situation of subvalvular narrowings, either congenital subvalvular membrane or muscular outflow tract stenosis in IHSS, this procedure is optimal for the evaluation of *supravalvular aortic stenosis*, a condition characterized by the presence of an aortic narrowing just above the aortic valve. This lesion may produce a tubular narrowing of the entire ascending aorta (Fig. 16–5), so-called ascending aorta hypoplasia, a thin membranous diaphragm, or an internally protruding circumferential ridge just above the sinuses of Valsalva. Although in these situations the aortic valve apparatus itself may be normal, concomitant valve abnormalities such as bicuspid anatomy are encountered frequently. Supravalvular aortic stenosis may be part of a congenital syndrome that also includes peripheral pulmonary artery stenosis, physical and mental retardation, hypocalcemia, and facial abnormalities.[15,16]

Aortic Valve Incompetence. Supravalvular

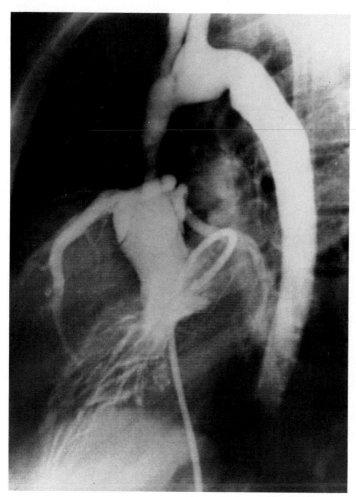

Fig. 16–5. Left lateral view of congenital supravalvular aortic stenosis. A transseptal catheter has been placed in the left ventricle. Contrast injection opacifies the left ventricular outflow tract, the coronary arteries, and the ascending and descending aorta. Note the long sequential narrowing of the entire ascending aorta, so-called hypoplasia, and the substantial dilation of the coronary arteries arising proximally to the narrowing.

injection of radiographic contrast during cine-angiography constitutes the most definitive diagnostic technique to assess aortic valve insufficiency. The sensitivity for detection of even small amounts of aortic regurgitation on the projected cineangiogram is high, and the possibility of erroneous overdiagnosis is real. Inappropriate technique, such as excessive injection volume and speed, catheter end-hole jet, mechanical catheter interference with the valve apparatus, simultaneous Valsalva maneuver, and transient bradycardia or premature beats may cause factitious angiographic appearance of aortic valve incompetence. On the other hand, an injection site too high in the upper portion of the ascending aorta, such that the root of the aorta is not filled completely, is inadequate for assessing aortic insufficiency.

The optimal technique is to inject through a closed-end straight catheter with multiple side holes[17,18] or a pigtail catheter advanced to the aortic valve and then withdrawn until it is positioned approximately 1 to 2 inches above the aortic valve. This approach minimizes the chance that catheter elongation during injection will advance the tip against the valve leaflets. Our own practice is to inject 40 to 50 ml of contrast media at a rate of 20 to 25 ml/sec. If displacement or recoil of the catheter detracts from the quality of the examination, a repeat injection following adjustment of the catheter position must be considered.

The concept of grading aortic insufficiency has to take several factors into consideration. Among these, the size and volume of the aorta, the concentration of contrast medium achieved by the injection, and the degree of dilatation and emptying capacity of the left ventricle rank highly. Technical factors of importance are the shape of the regurgitant jet of contrast medium which may be more impressive when seen tangentially in a particular projection, the type of exposure chosen, and the object density and the latitude of the film. It is advisable, therefore, that a particular laboratory develop a standard examination technique to achieve the greatest possible uniformity.

A common practice is to express the subjectively made observation of aortic valve incompetence in four degrees of severity (1 to 4 +). Minor variations in definition exist at the lower end of the scale because some authors tend to include findings that are most likely artifactual. A grade of 1 + aortic regurgitation signifies a minor degree of radiopaque reflux in diastole, dissipating in the left ventricular volume without resulting in a perceptible overall contrast increment of this chamber. A grade of 4 + aortic regurgitation denotes rapid and massive reflux within one diastole, resulting in fairly uniform opacification of the left ventricular chamber reaching a radiodensity similar to or greater than that of the ascending aorta. Grades 2 and 3 + are used to identify intermediate degrees of severity between these two extremes.

Comparison with clinical evidence of aortic valve incompetence has found good agreement in the majority of cases.[18] The radiologic contrast study was found to resolve clinical uncertainty in situations in which combined valve lesions made the clinical assessment difficult.

Comparison with observations at operation has also demonstrated the predictive value of cineaortography to be very reliable. Patients without evidence of regurgitation on cineaortography were subsequently found to have no more than mild regurgitation at operation, whereas all those identified as having 3 or 4 + regurgitation had severe incompetence.[18] The same angiographic approach can be used in the evaluation of a malfunctioning aortic valve prosthesis. Here, the possibility to differentiate on the cine films between valvular incompetence and paravalvular leak (Fig. 16–6) has to

be emphasized, and the difference can be distinguished on the angiographic study.

Aortic Aneurysms

Because a great proportion of the thoracic aorta's outer contours are seen on plain chest x-ray films, an aortic aneurysm is frequently suspected or diagnosed with this noninvasive test. Fluoroscopy, kymography, two-dimensional ultrasound, nuclear imaging, CT scanning, and magnetic resonance imaging (MRI) may be used for confirmation of the diagnosis. Thoracic aortography is, however, the most conclusive procedure because it renders the necessary details for potential surgical intervention. It is widely practiced both as an elective and an emergency procedure.

Both true and false aneurysms can occur in the thoracic aorta. The term *true aneurysm* implies that the outer wall of the aneurysm is composed of at least one of the three arterial wall layers, (intima, media, and adventitia) and the term *false aneurysm* signifies that the aortic wall actually has been perforated and the extravasating blood is contained by adjacent tissue and by thrombus formation. The most common true aneurysms are arteriosclerotic, luetic, or congenital in nature, whereas traumatic rupture and perforation are typical causes for false aneurysms.

Important information that can be gained from the angiographic procedure includes location and size of the aneurysm, relationship to origins of other vessels, proximity to other adjacent structures such as superior vena cava, trachea, or esophagus, and the characteristics of the aortic wall at the border of the aneurysm. These factors are all of importance in guiding the surgeon to choose the proper site for resection and to exclude the presence of unrecognized additional vascular pathology.

Arteriosclerotic Aneurysms. In the adult, particularly in the elderly, the most common type of thoracic aortic aneurysm by far is the arteriosclerotic type. The site of predilection is the distal arch or the descending aorta. The aneurysms are usually *fusiform* but may be *saccular.* As they are the result of wall weak-

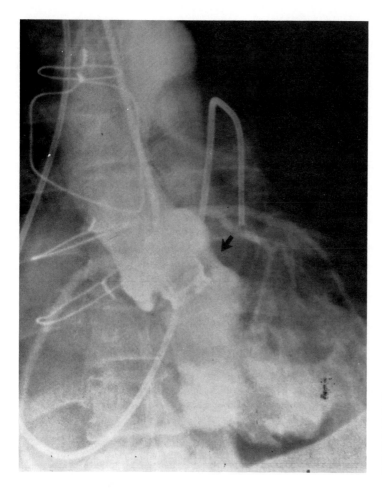

Fig. 16–6. Supravalvular aortogram in anteroposterior projection in a patient with an aortic valve prosthesis. Significant aortic regurgitation to the left ventricle occurred in paravalvular aortic position (arrow).

ening in the deeper portion of an atheromatous ulcer, one can expect the remaining wall of the aorta to show the typical changes of plaques and craters, and the aneurysms are frequently multiple.[19] The angiographic examination often demonstrates an increased distance between the inner contour and the outer wall (Fig. 16–7), which is related to the frequent occurrence of laminated thrombus and adventitial fibrosis.

Arteria Magna. An interesting and extreme form of this condition is the so-called arteria magna,[20] observed predominantly in the elderly and apparently caused by a profound diffuse loss of elastic tissue in the aortic media. In such cases the thoracic aorta becomes enormously widened and elongated. The risk of rupture is high, an event that in the thoracic region is most often fatal because of poor hem-

orrhage containment by adjacent organs. Fusiform and saccular aneurysms of the ascending aorta are less likely to be atherosclerotic. In the past, such aneurysms were most likely to be luetic, representing most often the late manifestation of syphilis. Typical and almost pathognomonic for these were linear calcifications in the ascending aortic wall, usually detectable on chest radiographs. This is a rare diagnosis today.

Other Types. A subclass of thoracic aortic aneurysms involves the sinuses of Valsalva. Commonly, the origin is congenital or idiopathic, and the aneurysm may involve all three sinuses. The underlying abnormality is medial necrosis with resultant weakness of the aortic wall. Specific examples include Marfan's syndrome, Ehlers-Danlos, and other connective tissue disorders. Incompetence of the aortic

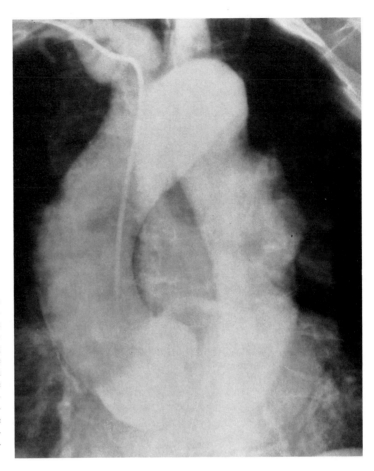

Fig. 16–7. Thoracic aortogram in anteroposterior projection illustrates general widening of the entire thoracic aorta. In the proximal portion of the descending aorta a large local contour bulge is noted, and the distance between the contrast-filled lumen and the outer contour of the distal descending aorta is increased. Operative findings confirmed the diagnosis of atherosclerotic aneurysm with marked wall thickening.

valve is frequently an associated finding. Less commonly, the origin may be acquired conditions such as bacterial endocarditis (e.g., occurring after cardiac surgical procedures such as aortic valve replacement[21]). Aneurysms of the sinus of Valsalva commonly rupture, resulting in fistulae with connections to other cardiac chambers, especially the right atrium and ventricle (Fig. 16–8).

Because many of the disease processes causing aortic aneurysms may also involve the major intrathoracic branches of the aorta, it is prudent to extend the angiographic examination to these vascular areas as well. In particular, the innominate and left subclavian arteries may be involved. Aneurysms of the left common carotid, intercostal, and brachial arteries, have also been described either as isolated findings or in combination with lesions in the aorta.

Traumatic Aneurysms. Post-traumatic an-

eurysms have increased in frequency. Rapid deceleration in conjunction with motor vehicle accidents explains their most frequent occurrence in the young and their localization to the isthmus of the aorta (Fig. 16–9), i.e., the border between the arch and the descending aorta where the inertia of the large column of blood exerts local wall stresses that may exceed elastic tolerance. Frequently the diagnosis of an aortic aneurysm is made after the acute phase, when during recovery of the severely injured victims a chest roentgenogram shows a bulge in the aortic contour. The underlying abnormality consists of a wall rupture with contained hematoma, thus representing a false aneurysm. Although the patient may be asymptomatic at the time when the diagnosis is made on chest roentgenogram, aortography and subsequent surgical repair are indicated because of the high risk of late rupture.[22]

Dissecting Aneurysm. Dissection of the

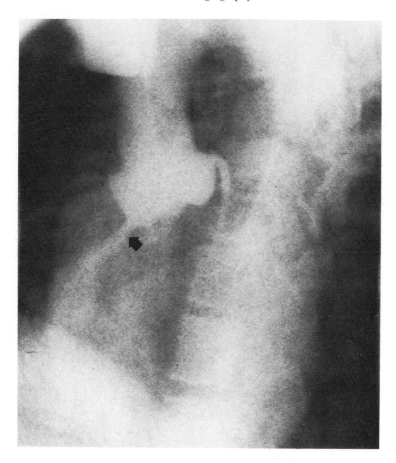

Fig. 16–8. Cineaortogram in LAO projection, demonstrating ruptured aortic sinus (sinus of Valsalva) aneurysm. The aneurysm formed from the wall of the right aortic sinus, just below the origin of the right coronary artery. Rupture (arrow) is into the right atrium.

aortic wall involves the thoracic aorta most frequently. Its high incidence in the male population between the ages of 50 and 70, particularly in patients with a history of systemic hypertension, makes it an important differential diagnosis to acute myocardial infarction. The initiating cause is an intimal tear with formation of intramural hematoma that extends along the weakened aortic media, which histologically shows signs of necrosis. Localization of the initial tear is important to determine patient risk and management. Application of the classification according to DeBakey is most useful in this respect. In this classification, type I describes a dissection whose initial tear is localized to the proximal portion of the ascending aorta, just above the aortic valve, with the false lumen extending around the arch (Fig. 16–10) to the descending aorta, not infrequently continuing to the abdominal portion of the aorta and the large pelvic arteries. A type II dissection is similar; however, the dissection terminates proximal to the first large arch vessel orifice. Type III dissection denotes a dissection that begins distal to the aortic arch (Fig. 16–11). Type III dissections generally involve less hazard because they do not directly affect the circulation to the most vital organs, the heart and the brain. Although less invasive approaches such as sequential chest roentgenograms, thoracic fluoroscopy, ultrasound, computerized tomography (CT), and MRI may render important clues, a thoracic aortogram is the definitive procedure in making an accurate diagnosis.

The optimal technical approach for a tho-

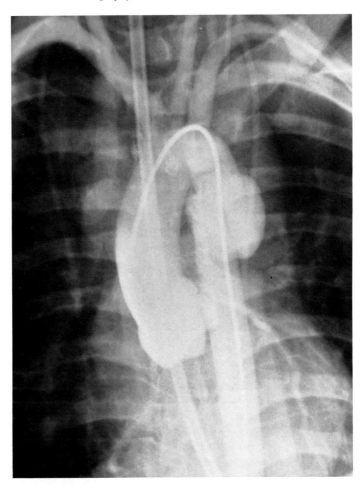

Fig. 16–9. Total rupture of the aorta at its isthmus by a rapid-deceleration vehicle accident. Note aortic wall contour defects and local bulbous accumulation of contrast medium, representing the false aneurysm contained by adjacent tissue. Surgical repair immediately following the angiogram was successful.

racic aortogram is retrograde from the femoral artery, preferably from the artery with the best pulsations. A nontraumatic catheter or soft J-tipped guide wire must be carefully guided by fluoroscopy and test injections. An increased distance between catheter and outer contour will alert the experienced angiographer to the presence of a dissection. Approach from brachial or axillary arteries is not necessary and probably inadvisable when intermittent or persistent pulse deficits exist. Whereas the angiographic identification of the false lumen itself, filling rapidly or slowly, is relatively easy on rapid film series, the precise localization of the tear and dislodged intimal flaps may be challenging. Additional injections at different sites within the aorta and using cineangiography for better identification of contrast flow pathways may be necessary. The same holds

true for evaluation of complicating events such as aortic valve incompetence, compromise of coronary orifices, and perforations, e.g., bleeding into the pericardial space. These considerations are strong arguments for a direct arterial approach as opposed to the less invasive intravenous injections. A similar approach is required for dissecting aneurysms that might be found in Marfan's syndrome or might be the result of iatrogenic trauma such as arterial catheterization, aortic valve replacement, or vascular surgery.

Aortic Coarctation

The diagnosis of aortic coarctation can be made by careful clinical examination in most cases. Signs of coarctation are a late systolic murmur in the typical location over the spine,

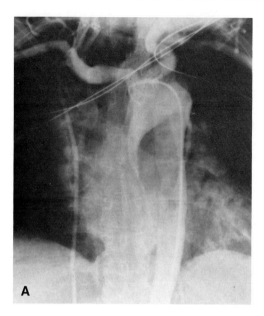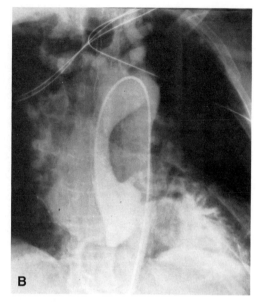

Fig. 16–10. Type I dissecting aortic aneurysm in a middle-aged patient with a history of hypertension. (A) Injection through a pigtail catheter was done at the aortic arch because further catheter advancement met resistance. Observe the marked narrowing of the ascending aorta, which is compromised by a large blood-distended and nonopacified false lumen. Large arch vessels are not compromised. (B) The aortic root was injected following careful advancement of the pigtail catheter. The injection demonstrates the large diameter of the false lumen. The dissection involves the aortic cusps, causing valve incompetence with contrast medium filling the left ventricle. Immediately after angiography the dissecting aneurysm and the regurgitant aortic valve were repaired surgically.

a pulse delay in the lower extremities, and a gradient of blood pressure readings between the upper and lower extremities. Not infrequently, however, the radiologist makes the diagnosis of aortic coarctation on chest roentgenograms by virtue of the impressively abnormal contour of the aortic arch and large vessels in the upper mediastinum, as well as rib notching and a hypertrophic rounded appearance of the left ventricular contour. Prominence of the ascending aorta is noted frequently, and is usually unrelated to the degree of hypertension. It suggests, however, the association of aortic valve abnormalities, such as bicuspid leaflets, present in up to a third of the cases of aortic coarctation.

Aortography again assumes an important diagnostic role and can differentiate the great variety of abnormal patterns (Fig. 16–12) which include complete aortic interruption, hypoplastic aortic segment, and the most common type, a stenosis of varying degrees at the site of the isthmus distal to the left subclavian

artery. Biplane AP and lateral (or RAO/LAO) aortography are undertaken initially, with contrast injection proximal to the coarctation (30 to 50 ml at 25 ml/sec) using either large-film or cineangiographic technique. If the anatomy of the coarctation is not well visualized, a second injection is done with either cranial or caudal angulation, depending on the findings of the first aortogram. An interesting associated finding in some cases is an aberrant right subclavian artery arising from the descending thoracic aorta distal to the coarctation and with lower pulse pressure in the right than in the left arm. Coarctation of the aorta sometimes may be seen in association with right-sided aortic arch.[23]

The retrograde catheter approach through the site of narrowing requires great caution. Not infrequently, collateral pathways entering into thin-walled poststenotic segments may be difficult to negotiate and definitely pose a hazard for inadvertent perforation. A brachial or axillary artery approach should be preferred

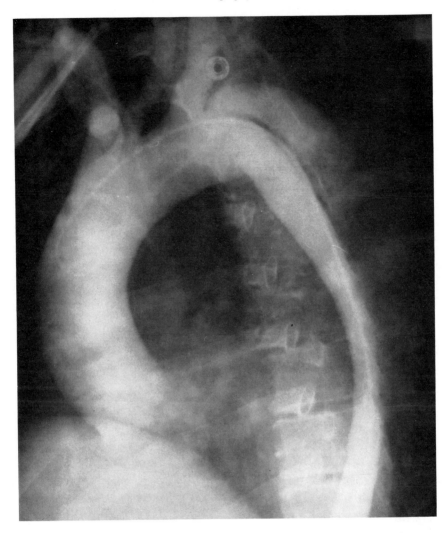

Fig. 16–11.   Type III dissecting aortic aneurysm in a 62-year-old man with previous hypertension. Aortogram in LAO projection shows faint opacification of the false lumen, which begins just after the origin of the left subclavian artery. A pigtail catheter was placed in the ascending aorta from the right groin and is in the true lumen. An intimal flap can be seen clearly dividing the true and false lumens in the descending thoracic aorta. The true lumen is compressed because of hematoma in the false lumen.

for entrance to the prestenotic aorta. In some situations the indirect angiographic approach, with injections into the central venous system or the pulmonary artery, may be a less hazardous alternative and may render sufficient information, particularly when image enhancement and subtraction techniques are used. If, however, the need for precise evaluation of hemodynamic changes exists, such as the exclusion of an aortic valve gradient or assessment of left ventricular function, cardiac catheterization is conveniently combined with selective angiography.

Patent Ductus Arteriosus

Thoracic aortography is a powerful diagnostic tool for identifying and evaluating a persistent ductus arteriosus. This lesion ranks high among congenital cardiovascular abnormalities with a prevalence of 1/5500 in the young population up to 14 years. If isolated, a patent ductus arteriosus carries a good prognosis, more than 95% of the patients reaching 18 years or older. In the child, typical symptoms and noninvasive findings may suffice to recommend surgical repair without the need

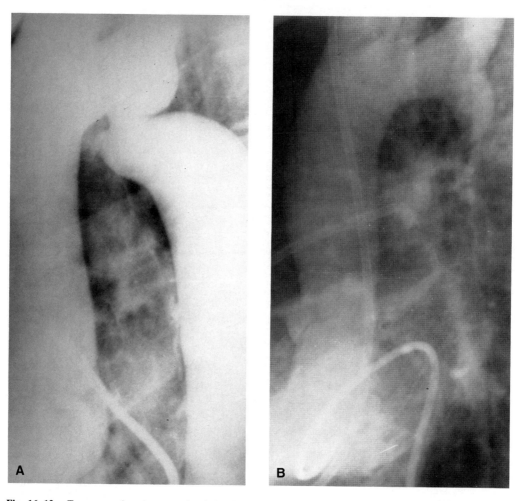

Fig. 16–12. Two cases of aortic coarctation in LAO projection. (A) Note marked distortion of the aortic arch with significant narrowing at the isthmus and poststenotic dilatation of the descending aorta. (B) The coarctation resulted in complete occlusion of the lumen.

for angiography. In the adult, subtle symptoms or combinations with other malformations increase the need for angiographic confirmation. Furthermore, differential diagnostic considerations in the presence of a continuous murmur in an adult should include conditions that have a longer natural history to full development, such as shunts by way of aberrant coronary arteries connecting with the pulmonary circulation, coronary artery fistulae or arteriovenous connections in the thoracic wall (e.g., laceration of the internal mammary artery following penetrating trauma). Selective aortic cineangiography with injection near the site of the expected arterial entrance is sensitive in demonstrating small shunts and surpasses the sensitivity of right heart catheterization with stepwise oximetry. Radionuclide tracer flow studies may match angiography in this respect; however, they are less conclusive with regard to topographic localization. Large shunts result in the typical appearance of increased pulmonary vascularity on the chest roentgenogram, and in such cases the aortogram may demonstrate a difference in caliber between the ascending and descending aorta. An aortogram is also able to establish the rare diagnosis of an aortopulmonary window, which has similar hemodynamic consequences to patent ductus arteriosus. In the event of secondary pulmo-

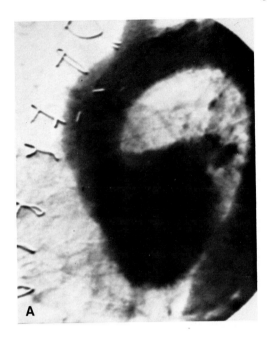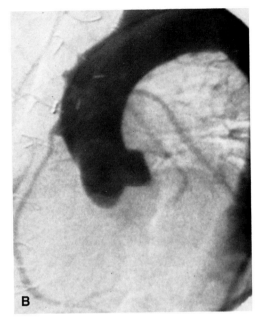

Fig. 16–13. Examples of digital angiography in patient with triple bypass surgery. (A) Following intravenous injection, contrast medium is seen in left ventricle and thoracic aorta, both viewed in LAO projection. Faint opacification of saphenous vein bypass graft segments can be seen between inner contour of ascending aorta and contrast-filled left ventricle. (B) Following direct injection of the aortic root, the three grafts can be clearly identified. Motion artifacts at distal grafts caused by cardiac activity and overlapping with contrast medium in ascending aorta of proximal graft portions limit significantly the diagnostic information. (Courtesy of D. Kim, M.D.)

nary hypertension with equilibrated resistance, the shunt may be reversed, resulting in a corresponding negative contrast defect by the unopacified blood in the contrast column.

Coronary Bypass Grafts

The current need for postoperative demonstration of aortocoronary venous bypass grafts exists primarily in patients with recurrence of angina pectoris. Selective injections into the individual grafts are generally performed in conjunction with a repeat selective coronary arteriogram of the native circulation. Although this selective approach is successful in most cases, difficulties may be encountered when the proximal graft anastomosis is in an unusual position or when a "flush" proximal occlusion has to be documented. As a last resort, a nonselective, large bolus of contrast medium may be injected into the ascending aorta. The results of such injections are frequently disappointing. Complete absence of filling following rapid injection (20 ml/sec or more) of 40 to 50 ml of contrast agent into the ascending aorta, however, is reasonably good evidence for graft occlusion. If filling of the graft in question is noted, the diagnosis of a stenosis or impaired flow must be made cautiously. Digital subtraction technique enhances contrast and is therefore recommended.[24]

Frequently the results of the selective angiogram of the native coronary arteries give indirect but important clues, such as retrograde filling of the distal graft and/or persistence or recurrence of collaterals directed to the bypassed coronary artery branch. Intravenous digital angiography has been advocated for the demonstration of coronary artery bypass grafts, but is even less likely to cope with the above mentioned difficulties (Fig. 16–13). The same holds for the use of CT scanning, advocated by some to identify the proximal grafts in transectional fashion without demonstrating localized narrowing unless by serendipity. Modern high-speed dynamic CT scanners presently being developed offer some promise because they may be used to determine the rate of contrast turnover possibly reflecting regional flow impairment.

REFERENCES

1. Forssmann W: Die Sondierung des rechten Herzens. Klin Wochenschr 8:2085, 1929.
2. dos Santos R, Lamas AC, Pereira-Caldas J: Arteriografia da aorta e dos vasos abdominalis. Med Contemp 47:93, 1929.
3. Nuvoli I: Arteriografia dell' aorta ascendente o del ventriculo. Policlinico (Prat) 43:227, 1936.
4. Seldinger SI: Catheter replacement of the needle in percutaneous arteriography: A new technique. Acta Radiol (Stockh) 39:368, 1953.
5. Hanafee W: Axillary artery approach to carotid, vertebral abdominal aorta, and coronary angiography. Radiology 81:559, 1963.
6. Roy P: Percutaneous catheterization by the axillary artery. AJR 94:1, 1965.
7. Boijsen E: Selective visceral angiography using a percutaneous axillary technique. Br J Radiol 39:414, 1966.
8. Dudrick S, Masland W, Mishkin M: Brachial plexus injury following axillary artery puncture. Radiology 88:271, 1967.
9. Molnar W, Paul DJ: Complication of axillary arteriotomies: Analysis of 1762 consecutive studies. Radiology 104:269, 1972.
10. Maxwell DD, March HB, Mispireta LA: Translumbar selective coronary arteriography. Cardiovasc Intervent Radiol 5:157, 1982.
11. Gishen P, Lakier JB: The ascending aorta in aortic stenosis. Cardiovasc Radiol 2:85, 1979.
12. Paulin S: Contrast agents for selective coronary arteriography. Cathet Cardiovasc Diagn 10:425, 1984.
13. Contrast Material Symposium, San Francisco, CA, October 22–23, 1983. Investigative Radiol 19:Suppl 4, 1984.
14. Nordenstrom B, Ovenfors CO, Westberg G: Experimental stereoangiography of the coronary and bronchial arteries. Acta Chir Scand Suppl 245, 1959.
15. Beuren AJ, et al: The syndrome of supravalvular aortic stenosis, peripheral pulmonary stenosis, mental retardation and similar facial appearance. Am J Cardiol 13:471, 1964.
16. Williams JCP, Barratt-Boyes BG, Lowe JB: Supravalvular aortic stenosis. Circulation 24:1311, 1961.
17. Taubman JO, Goodman DJ, Steiner RE: The value of contrast studies in the investigation of aortic valve disease. Clin Radiol 17:23, 1966.
18. Cohn LH, et al: Preoperative assessment of aortic regurgitation in patients with mitral valve disease. Am J Cardiol 19:177–182, 1967.
19. Sprayregen S: Radiologic spectrum of arteriosclerotic aneurysms of aortic arch. NY State J Med 78:2198, 1978.
20. Randall PA, et al: Arteria magna revisited. Radiology 132:295, 1979.
21. Holmes EC, Bredenberg CE, Brawley RK: Aneurysm of the sinus of Valsalva resulting from bacterial endocarditis. Ann Thorac Surg 15:1628, 1973.
22. Bennett DE, Cherry JK: The natural history of traumatic aneurysms of the aorta. Surgery 6:15, 1967.
23. Edelman RR, Weintraub R, Paulin S: Coarctation of the aorta with right aortic arch of the mirror-image type. AJR 140:1135, 1983.
24. Guthaner D, et al: A comparison of digital subtraction techniques in the evaluation of coronary graft patency. (Abstract) Presented at the American College of Cardiology Meeting, March 1984, Dallas, Texas.

Part V

Evaluation of Cardiac Function

17

Dynamic and Isometric Exercise During Cardiac Catheterization

BEVERLY H. LORELL and WILLIAM GROSSMAN

Patients with significant heart disease may have entirely normal hemodynamics measured in the resting state during cardiac catheterization. Because most cardiac symptoms are precipitated by exertion or some other stress, however, it is often important that hemodynamic performance be assessed both at rest and during some form of stress such as muscular exercise, pharmacologic intervention, or pacing-induced tachycardia. Such an evaluation enables the physician to assess both the level of cardiovascular reserve and the relationship (if any) of specific symptoms to hemodynamic impairment. Physiologic information so obtained is often valuable in prescribing specific medical therapy, selecting patients for corrective cardiac surgery, and estimating prognosis.

Muscular exercise, both dynamic and isometric, has been studied extensively, and the normal hemodynamic responses are reasonably well understood. In the cardiac catheterization laboratory, muscular exercise may be used in the hemodynamic evaluation of patients with heart disease. There are major differences between the hemodynamic responses to dynamic exercise done either in the *supine* or *erect* position and static, isometric exercise, and each type of exercise will be discussed separately.

DYNAMIC EXERCISE

Dynamic exertion is the major form of exertion in everyday activity. During dynamic exertion, skeletal muscles are actively contracting and developing force that is translated into motion and work. This is accompanied by an increase in the amount of oxygen taken up by pulmonary capillary blood in the lungs and transported by arterial blood to working skeletal muscles. In normal sedentary individuals, the level of oxygen consumption during maximal exercise ($\dot{V}O_2$ max) can increase about twelve-fold in comparison to that during the resting state.[1] Additional factors influencing $\dot{V}O_2$ max include gender, oxygen tension of inspired air, ambient and body temperature, and the blood hemoglobin content. Age and fitness also modify $\dot{V}O_2$ max because there is about a 5% decrease in $\dot{V}O_2$ max per decade during aging. During athletic training, $\dot{V}O_2$ max increases because of both cardiovascular and skeletal muscle adaptation. In marathon runners and Olympic class athletes, $\dot{V}O_2$ max may represent an 18-fold increase in oxygen consumption above the resting state. In any individual, the $\dot{V}O_2$ max depends on the integration of cardiac, metabolic, vascular, and pulmonary responses. The increased oxygen requirements of muscular exercise are met by both an increase in the cardiac output and an increased extraction of oxygen from arterial blood by skeletal muscle, which causes widening of the arteriovenous oxygen difference. The ability of the heart to increase its output appropriately for the increase in oxygen consumption at any level of exercise is met by an increase in *heart rate* and by an increase in *stroke volume*. The *relative contributions of heart rate and stroke volume* depend on the type of exercise (supine versus upright), the level of exercise, the limitation of diastolic filling at high heart rates, and the response to sympathetic stimulation. Metabolic adaptations of exercising muscle include a switch from utilization of free fatty acids at rest to an accelerated breakdown of muscle glycogen stores and enhanced uptake of blood-borne glucose, which is supplied by increased hepatic gluconeogenesis. Because carbohydrate metabolism produces more carbon dioxide than fat metabolism, the *respiratory quotient* (ratio of CO_2 production to O_2 consumption) rises from a resting value of about 0.7 toward 1.0.[2] The delivery of blood-borne oxygen and glucose to working skeletal muscle is enhanced in the presence of normal vasculature by a reduction in skeletal muscle vascular resistance mediated by metabolic byproducts and by sympathetically mediated vasoconstriction elsewhere, which cause a redistribution of blood away from the renal and splanchnic beds to exercising muscle.

In addition, exercise depends on the ability of the respiratory mechanism to increase oxygen supply. During progressive exercise, there is a linear increase in minute ventilation relative to the increase in oxygen consumption. When such a level of exercise is reached that insufficient oxygen is delivered to exercising muscle, anaerobic metabolism of glycogen and glucose develops causing metabolic acidosis and an increase in respiratory quotient to values ≥ 1.0 such that minute ventilation increases out of proportion to oxygen consumption.[3] Beyond this **anaerobic threshold** the accumulation of hydrogen ions usually causes skeletal muscle weakness, pain, and severe breathlessness, followed by exhaustion and cessation of exercise. The factors determining

the duration and workload of exercise beyond the anaerobic threshold that can be endured by some subjects are poorly understood.

As will be discussed below, we usually structure exercise studies in the catheterization laboratory so that the patient reaches a *steady-state level of submaximal exercise* below the anaerobic threshold and exercise can be sustained for several minutes. The approach permits a critical examination of cardiovascular reserve; that is, is the increase in cardiac output appropriate for the increase in oxygen consumption occurring at that particular level of exercise?

Oxygen Uptake and Cardiac Output

There is a linear relationship between oxygen consumption and increasing workload. Oxygen uptake as measured from expired air collections increases abruptly after initiation of dynamic exercise reflecting additional work to overcome inertia of the legs and then increases steadily over a few minutes to reach a new steady state that is directly related to the level of exercise.[4,6] Data illustrating these changes are shown in Figure 17–1. Simultaneously, the mixed venous blood oxygen saturation decreases to a lower steady level related to the intensity of exercise, producing an

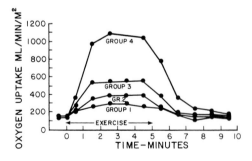

Fig. 17–1. Oxygen consumption in normal subjects during exercise. Each group represents a different level of exercise, with the most intense exercise being performed by Group 4. Note the prompt increase and establishment of a new steady state in oxygen uptake that is directly related to the intensity of the exercise. (From Donald KW, et al: The effect of exercise on the cardiac output and circulatory dynamics of normal subjects. Clin Sci 14:37, 1955. Used with permission of the publisher.)

increase in the arteriovenous oxygen difference.

The cardiac output increases linearly with increasing workload during both supine and upright exercise in normal subjects.[4–7] Dexter and his colleagues,[4] who studied the effect of exercise on circulatory dynamics in seven normal individuals, found that the relationship between cardiac output and oxygen consumption is predictable (Fig. 17–2). As can be seen from the regression equation for this relationship, for each increment of 100 ml/min/m² of oxygen consumption during exercise, there is an increase in cardiac output of 590 ml/min/m².

The linear relationship between oxygen uptake and cardiac output response during exercise, illustrated in Figure 17–2, may be used to assess whether the cardiac output response measured in an individual patient is appropriate to the level of exercise and increased oxygen uptake. The regression formula: cardiac index (L/min/m²) = 0.0059X + 2.99 where X = O_2 consumption in ml/min/m², may be used to calculate the *predicted cardiac index* for a given level of O_2 consumption (X), and the predicted cardiac index may then be compared to the measured cardiac index. Note that this assessment can be performed at any steady-state level of exercise, and does not depend on achieving any specific "target" level of exertion. This equation can be used to calculate a predicted cardiac index by measuring oxygen consumption during dynamic exercise. The patient's actual measured cardiac index during exercise is then divided by the predicted cardiac index to determine the deviation from normal. We have termed this ratio the **"exercise index,"** since it allows expression of exercise capacity as a percentage of the normal response. An exercise index of:

$$\frac{\text{measured cardiac index}}{\text{predicted cardiac index}} \geqq 0.8$$

indicates a normal cardiac output response to exercise.

Another way of using this same relationship between cardiac output and oxygen consumption involves calculation of the **"exercise factor,"** which is the *increase* in cardiac output with exercise divided by the corresponding *increase* in oxygen consumption. A normal exercise factor would be an increase of $\geqq 600$ ml/min in cardiac output per 100 ml/min increase in oxygen consumption.[5,8] An exercise factor less than

$$\frac{600 \text{ ml/min cardiac output}}{100 \text{ ml/min } O_2 \text{ consumption}}$$

indicates a subnormal response in cardiac output; like an exercise index of $\leqq 0.8$, it suggests some pathologic process limiting the heart's ability to meet the exercise-induced increase in oxygen consumption with an appropriate increase in cardiac output and an excessive reliance on arterial oxygen extraction and widening of the arteriovenous oxygen difference.

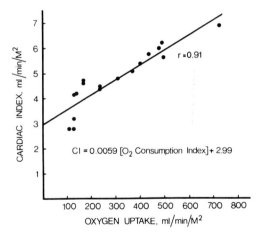

Fig. 17–2. The relationship between cardiac output and oxygen consumption (both indexed for body surface area) during supine dynamic exercise of varying intensity in normal subjects, based on the data of Dexter.[1] As can be seen from the regression equation for this relationshp, for each increment of 100 ml/min/m² of oxygen consumption, there is an increase in cardiac output of 0.59 liters/min/m² or 590 ml/min/m².

Systemic and Pulmonary Arterial Pressure and Heart Rate

Systemic arterial pressure and mean arterial pressure also increase linearly in relation to oxygen consumption during dynamic exercise in the supine or upright position in the normal subject, although the response is somewhat variable.[6,8–11] In spite of this increase in pressure, systemic vascular resistance decreases substantially during dynamic exercise, indicating that the elevated arterial blood pressure is secondary to increased cardiac output. Patients who are unable to generate an adequate increase in cardiac output during dynamic exercise may also increase their arterial pressure, but in this circumstance, systemic vascular resistance does not decline and may actually increase.

The behavior of the pulmonary circulation in response to dynamic exercise is different from that of the systemic circulation in normal individuals. Mean pulmonary artery pressure increases nearly proportionally with cardiac output (pulmonary blood flow) so that there is only a slight decrease in pulmonary vascular resistance in contrast to the normal substantial decrease in resistance of the systemic vasculature.

Heart rate increases consistently during both supine and upright dynamic exercise, and it increases linearly in relation to oxygen consumption. During dynamic *supine exercise* in the catheterization laboratory, tachycardia is the predominant factor in increasing cardiac output. Tachycardia exerts a positive inotropic effect (the so-called Treppe phenomenon), but increased sympathetic nervous system activity appears to be the most significant factor leading to enhanced myocardial contractility.[8,9] In most normal subjects, supine bicycle exercise is accompanied by an increase in ejection fraction and other ejection indices of left ventricular systolic function with a decrease in left ventricular end-systolic volume.[8,12]

In the supine position in normal subjects, left ventricular end-diastolic volume at rest is nearly maximal and substantially larger than end-diastolic volume during peak upright exercise; thus, during supine exercise there is no change or, more commonly, a decrease in end-diastolic volume.[6,13] Thus, the net effect of the decrease in left-ventricular end-diastolic volume and the increase in ejection fraction is that stroke volume shows only minor (if any) increase during vigorous supine exercise. Several investigators[4,5,8–11] have examined the re-

sponse of cardiac output, stroke volume, and heart rate to a given level of supine exercise in normal subjects and shown that the increase in cardiac output is caused primarily by an increase in heart rate with a negligible contribution by increased stroke volume. During repeat exercise when heart rate is held constant, there is a comparable increase in cardiac output caused by a marked increase in stroke volume.[10] When heart rate is artificially increased by electrical pacing in the absence of dynamic exercise, however, a major fall in stroke volume occurs,[10] indicating that further cardiovascular adjustments are required for an adequate hemodynamic response to dynamic exercise.

Thus, to adequately interpret the response to *supine exercise* in the catheterization laboratory, it is important to recognize that the increase in cardiac output in normal young subjects is caused by a proportionate increase in heart rate. As will be discussed below, when chronotropic reserve is depressed, an appropriate increase in cardiac output relative to oxygen consumption depends on the capacity to augment left ventricular diastolic filling and end-diastolic fiber tension, leading to an increase in stroke volume by means of the Frank-Starling mechanism.

Upright versus Supine Exercise

The contributions of heart rate and stroke volume to cardiac output differ from supine to upright bicycle exercise. End-diastolic volume at rest is near maximum when a normal subject is supine, smaller when he is sitting, and smallest when he is standing.[6,13] When he is in the upright position, left ventricular end-diastolic volume, cardiac output, and stroke volume are lower than when he is in the supine position.[6,11,14,15] During erect bicycle exercise, most normal subjects demonstrate an increase in ejection fraction and reduction in end-systolic volume, some enhancement of left ventricular end-diastolic volume, and an increase in stroke volume as well as heart rate.[6,11,13,16] Left ventricular end-diastolic volume and stroke volume tend to increase up to about 50%

of peak oxygen consumption and then to plateau or actually decrease at high levels of exercise.[6] At high levels of exercise and fast heart rates, recruitment of the Frank-Starling mechanism may be blunted by the effects of tachycardia and limitation of diastolic filling due to shortening of diastole. Thus, at high levels of upright exercise, stroke volume is preserved by a progressive decrease in end-systolic volume and increase in ejection fraction in the presence of a constant or decreased left ventricular end-diastolic volume.[6,7]

Caution must be used in interpreting the relative contributions of "inotropic reserve" and utilization of the Frank-Starling mechanism in patients studied during dynamic exercise in the catheterization laboratory.[17] The effects of *advancing age* profoundly alter the exercise response. In healthy subjects, there appear to be no age-related changes in resting cardiac output, ejection fraction, end-systolic or end-diastolic volumes.[18] With age, there is a reduction in both peak oxygen consumption and cardiac output during exercise. Further, with advancing age there is a reduction in the heart rate and contractility response during exercise, so that the increase in cardiac output at any level of exercise is accomplished by a significant increase in end-diastolic volume and in stroke volume.[18,19] Thus, as discussed above, studies of the effects of dynamic supine bicycle exercise in young adults have generally shown no change or a fall in left ventricular end-diastolic pressure and volume during exercise. In contrast, studies of older normal subjects or patients with atypical chest pain and normal coronary arteries have generally shown that both dynamic supine and upright bicycle exercise are associated with a slight increase in left ventricular end-diastolic pressure,[11,12,20,21] which is consistent with an age-dependent reliance on an increase in preload during exercise. For example, in a group of 10 sedentary men whose average age was 46 years, there was a rise in left ventricular end-diastolic pressure from 8 ± 1 to 16 ± 2 mmHg during supine bicycle exercise, and a rise from 4 ± 1 to 11 ± 1 mmHg during upright bicycle exercise.[11] The diminished heart rate and con-

tractility responses during exercise and resultant increased dependence on the Frank-Starling mechanism with aging may reflect an age-related decrease in responsiveness to beta-adrenergic stimulation.[22-24] There are also *gender*-related differences in the normal response to exercise. Normal men and women can achieve comparable increases in weight-adjusted peak oxygen consumption, heart rate, and blood pressure. Normal women, however, generally achieve increases in stroke volume during upright exercise through an increase in end-diastolic volume without an increase in ejection fraction, whereas normal men exhibit a progressive increase in ejection fraction to peak exercise.[25]

The interpretation of normal versus abnormal left ventricular systolic performance during dynamic exercise may also be complicated by the effects of *chronic β-adrenergic blockade*. Studies of the hemodynamic effects of chronic beta-adrenergic blockade on graded exercise in hypertensive but otherwise healthy young adults have shown that no impairment of maximal exercise capacity (maximal oxygen consumption) or cardiac output response occurs during chronic β-adrenergic blockade.[26] Beta-blockade, however, causes a reduction in heart rate at any level of exercise, and this relative reduction in heart rate is compensated for by both a widening of the arteriovenous O_2 difference and an increase in stroke volume, associated with an increased left ventricular end-diastolic volume and a reduced arterial blood pressure (impedance to ejection).[26,27]

In normal β-blocked subjects, increases in cardiac output during exercise depend on increasing stroke volume by means of the Frank-Starling mechanism. Thus, the dynamic exercise response of a patient on chronic β-adrenergic blocking therapy may be associated with an "inappropriately" low increase in cardiac output relative to oxygen consumption accompanied by excessive widening of the arteriovenous oxygen difference with an increased reliance on an increase in left ventricular end-diastolic volume. During dynamic supine exercise in the catheterization laboratory, the finding that an increase in cardiac output depends on an increase in left ventricular end-diastolic volume (and pressure) could be caused by either β-adrenergic blockade per se or intrinsic impairment of left ventricular systolic function. For these reasons, strong consideration should be given to discontinuation of β-adrenergic blocking drugs at least 24 hours before catheterization if the hemodynamic response to dynamic exercise is planned to assess the adequacy of cardiovascular reserve.

Left Ventricular Diastolic Function

The interpretation of the changes in left ventricular diastolic pressure that occur during exercise depends greatly on an appreciation of the adaptations in diastolic function which occur during exercise. In normal subjects, multiple adjustments occur to accommodate an increased transmitral flow into the left ventricle in the face of an abbreviated diastolic filling period and to maintain low pressures throughout diastole. In normal subjects, exercise is associated with a progressive acceleration of isovolumetric relaxation so that enhanced diastolic filling occurs with minimal change in mitral valve opening pressure.[28] The exercise-induced enhancement of diastolic relaxation and filling is probably modulated by both β-adrenergic stimulation and increased heart rate.

In normal subjects, there is either no change or a downward shift in the left ventricular diastolic pressure-volume relation during exercise (Fig. 17–3). In the presence of ischemia or cardiac hypertrophy, however, exercise may provoke an upward shift in the left ventricular diastolic pressure-volume relationship, so that any level of left ventricular end-diastolic volume is associated with a much higher left ventricular end-diastolic pressure (LVEDP). In such patients, the left ventricle may be regarded as exhibiting increased chamber stiffness (decreased distensibility) during exercise. In patients with coronary artery disease, a transient but striking upward shift in the left ventricular diastolic pressure-volume

relation is common during episodes of ischemia.[29] Such patients with coronary artery disease who develop angina during dynamic exercise in the catheterization laboratory commonly show a marked rise in left ventricular end-diastolic pressure such as the rise in LVEDP from 9.8 ± 2.5 to 31.2 ± 6.5 mmHg reported by Parker et al. in a group of 24 patients who developed angina during supine bicycle exercise,[20] and seen by others during supine[21] and upright bicycle exercise.[30] A careful study of the dynamics of left ventricular diastolic filling during exercise in patients with coronary artery disease has been reported by Carroll and co-workers.[31] These authors studied left ventricular diastolic pressure-volume relations in 34 patients with coronary disease who developed ischemia during exercise and compared the finding to those in 5 patients with minimal cardiovascular disease (control) and 5 patients with an akinetic area at rest (scar group) from a prior infarction, but no active ischemia during exercise. There was an upward shift in the left ventricular diastolic pressure-volume relationship during exercise-induced ischemia, which was not seen in either the scar or the control group (Fig. 17–3). Therefore, interpretation of an exercise-induced rise in left ventricular end-diastolic pressure in patients with coronary artery disease is complex and may be related both to a decrease in left ventricular chamber distensibility, and to an increase in left ventricular end-diastolic volume secondary to a reduction in ejection fraction.[12,16,20,21,30,31]

The presence of cardiac hypertrophy is frequently characterized by depression of the rates of left ventricular relaxation and diastolic filling at rest, which profoundly impedes left ventricular filling during exercise-induced tachycardia.[28] In patients with conditions such as hypertrophic cardiomyopathy or hypertensive hypertrophic cardiomyopathy in whom baseline left ventricular end-systolic volumes are small, there is no reserve to further enhance systolic shortening and abnormal diastolic properties limit the capacity to recruit the Frank-Starling mechanism during exercise. Furthermore, tachycardia may provoke ische-

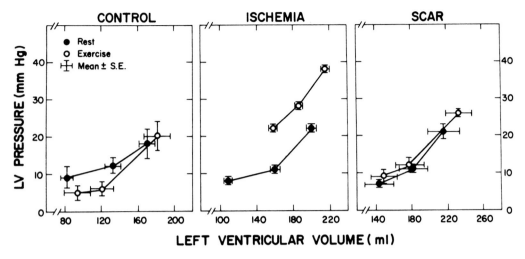

Fig. 17–3. Left ventricular (LV) diastolic pressure-volume relations at rest and during exercise in patients without heart disease (control), compared to patients with coronary disease who developed ischemia during exercise (ischemia) and patients with akinetic areas due to previous infarction but no active ischemia during exercise (scar). Pressure and volume are averaged at three diastolic points: early diastolic pressure nadir, mid-diastole, and end diastole. The control group had a downward shift of the early diastolic pressure-volume relation, but the ischemia group showed an upward and rightward shift. (Reproduced with permission from Carroll J.D., Hess OM, Hirzel HO, Krayenbuehl HP: Dynamics of left ventricular filling at rest and during exercise. Circulation 68:59, 1983.)

mia (due to impaired coronary vasodilator reserve) accompanied by an upward shift in the diastolic pressure-volume relationship. These findings with exercise-induced tachycardia in patients with coronary disease and/or advanced left ventricular hypertrophy are remarkably similar to the changes in diastolic function seen during angina induced by pacing tachycardia, as described in Chapter 18.

Evaluation of Left Ventricular Failure

Examples of the hemodynamic changes that can occur during supine bicycle exercise are

shown in Tables 17–1 and 17–2. Table 17–1 illustrates the response to 6 minutes of supine bicycle exercise of a 36-year-old woman with an idiopathic dilated cardiomyopathy (ejection fraction 40%) whose major symptom was exertional dyspnea. Because her ejection fraction was only moderately depressed and her hemodynamics were nearly normal at rest, resting hemodynamic data alone did not clarify whether her cardiovascular reserve was impaired and whether her exertional dyspnea was likely to be cardiac in origin. During exercise, the cardiac index increased appropriately rel-

Table 17–1. *Response to Supine Bicycle Exercise in a 36-Year-Old Woman with Dilated Cardiomyopathy*

	Resting	Exercise (6 minutes)
O$_2$ consumption index (ml/min/m^2)	117	504
AV O$_2$ difference (ml/L)	34	75
Cardiac index (L/min/m^2)	3.4	6.7
Heart rate (beats/min)	80	140
Systemic arterial pressure (mmHg), systolic/diastolic (mean)	130/70 (95)	142/83 (110)
Right atrial mean pressure (mmHg)	6	7
Pulmonary capillary wedge mean pressure (mmHg)	11	27
Left ventricular pressure (mmHg)	130/17	142/28
Exercise index	—	1.1
Exercise factor	—	8.5

Table 17–2. *Response to Supine Bicycle Exercise in a 60-Year-Old Man with Dilated Cardiomyopathy*

	Resting	Exercise (6 minutes)
O_2 consumption index (ml/min/m²)	128	469
AV O_2 difference (ml/L)	40	96
Cardiac index (L/min/m²)	3.2	4.9
Heart rate (beats/min)	90	141
Systemic arterial pressure (mmHg), systolic/diastolic (mean)	91/62 (73)	107/67 (88)
Right atrial mean pressure (mmHg)	5	20
Pulmonary capillary wedge mean pressure (mmHg)	12	34
Left ventricular pressure (mmHg)	91/16	107/34
Exercise index	—	0.85
Exercise factor	—	4.9

ative to the increase in oxygen consumption, yielding an exercise index of 1.1 and an exercise factor of

$$\frac{3300 \text{ ml/min/m}^2, \, \Delta \text{ cardiac index}}{387 \text{ ml/min/m}^2, \, \Delta \text{ O}_2 \text{ cons. index}} = 8.5$$

The increase in cardiac output, however, was accomplished at the cost of a substantial increase in mean pulmonary capillary wedge pressure, which rose from 11 to 27 mmHg. These data suggest that she had some limitation of inotropic reserve and that her ability to increase cardiac output depended heavily on utilization of the Frank-Starling mechanism. Thus, her dyspnea can be considered to be of cardiac origin.

A patient with more severe impairment of cardiovascular reserve is illustrated in Table 17–2, which shows the response to 6 minutes of supine bicycle exercise of a 60-year-old man with idiopathic dilated cardiomyopathy and symptoms of marked fatigue and dyspnea with minimal exertion. His chest roentgenogram showed cardiomegaly with no evidence of pulmonary edema, and his rest hemodynamics were nearly normal. Supine bicycle exercise, however, was associated with a marked rise in both left and right heart filling pressures, and a marginal ability to increase cardiac output appropriately relative to his increase in

oxygen consumption. His exercise index was 0.85 with a low exercise factor at

$$\frac{1700 \text{ ml/min/m}^2, \, \Delta \text{ cardiac index}}{341 \text{ ml/min/m}^2, \, \Delta \text{ O}_2 \text{ cons. index}} = 4.9$$

The cause of exercise intolerance in most patients with left ventricular failure is diminished cardiovascular reserve so that inadequate oxygen is delivered to working skeletal muscle to meet the demands of aerobic metabolism. As illustrated in the above examples, the relative contributions of the inability of the heart to augment cardiac output versus an exercise-induced rise in pulmonary capillary wedge pressure that could impair gas exchange are controversial. Exercise tolerance in patients with congestive heart failure is highly variable and correlates poorly with ejection fraction. Studies of the hemodynamic and ventilatory response to exercise have shown that as the clinical severity of congestive heart failure worsens, there is a progressive decrease in maximal oxygen consumption, the premature onset of the anaerobic threshold, and the decline of both maximal cardiac output and the cardiac output achieved at levels of submaximal oxygen consumption.[32–35] Studies of *brief exercise* performed by patients with chronic congestive heart failure have shown that arterial oxygen saturation usually increases (presumably due to increased ventilation) despite elevation of the pulmonary capillary wedge pressure, maximal oxygen extraction is normal, and ventilatory mechanisms do not limit maximum oxygen consumption so that both symptomatic limitation and the inability to normally increase oxygen delivery are caused by the failure to adequately increase cardiac output.[33–35] Conversely, in patients with depressed left ventricular ejection fraction who can achieve normal levels of exercise, factors that contribute to normal exercise capacity include normal augmentation of heart rate, the ability to increase cardiac output through further increases in left ventricular end-diastolic volume and stroke volume, and tolerance of a high pulmonary venous pressure, possibly because of enhanced lymphatic drainage.[36]

Thus, in patients with severe depression of left ventricular ejection fraction who cannot increase left ventricular ejection fraction during exercise, the failure to increase cardiac output normally appears to be related both to the inability to increase stroke volume through an increase in left ventricular end-diastolic volume and the inability to increase heart rate relative to age-matched subjects.[32,33,37,38] This **impaired chronotropic response** appears to be caused by an impaired postsynaptic response to β-adrenergic stimulation that may be related to several defects, including a reduced cardiac beta receptor density, a blunted upregulation of beta-receptor density during exercise, "uncoupling" of the beta-receptor and adenylate cyclase activity, and deficient production of cyclic AMP.[38–41] An insufficient exercise heart rate alone is not the only critical factor, because an inability to increase stroke volume may also contribute to the abnormal cardiac reserve during exercise. The factors responsible for inadequate stroke volume reserve in patients with severe depression of left ventricular ejection fraction are controversial, but may include the inability to increase the rate and extent of left ventricular diastolic filling because of impairment of sympathetically-mediated acceleration of myocardial relaxation, loss of ventricular distensibility due to underlying fibrosis or hypertrophy, inadequate systemic vasodilator capacity, and impaired right ventricular function.[31,34,37,42]

Evaluation of Valvular Heart Disease

Valvular Stenosis. Exercise may also be used in the cardiac catheterization laboratory to evaluate valvular heart disease. Gradients across the atrioventricular and semilunar valves may become apparent during exercise and may reach levels that account for the clinical symptoms of the patient. Exercise hemodynamics are especially useful when the resting transvalvular gradient or estimated valve area has borderline significance.

An example of the hemodynamic changes in moderate mitral stenosis during supine dynamic exercise is shown in Figure 17–4. As the result of increased mitral valve flow and a decreased diastolic filling period, the pressure gradient has to increase significantly, producing left atrial pressures of sufficient magnitude to cause clinical symptoms. Cardiac output increased significantly, yielding an exercise index of 1.2 and an exercise factor of

$$\frac{2800 \text{ ml/min, } \Delta \text{ cardiac output}}{481 \text{ ml/min, } \Delta \text{ O}_2 \text{ consumption}} = 5.8$$

These data are compatible with mild mitral stenosis and illustrate the changes in a diastolic pressure gradient across the mitral valve required to produce an increase in cardiac output appropriate to the increased oxygen requirements of strenuous exercise.

In evaluating hemodynamic changes across *stenotic valves* during exercise, it is often found that the calculated valve area during exercise may vary somewhat (it is usually slightly larger) from that calculated on the basis of resting data. This variance is generally small and may be related to actual changes in the degree of valvular obstruction (a higher gradient and greater flow may force the stenotic leaflets to open farther), deficient data, or computational errors inherent in the assumptions applied to the equation for calculating valve orifice size.[43]

Supine dynamic exercise is also useful as a tool to study the efficacy of *balloon mitral valvuloplasty* in lowering left atrial pressure and the transmitral gradient to determine the need for further dilatation during the procedure. Following performance of transseptal catheterization by the usual method, the Mullins sheath is positioned in the left atrium. A 7 Fr Critikon balloon flotation catheter is advanced through the Mullins sheath into the left

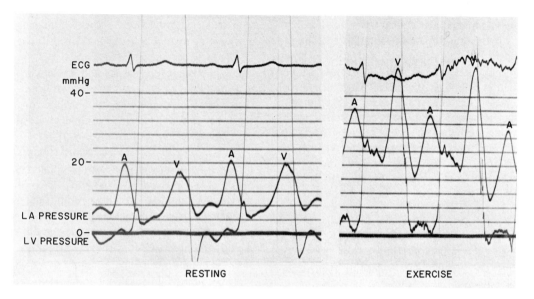

Fig. 17–4. Simultaneous pressure recordings from left atrium and left ventricle at rest and at five minutes of bicycle ergometer exercise in a patient with mitral stenosis. The following hemodynamic data were obtained:

	Resting	Exercise
Left atrium pressure (mmHg)		
A	20	34
V	18	46
mean diastolic	10	26
Left ventricle mean diastolic pressure (mmHg)	1	4
O_2 consumption (ml/min)	207	688
AV O_2 difference (ml/min)	31	74
Cardiac output (L/min)	6.5	9.3
Heart rate (beat/min)	72	108
Mitral valve area (cm²)	1.6	1.8
Exercise index		1.2
Exercise factor		5.9

atrium. The balloon is inflated, and the Critikon catheter is advanced across the mitral valve into the left ventricle. The Mullins sheath is then advanced carefully over the Critikon catheter (with balloon still inflated) into the left ventricle. The Critikon balloon is deflated and the catheter is removed; next, two 0.038-inch exchange length J-tipped guide wires are advanced into the left ventricle, where they are coiled in the left ventricular apex. The Mullins sheath is next removed, leaving the two wires in the left ventricle. A 7 Fr Critikon balloon flotation catheter is then advanced across each of the two exchange length wires, with one balloon catheter being positioned in the left ventricle, and the other being positioned in the left atrium. The guide wires are removed, leaving a balloon flotation catheter in the left atrium and one in the left ventricle. These catheters are used to measure simultaneous left ventricular and left atrial pressures simultaneously with measurements of oxygen consumption at baseline and during dynamic exercise, which can be performed before and after mitral valve dilatation.

Valvular Insufficiency. The hemodynamic consequences of *valvular insufficiency* with ventricular volume overload may be subtle at rest. Dynamic exercise, by calling upon the heart to substantially augment its forward cardiac output, may elicit changes in left ventricular end-diastolic pressure and volume (preload) and in systemic vascular resistance (afterload) that are useful in assessing the cardiovascular limitations imposed by the valve lesion. Of particular importance here is the inability of many patients with valvular insufficiency to increase forward cardiac output in an appropriate manner, resulting in a low exercise index and an abnormal exercise factor. Dynamic exercise is especially valuable in such patients because the qualitative assessment of valvular insufficiency from angiograms may be unreliable and does not correlate well with the extent of functional impairment.

Figure 17–5 shows the effects of dynamic bicycle exercise in a 55-year-old man with rheumatic heart disease and mitral regurgitation. The patient was able to increase cardiac output normally, but as seen in Figure 17–5, mean pulmonary capillary wedge pressure in-

creased from 18 mmHg to 30 mmHg, with V waves to 60 mmHg, during 6 minutes of supine bicycle exercise. This patient had successful mitral valve replacement, with relief of symptoms.

Performing a Dynamic Exercise Test

Dynamic exercise during cardiac catheterization is easily performed with a bicycle ergometer while the patient is supine. A protocol detailing the exercise test should be prepared before the test to ensure that all essential data are obtained. Pressures should be obtained so that the appropriate valve gradients can be evaluated, and left ventricular pressure should

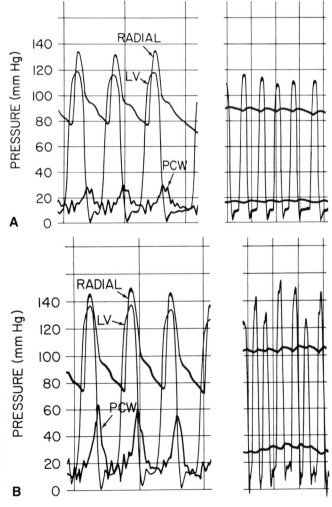

Fig. 17–5. Hemodynamic findings during exercise in a 55-year-old man with mitral regurgitation. Left ventricular (LV), pulmonary capillary wedge (PCW), and radial artery pressure tracings are shown before (A) and during (B) the sixth minute of supine bicycle exercise. PCW mean pressure and V wave increased substantially with exercise.

be monitored if left ventricular performance is in question.

Supine bicycle exercise tests are performed most easily when catheterization is by the arm approach. Supine bicycle exercise tests, however, can also be done with safety when catheterization is by the femoral approach if care is taken to place the right and left heart manifolds and transducers in a stable and accessible position on the chest away from leg motion artifact and if the femoral venous and arterial sheaths are visualized and secured in place by the hand of one operator during exercise to ensure that catheters and sheaths are not displaced during leg movement.

We usually carry out a supine bicycle exercise test immediately after baseline hemodynamics and cardiac output have been measured, before contrast angiography. The patient's feet are secured in the bicycle stirrups, and the right heart, left heart, and systemic arterial catheters and attached manifolds are positioned so that they are not kinked or under tension and will not be disturbed during the exercise. Next, the system for measuring oxygen consumption is put in place (see Chapter 8). As an alternative to Douglas bag air collection, we have used the MRM-2 (Waters Instruments, Inc., Rochester, MN), which gives oxygen consumption readings using a polarographic oxygen sensor continuously during dynamic exercise and allows assessment of whether a steady state has been achieved (Fig. 17–1). This instrument, which has a response time of 10 seconds in detecting a step change in oxygen consumption, is ideal for making $\dot{V}O_2$ measurements during sustained effort. This device has advantages for dynamic exercise in the catheterization laboratory in that: (1) the clear plastic faceplate can be worn comfortably during exercise without the need for a mouthpiece or noseclip and adds no respiratory burden, and (2) it permits a continuous display of time-averaged $\dot{V}O_2$ during exercise so that both the level of exercise and establishment of a steady state can be monitored. Alternatively, cardiac output can be assessed using an indicator-dilution technique (e.g., thermodilution, indocyanine

green dye), and oxygen consumption can be estimated as the quotient of cardiac output and arteriovenous oxygen difference.

Before beginning exercise, the patient is instructed that he or she will be coached to achieve a certain level of submaximal exercise over the first minute of exercise that can be sustained for an additional 4 to 6 minutes. This detailed patient instruction is useful because some patients may be accustomed to the different format of progressively graded exercise aimed at achieving a transient level of maximal exhaustion-limited exercise used in upright treadmill tests. A sufficient number of syringes for measuring systemic arterial and mixed venous (pulmonary artery) blood oxygen saturation content should be at hand.

With the patient resting quietly and feet positioned on the bicycle, all pressures are zeroed, phasic and mean pressures are recorded at 25 or 50 mm/sec paper speed and at the gain to be used in exercise, and cardiac output measurements are repeated to obtain an accurate pre-exercise baseline with legs elevated in the stirrups. Pressures are zeroed once again, *all* pressures are then redisplayed, and paper speed is slowed (5 to 10 mm/sec). Exercise is then begun with *all pressures displayed continuously* on the monitor and recorded at slow speed. We generally record LV phasic pressure, systemic arterial (e.g., radial or femoral artery) mean pressure, and pulmonary capillary mean pressure simultaneously. Using a PPG Biomedical Systems EVR with an HTR-12 multichannel recorder, we generally record at 100 or 200 gain for *all pressures*, so that all pressures may be visualized simultaneously (as shown in Fig. 17–5). Each minute, a brief recording of all three pressures on phasic at 25 to 50 mm/sec paper speed is accomplished, after which the pulmonary capillary and systemic arterial pressures are returned to "mean," and the paper speed slowed to 5 to 10 mm/sec. The continuous observation and recording of pressures is important because it permits the accurate monitoring of any rise in filling pressure or fall in arterial pressure during exercise and ensures that catheters remain in correct position for measurements at peak exercise. After the patient has achieved a steady-state level of exercise for 4 minutes, simultaneous LV-systemic arterial, LV-PCW, and PCW-to-PA pullback pressures are recorded during minutes 4 to 6, after increasing the recorder speed to 50 mm/sec without attempting to rezero the transducers. The right heart catheter is pulled back to the pulmonary artery and exercise cardiac output is measured by Fick or thermodilution technique, at which time arterial and pulmonary artery blood samples are drawn for measurement of oxygen saturation. Expired air is collected or MRM continuous $\dot{V}O_2$ measurements are recorded starting at the fourth minute into exercise, at which time a steady state has been established (see Fig. 17–1).

Precautions should be taken during exercise to ensure patient safety. The duration and intensity of the exercise must be tailored to fit the needs of the individual patient. The electrocardiogram should be monitored constantly to avert serious arrhythmias, and exercise should be terminated if significant symptoms or greatly abnormal hemodynamic alterations occur. Little additional diagnostic information can be obtained by continuing the exercise to the point of producing pulmonary edema.

ISOMETRIC EXERCISE

Lind and his colleagues reported more than 20 years ago that sustained isometric contraction of the forearm flexor muscles produces a cardiovascular reflex consisting of increases in heart rate, arterial blood pressure, and cardiac output.[44] The precise nature of this reflex is not completely understood, but it appears to require afferent neural impulses from the exercising extremity and may be related to inhibition of vagal activity.[44,45] Although the cardiac output response may be blunted, the anticipated responses in heart rate and blood pressure are not blocked by administration of propranolol, indicating that more is involved than a simple increase in beta-adrenergic stimulation.[46]

Hemodynamic Response

The hemodynamic response to isometric handgrip exercise has been studied in a series of normal subjects and patients with heart disease.[47–49] In normal adult subjects, heart rate, systemic arterial pressure, and cardiac output increase, whereas systemic vascular resistance shows no change, indicating that the increase in systemic arterial pressure is caused by the increased cardiac output rather than by a vasoconstrictor response. No significant or consistent change in left ventricular end-diastolic pressure or stroke volume occurs, whereas stroke work, a function of both arterial pressure and stroke volume, generally increases. Contrast ventriculography studies in normal subjects have shown that handgrip exercise results in a decrease in left ventricular end-systolic and end-diastolic volumes and a slight increase in ejection fraction. The augmentation of left ventricular performance during isometric exercise may be caused by both increased left ventricular myocardial contractility and the Frank-Starling mechanism. Studies of myocardial mechanics performed during isometric exercise reveal increases in V_{max}, the theoretic maximal velocity of contractile element shortening at zero load, and in left ventricular peak dP/dt.[47,49]

Patients with heart disease and decreased left ventricular function or inotropic reserve commonly show an abnormal hemodynamic and contractile response to isometric exercise.[47] Although left ventricular peak dP/dt may increase in diseased hearts, changes are of less magnitude than in normal subjects. Left ventricular stroke work may increase, remain unchanged, or decrease in response to isometric exercise in pathologic states. This may itself be evidence of compromised left ventricular function, but is more apparent when the change in stroke work is compared to the change in left ventricular end-diastolic pressure. Significant increases in left ventricular end-diastolic pressure are seen commonly in the abnormal response to isometric exercise[47] and indicate decreased inotropic reserve and dependence on the Frank-Starling mechanism in order to augment left ventricular perform- ance. In decompensated hearts, stroke work may not increase and may actually fall despite increased left ventricular filling pressures. This is an abnormal response, indicating poor left ventricular performance, and may be accom- panied by a decrease in cardiac output and an increase in systemic vascular resistance.

Performing an Isometric Exercise Test

Isometric exercise is most commonly per- formed as sustained handgrip. The subject is first tested to evaluate his maximal voluntary contraction. A partially inflated sphygmoma- nometer cuff or a specially designed handgrip dynamometer may be used. This testing may be done before cardiac catheterization and should be done well before the actual handgrip test. The patient must be coached and en- couraged to grip as hard as possible at the time maximal voluntary contraction strength is de- termined. Baseline resting hemodynamic data should include heart rate, systemic arterial pressure (phasic and mean), left ventricular pressure, and cardiac output. Cardiac output is most easily determined for this form of ex- ercise using the indicator dilution method (e.g., thermodilution, indocyanine green dye), or the Fick method with the continuous oxygen consumption measurement (MRM) technique.

Once baseline data are collected, the subject is asked to grip the dynamometer at a level of 30% to 50% of his previously determined max- imal voluntary contraction. Some coaching is usually required to ensure that the patient sus- tains the grip. It is important that the patient not do a Valsalva maneuver during handgrip exercise, and the respiratory pattern should be closely observed. Valsalva maneuver may be avoided simply by engaging the patient in con- versation during the test. We have used 50% maximal voluntary contraction for 3 minutes, and begin repeat measurements of pressures and cardiac output at 2 minutes and 30 sec- onds, so that measurements are completed at 3 minutes and the test may be terminated. The electrocardiogram should be monitored con- tinuously to exclude the appearance of ar- rhythmias.

ISOPROTERENOL STRESS TEST

The infusion of the beta-agonist isoproter- enol has been advocated as an alternative to dynamic or isometric exercise in the catheter- ization laboratory for evaluation of hemody- namic reserve during stress. The cardiovas- cular responses to isoproterenol infusion in normal subjects are similar to those of supine dynamic exercise and include an increase in heart rate and left ventricular systolic pressure, a fall in systemic vascular resistance, an in- crease in cardiac output, and an increase in left ventricular ejection fraction with a reduc- tion of end-systolic and end-diastolic vol- umes.[10,50] The increase in cardiac output is largely met by an increase in heart rate with minimal change in stroke volume; however, if heart rate is held constant, the increase in car- diac output is accomplished by an augmenta- tion of stroke volume.[10] In patients with severe left ventricular failure, the chronotropic and cardiac output response to isoproterenol is blunted because of postsynaptic desensitiza- tion of the beta receptor pathway.[38] Further- more, we have found that even low doses of isoproterenol infusion are frequently associ- ated with distress caused by sweating, a sen- sation of anxiety, and disturbing "palpita- tions" accompanying marked tachycardia in the absence of exertion. For these reasons, we generally prefer the stresses of dynamic or iso- metric exercise.

REFERENCES

1. Weiner DA: Normal hemodynamic, ventilatory, and metabolic response to exercise. Arch Intern Med 143:2173, 1983.
2. Felig P, Wahren J: Fuel homeostasis in exercise. N Engl J Med 293:1078, 1975.
3. Wasserman K: Breathing during exercise. N Engl J Med 298:780, 1978.
4. Dexter L, et al: Effects of exercise on circulatory dynamics of normal individuals. J Appl Physiol 3:439, 1951.
5. Donald KW, Bishop JM, Cumming G, Wade OL: The effect of exercise on the cardiac output and cir-

culatory dynamics of normal subjects. Clin Sci 14:37, 1955.

6. Higginbotham MB, et al: Regulation of stroke volume during submaximal and maximal upright exercise in normal man. Circ Res 58:281, 1986.

7. Plotnick GD, et al: Use of the Frank-Starling mechanism during submaximal versus maximal upright exercise. Am J Physiol 251:H1101, 1986.

8. Sonnenblick EH, Braunwald E, Williams JF Jr, Glick G: Effects of exercise on myocardial force-velocity relations in intact unanesthetized man. Relative roles of changes in heart rate, sympathetic activities and ventricular dimensions. J Clin Invest 44:2051, 1965.

9. Braunwald E, Sonnenblick EH, Ross J Jr, Glick G, Epstein S: An analysis of the cardiac response to exercise. Circ Res 20 (Suppl I):44, 1967.

10. Ross J Jr, Linhart JW, Braunwald E: Effects of changing heart rate in man by electrical stimulation of the right atrium; studies at rest, during exercise, and with isoproterenol. Circulation 32:549, 1965.

11. Thadani U, Parker JO: Hemodynamics at rest and during supine and sitting bicycle exercise in normal subjects. Am J Cardiol 41:52, 1978.

12. Tebbe V, et al: Peak systolic blood pressure/end-systolic function in coronary artery disease with and without angina pectoris assessed from exercise ventriculography. Clin Cardiol 3:19, 1980.

13. Crawford M, White D, Amon K: Echocardiographic evaluation of left ventricular size and performance during hand-grip and supine and upright bicycle exercise. Circulation 59:1188, 1979.

14. Bevegard S, Holgren A, Jonsson B: The effect of body position on the circulation at rest and during exercise with special reference to the influence on stroke volume. Acta Physiol Scand 49:279, 1960.

15. Wilson M: Left ventricular diameter, posture and exercise. Circ Res 11:90, 1962.

16. Rerych R, et al: Cardiac function at rest and during exercise in normals and patients with coronary heart disease. Ann Surg 187:449, 1978.

17. Ross J Jr, et al: Left ventricular performance during muscular exercise in patients with and without cardiac dysfunction. Circulation 34:597, 1966.

18. Rodeheffer RJ, et al: Exercise cardiac output is maintained with advancing age in healthy human subjects: cardiac dilatation and increased stroke volume compensated for a diminished heart rate. Circulation 69:203, 1984.

19. Port S, Cobb FR, Coleman RE, Jones RH: Effect of age on the response of the left ventricular ejection fraction to exercise. N Engl J Med 303:133, 1980.

20. Parker JO, Di Georgi S, West RO: A hemodynamic study of acute coronary insufficiency precipitated by exercise. Am J Cardiol 17:470, 1966.

21. McAllister BD, et al: Left ventricular performance during mild supine leg exercise in coronary artery disease. Circulation 37:922, 1968.

22. Kuramoto K, et al: Comparison of hemodynamic effects of exercise and isoproterenol infusion in normal young and old men. Jpn Cir J 43:71, 1979.

23. Lakatta EG: Age-related alterations in the cardiovascular response to adrenergic mediated stress. Fed Proc 39:3173, 1980.

24. Gerstenblith D, Renlund DG, Lakatta EG: Cardio-vascular response to exercise in younger and older men. Fed Proc 46:1834, 1987.

25. Higginbotham MB, et al: Sex-related differences in the normal cardiac response to upright exercise. Circulation 70:357, 1984.

26. Reybrouck T, Amery A, Billiet L: Hemodynamic response to graded exercise after chronic beta-adrenergic blockage. J Appl Physiol 42:133, 1977.

27. Bevilacqua M, et al: Role of the Frank-Starling mechanism in maintaining cardiac output during increased levels of treadmill exercise in beta-blocked normal men. Am J Cardiol 63:853, 1989.

28. Murgo JP, Craig WE, Pasipoularides A: Evaluation of time course of left ventricular isovolumic relaxation in man. (1986) *In* Grossman W, Lorell BH (eds): Diastolic Relaxation of the Heart. Boston: Martinus Nijhoff, pp 217–229.

29. Grossman W, Barry WH: Diastolic pressure-volume relations in the diseased heart. Fed Proc 1980:148.

30. Thadani U, West RO, Mathew TM, Parker JO: Hemodynamics at rest and during supine and sitting bicycle exercise in patients with coronary artery disease. Am J Cardiol 39:776, 1977.

31. Carroll JD, Hess OM, Krayenbuehl HP: Diastolic function during exercise-induced ischemia in man. (1986) *In* Grossman W, Lorell BH (eds): Diastolic Relaxation of the Heart. Boston: Martinus Nijhoff, pp 217–229.

32. Epstein SE, et al: Characterization of the circulatory response to maximal upright exercise in normal subjects and patients with heart disease. Circulation 35:1049, 1963.

33. Higginbotham MB, et al: Determinants of variable exercise performance among patients with severe left ventricular dysfunction. Am J Cardiol 51:52, 1983.

34. Weber KT, Kinasewitz GT, Janicki JS, Fishman AP: Oxygen utilization and ventilation during exercise in patients with chronic cardiac failure. Circulation 65:1213, 1982.

35. Franciosa JA, Leddy CL, Wilen M, Schwartz DE: Relation between hemodynamic and ventilatory responses in determining exercise capacity in severe congestive heart failure. Am J Cardiol 53:127, 1984.

36. Litchfield RL, et al: Normal exercise capacity in patients with severe left ventricular dysfunction: compensatory mechanisms. Circulation 66:129, 1982.

37. Szlachcic J, et al: Correlates and prognostic implication of exercise capacity in chronic congestive heart failure. Am J Cardiol 55:1037, 1985.

38. Colucci WS, et al: Impaired chronotropic response to exercise in patients with congestive heart failure. Circulation 80:314, 1989.

39. Bristow MR, et al: Decreased catecholamine sensitivity and B-adrenergic receptor density in failing human hearts. N Engl J Med 307:205, 1982.

40. Mancini DM, et al: Characterization of lymphocyte beta-adrenergic receptors at rest and during exercise in ambulatory patients with chronic congestive heart failure. Am J Cardiol 63:307, 1989.

41. Feldman MD, et al: Deficient production of cyclic AMP: Pharmacologic evidence of an important cause of contractile failure in patients with end-stage heart failure. Circulation 75:331, 1987.

42. Latham RD, Thorton JW, Mulrow JP: Cardiovascular reserve in idiopathic dilated cardiomyopathy as de-

termined by exercise response during cardiac catheterization. Am J Cardiol 59:1375, 1987.

43. Richardson JW, Anderson FL, Tsargaris TJ: Rest and exercise hemodynamic studies in patients with isolated aortic stenosis. Cardiology 64:1, 1979.

44. Lind AR, et al: Circulatory effects of sustained voluntary muscle contraction. Clin Sci 27:229, 1964.

45. Donald KW, et al: Cardiovascular responses to sustained (static) contractions. Circ Res 20 (Suppl. 1):15, 1967.

46. MacDonald HR, Sapru RP, Taylor SH, Donald KW: Effect of intravenous propranolol on the systemic circulatory response to sustained handgrip. Am J Cardiol 18:333, 1966.

47. Grossman W, et al: Changes in the inotropic state of the left ventricle during isometric exercise. Br Heart J 35:697, 1973.

48. Flessas AP, Ryan TJ: Cardiovascular responses to isometric exercise in patients with mitral stenosis. Comparison with normal subjects and patients with depressed ejection fraction. Arch Intern Med 142:1629, 1982.

49. Krayenbuehl HP, Rutishauser W, Schoenbeck M, Amende I: Evaluation of the left ventricular function from isovolumic pressure measurements during isometric exercise. Am J Cardiol 29:323, 1972.

50. Krasnow N, et al: Isoproterenol and cardiovascular performance. Am J Med 37:514, 1964.

18

Hemodynamic Stress Testing Using Pacing Tachycardia

RAYMOND G. MCKAY and WILLIAM GROSSMAN

G raded tachycardia using atrial pacing was first introduced in 1967 by Sowton and co-workers[1] as a stress test which could be used in the cardiac catheterization laboratory to evaluate patients with ischemic heart disease. Sowton noted that artificially increasing the heart rate by pacing the right atrium could usually induce angina in patients with symptomatic coronary artery disease. Moreover, he found that the degree of pacing stress needed to produce ischemia, defined in terms of the pacing rate and duration, was more or less reproducible in any given patient. Since Sowton's original description, numerous investigators have described characteristic pacing-induced electrocardiographic changes,[2–8] derangements of myocardial lactate metabolism,[3–4] hemodynamic abnormalities,[9–18] regional wall motion abnormalities,[19–20] and defects in thallium scintigraphy.[21–24] Although agreement on the overall usefulness of atrial pacing has not been uniform, it is clear that the technique can safely and reliably induce ischemia in most patients with coronary artery disease and that information obtained during the pacing-induced ischemic state can often be helpful in the diagnosis and treatment of the patient's underlying disease.

HEMODYNAMIC EFFECTS OF PACING TACHYCARDIA

The principal form of stress that accompanies pacing tachycardia is an increase in myocardial oxygen consumption secondary to the increased heart rate and an increase in myocardial contractility because of a Treppe effect.[25] Associated with this increase in myocardial oxygen consumption is a reflex coronary vasodilatation with an increase in myocardial blood flow.[26] Apart from these changes in oxygen demand and supply, pacing tachycardia appears to be associated with no major hemodynamic stress, at least in patients with normal coronary arteries. Artificially increasing the heart rate by pacing the right atrium is accompanied by a concomitant decrease in ventricular stroke volume, with little or no overall change in cardiac output. Moreover, there appears to be no significant change in ventricular afterload, venous return, or circulating catecholamines during pacing tachycardia. The physiology of pacing is thus distinctly different from that of dynamic or isometric exercise, where there is not only an increase in heart rate and in myocardial contractility, but also major changes in ventricular loading conditions and cardiac output in re-

283

sponse to increased metabolic demands from the periphery.

Because of the differences in physiology between atrial pacing and exercise, each technique has relative advantages and disadvantages as a form of stress testing in the catheterization laboratory. Unlike pacing, exercise is associated with an increase in both heart rate and systolic blood pressure. As a result, exercise is usually capable of achieving a higher rate-pressure product (i.e., heart rate × peak systolic pressure) and represents a more severe form of stress with greater increases in myocardial oxygen consumption. On the other hand, pacing is not associated with exercise-induced changes in cardiac output or ventricular loading conditions, and the characterization of ventricular function is subsequently easier. In addition, atrial pacing is superior to exercise for evaluating myocardial metabolic function because the rapid rise in arterial lactate levels that accompanies exercise may obscure abnormal patterns of myocardial lactate metabolism. Finally, unlike exercise, with the termination of pacing and the rapid diminution of myocardial oxygen requirement, myocardial ischemia almost always resolves rapidly (e.g., within 1 to 2 minutes) in the immediate post-pacing period. As a result, the physician has slightly more control over the amount of stress that the patient experiences, with very little chance of prolonged ischemia occurring in the post-stress period.

Pacing has been used as a form of stress testing in patients with heart disease for over 15 years. Although the technique has been most useful in the assessment of patients with coronary artery disease, there have been isolated reports on the utility of the technique in patients with other forms of cardiac disease including valvular heart disease and cardiomyopathy. This chapter will focus primarily on the pathophysiology of pacing-induced ischemia and will touch only briefly on the potential use of the method in evaluating patients with other forms of cardiac dysfunction.

METHOD FOR A PACING STRESS TEST

Atrial pacing protocols can usually be conducted in the cardiac catheterization laboratory without undue prolongation of the routine catheterization procedure or significant added risk to the patient. In our experience, pacing is best conducted following the routine diagnostic aspects of catheterization and usually extends the procedure by no more than 15 to 30 minutes, depending on the details of the protocol. It is important that detailed planning of the protocol be made before the catheterization is begun to help incorporate the atrial pacing into the routine catheterization as much as possible without unnecessary repetition of maneuvers and excessive prolongation of arterial time. Thus, if pacing is to be conducted with monitoring of right-sided pressure and cardiac output, two sites of venous access may need to be obtained at the beginning of the catheterization before systemic heparinization is achieved. Likewise, if pacing is to be conducted with simultaneous monitoring of left ventricular pressures, then coronary angiography should be performed before left ventriculography so that the left heart catheter can be left in place following the contrast ventriculogram, rather than in the reverse order so that the left ventricular catheter needs to be reinserted for the atrial pacing protocol.

The type of pacing catheter used for the pacing protocol can vary depending on the type of information that is to be evaluated during the pacing procedure. In general, the pacing catheter can be either unipolar or bipolar. If pacing is to be conducted with simultaneous myocardial metabolic assessment, a Gorlin pacing catheter that provides simultaneous pacing and coronary sinus lactate sampling is ideal for placement in the coronary sinus. Similarly, if assessment of myocardial oxygen consumption is to be made, a coronary sinus pacing catheter with the capability of measuring coronary blood flow, such as the Baim catheter (Elecath, Rahway, NJ), may be used. If pacing is to be conducted with simultaneous measurement of left heart filling pressures and cardiac output, then both a pacing catheter and a second right heart catheter (typically, a thermodilution flow-directed catheter) may be inserted into the right heart.

The pacing catheter may be inserted by either venous cutdown or percutaneous technique from the groin, the antecubital fossa, or the neck. Use of a coronary sinus pacing catheter usually requires a neck or arm approach for easier access into the coronary sinus.

Perhaps the most critical part of the atrial pacing technique is proper placement of the pacing lead, because accidental displacement of the pacing tip during pacing can disrupt the protocol. The pacing lead can be placed either at the superior vena cava-right atrial junction, at the lateral right atrial wall, or in the coronary sinus. Placement of the pacing lead is most stable either at the superior vena cava-right atrial junction or in the coronary sinus because displacement of the lead commonly occurs from the lateral atrial wall during spontaneous respiration. Stimulation on the phrenic nerve with subsequent diaphragmatic stimulation also occurs commonly with placement of the catheter against the lateral atrial wall. To avoid problems with displacement of the pacing tip, we have used a bipolar flared pacing catheter (Atri-pace I, Mansfield Scientific, Mansfield, MA). As shown in Figure 18–1, this catheter has two pacing leads that flare out in a V shape. At any given time, at least one of the tips is in contact with the atrial wall, and therefore

disruption of the pacing caused by respiration or the patient's motion is very unlikely.

Once the pacing catheter is positioned in the right atrium, it is connected to the pulse generator unit. This unit should be equipped with a fixed rate mode, pacing at least to rates of 170 beats per minute, and a variable output from 0.5 to 10 milliamperes. Bipolar pacing catheters may be connected directly to the pacemaker unit or attached through extension wires with alligator clamps. Unipolar catheters should have their negative pole grounded to the skin using either a needle electrode or standard electrocardiographic plates.

Once the pacing catheter has been positioned properly and connected to the pulse generator, the ability of the pacemaker to stimulate the atrium and to control ventricular rate should be assessed. Initially, the output of the generator is set at 2 to 3 milliamperes, and the pacing rate is adjusted to 10 beats above the sinus rate. Pacing is then begun, and if there is ventricular capture, the pacing rate is increased by 10 beats per minute every 5 seconds until a rate of 150 to 160 beats per minute is reached. Inadequate pacing may be secondary to an inadequate output of the pulse gen-

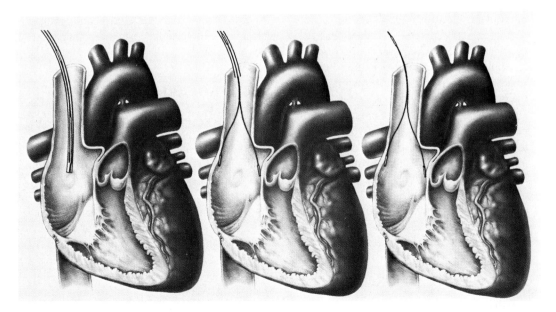

Fig. 18–1. Placement of the Mansfield Atri-Pace I, a bipolar flared pacing catheter that is useful for performing pacing stress tests. Stability of electrical capture is a strong point of this catheter.

erator, improper lead positioning, or the development of atrioventricular block. The output of the pulse generator may be increased, but in general, stimulating energies in excess of 7 to 8 milliamperes frequently result in painful phrenic nerve stimulation. If excessively high energies are required for capture, the electrode lead should be repositioned. If atrioventricular block develops at higher stimulatory rates, 1 mg of intravenous atropine may be administered: this generally ensures adequate atrioventricular conduction up to rates ≥ 140 beats/minute.

Following proper lead positioning and an adequate trial of pacing to assess capture, the actual pacing protocol may be done. In our laboratory, a pacing stress test is usually begun approximately 20 beats per minute above the baseline rate, with increases in the pacing rate by 20 beats per minute every 2 minutes, until angina pectoris or characteristic hemodynamic alteration occurs or until 85% of maximum age-predicted heart rate is achieved. Placement of a thermodilution balloon-tip flow-directed catheter, a left heart catheter, and a radial arterial cannula before pacing allows simultaneous assessment of right and left heart pressures, cardiac output measurement by thermodilution and/or Fick method, and determination of systemic and pulmonary vascular resistances. Assessment of left ventricular volumes may also be accomplished with standard angiographic, echocardiographic, or radionuclide techniques.

Following the induction of chest pain during pacing tachycardia, pacing may be continued at the same heart rate safely for up to 3 to 5 minutes, during which hemodynamic, metabolic, and electrocardiographic data may be obtained. Following the cessation of pacing, chest pain usually resolves quickly but may occasionally persist for up to 1 to 2 minutes after the return to sinus rhythm.

PACING-INDUCED ANGINA

Initial reports on the use of atrial pacing suggested that pacing-induced angina was a sensitive marker for the presence of ischemic heart disease and could serve as a suitable ischemic endpoint of pacing protocols.[1] Specifically, the induction of angina was thought to mark a highly reproducible anginal threshold defined in terms of the pacing rate and duration. Subsequent investigators have found, however, that chest pain is neither a sensitive nor a specific indicator of the presence of coronary artery disease. Robson et al.,[6] for example, demonstrated that chest pain could be elicited in 80% of patients with normal coronary arteries if they were paced at extremely high rates (in excess of 180 beats per minute). Moreover, Chandraratna[27] and others[7] have demonstrated the absence of angina in some patients with coronary artery disease who were stressed with pacing tachycardia at a significantly high rate. Similarly, in terms of defining anginal threshold according to the pacing rate and duration, as many as 20% of individuals have been shown to have considerable variation in these parameters.[28] In view of these results, it is clear that chest pain alone should not be used as a reliable marker for the presence of pacing-induced ischemia. Improved sensitivity and specificity of pacing-induced chest pain, however, are noted when additional evidence of ischemia, such as pacing-induced electrocardiographic changes or myocardial metabolic abnormalities, are noted.

ELECTROCARDIOGRAPHIC CHANGES IN RESPONSE TO A PACING STRESS TEST

Like pacing-induced angina, the presence of ischemic ST segment depression during pacing tachycardia has not been regarded previously as a sensitive or specific marker for the presence of coronary artery disease. For example, in terms of sensitivity, Rios and Hurwitz compared pacing tachycardia and exercise in 50 patients and found diagnostic ECG changes with pacing in only 20% of patients in comparison to 83% of patients with exercise.[5] Similarly, in terms of specificity, Robson reported ST segment depression of 1.5 mm or more during pacing tachycardia in as many as 80%

of patients with normal coronary arteries.[6] In addition to poor overall sensitivity and specificity, pacing tachycardia is associated with certain distortions of the electrocardiogram that sometimes make interpretation of ischemic ST segment changes difficult or impossible. Pacing is associated with prolongation of the PR interval in most patients and extreme prolongation of this interval can cause the pacemaker spike to fall within the ST segment of the preceding paced complex and thus obscure potential ST segment changes.

In spite of the previously reported poor utility of pacing-induced ECG changes, work from our laboratory has suggested an improved sensitivity and specificity of ischemic ST segment depression during pacing tachycardia *if certain technical guidelines of the pacing protocol are followed.*[7] Several earlier pacing trials that reported a low sensitivity of pacing ECG changes used only limited three-lead recording, and it is clear, at least with standard exercise testing, that sensitivity can be improved substantially with full 12-lead monitoring.[29,30] Other pacing trials reporting low sensitivity have used the induction of chest pain as an endpoint for the pacing stimulus; as previously mentioned, chest pain alone is not a reliable marker for pacing-induced ischemia. In terms of poor specificity, it is notable that pacing trials that have reported the presence of ST segment depression in patients with normal coronary arteries reported these changes at very high pacing rates, in excess of 180 beats per minute.

To re-evaluate the potential utility of pacing-induced ECG changes, pacing trials should be conducted using the following guidelines. *First,* a 12-lead ECG is used for monitoring, and the ECG is regarded as positive for myocardial ischemia if at least 1 mm or more of horizontal or downsloping ST segment depression is produced. *Second,* pacing tachycardia is terminated when 85% of maximal age-predicted heart rate is achieved or when typical ischemic chest pain is accompanied by diagnostic ECG changes. *Finally,* if marked prolongation of the PR interval distorts the preceding ST segment changes, the ECG is considered positive for ischemia only if there is ST segment depression in the first five beats following the discontinuation of the pacing stimulus.

Using these guidelines, actual pacing protocols conducted in our experience have had an overall sensitivity and specificity of 94% and 83%, respectively, with regard to pacing-induced electrocardiographic changes. In addition, distortion of the ST segment by the pacing stimulus because of marked prolongation of the PR interval appears to occur infrequently when the peak pacing rate is no higher than 85% of the maximum age predicted heart rate. Moreover, in at least one subgroup of patients who were tested with both atrial pacing and standard treadmill exercise,[7] the concordance between pacing-induced and exercise-induced electrocardiographic changes was 90%. Examples of pacing-induced and exercise-induced electrocardiographic changes are shown for a patient with normal coronary arteries in Figure 18–2A and for a patient with coronary artery disease in Figure 18–2B.

A more recent study has suggested that the sensitivity of pacing-induced electrocardiographic changes may be further improved with the use of endocardial electrograms obtained during the pacing stress test. Nabel et al.[8] reported on the use of local unipolar electrograms recorded from the tip of a 0.064 cm diameter guide wire positioned against the endocardial surface of potentially ischemic regions. Endocardial electrograms, left ventricular end-diastolic pressure and multiple surface ECG leads were recorded during and after rapid atrial pacing in 21 patients with coronary artery disease. Before pacing, endocardial electrograms in all 21 patients were free of ST segment elevation. After rapid atrial pacing, marked ST segment elevation was apparent in 17 of the 21 patients. This ST segment elevation could be abolished in all patients with the use of nitroglycerin. Moreover, in several patients, endocardial ST elevation after pacing was abolished by successful percutaneous coronary angioplasty of the critically stenosed artery supplying the ischemic region of myocardium. The authors concluded

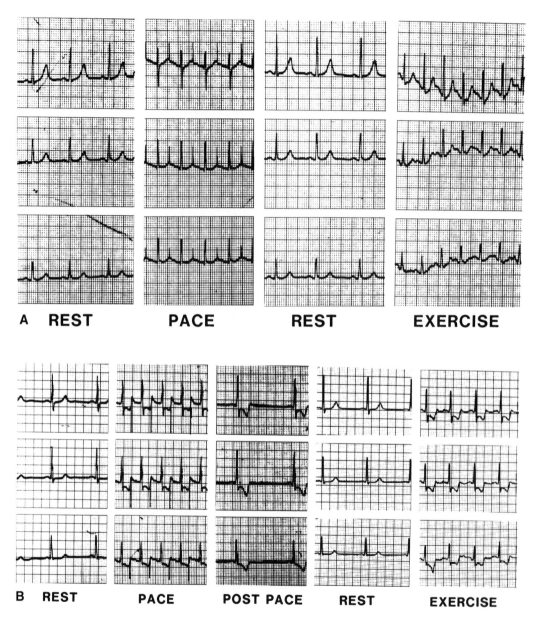

Fig. 18–2. (A) Electrocardiographic response to atrial pacing and exercise stress in a man with normal coronary arteries. From top to bottom, leads V4, V5, and V6 are monitored. (B) Comparison of electrocardiographic response to atrial pacing and exercise stress in a man with severe three-vessel coronary artery disease. Leads V4, V5, and V6 are monitored (top to bottom) as in A. ST depression occurs to the same degree with both types of stress. (Reprinted with permission from Heller GV, et al: The pacing stress test: a reexamination of the relation between coronary artery disease and pacing induced electrocardiographic changes. Am J Cardiol 54:50, 1984.)

that endocardial electrographic changes are a reliable marker of pacing-induced myocardial ischemia, and may be more sensitive than angina, pacing-induced hemodynamic changes, or ST segment depression on the surface ECG.

MYOCARDIAL METABOLIC CHANGES INDUCED BY A PACING STRESS TEST

Abnormal myocardial metabolism has been documented during pacing-induced ischemia by means of coronary sinus sampling and the subsequent measurement of coronary arterial and venous blood lactate. Because lactate production is a byproduct of anaerobic glycolysis, its production by the heart and appearance within the coronary sinus is a sign of myocardial ischemia. Previous investigators have noted rapid increases in coronary sinus lactate during pacing tachycardia in patients with coronary artery disease, often before the appearance of angina.[3,4] With cessation of pacing, the elevated coronary sinus lactates fall rapidly, representing a washout of the accumulated myocardial lactate and diminished lactate production as normal oxygenation is restored. Monitoring of arterial lactate levels while coronary sinus lactate levels are rising usually shows little or no elevation, in marked contrast to arterial lactate levels during exercise. As a result, atrial pacing is superior to exercise for evaluating abnormal myocardial metabolic function because rapidly rising arterial lactate levels during exercise may obscure abnormal patterns of myocardial lactate metabolism.

Monitoring of coronary sinus lactate during pacing protocols is most easily accomplished with a Gorlin pacing catheter. Placement of the Gorlin catheter in the coronary sinus can usually be confirmed by injection of a small amount of contrast medium. Care must be taken not to perforate either the coronary sinus or the great cardiac vein, as well as not to place the pacing tip of the catheter too distally, because placement of the distal catheter into the great cardiac vein may result in ventricular rather than atrial pacing.

Arterial and coronary venous blood lactate concentrations in response to a pacing stress test are illustrated in Figure 18–3. As can be seen, in the control state the concentration of coronary sinus blood lactate is lower than lactate concentration in arterial blood, reflecting the fact that the heart normally consumes lactate as a fuel. During pacing tachycardia, coronary sinus blood lactate concentration rises progressively and exceeds arterial blood lactate concentration, reflecting a shift to anaerobic metabolism of the ischemic myocardium. The lactate falls rapidly after discontinuation of pacing, because the heart rate returns to control immediately.

HEMODYNAMIC CHANGES DURING A PACING STRESS TEST

Previous investigators have described hemodynamic alterations associated with the pacing-induced ischemic state and have contrasted the hemodynamic changes seen in patients with normal coronary arteries with those observed in patients with significant coronary obstructive disease.[9–18]

Patients without ischemic heart disease who are stressed by atrial-paced tachycardia generally demonstrate no significant change in cardiac output, mean arterial pressure, arteriovenous oxygen difference, and systemic vascular resistance. Left ventricular end-diastolic pressure and pulmonary capillary wedge pressure generally fall during pacing tachycardia and then return toward prepacing baseline levels in the immediate post-pacing period. Left ventricular end-diastolic and end-systolic volumes fall during pacing tachycardia with a decrease in stroke volume and no significant change in ejection fraction.

Patients with coronary artery disease who are paced to ischemia likewise manifest no significant change in cardiac output, mean arterial pressure, arteriovenous oxygen difference, or systemic vascular resistance. Some investigators have documented slight decreases in cardiac output with slight increases in mean arterial pressure, arterial venous oxygen difference and system resistance. These

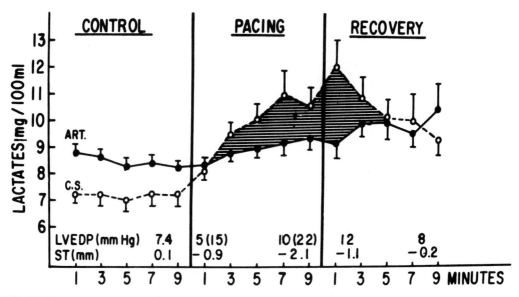

Fig. 18–3. Mean values for arterial (ART.) and coronary sinus (C.S.) blood lactate concentrate before (control), during and after tachycardia in 17 patients with coronary artery disease. Left ventricular end-diastolic pressure (LVEDP) changes little during pacing tachycardia, but is elevated during brief periods of interruption of pacing (values in parentheses). ST segment depression developed progressively during pacing tachycardia and resolved in recovery. Lactate extraction shifted to lactate production during ischemia, and this persisted into recovery for a brief period. (Reproduced with permission from Parker JO, Chiong MA, West RO, Case RB: Sequential alterations in myocardial lactate metabolism, S-T segments, and left ventricular function during angina induced by atrial pacing. Circulation 40:113, 1969.)

dfferences, however, probably are related to the intensity of pacing-induced ischemia, its duration before the measurement of hemodynamic variables, and the amount of myocardium that has become ischemic, with more extensive hemodynamic abnormalities occurring in the setting of more extensive myocardial ischemia. The most dramatic differences in pacing hemodynamics between patients with normal coronary arteries and those with coronary artery disease are seen in terms of left ventricular pressure-volume relationships during pacing tachycardia and in the immediate post-pacing period. Of note, left ventricular filling pressures do not show the progressive decrease seen in nonischemic patients, and elevations in pulmonary capillary wedge, mean pulmonary artery, and occasionally left ventricular end-diastolic pressure occur at maximum pacing. Most important, there is an abrupt rise in left ventricular end-diastolic pressure in the immediate post-pacing period. Similarly, ventricular end-diastolic and end-systolic volumes decrease less during pacing-

induced tachycardia in patients with ischemic heart disease in comparison to normal subjects, and there is often a significant decrease in left-ventricular ejection fraction.

A study looking at pressure-volume relationships during pacing tachycardia conducted by us illustrates well the differences between nonischemic and ischemic hemodynamic responses to pacing.[31] In this study, 22 patients, including 11 patients with normal coronary arteries and 11 patients with significant coronary artery disease, underwent sequential atrial pacing with simultaneous monitoring of left ventricular pressure and ventricular volume measured from gated radionuclide ventriculography. Using synchronized left ventricular pressure tracings and radionuclide time-activity volume curves, three sequential pressure-volume diagrams were constructed for each patient corresponding to baseline, intermediate, and maximum pacing levels. All 11 patients with coronary artery disease demonstrated angina and significant ST segment depression at maximum pacing, but none of the 11 patients with normal coronary arteries showed any evidence of pacing-induced ischemia.

Figure 18–4 shows typical left ventricular pressure-volume curves for a patient with normal coronary arteries, stressed with pacing tachycardia. Notably, there is a progressive leftward shift for the loop with an increased heart rate and a progressive downward shift in the left ventricular diastolic pressure-volume limb of each pressure-volume curve. It is clear that changes in both systolic and diastolic function have occurred in these patients during pacing tachycardia. In terms of systolic function, the progressive leftward shift of the end-systolic portion of the loop presumably represents increased contractility secondary to a Treppe effect. Other investigators have likewise demonstrated a positive inotropic stimulus in response to increased heart rate, with increases in isovolumetric contraction indices (e.g., dP/dt) and ejection phase indices (e.g., circumferential fiber shortening) during pacing tachycardia.[25] With respect to diastolic function the progressive downward shift of the diastolic limbs in Figure 18–4 suggests that left ventricular distensibility has increased slightly during pacing tachycardia. Whether this down-

ward shift is related to an increase in myocardial relaxation, an alteration in viscoelastic properties, or a change in factors extrinsic to the myocardium (e.g., right ventricle, pericardium) is not known. It is notable that some investigators have documented mild chronotropic increases in markers of diastolic relaxation such as peak negative dP/dt[32] and the time constant tau[33] in animals, and more recently the peak rate of posterior wall thinning[34] and left ventricular internal dimension change[35] in man.

In comparison to Figure 18–4, Figure 18–5 shows sequential left ventricular pressure-volume diagrams for a patient with coronary artery disease who was paced to ischemia. All patients in our study who developed chest pain and ischemic ECG changes demonstrated a similar pressure-volume pattern with an initial shift of the pressure-volume loop to the left at an intermediate heart rate, followed by a rightward shift at peak pacing when ischemia developed. In terms of systolic function, it is clear that pacing resulted in an initial Treppe effect with a leftward shift of the end systolic portion of the diagram at intermediate pacing, followed by systolic failure at peak pacing with an increase in ventricular volumes and a right-

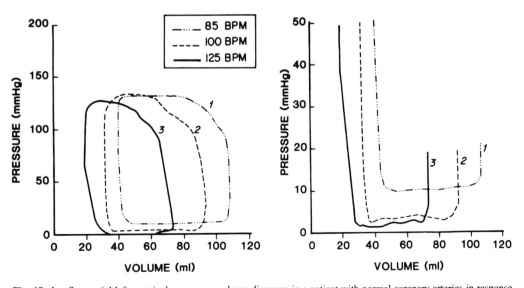

Fig. 18–4. Sequential left ventricular pressure-volume diagrams in a patient with normal coronary arteries in response to atrial pacing tachycardia at 3 increasing heart rates. See text for discussion. (Reproduced with permission from Aroesty JM, et al: Simultaneous assessment of left ventricular systolic and diastolic dysfunction during pacing-induced ischemia. Circulation 71:889, 1985.)

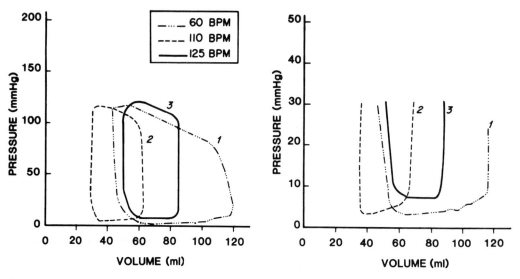

Fig. 18–5. Sequential left ventricular pressure-volume diagrams in a patient with three-vessel coronary artery disease who was paced at 3 increasing heart rates. The patient developed angina and ischemic S-T depression at peak pacing. See text for discussion. (Reproduced with permission from Aroesty, JM, et al.: Simultaneous assessment of left ventricular systolic and diastolic dysfunction during pacing-induced ischemia. Circulation 71:889, 1985.)

ward shift in the end-systolic portion of the curve. Similarly, in terms of diastolic function, it is evident that the patient did not show a progressive downward shift of the diastolic limb of the left ventricular pressure-volume curve but actually experienced an upward shift at intermediate and peak pacing. In part, the increase in LVEDP at peak pacing is related to systolic failure with an increase in ventricular volume. Because the patient did not experience evidence of systolic failure at the intermediate pacing level, however, it is also clear that this patient has experienced a primary decrease in left ventricular diastolic distensibility so that pressure is higher at any given chamber volume throughout diastole.

Speculation has continued over the last two decades as to whether the increase in diastolic pressures during pacing-induced ischemia is related to a primary decrease in distensibility or is secondary to systolic failure with increases in ventricular volume. At present, it seems clear that both mechanisms play some role in the elevated diastolic pressures. The evidence, however, suggests that changes in diastolic distensibility actually precede altered systolic function.[31]

The cause of the altered diastolic distensi-

bility during pacing-induced ischemia has been debated, and a number of different mechanisms[14–17,36,37] have been proposed, including incomplete myocardial relaxation, altered diastolic tone, partial ischemic contracture of some myofibrils within the distribution of the stenotic or occluded coronary artery, altered right ventricular loading, and influence of the pericardium. At the present, it seems likely that relaxation of myocardial cells within the reversibly ischemic region is slowed and does not proceed to completion by end diastole.[36,37] This may be related to impaired diastolic calcium sequestration by sarcoplasmic reticulum, but data are insufficient to permit a firm conclusion.

The post-pacing rise in left ventricular end-diastolic pressure is perhaps the most concrete evidence of pacing-induced ischemia during atrial pacing protocols. In our protocols, this post-pacing rise is calculated on beats numbers 5 through 15 after discontinuation of pacing, with greater than a 5 mmHg increase in LVEDP in comparison to the prepacing baseline being considered abnormal. Figure 18–6 shows a typical post-pacing rise in LVEDP in a patient who experienced angina. Figures 18–7 and 18–8 summarize hemodynamic

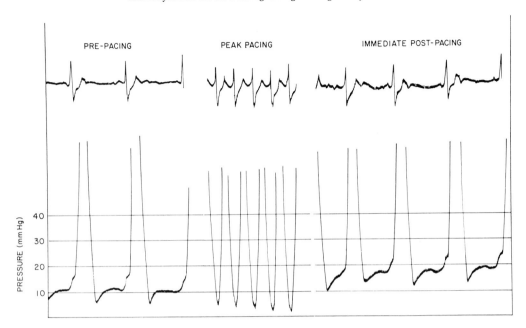

Fig. 18–6. Left ventricular end-diastolic pressure during atrial pacing tachycardia and in the immediate postpacing period. Left ventricular end-diastolic pressure increases substantially with resumption of sinus rhythm in this patient with coronary artery disease, who developed myocardial ischemia in response to pacing-induced tachycardia.

changes in patients with normal coronary arteries and those with ischemic heart disease in response to a pacing stress test.

The hemodynamic alterations induced by pacing tachycardia in patients with normal coronary arteries and those with ischemic heart disease have also been useful, by means of comparison, in assessing myocardial performance in patients with other forms of cardiac disease. Feldman et al.[38] have examined the utility of atrial pacing tachycardia in evaluating the systolic and diastolic myocardial re-

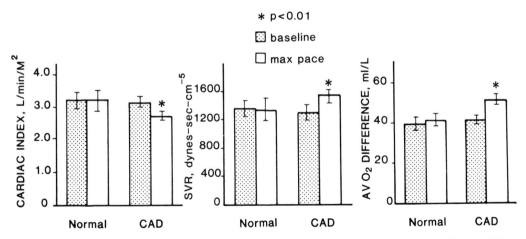

Fig. 18–7. Changes in cardiac index, systemic vascular resistance (SVR), and arteriovenous oxygen difference (AVO_2) in 5 patients with normal coronary arteries and 20 patients with coronary artery disease during pacing tachycardia. Patients with coronary disease showed a significant decrease in cardiac index and increase in SVR and AVO_2 difference during maximum pacing tachycardia. (Reprinted with permission from McKay RG, et al: The pacing stress test reexamined: Correlation of pacing-induced hemodynamic changes with the amount of myocardium at risk. J Am Coll Cardiol 3:1469, 1984.)

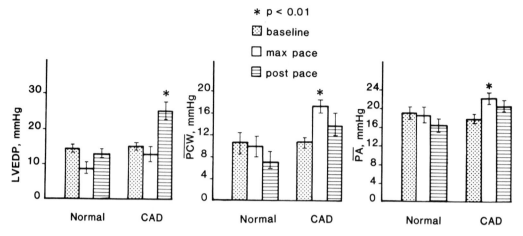

Fig. 18–8. Changes in left ventricular end-diastolic pressure (LVEDP), mean pulmonary capillary wedge pressure (PCW), and mean pulmonary artery pressure (PA) in 5 patients with normal coronary arteries and 20 patients with coronary artery disease during maximum pacing tachycardia and immediately after pacing. Patients with coronary disease showed significant elevation of PA and PCW at maximum pacing, and of LVEDP immediately after pacing. (Reprinted with permission from McKay RG, et al: The pacing stress test reexamined: Correlation of pacing-induced hemodynamic changes with the amount of myocardium at risk. J Am Coll Cardiol 3:1469, 1984.)

serve of patients with dilated cardiomyopathy. Pacing-induced changes in left ventricular pressure and volume were compared in seven patients with a dilated cardiomyopathy (mean left ventricular ejection fraction 19%) with findings in six patients with normal coronary arteries and normal left ventricular function (mean left ventricular ejection fraction 69%). The patients with normal left ventricular function demonstrated significant increases in left ventricular peak-positive dP/dt, the left ventricular end-systolic pressure-volume ratio, and left ventricular peak filling rate during graded increases in heart rate with atrial pacing. They also exhibited a progressive leftward and downward shift of their pressure-volume diagrams, compatible with increased contractility and diastolic distensibility in response to pacing tachycardia. In contrast, patients with dilated cardiomyopathy demonstrated no increase in either left ventricular peak-positive dP/dt or the end-systolic pressure-volume ratio, and absence of a progressive leftward shift of their pressure-volume diagrams. Moreover, patients with dilated cardiomyopathy demonstrated no increase in left ventricular peak filling rate and a blunted downward shift of the diastolic limb of their pressure-volume diagrams. These data suggest that patients with

dilated cardiomyopathy demonstrate little or no enhancement of systolic and diastolic function during atrial pacing tachycardia, indicating a depression of both inotropic and lusitropic reserve.

REGIONAL WALL MOTION ABNORMALITIES DURING A PACING STRESS TEST

Regional wall motion abnormalities during pacing-induced ischemia have been noted with both contrast ventriculography and gated radionuclide ventriculography. Using contrast ventriculography, Dwyer studied 8 patients with coronary artery disease who were paced to angina and found that three developed regional hypokinesis in one area, while the remaining five developed at least two separate areas of hypokinesis or akinesis.[19] In all cases, an associated coronary artery lesion could be identified in the vessel that supplied the area of the new regional wall motion abnormality. Similarly, Tzivoni et al., using radionuclide ventriculography, found that 9 out of 11 patients developed new regional wall motion abnormalities in response to pacing-induced ischemia.[20] The overall specificity and sensitivity of pacing-induced regional wall motion abnormalities have not been documented, however.

THALLIUM SCINTIGRAPHY AND THE PACING STRESS TEST

A recent development that has improved the overall utility of atrial pacing as a stress test has been the incorporation of thallium scintigraphy into pacing protocols. In patients with normal coronary arteries, pacing tachycardia is associated with a homogeneous increase in myocardial oxygen consumption and a secondary increase in coronary blood flow. In patients with coronary artery disease, however, regional increases in myocardial blood flow may be limited by critical coronary stenoses. Because initial myocardial uptake of thallium-201 has been shown to reflect myocardial perfusion, myocardial ischemia induced by pacing tachycardia should theoretically be detectable by thallium scintigraphy. Although early reports on the simultaneous use of atrial pacing and thallium scintigraphy suggested serious limitations,[20,21] studies with improved methodology indicate that this approach is successful in detecting both reversible ischemia and infarcted myocardium.[22-24] For example, Weiss et al. have reported an overall sensitivity of 100% of atrial pacing protocols utilizing thallium scintigraphy for detection of significant coronary stenoses.[22] Moreover, the authors noted that the technique could accurately demonstrate the site, extent, and severity of coronary artery disease.

To assess further the utility of combined atrial pacing and thallium scintigraphy, our laboratory examined the correlation between pacing-induced and exercise-induced thallium defects in patients referred for evaluation of chest pain.[23] The overall sensitivity and specificity of thallium imaging after atrial pacing were excellent. Moreover, segment-by-segment comparison of the thallium scans after either pacing or exercise stress testing revealed a correlation of 83%.

Simultaneous use of thallium scintigraphy and atrial pacing tachycardia can be accomplished by injection of 1.5 to 2.0 mCi of thallium-201 at peak pacing followed by continued pacing for at least an additional 5 minutes. In routine thallium-exercise testing, exercise is maintained for only 30 to 60 seconds after the injection of the radionuclide to allow the thallium to reach the myocardium. Because of the rapid decrease in heart rate after the discontinuation of pacing and the subsequent rapid diminution of myocardial oxygen requirements, however, pacing is extended to 5 minutes. Following discontinuation of the pacing stimulus, while the patient is in the supine position, standard anterior, 40-degree left anterior oblique and 70-degree left anterior oblique views are obtained immediately in the catheterization laboratory with a mobile scintillation camera. Repeat standard views are obtained subsequently 4 hours after the termination of the pacing protocol.

Figure 18–9 shows the arterial blood thal-

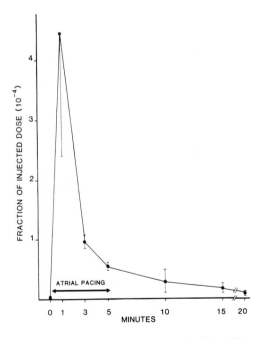

Fig. 18–9. Fraction of injected dose of thallium-201 in the arterial blood as a function of time after injection in 7 patients stressed with pacing tachycardia. Pacing was continued for the first 5 minutes of the sample collections. By 5 minutes, the arterial activity decreases to less than one tenth of the peak value. (Reprinted with permission from Heller GV, et al: The pacing stress test: thallium-201 myocardial imaging after atrial pacing. J Am Coll Cardiol 3:1197, 1984.)

lium activity curve obtained in patients during pacing tachycardia and the first 15 minutes after the discontinuation of pacing. The arterial activity is highest during the first minute after injection and decreases to approximately one tenth of the peak level within 5 minutes. The highest blood activity of thallium thus occurs well within the 5-minute pacing period following injection.

Figures 18–10, 18–11, and 18–12 show examples of pacing thallium scans in a patient with normal coronary arteries and in patients with coronary artery disease.

NONINVASIVE EXTERNAL CARDIAC PACING

An innovative development in the field of pacing stress tests has been the refinement of noninvasive external cardiac pacing and the incorporation of this pacing modality into pacing stress protocols. Noninvasive external car-

diac pacing was first introduced by Zoll in 1952 and represented the first successful cardiac stimulation during asystole or bradycardia in humans.[39] Although effective, the electrical shock and skeletal muscle stimulation caused by the original Zoll pacemaker often resulted in severe discomfort. Modifications of this pacing mode, however, have led to more reliable cardiac stimulation and reduced discomfort.

The hemodynamic responses to noninvasive external cardiac pacing have been reported by Feldman et al.[40] in 16 patients undergoing cardiac catheterization, including 13 patients with significant coronary artery disease and three with normal coronary arteries. All patients had noninvasive pacing at increasing heart rates to 85% of age-predicted maximal heart rate. At maximal pacing, all patients demonstrated a rise in right atrial, pulmonary artery, and mean aortic pressures. Cardiac index remained unchanged, reflecting parallel increases in arte-

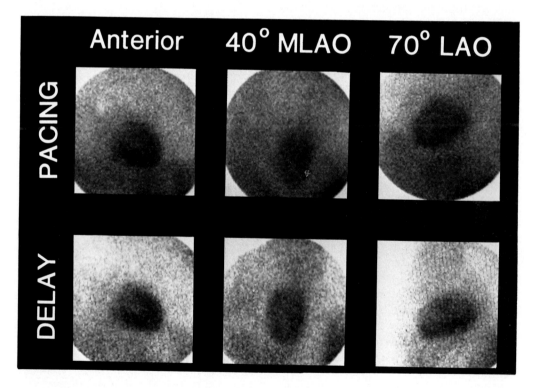

Fig. 18–10. Thallium scan during a pacing stress test in a patient with normal coronary arteries who was paced to a heart rate of 160 beats per minute. The patient did not develop chest pain or electrocardiographic changes. The thallium scintigram during pacing is identical with that at 4 hours later (Delay).

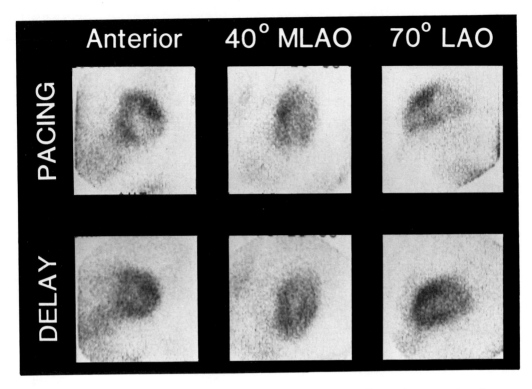

Fig. 18–11. Pacing thallium scan in a patient with three-vessel coronary artery disease who was paced to a heart rate of 150 beats per minute and who developed angina and electrocardiographic changes of ischemia. Scans show an inferoapical thallium defect that fills in 4 hours later (Delay).

riovenous oxygen difference and oxygen consumption. One minute after cessation of pacing, pulmonary artery pressure and oxygen consumption remained elevated, whereas arteriovenous oxygen difference returned to baseline with a subsequent rise in cardiac index. Angina occurred in eight patients with coronary artery disease at peak pacing and was accompanied by a rise in left ventricular end-diastolic pressure after pacing. In the remaining eight patients without pacing-induced angina, including the three patients with normal coronary arteries, there was no significant change in left ventricular end-diastolic pressure. The authors concluded that noninvasive external cardiac pacing produces a rise in both right and left heart filling pressures and in oxygen consumption that persist after pacing, and may provoke angina and hemodynamic alterations consistent with myocardial ischemia. Moreover, this mode of pacing appeared hemodynamically safe.

Feldman further extended his observations on noninvasive pacing by incorporating thallium scintigraphy in noninvasive stress-testing protocols.[41] In 14 patients who underwent noninvasive pacing stress tests with simultaneous hemodynamic monitoring and thallium scintigraphy, reversible thallium defects corresponding to significant coronary artery stenoses seen on coronary angiography were induced in 12 patients. In nine of these patients who underwent both noninvasive pacing protocols and standard exercise thallium stress tests, thallium scintigraphy at peak pacing and during delayed views did not differ significantly from exercise thallium scintigraphy. The authors concluded that noninvasive external cardiac pacing in combination with thallium scintigraphy is capable of detecting significant coronary artery disease and may be comparable to routine exercise thallium stress testing. One limitation associated with the technique, however, was local pacing-induced

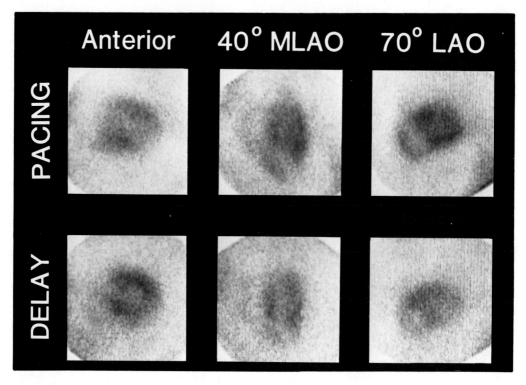

Fig. 18–12. Pacing thallium scan in a patient with a prior apical infarction who was paced to a heart rate of 150 beats per minute. The patient did not develop chest pain or electrocardiographic changes at maximum pacing. The scans show a fixed apical defect.

patient discomfort, which occurred to some degree in all patients.

CLINICAL USES OF ATRIAL PACING

The complete evaluation of a patient's cardiac function in the catheterization laboratory often requires an examination of the patient's performance under stressed conditions when electrocardiographic, metabolic, and hemodynamic abnormalities may manifest themselves fully. The role of stress testing is particularly important in the evaluation of patients with ischemic heart disease where, for example, it may be necessary to determine a patient's anginal threshold, the magnitude of hemodynamic impairment during ischemia, the efficacy of antianginal therapy, and a need for intervention therapy such as percutaneous coronary angioplasty or coronary bypass surgery. Although standard dynamic and isomet-

ric exercise may serve as a form of stress for many patients, not all patients are able to exercise because of physical disabilities, old age, pulmonary disease, peripheral vascular disease, and possibly β blockade. In each of these situations, atrial pacing may be used as a suitable form of stress.

REFERENCES

1. Sowton GE, Balcon R, Cross D, Frick MH: Measurement of the angina threshold using atrial pacing. Cardiovasc Res 1:301, 1967.
2. Lau SH, et al: Controlled heart rate by atrial pacing in angina pectoris: a determinant of electrocardiographic S-T depressions. Circulation 38:711, 1968.
3. Parker JO, Chiong MA, West RO, Case RB: Sequential alterations in myocardial lactate metabolism, S-T segments, and left ventricular function during angina induced by atrial pacing. Circulation 40:113, 1969.
4. Helfant RH, et al: Differential hemodynamic, metabolic, and electrocardiographic effects in subjects with and without angina pectoris during atrial pacing. Circulation 42:601, 1970.

5. Rios JC, Hurwitz LE: Electrocardiographic responses to atrial pacing and multistage treadmill exercise testing. Correlation with coronary anatomy. Am J Cardiol 34:986, 1976.

6. Robson RH, Pridie R, Fluck DC: Evaluation of rapid atrial pacing in diagnosis of coronary artery disease. Evaluation of atrial pacing test. Br Heart J 38:986, 1976.

7. Heller GV, et al: The pacing stress test: a reexamination of the relation between coronary artery disease and pacing induced electrocardiographic changes. Am J Cardiol 54:50, 1984.

8. Nabel EG, et al: Detection of pacing-induced myocardial ischemia by endocardial electrograms recorded during cardiac catheterization. J Am Coll Cardiol 11:983, 1988.

9. Parker JO, Ledwich JR, West RO, Case RB: Reversible cardiac failure during angina pectoris. Circulation 34:745, 1969.

10. Linhart JW, Hildner FJ, Barold SS: Left heart hemodynamics during angina pectoris induced by atrial pacing. Circulation 40:483, 1969.

11. Khaja F, et al: Assessment of ventricular function in coronary artery disease by means of atrial pacing and exercise. Am J Cardiol 26:107, 1970.

12. Parker JO, Khaja F, Case RB: Analysis of left ventricular function by atrial pacing. Circulation 43:241, 1971.

13. McCans JL, Parker JO: Left ventricular pressure-volume relationships during myocardial ischemia in man. Circulation 48:775, 1973.

14. McLaurin LP, Rolett EL, Grossman W: Impaired left ventricular relaxation during pacing induced ischemia. Am J Cardiol 32:751, 1973.

15. Mann T, Brodie BR, Grossman W, McLaurin LP: Effect of angina on the left ventricular diastolic pressure-volume relationship. Circulation 55:761, 1977.

16. Barry WH, Brooker JZ, Alderman EL, Harrison DC: Changes in diastolic stiffness and tone of the left ventricle during angina pectoris. Circulation 49:225, 1974.

17. Mann T, Goldberg S, Mudge GH, Grossman W: Factors contributing to altered left ventricular diastolic properties during angina pectoris. Circulation 59:14, 1979.

18. Thadani U, et al: Clinical hemodynamic and metabolic responses during pacing in the supine and sitting postures in patients with angina pectoris. Am J Cardiol 44:249, 1979.

19. Dwyer EM: Left ventricular pressure-volume alterations and regional disorders of contraction during myocardial ischemia induced by atrial pacing. Circulation 42:1111, 1970.

20. Tzivoni D, et al: Diagnosis of coronary artery disease by multi-gated radionuclide angiography during right atrial pacing. Chest 80:562, 1981.

21. Vrobel TR, et al: Insensitivity of thallium 201 imaging in detecting pacing-induced myocardial ischemia (abstr.). Circulation 59 (suppl II):II, 1979.

22. Weiss AT, et al: Atrial pacing thallium scintigraphy in the evaluation of coronary artery disease. Isr J Med Sci 19:495, 1983.

23. Heller GV, et al: The pacing stress test: thallium-201

24. McKay RG, et al: The pacing stress test reexamined: Correlation of pacing-induced hemodynamic changes with the amount of myocardium at risk. J Am Coll Cardiol 3:1469, 1984.

25. Ricci D, Orlick A, Alderman E: Role of tachycardia as an inotropic stimulus in man. J Clin Invest 63:695, 1979.

26. Holmberg S, Varnauskas E: Coronary circulation during pacing-induced tachycardia. Acta Med Scand 190:491, 1971.

27. Chandraratna PAN, et al: Spectrum of hemodynamic responses to atrial pacing in coronary artery disease. Br Heart J 35:1033, 1973.

28. Thadani U, et al: Are the clinical and hemodynamic events during pacing in patients with angina reproducible? Circulation 60:1036, 1979.

29. Chaitman BR, et al: Improved efficiency of treadmill exercise testing using multiple lead ECG system and basic hemodynamic exercise response. Circulation 57:71, 1978.

30. Chaitman BR, et al: The importance of clinical subsets in interpreting maximal treadmill exercise test results: the role of multiple lead ECG systems. Circulation 59:560, 1979.

31. Aroesty JM, et al: Simultaneous assessment of left ventricular systolic and diastolic dysfunction during pacing-induced ischemia. Circulation 71:889, 1985.

32. Karliner JS, et al: Pharmacological and hemodynamic influences on the rate of isovolumetric left ventricular relaxation in the conscious dog. J Clin Invest 60:511, 1977.

33. Weiss JL, Fredericksen JW, Weisfeldt ML: Hemodynamic determinants of the time-course of fall in canine left ventricular pressure. J Clin Invest 58:751, 1976.

34. Fifer MA, Borow KM, Colan S, Lorell BH: Left ventricular diastolic filling; contributions of heart rate, age, and extent of systolic shortening. Circulation 68 (III): III, 1983.

35. Bahler RC, Vrobel TR, Martin P: The relation of heart rate and shortening fraction to echocardiographic indexes of left ventricular relaxation in normal subjects. J Am Coll Card 2:926, 1983.

36. Grossman W: Why is the left ventricular diastolic pressure increased during angina pectoris? J Am Coll Cardiol 5:607, 1985.

37. Sasayama et al: Changes in diastolic properties of the regional myocardium during pacing-induced ischemia in human subjects. J Am Coll Cardiol 5:599, 1985.

38. Feldman MD, Alderman JD, Aroesty JM, Royal HD, Ferguson JJ, Owen RM, Grossman W, McKay RG: Depression of systolic and diastolic myocardial reserve during atrial pacing tachycardia in patients with dilated cardiomyopathy. J Clin Invest 82:1661, 1988.

39. Zoll PM: Resuscitation of the heart in ventricular standstill by external electrical stimulation. N Engl J Med 248:768, 1952.

40. Feldman MD, Zoll PM, Aroesty JM, et al: Hemodynamic responses to noninvasive external cardiac pacing. Am J Med 84:395, 1988.

41. Feldman MD, Warren SE, Gervino EV, et al: Noninvasive external cardiac pacing for thallium-201 scintigraphy. Am J Physiol Imaging 3:172, 1988.

myocardial imaging after atrial pacing. J Am Coll Cardiol 3:1197, 1984.

19

Measurement of Ventricular Volumes, Ejection Fraction, Mass, Wall Stress, and Regional Wall Motion

MICHAEL A. FIFER and WILLIAM GROSSMAN

C ardiac angiography was introduced initially to provide qualitative information regarding anatomic abnormalities of the cardiovascular system. Subsequently, it became apparent that quantitative information derived from cineangiography could provide insight into *functional* abnormalities of the heart as well. Direct measurement of ventricular dimension, area, and wall thickness allows calculation of volume, ejection fraction, mass, and wall stress. Assessment of volume-time, pressure-volume, and stress-volume relationships provides additional information regarding systolic and diastolic function of the ventricular chambers. Finally, techniques developed to assess *regional* left ventricular wall motion have proved useful in the evaluation of patients with coronary artery disease. The ventricular angiograms obtained by the techniques described in Chapter 14 can be used to derive quantitative descriptors of ventricular chamber size, mass, wall stress, and systolic and diastolic function.

VOLUMES

Technical Considerations

As discussed in detail in Chapter 14, ventriculograms are generally recorded on cine triculograms are generally recorded on cine

film at 30 to 60 frames/sec, and radiographic contrast agent is usually injected into the left ventricle at rates of 7 to 15 ml/sec for a total volume of 35 to 50 ml. Alternatively, the left ventricle may be visualized from contrast injections into the pulmonary artery, the left atrium (by the transseptal technique), or, in cases of severe aortic insufficiency, the aortic root. Attention to catheter position and injection rate minimizes the occurrence of ventricular ectopy during contrast studies; this is important because analysis of extrasystoles and post-extrasystolic beats cannot be used for proper assessment of basal ventricular function.

In the first step in calculating left ventricular chamber volume, the left ventricular outline or silhouette is traced. The ventricular silhouette should be traced at the *outermost margin of visible radiographic contrast* so as to include trabeculations and papillary muscles within the perimeter (Fig. 19–1). The aortic valve border is defined as a line connecting the inferior aspects of the sinuses of Valsalva.

To facilitate the calculation of left ventricular volume, the ventricle is usually approximated by an ellipsoid.[1,2] Alternatively, techniques based on Simpson's rule, which is

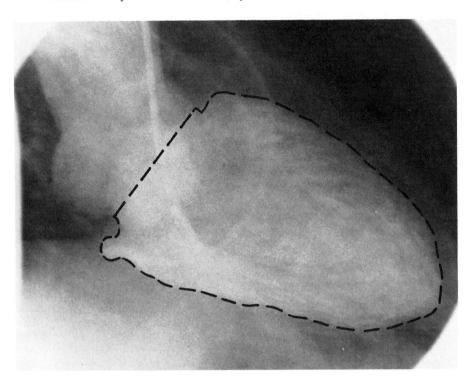

Fig. 19–1. Left ventriculogram in the 30-degree right anterior oblique projection. The ventricular outline has been traced, as indicated by the broken line.

independent of assumptions regarding ventricular shape, may be used;[3] these, however, are considerably more laborious unless computer techniques are used. Because the x rays emanate from a point source, they are nonparallel; correction must therefore be made for magnification of the ventricular image onto the image intensifier. A further complicating factor is so-called pincushion distortion, i.e., greater magnification at the periphery than in the center of the image, resulting from spherical aberration of the electromagnetic lens system.[4] Finally, ventricular volumes calculated by most mathematical techniques overestimate true ventricular chamber volume, and regression equations must be used to correct for the overestimation.

Biplane Formula

Biplane left ventriculography may be performed in the anteroposterior (AP) and lateral,[2] 30-degree right anterior oblique (RAO) and 60-degree left anterior oblique (LAO),[5] or angulated (e.g., 45-degree RAO and 60-degree LAO—25-degree cranial)[6] projections. Although a complex geometric shape, the left ventricle can be approximated with considerable accuracy by an ellipsoid[2] (Fig. 19–2). The volume of an ellipsoid is given by the equation:

$$V = \frac{4}{3} \pi \frac{L}{2} \frac{M}{2} \frac{N}{2} = \frac{\pi}{6} LMN \qquad (1)$$

where V is volume, L is the long axis, and M and N are the short axes of the ellipsoid. The long axis, L, is taken practically to be L_{max}, the longest chord that can be drawn within the ventricular silhouette in either projection. To determine M and N, each of the biplane projections of the left ventricle is approximated by an ellipse. M and N are taken to be the minor axes of these ellipses and have been drawn by hand by some investigators as perpendicular lines bisecting the long axes.[4] Alternatively, the *area-length method*, as intro-

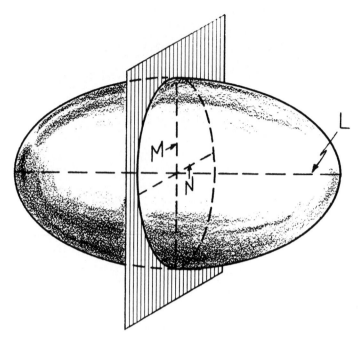

Fig. 19–2. Ellipsoid used as reference figure for the left ventricle. The long axis, L, and the short axes, M and N, are shown.

duced by Dodge and coworkers,[2] calculates M and N from the silhouette areas and long axis lengths in each projection, using the standard geometric formula for the area of an ellipse as a function of its major and minor axes. Thus, for biplane oblique (RAO/LAO) left ventriculography the areas of the two ventricular silhouettes are given as:

$$A_{RAO} = \pi \frac{L_{RAO}}{2} \frac{M}{2} \text{ and } A_{LAO} = \pi \frac{L_{LAO}}{2} \frac{N}{2}$$

L_{RAO} and L_{LAO} are the longest chords that can be drawn in the RAO and LAO silhouettes, respectively. The area of each traced silhouette (e.g., Fig. 19–1) is obtained by planimetry, and M and N are calculated by rearrangement as:

$$M = \frac{4A_{RAO}}{\pi L_{RAO}} \text{ and } N = \frac{4A_{LAO}}{\pi L_{LAO}} \quad (2)$$

Combining equations 1 and 2:

$$V = \frac{\pi}{6} L_{max} \left(\frac{4A_{RAO}}{\pi L_{RAO}} \right) \left(\frac{4A_{LAO}}{\pi L_{LAO}} \right)$$

$$= \frac{8}{3\pi} \frac{A_{RAO} A_{LAO}}{L_{min}} \quad (3)$$

where L_{min} is the shorter of L_{RAO} and L_{LAO}. Because L_{RAO} is nearly always greater than L_{LAO}, L_{LAO} is usually substituted for L_{min}.

Equation 3 is derived for projections at right angles, or *orthogonal* projections, and is applicable to biplane oblique ventriculography in the 30-degree RAO and 60-degree LAO views, as just described, or for the older AP and lateral format. While it is not valid theoretically for nonorthogonal projections (e.g., RAO and angulated LAO), it has been demonstrated empirically to be useful in this situation as well.[6]

Right ventricular volumes have been calculated from biplane AP and lateral films using a modification of the Dodge area-length technique[7,8] or Simpson's rule.[8–10] Because right ventricular volumes are rarely calculated from cineangiographic studies today, the reader is referred elsewhere for methodologic details.[7–10]

Single-Plane Formula

The area-length ellipsoid method for estimating left ventricular chamber volume has been modified for use when only single-plane measurements obtained in the AP or RAO projection are available.[4,11–13] Inherent in single-plane methods is the assumption that the left ventricular shape may be approximated by a prolate spheroid,[12] i.e., an ellipsoid in which the two minor axes are equal. Thus, it is assumed that the minor axis of the ventricle in the projection used is equal to the minor axis in the orthogonal plane, which was not filmed. Recalling equation 1 for the general case of an ellipsoid:

$$V = \frac{\pi}{6} LMN$$

If only single-plane (e.g., RAO) ventriculography is done, we assume that $M = N$, and that L in the plane presented is the true long axis of the ellipsoid. M is calculated from the single-plane silhouette area (A) and L by the area-length method as $M = 4A/\pi L$. Thus, the single-plane volume calculation becomes:

$$V = \frac{\pi}{6} LM^2 = \frac{\pi}{6}L \left(\frac{4A}{\pi L}\right)^2 = \frac{8A^2}{3\pi L} \quad (4)$$

Magnification Correction: Single-Plane

When large cut film was used for angiocardiography, the degree of magnification of the ventricle on the film could be predicted if the x-ray-tube-to-ventricle and ventricle-to-film distances were known.[2] The techniques for calculation of ventricular volume and correction for magnification using large cut or roll film, rarely used today, were described in detail in the second edition of this textbook, and the interested reader is referred to that source for reference.

For cine techniques, the overall correction factor must account for a three-step process: magnification of the ventricle onto the surface of the image intensifier, minification of the image when recorded on 35 mm film, and re-magnification of the image onto the screen of the cine projector. Correction for overall change in image size is best accomplished by filming a calibrated grid at the estimated level of the ventricle[11] and submitting the grid to the same three-step process.

The introduction of x-ray systems in which the center of the ventricle can be positioned at a fixed point ("isocenter"), around which the x-ray tubes and image intensifiers rotate, has facilitated accurate determination of the magnification factors. With techniques in which isocenter is not determined, it is difficult to locate precisely the center of the ventricle; thus, the correction factor is only approximate. Correction is usually accomplished by filming the grid at the estimated height of the center of the ventricle, usually approximated as mid-chest level. If the ventriculogram is filmed in the RAO projection, and the grid is filmed with the x-ray tube and the image intensifier in the vertical position, some error will be introduced because, in the absence of an isocenter system, the distances between tube, ventricle, and image intensifier do not remain constant during rotation.

In an isocenter system, the tube is rotated to the 90-degree lateral position and the x-ray table is raised or lowered until the left ventricle is centered on the fluoroscopic screen. The table height is fixed in position for left ventriculography. The tube and image intensifier are then rotated to the appropriate projection (e.g., 30 degrees RAO). The left ventricle is now at isocenter. After ventriculography, the tube and image intensifier are returned to 0 degrees and swung out to the side of the patient. The grid is filmed at the height of the middle of the image intensifier when it has been in the 90-degree lateral position; this height is the same for all patients. Equipment design ensures that, because the left ventricle was at isocenter when filmed, rotation of the tube and image intensifier before filming the grid does not affect the distances between tube, ventricle, and image intensifier.

The use of a calibrated grid is illustrated in Figure 19–3. For calculation of the correction factor, the traced silhouette of the ventricle is placed over the projected image of the grid (which in Figure 19–3 consists of squares 1 cm^2 in area), and the squares that are closest to the image of the ventricle are planimetered (Fig. 19–3). The choice of squares near the projected image of the ventricle helps to cor-

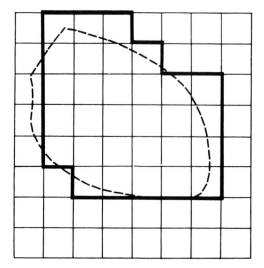

Fig. 19–3. Correction for magnification by use of a calibrated grid. The grid may be filmed at the level of the left ventricle (see text) after ventriculography is completed. For calculation, the grid (which consists of squares exactly 1 cm² in area) is traced from its projected image, and the squares that are closest in position to the image of the left ventricle on the left ventricular cineangiogram are planimetered. In this example, the left ventricular silhouette has been sketched in dotted lines for reference. As can be seen (bold outline), 30 squares were planimetered. See text for discussion and method of calculating the correction factor.

rect for pincushion distortion at the edges of the cine frame. In the example shown in the figure, 30 squares were planimetered. If the projected (planimetered) area is A_p, and the actual area (number of squares) is A_{true}, then the linear correction factor (CF) is:

$$CF = \sqrt{A_{true}/A_p}$$

In the example in Figure 19–3, 30 squares were planimetered, so that $A_{true} = 30$ cm². In the single-plane formula, the cube of the linear correction fraction adjusts the volume for magnification:

$$V = \frac{8}{3\pi} (CF)^3 \frac{A^2}{L}$$

The use of grids and other means of calculating magnification correction factors has been reassessed by Sheehan and Mitten-Lewis.[14] They found that the error introduced by considering a large central square area of

the grid rather than the portion encompassing a particular ventricular silhouette was negligibly small. Replacement of the grid by a circular disk did not significantly alter the calculated correction factor. Finally, the use of catheters with radiopaque markers separated by 1 cm also yielded accurate correction factors.

Magnification Correction: Biplane

In biplane studies, a correction factor must be calculated separately for each projection, yielding CF_{RAO} and CF_{LAO} in biplane oblique cineangiography. The linear correction factor is multiplied by the measured lengths, and the square of this correction factor is multiplied by planimetered areas to convert to true lengths and areas. Accordingly, the corrected volume of the ventricle is:

$$V = \frac{8}{3\pi} \frac{(CF_{RAO})^2(CF_{LAO})^2}{CF_{LAO}} \frac{A_{RAO}A_{LAO}}{L_{LAO}}$$

$$= \frac{8CF_{RAO}^2CF_{LAO}}{3\pi} \frac{A_{RAO}A_{LAO}}{L_{LAO}} \qquad (5)$$

Magnification Correction without Grids

With isocenter systems, equipment design facilitates calculation of the correction factors. When the ventricle is centered in both x-ray beams in such a system, its position in space is fixed (at isocenter). In one such system, illustrated in Figure 19–4, the horizontal tube-to-ventricle and ventricle-to-image intensifier distances are fixed, and remain constant despite rotation and/or angulation of the beam. The vertical tube-to-ventricle distance is fixed, but movement of the vertical image intensifier allows variation in the ventricle-to-image intensifier distance.

As seen in Figure 19–4, for the horizontal image, the degree of magnification (projected length, l_p, relative to true length, l_{true}) of the ventricle onto the image intensifier is given by $(a + b)/a$, and will be the same for all patients (as will, of course, the minification of the image onto the film and the remagnification

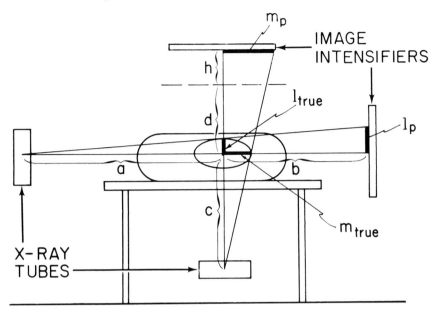

Fig. 19–4. Biplane isocenter system. When the patient is moved into a position that places the left ventricle at the isocenter, then the relationships between x-ray tubes, ventricle, and image intensifiers are fixed (as indicated by letters a to d), with the exception of h, the height of the vertical image intensifier above its lowest position. If h is known, the horizontal and vertical correction factors can then be calculated without the use of grids. See text for further explanation.

onto the projector screen). Thus, the horizontal or "lateral" CF can be determined once, and the same correction can be used for all patients (provided that no changes are made in the x-ray equipment or projector). For the vertical image, the degree of magnification is (c + d + h)/c; only h, the distance of the image intensifier above its lowest position, varies from patient to patient. The vertical CF may be determined once for several values of h, and a chart may be constructed listing values of CF for each value of h. If h is measured during each patient study, the vertical CF is known. Thus, if an isocenter biplane system is used and this approach is followed, it is unnecessary to film grids with each case.

This approach is based on the assumption that the effects of pincushion distortion do not vary significantly with differences in ventricular size and shape. It may be used for either single-plane or biplane ventriculography as long as the ventricle is positioned at isocenter at the time of filming. In some biplane isocenter systems, both the vertical and horizontal image intensifiers are mobile, so that allowance must be made for the positions of both image intensifiers in the calculation of the correction factors.

Regression Equations

Postmortem studies of hearts injected with contrast material have demonstrated that angiographic volumes calculated by equation 5 overestimate true left ventricular cavity volumes.[2,4,5] This overestimation is due in large part to the papillary muscles and trabeculae carneae, which do not contribute to blood volume but are nevertheless included within the traced left ventricular silhouette. Regression equations derived from these studies are used to adjust the calculated volumes. A list of the most commonly used regression equations is given in Table 19–1. For biplane studies in AP and lateral projections using large film techniques, the regression equation of Dodge and Sandler[15] (Table 19–1) is used. For children (in whom this regression equation may yield a negative volume), another formula has been suggested[16] (Table 19–1). For cine studies in the 60-degree RAO/30-degree LAO projections, Wynne et al. used postmortem casts,

Table 19–1. *Regression Equations to Correct for Overestimation in Calculation of Left Ventricular Volumes*

Investigator	Angiographic Method	Age Group	Regression Equation
Wynne et al.[5]	Biplane cine RAO and LAO	Adults	$V_A = 0.989C_C - 8.1$
	Single-plane cine RAO	Adults	$V_A = 0.938V_C - 5.7$
Kennedy et al.[13]	Single-plane cine RAO	Adults	$V_A = 0.81V_C + 1.9$
Dodge et al.[2,15]	Biplane serial AP and lateral	Adults	$V_A = 0.928V_C - 3.8$
Graham et al.[16]	Biplane cine AP and lateral	Children	$V_A = 0.733V_C$
Sandler et al.[12]	Single-plane serial AP	Adults	$V_A = 0.951V_C - 3.0$

V_A = actual volume.
V_C = calculated volume.

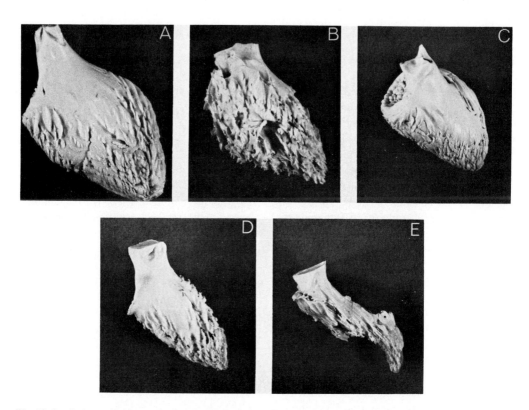

Fig. 19–5. Left ventricular casts made from fresh postmortem specimens of human hearts, using an encapsulant mixed with barium sulfate powder. The shape of the left ventricle only roughly approximates an ellipsoid of revolution; nevertheless, amazingly good correlation was obtained between true volume of these casts (measured by water displacement of the actual cast) and calculated volume (Fig. 19–6.) (From Wynne J, et al: Estimation of left ventricular volumes in man from biplane cineangiograms filmed in oblique projections. Am J Cardiol 41:726, 1978.)

as shown in Figure 19–5, to derive the regression equation illustrated in Figure 19–6.[5]

Single-plane techniques tend to overestimate volume significantly as compared to biplane methods, and this is reflected in the single-plane regression equations (Table 19–1).

EJECTION FRACTION AND REGURGITANT FRACTION

Visual inspection of the cine film generally allows selection of frames depicting maximum (end-diastolic) and minimum (end-systolic)

ventricular volume. Ejection fraction (EF) is then calculated as:[17,18]

$$EF = (EDV - ESV)/EDV = SV/EDV \tag{6}$$

where SV is the angiographic stroke volume.

In patients with aortic and/or mitral regurgitation, comparison of the angiographically determined stroke volume with the forward stroke volume determined by the Fick, indocyanine green dye, or (in the absence of concomitant tricuspid regurgitation) thermodilution technique yields the regurgitant stroke volume, that portion of the ejected volume that

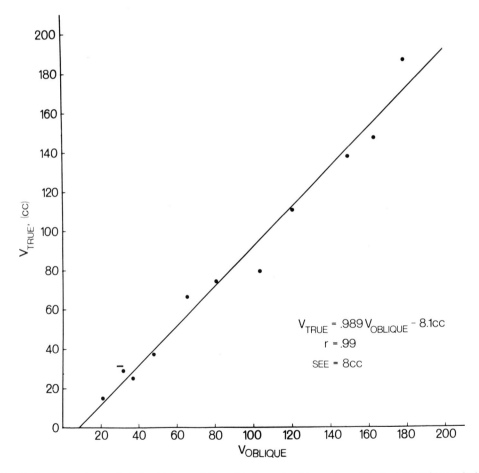

Fig. 19–6. Regression analysis for 11 human left ventricular casts of true volume (V_{true}) versus volume calculated from biplane oblique cine films of each cast ($V_{oblique}$), using equation 4. As can be seen, $V_{oblique}$ slightly overestimated V_{true}, although the correlation was excellent. (From Wynne J, et al: Estimation of left ventricular volumes in man from biplane cineangiograms filmed in oblique projections. Am J Cardiol 41:726, 1978.)

is regurgitated and thus does not contribute to the net cardiac output.[15] The regurgitant fraction (RF) is defined as:[17–19]

$$RF = \frac{SV_{angiographic} - SV_{forward}}{SV_{angiographic}} \quad (7)$$

An assumption of this calculation is constancy of heart rate between determination of forward cardiac output and performance of left ventriculography. If the heart rate is substantially different at these times, a modified method for calculating RF must be used where the angiographic minute output ($SV_{angiographic} \cdot HR$) is substituted for angiographic stroke volume, and the forward minute output or cardiac output is substituted for the forward stroke volume. This calculation is based on the assumption that cardiac output is independent of heart rate to a first approximation.

Because derivation of RF involves the difference between the two stroke volume measurements, both of which contain some degree of error, the error in RF itself may be significant; interpretation of this number should be influenced by qualitative assessment of the degree of regurgitation seen on the angiogram. In cases of combined aortic and mitral regurgitation, estimation of the relative contribution of the two lesions must be made from the cineangiograms.

OTHER TECHNIQUES FOR MEASURING VENTRICULAR VOLUME AND EJECTION FRACTION: DIGITAL SUBTRACTION ANGIOGRAPHY AND THE IMPEDANCE CATHETER

Image enhancement by computerized digital subtraction techniques can be used to obtain left ventriculograms after peripheral intravenous administration of contrast material.[20,21] Peripheral injection of the contrast agent eliminates the problem of ventricular extrasystoles sometimes associated with direct injection of contrast material into the ventricular chamber. Alternatively, the image enhancement provided by the digital subtraction process permits

direct left ventricular injections with small volumes of contrast agents,[20] possibly allowing multiple ventriculograms under varying conditions during a single catheterization procedure. Ventricular volume and ejection fraction may be calculated from digital subtraction ventriculograms using the area-length method[20] as described for standard ventriculograms. Alternatively, ejection fraction may be determined by computer analysis of the attenuation of x rays by the contrast agent within the ventricle.[21,22] This technique is independent of geometric assumptions regarding the shape of the ventricle.

A multielectrode catheter capable of measuring intracavitary electrical impedance has been introduced,[23,24] and may prove useful for the measurement of ventricular volume and ejection fraction without the use of contrast agents. The catheter is shown in Figure 19–7 and consists of 12 platinum ring electrodes mounted at 1 cm intervals along the distal end of an 8 or 9F end-hole catheter. A 4μA current flows through the blood of the ventricular chamber between selected ring electrodes, and the voltage needed to drive this current reflects the instantaneous electrical impedance of the blood, which has been shown to be a direct function of the blood volume. Validation studies[23,24] indicate that both LV and RV volumes can be measured by this technique. An illustration of the potential usefulness of this catheter in assessing LV pressure-volume-relationship is shown in Figure 19–8.

LEFT VENTRICULAR MASS

Measurement of left ventricular wall thickness, in addition to the parameters measured for volume determination, allows calculation of left ventricular wall volume and estimation of left ventricular mass (LVM). For these calculations, it is assumed that wall thickness is uniform throughout the ventricle. Wall thickness (h) is measured at end-diastole at the left ventricular free wall roughly two thirds of the distance from the aortic valve to the apex in the AP[25] or RAO[13] projection. Appropriate magnification correction is applied. The total

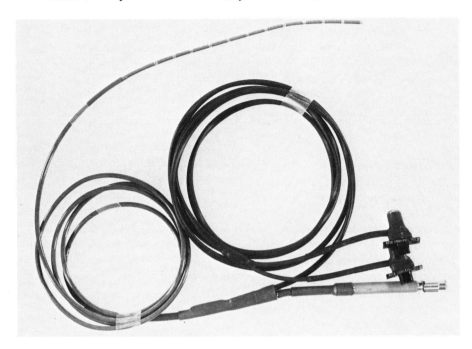

Fig. 19–7.   Multielectrode impedance catheter for measurement of instantaneous chamber blood volume.[23] See text for description.

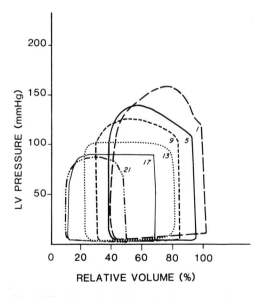

Fig. 19–8.   Use of multielectrode impedance catheter, shown in Figure 19–7, to obtain LV pressure-volume loops every fourth beat during inhalation of amyl nitrite. (Reproduced with permission from McKay RG, et al: Instantaneous measurement of left and right ventricular stroke volume and pressure-volume relationships with an impedance catheter. Circulation 69:703, 1984.)

volume of left ventricular chamber and wall, V_{c+w}, is approximated by that of the corresponding ellipsoid:

$$V_{c+w} = \frac{4}{3} \pi \left(\frac{L+2h}{2}\right)\left(\frac{M+2h}{2}\right)\left(\frac{N+2h}{2}\right)$$

$$= \frac{\pi}{6}(L+2h)\left(\frac{4A_{RAO}}{\pi L_{RAO}} + 2h\right)$$

$$\cdot \left(\frac{4A_{LAO}}{\pi L_{LAO}} + 2h\right) \qquad (8)$$

for biplane methods. As with h, appropriate correction for magnification must be applied to A and L so that V_{c+w} represents the total volume of the left ventricular chamber and wall corrected for magnification. For single-plane methods, it is assumed that $M = N$, yielding the single-plane formula:

$$V_{c+w} = \frac{\pi}{6}(L + 2h)\left(\frac{4A}{\pi L} + 2h\right)^2 \qquad (9)$$

The volume of the chamber is calculated by the biplane or single-plane technique. In order to exclude the volume of the papillary muscles and trabeculae from the chamber volume (and thus include their mass in LVM), the appropriate regression equation is applied, so that V_c is the *regressed value* for chamber volume. Left ventricular mass, then, is calculated as:

$$LVM = 1.050V_w = 1.050(V_{c+w} - V_c)$$ (10)

where V_w is wall volume, and 1.050 is the specific gravity of heart muscle. This method has been validated by postmortem examination of hearts[25,26]; however, it may not be accurate in the presence of marked right ventricular hypertrophy or pericardial effusion or thickening, where the accurate measurement of wall thickness from the RAO silhouette may be impossible. The left ventricular wall thickness may sometimes be seen well in the LAO projection in the region of the posterior wall, or may be measured accurately by echocardiography, computerized tomography, or magnetic resonance imaging. Values obtained by any of these methods may be used for calculation of left ventricular mass.

NORMAL VALUES

A number of investigators have reported normal values in adults and children for left ventricular volume, ejection fraction, wall thickness, and mass.[5,16,27–29] These are summarized in Table 19–2.

WALL STRESS

While consideration of ventricular pressure and volume is useful for assessment of *ventricular* performance, direct evaluation of *myocardial* function requires attention to forces acting at the level of the individual myocardial fiber. In particular, correction must be made for differences in ventricular wall thickness and chamber radius (R), which modify the extent to which intraventricular pressure (P) is borne by the individual fiber; this is especially important in disease states characterized by ventricular hypertrophy or dilatation or both. Such a correction may be achieved by consid-

eration of wall stress (σ).[30–33] Several formulae are commonly used to calculate stress, all related to the basic Laplace relation:

$$\sigma = \frac{PR}{2h}$$ (11)

Assumptions of the shape of the ventricular chamber and the properties of the ventricular wall have led to a number of such formulae for wall stress components in the circumferential, meridional, and radial directions (Fig. 19–9). Consideration of circumferential and meridional stress has been particularly useful for clinical applications. A representative formula for calculation of circumferential stress, σ_c,[31] is:

$$\sigma_c = \frac{Pb}{h}\left(1 - \frac{h}{2b}\right)\left(1 - \frac{hb}{2a^2}\right)$$ (12)

where a and b are the major and minor semi-axes, respectively, at the midwall. Meridional stress, σ_m, may be calculated as:[32]

$$\sigma_m = \frac{PR}{2h(1 + h/2R)}$$ (13)

where R is the internal chamber radius as bounded by the endocardial surface. For more detailed consideration of wall stress formulae, the reader is referred to reviews of the subject.[31,33]

Calculation of wall stress in disease states has provided information not apparent from consideration of pressure and volume data alone. For example, it has been demonstrated that peak stress does not necessarily occur at the same time in the cardiac cycle as does peak pressure and that, in "compensated" pressure overload, the increase in ventricular pressure is offset by a proportional increase in wall thickness, so that wall stress remains normal (Fig. 19–10).[32]

VOLUME-TIME AND PRESSURE-VOLUME CURVES

Left ventriculography performed with rapid filming rates has permitted construction of the ventricular volume-time curve[3,34] (Fig.

Table 19–2. *Normal Average Values for Left Ventricular Parameters by Angiocardiography*

Investigator	Angiographic Method	Number of Patients	Age Group	End-Diastolic Volume (ml/m²)	End-Systolic Volume (ml/m²)	Ejection Fraction	Wall Thickness (mm)	Mass (g)
Wynne et al.[5]	Biplane cine RAO-LAO	17	Adults	72 ± 15	20 ± 8	0.72 ± 0.08	—	—
Kennedy et al.[27]	Biplane serial AP and Lat	16	Adults	70 ± 20	24 ± 10	0.67 ± 0.08	10.9 ± 2.0	167 ± 42
Hood[28]	Biplane serial AP and Lat	6	Adults	79 ± 11	28 ± 6	0.67 ± 0.07	8.5 ± 1.3	164 ± 35
Hermann and Bartle[29]	Biplane serial AP and Lat	6	Adults	71 ± 20	30 ± 10	0.58 ± 0.05	—	—
Graham et al.[16]	Biplane cine AP and Lat	19	Children less than 2 yr	42 ± 10	—	0.68 ± 0.05	—	96 ± 11*
Graham et al.[16]	Biplane cine AP and Lat	37	Children older than 2 yr	73 ± 11	—	0.63 ± 0.05	—	86 ± 11*

Mean ± SD
*gm/m²

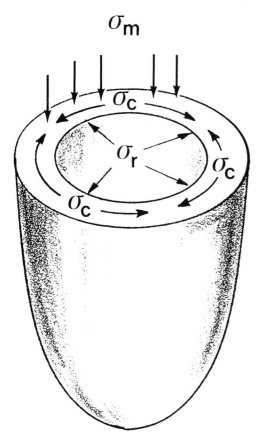

Fig. 19–9. Circumferential (σ_c), meridional (σ_m), and radial (σ_r) components of left ventricular wall stress for an ellipsoid model. The three components of wall stress are mutually perpendicular.

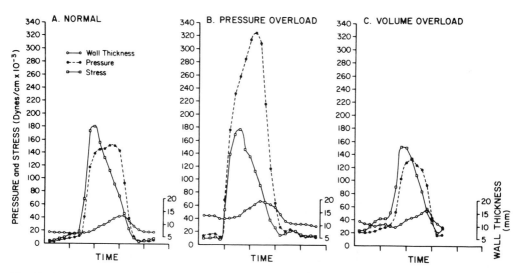

Fig. 19–10. A comparison of changes in left ventricular pressure (solid dots), wall thickness (open dots), and meridional stress (open squares) throughout the cardiac cycle for representative normal, pressure-overloaded, and volume-overloaded ventricles. These parameters are plotted at 40-msec intervals. In all three types of ventricles, peak stress occurs earlier than peak pressure. In the pressure-overloaded ventricle (B), peak pressure is markedly elevated, but peak systolic stress and end-diastolic stress are normal. In the volume-overloaded ventricle (C), peak systolic stress is normal, but end-diastolic stress is elevated. (Reproduced with permission from Grossman W, Jones D, McLaurin LP: Wall stress and patterns of hypertrophy in the human left ventricle. J Clin Invest 56:56, 1974.)

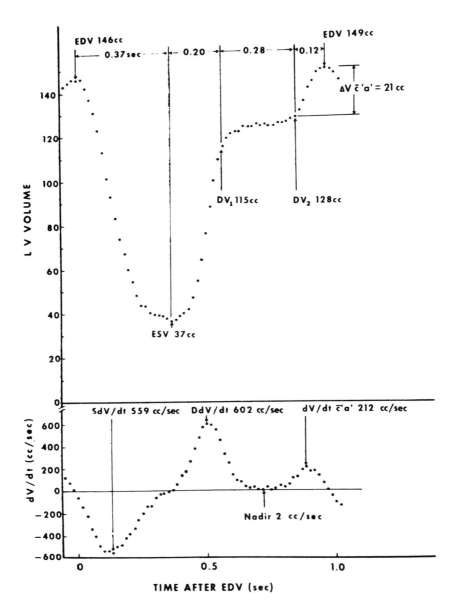

Fig. 19–11. Plots of left ventricular (LV) volume and the rate of change of volume (dV/dt) versus time calculated from a single-plane cineangiogram in a normal subject. The maximum value of dV/dt during diastole, i.e., the peak rate of diastolic filling (D dV/dt) of the ventricle, has been proposed as an index of early diastolic function. End-diastolic (EDV) and end-systolic (ESV) volumes are indicated. (Reproduced with permission from Hammermeister KE, Warbasse JR: The rate of change of left ventricular volume in man. Circulation 49:739, 1974.)

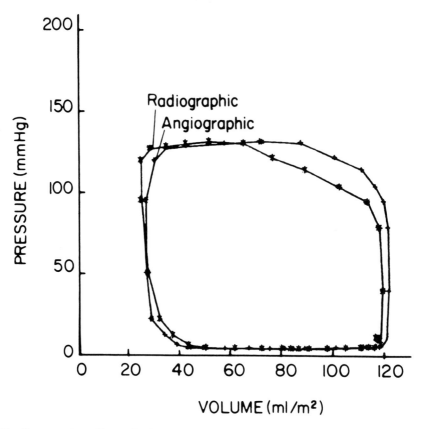

Fig. 19–12. Pressure-volume diagram for the left ventricle. In this example, the diagram derived from single-plane cineangiography is compared to that constructed from radionuclide volume data. (Reproduced with permission from McKay RG, et al: Left ventricular pressure-volume diagrams and end-systolic pressure-volume relations in human beings. J Am Coll Cardiol 3:301, 1984.)

19–11). Calculation of the maximum slope of the early diastolic portion of the curve, i.e., the peak rate of early diastolic filling of the ventricle, has been suggested as an index of early diastolic function.[34]

Simultaneous measurement of ventricular pressure and volume allows construction of the pressure-volume diagram (Fig. 19–12).[35–38] The position and slope of the diastolic portion of the pressure-volume curve provide information regarding diastolic properties of the ventricle.[36,39] Construction of the systolic portion of the curve is useful for analysis of the end-systolic pressure-volume relation, a measure of ventricular contractile function (see Chapter 20).

REGIONAL LEFT VENTRICULAR WALL MOTION

The recognition that left ventricular regional dyssynergy is a more sensitive marker of coronary artery disease than is depression of global function has led to attempts to quantify abnormalities of regional wall motion. Left ventriculography is performed in the RAO or RAO and LAO projections. The ventricle is divided into regions by one of two methods: (1) construction of lines perpendicular to the major axis that divide the major axis into equal segments[40,41] or (2) construction of lines drawn from the midpoint of the major axis to the ventricular outline at intervals of a fixed number of degrees. Extent of inward (or out-

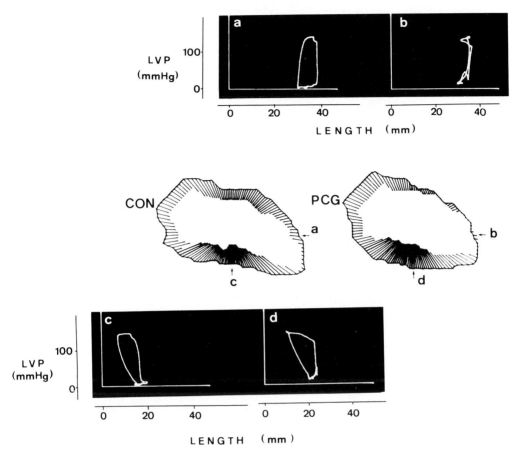

Fig. 19–13. Assessment of regional wall motion in the control state (CON) and after induction of angina pectoris by atrial pacing tachycardia (PCG). Left ventricular pressure (LVP)-length loops are plotted for a myocardial region distal to a stenotic coronary artery (a and b) and for a normally perfused region (c and d). (Reproduced with permission from Sasayama S, et al: Changes in diastolic properties of the regional myocardium during pacing-induced ischemia in man. J Am Coll Cardiol 5:599, 1985.)

ward) movement of individual segments can then be measured, generally with the aid of computer techniques, providing quantitative measures of hypokinesis, akinesis, and dyskinesis. It has been proposed that densitometric analysis of digital subtraction ventriculograms further refines measures of regional function.[42]

An automated method of processing the left ventricular cineangiogram has been reported by Sasayama and co-workers.[43–45] End-diastolic and end-systolic ventricular silhouettes are superimposed (Fig. 19–13), and 128 radial grids are drawn from the center of gravity of the end-diastolic silhouette to the endocardial margins. Measurement of the length of each radial grid between end-diastolic and end-sys-

tolic silhouettes measures segmental systolic and diastolic function. Figure 19–13 illustrates this technique in a patient with coronary disease before (CON) and after (PCG) induction of angina pectoris by rapid atrial pacing. Simultaneously measured LV pressure (LVP) permits construction of segmental LV pressure-length loops for the normally perfused myocardial region (c and d), as well as for a region perfused by a stenotic coronary artery (a and b). Depressed wall motion develops during angina in region a/b, and compensatory hyperkinesis develops in region c/d.

Another approach has been used by Sheehan and colleagues at the University of Washington in Seattle.[46,47] In this approach, wall motion

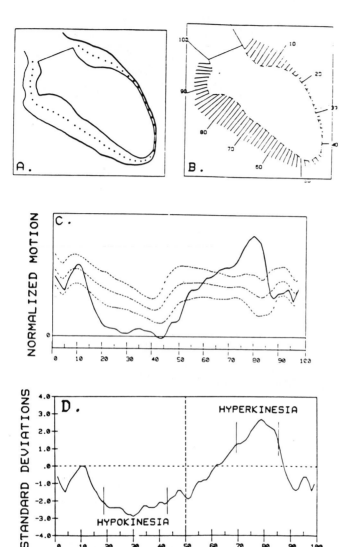

Fig. 19–14. Wall motion as assessed by the center line method. The center line (dotted line in panel A) is constructed midway between the end-systolic and end-diastolic silhouettes. In panel B, chords are drawn at right angles to the center line. The percentage of systolic shortening along each chord is plotted (solid line in panel C) and compared to normal mean and standard deviation values (dashed and dotted lines). Deviation from normal is replotted in panel D. (Reproduced with permission from Sheehan FH, Bolson EL, Dodge HT, Mathey DG, Schofer J, Woo H: Advantages and applications of the center line method for characterizing regional ventricular function. Circulation 74:293, 1986.)

is measured along 100 chords constructed as perpendiculars to a line drawn midway between the end-diastolic and end-systolic left ventricular contours (Fig. 19–14). The motion of each chord is compared to a normal range established from analysis of ventriculograms from patients without heart disease. Deviations from the normal range indicate hypokinesis or hyperkinesis. In studies of wall motion following thrombolysis, availability of the LAO in addition to the RAO projection proved particularly useful in patients with left circumflex coronary artery thrombosis.[47]

REFERENCES

1. Arvidsson H: Angiocardiographic observations in mitral disease. Acta Radiol suppl 158, 1958.
2. Dodge HT, Sandler H, Ballew DW, Lord JD Jr.: The use of biplane angiocardiography for the measurement of left ventricular volume in man. Am Heart J 60:762, 1960.
3. Chapman CB, Baker O, Reynolds J, Bonte FJ: Use of biplane cinefluorography for measurement of ventricular volume. Circulation 18:1105, 1958.
4. Greene DG, Carlisle R, Grant C, Bunnell IL: Estimation of left ventricular volume by one-plane cineangiography. Circulation 35:61, 1967.
5. Wynne J, et al: Estimation of left ventricular volumes in man from biplane cineangiograms filmed in oblique projections. Am J Cardiol 41:726, 1978.

6. Rogers WJ, et al: Quantitative axial oblique contrast left ventriculography: validation of the method by demonstrating improved visualization of regional wall motion and mitral valve function with accurate volume determinations. Am Heart J 103:185, 1982.

7. Arcilla RA, Tsai P, Thilenius O, Ranninger K: Angiographic method for volume estimation of right and left ventricles. Chest 60:446, 1971.

8. Graham TP Jr., Jarmakani JM, Atwood GF, Canent RV Jr.: Right ventricular volume determinations in children. Normal values and observations with volume or pressure overload. Circulation 47:144, 1973.

9. Goerke RJ, Carlsson E: Calculation of right and left cardiac ventricular volumes. Method using standard computer equipment and biplane angiocardiograms. Invest Radiol 2:360, 1967.

10. Gentzler RD, Briselli MF, Gault JH: Angiographic estimation of right ventricular volume in man. Circulation 50:324, 1974.

11. Kasser IS, Kennedy JW: Measurement of left ventricular volumes in man by single-plane cineangiocardiography. Invest Radiol 4:83, 1969.

12. Sandler H, Dodge HT: The use of single plane angiocardiograms for the calculation of left ventricular volume in man. Am Heart J 75:325, 1968.

13. Kennedy JW, Trenholme SE, Kasser IS: Left ventricular volume and mass from single-plane cineangiocardiogram. A comparison of anteroposterior and right anterior oblique methods. Am Heart J 80:343, 1970.

14. Sheehan FH, Mitten-Lewis S: Factors influencing accuracy in left ventricular volume determination. Am J Cardiol 64:661, 1989.

15. Sandler H, Dodge HT, Hay RE, Rackley CE: Quantitation of valvular insufficiency in man by angiocardiography. Am Heart J 65:501, 1963.

16. Graham TP Jr., Jarmakani JM, Canent RV Jr., Morrow MN: Left heart volume estimation in infancy and childhood. Reevaluation of methodology and normal values. Circulation 43:895, 1971.

17. Arvidsson H, Karnell J: Quantitative assessment of mitral and aortic insufficiency by angiocardiography. Acta Radiol 2:105, 1964.

18. Miller GAH, Brown R, Swan HJC: Isolated congenital mitral insufficiency with particular reference to left heart volumes. Circulation 29:356, 1964.

19. Jones JW, et al: Left ventricular volumes in valvular heart disease. Circulation 29:887, 1964.

20. Sasayama S, et al: Automated method for left ventricular volume measurement by cineventriculography with minimal doses of contrast medium. Am J Cardiol 48:746, 1981.

21. Nissen SE, Elion JL, Grayburn P, et al: Determination of left ventricular ejection fraction by computer densitometric analysis of digital subtraction angiography: experimental validation and correlation with area-length methods. Am J Cardiol 59:675, 1987.

22. Tobis J, et al: Measurement of left ventricular ejection fraction by videodensitometric analysis of digital subtraction angiograms. Am J Cardiol 52:871, 1983.

23. McKay RG, et al: Instantaneous measurement of left and right ventricular stroke volume and pressure-volume relationships with an impedance catheter. Circulation 69:703, 1984.

24. Kass DA, Midei M, Graves W, et al: Use of a con-ductance (volume) catheter and transient inferior vena caval occlusion for rapid determination of pressure-volume relationships in man. Cathet Cardiovasc Diagn 15:192, 1988.

25. Rackley CE, Dodge HT, Coble YD Jr, Hay RE: A method for determining left ventricular mass in man. Circulation 29:666, 1964.

26. Kennedy JW, Reichenbach DD, Baxley WA, Dodge HT: Left ventricular mass. A comparison of angiocardiographic measurements with autopsy weight. Am J Cardiol 19:221, 1967.

27. Kennedy JW, et al: Quantitative angiocardiography. I. The normal left ventricle in man. Circulation 34:272, 1966.

28. Hood WP Jr: Wall stress in the normal and hypertrophied human left ventricle. Am J Cardiol 22:550, 1968.

29. Hermann HJ, Bartle SH: Left ventricular volumes by angiocardiography: comparison of methods and simplification of techniques. Cardiovasc Res 4:404, 1968.

30. Sandler H, Dodge HT: Left ventricular tension and stress in man. Circ Res 13:91, 1963.

31. Mirsky I: Review of various theories for the evaluation of left ventricular wall stresses. *In* Mirsky I, Ghista DN, Sandler H (eds): Cardiac Mechanics. New York, John Wiley & Sons, Inc., 1974, p. 381.

32. Grossman W, Jones D, McLaurin LP: Wall stress and patterns of hypertrophy in the human left ventricle. J Clin Invest 56:56, 1974.

33. Yin FCP: Ventricular wall stress. Circ Res 49:829, 1981.

34. Hammermeister KE, Warbasse JR: The rate of change of left ventricular volume in man. II. Diastolic events in health and disease. Circulation 49:739, 1974.

35. Arvidsson H: Angiocardiographic determination of left ventricular volume. Acta Radiol 56:321, 1961.

36. Dodge HT, Hay RE, Sandler H: Pressure-volume characteristics of diastolic left ventricle of man with heart disease. Am Heart J 64:503, 1962.

37. Bunnell IL, Grant C, Greene DG: Left ventricular function derived from the pressure-volume diagram. Am J Med 39:881, 1965.

38. McKay RG, et al: Left ventricular pressure-volume diagrams and end-systolic pressure-volume relations in human beings. J Am Coll Cardiol 3:301, 1984.

39. Grossman W: Relaxation and diastolic distensibility of the regionally ischemic left ventricle. *In* Grossman W, Lorell BH (eds): Diastolic Relaxation of the Heart. Boston, Martinus Nijhoff Publishing, 1988, 193–203.

40. Herman MV, Heinle RA, Klein MD, Gorlin R: Localized disorders in myocardial contraction. Asynergy and its role in congestive heart failure. N Engl J Med 277:222, 1967.

41. Sniderman AD, Marpole D, Fallen EL: Regional contraction patterns in the normal and ischemic left ventricle in man. Am J Cardiol 31:484, 1973.

42. Chappuis F, Widmann T, Guth B, et al: Quantitative assessment of regional left ventricular function by densitometric analysis of digital-subtraction ventriculograms: correlation with myocardial systolic shortening in dogs. Circulation 77:457, 1988.

43. Sasayama, S, Nonogi H, Kawm C: Assessment of

left ventricular function using an angiographic method. Jpn Circ J 46:1177, 1982.

44. Fujita M, et al: Automatic processing of cine ventriculograms for analysis of regional myocardial function. Circulation 63:1065, 1981.

45. Sasayama S, et al: Changes in diastolic properties of the regional myocardium during pacing-induced ischemia in human subjects. J Am Coll Cardiol 5:599, 1985.

46. Sheehan FH, Bolson EL, Dodge HT, et al: Advantages and applications of the centerline method for characterizing regional ventricular function. Circulation 74:293, 1986.

47. Sheehan FH, Schofer J, Mathey DG, et al: Measurement of regional wall motion from biplane contrast ventriculograms: A comparison of the 30 degree right anterior oblique and 60 degree left anterior oblique projections in patients with acute myocardial infarction. Circulation 74:796, 1986.

20

Evaluation of Systolic and Diastolic Function of the Myocardium

WILLIAM GROSSMAN

A critical aspect of most cardiac catheterization procedures is the evaluation of myocardial function. At its simplest, this consists of a visual assessment of the left ventricular (LV) contractile pattern from the left ventriculogram, together with measurements of LV end-diastolic pressure. In laboratories such as ours, where most patients have right heart catheterization and cardiac output measurement as part of a standard cardiac catheterization procedure, additional information about LV function may be gleaned from the cardiac output, stroke volume, and pulmonary capillary wedge pressure, whereas right ventricular (RV) function is reflected in the values for right ventricular end-diastolic pressure (RVEDP) and right atrial pressure. Measurements of pressures and cardiac output give important information about overall cardiac function, but may shed little light on the question as to whether dysfunction is due to abnormal systolic or diastolic myocardial performance. This chapter describes some of the specific methods that can be used in the cardiac catheterization laboratory to examine myocardial performance in systole and diastole.

SYSTOLIC FUNCTION

Preload, Afterload, and Contractility

Systolic function of the myocardium is a reflection of the interaction of myocardial pre-load, afterload, and contractility. **Preload** is the load that stretches myofibrils during diastole and determines the end-diastolic sarcomere length. For the left ventricle, this load is often quantified as the LV end-diastolic pressure (EDP). This pressure, taken together with LV wall thickness (h) and radius (R), determines LV end-diastolic *wall stress* ($\sigma \sim PR/h$), which is an estimate of the force stretching the myocardial fibers at end-diastole. The end-diastolic stress or "stretching force" is resisted by the intrinsic stiffness or elasticity of the myocardium, and the interaction of end-diastolic stretching force and myocardial stiffness determines the extent of end-diastolic sarcomere stretch. Thus, if the myocardium is diffusely fibrotic or infiltrated with amyloid, a very high end-diastolic stretching force may be required to produce even a normal end-diastolic sarcomere length. In such a case, LVEDP may be very high (e.g., >25 mm Hg), and attempts to lower it by diuretic or veno-dilator therapy lead to reduction in end-diastolic sarcomere stretch to subnormal values and a concomitant fall in cardiac output.

Changes in preload influence both the extent and velocity of myocardial shortening in experiments using isolated cardiac muscle preparations. Increased preload augments the extent and velocity of myocardial shortening at any given afterload. In the intact heart, the relationship is more complex because increases in preload generally produce increases in LV chamber size and LV systolic pressure. Thus, *afterload* (the force resisting systolic shortening) is also increased, and this increase tends to blunt the increases in extent and velocity of myocardial shortening due to increased diastolic fiber stretch. This point will be discussed in more detail later in this chapter, under the section on ejection phase indexes of systolic function.

Afterload, the force resisting systolic shortening of the myofibrils, varies throughout systole as the ventricular systolic pressure rises and blood is ejected from the ventricular chamber. LV systolic stress approximates the force resisting myocardial fiber shortening within the wall of the ventricle. The theory and methods for calculation of wall stress are described in Chapter 19. End-systolic wall stress is considered by many to be the final afterload that determines the extent of myocardial fiber shortening, when preload and contractility are constant. Thus, an increase in end-systolic wall stress results in a decrease in myocardial fiber shortening. For the intact ventricle, an increase in afterload (end-systolic wall stress) results, therefore, in a fall in stroke volume and ejection fraction.

Contractility refers to the property of heart muscle that accounts for alterations in performance induced by biochemical and hormonal changes, and has classically been regarded as independent of preload and afterload. Contractility is generally used as a synonym for *inotropy:* both terms refer to the level of activation of cross-bridge cycling during systole. Contractility changes are assessed in the experimental laboratory by measuring myocardial function (extent or speed of shortening, maximum force generation) while preload and afterload are held constant. In contrast to skeletal muscle, the strength of contraction of heart muscle can be increased readily by a variety of biochemical and hormonal stimuli, some of which are listed in Table 20–1.

Increased myocardial contractility may be present in patients with hyperadrenergic states, thyrotoxicosis, and hypertrophic cardiomyopathy and in response to a variety of drugs. It is manifest by an increase in the speed and extent of myocardial contraction at constant afterload and preload.

In recent years, fundamental experiments in isolated myocardial tissue have demonstrated that contractility is not truly preload-independent. Increased end-diastolic sarcomere stretch leads to an immediate increase in the strength of contraction due to the Frank-Starling mechanism, followed by a gradual further increase in contractile strength over the subsequent 5 to 10 minutes.[1–3] Evidence supports a role for both increased intracellular Ca^{++} release and increased myofilament sensitivity to any given level of cytosolic Ca^{++} as underlying the length-dependent activation seen with increased preload.[2]

Assessment of systolic function requires consideration of the simultaneous influence of afterload, preload, and contractility. Systolic function should *not* be regarded as synonymous with contractility. Major depression of systolic function may occur with normal contractility, as in conditions with so-called afterload excess discussed later in this chapter.

Isovolumic Indices

One of the oldest and most widely used measures of myocardial contractility is the maximum rate of rise of LV systolic pressure, dP/dt. It was noted more than 50 years ago by Wiggers that in animal experiments the failing ventricle showed a reduction in the steepness of the upslope of the ventricular pressure pulse.[4] In 1962, Gleason and Braunwald first reported measurement of dP/dt in man.[5] They studied 40 patients with micromanometer catheters and found that maximum dP/dt in patients without hemodynamic abnormalities ranged from 841 to 1696 mm Hg/sec in the left ventricle, and 223 to 296 mm Hg/sec in the right ventricle. Interventions known to increase myocardial contractility, such as exercise and infusion of norepinephrine or isoproterenol, caused major increases in dP/dt. Increased

Table 20–1. *Hormones and Drugs That Influence Myocardial Contractility*

	Presumed Mechanism	Influence on Contractility
1. Catecholamines with β agonist activity	β receptor stimulation → ↑ adenylate cyclase activity → ↑ cyclic AMP → ↑ Ca^{++} influx through sarcolemma → ↑ cytosolic Ca^{++}	+
2. Digitalis glycosides	Inhibition of Na^+-K^+ ATPase → ↑ intracellular Na^+ → ↑ Na^+/Ca^{++} exchange → ↑ cytosolic Ca^{++}	+
3. Calcium salts	↑ Extracellular Ca^{++} → ↑ Ca^{++} influx via slow channels and Na^+/Ca^{++} exchange → ↑ cytosolic Ca^{++}	+
4. Caffeine	Multiple actions: (1) local release of catecholamines (2) inhibition of sarcoplasmic reticular Ca^{++} uptake (3) inhibition of phosphodiesterase → ↑ cyclic AMP (4) ↑ sensitivity of contractile proteins to Ca^{++}	+
5. Milrinone, amrinone, other bipyridines	Phosphodiesterase inhibition → ↑ cyclic AMP → ↑ cytosolic Ca^{++}	+
6. Thyroid hormone	Increases myosin ATPase activity by altering production of certain myosin isozymes	+
7. Calcium-blocking agents (verapamil, nifedipine, D600, diltiazem)	Block Ca^{++} entry via slow channels	−
8. Barbiturates, ethanol	Depress contractility by unknown mechanism	−

heart rate produced by intravenous atropine also caused a rise in maximum dP/dt, and the authors attributed this to the ''treppe'' phenomenon described by Bowditch. Acute increases in arterial pressure and afterload produced by infusion of the α-adrenergic vasoconstricting agent methoxamine produced little change in dP/dt. These points are illustrated in Figures 20–1 and 20–2.

In normal subjects and in patients with no significant cardiac abnormality, maximum dP/dt increases significantly in response to isometric exercise,[6] dynamic exercise,[5] tachycardia by atrial pacing[7,8] or atropine,[5] β-agonists,[5] and digitalis glycosides.[9] Relatively few studies have been done in humans assessing the changes in dP/dt induced by alterations in afterload and preload, but studies that have been done indicate that maximum posi-

tive dP/dt tends to increase slightly (6 to 8%) with moderate increases in LV preload[10] and shows little change with methoxamine-induced increases[5] or nitroprusside-induced decreases[11] in mean arterial pressure of 25 to 30 mm Hg. Extensive studies in animals have examined the influence of changes in afterload, preload, and contractility on maximum dP/dt.[10,12–15] These studies generally show that maximum dP/dt rises with increases in afterload and preload, but the changes were quite small (<10%) in the physiologic range.

As discussed in Chapter 9, accurate measurement of dP/dt requires a pressure measurement system with excellent frequency-response characteristics. Micromanometer catheters are generally required to achieve this frequency-response range.[16] Differentiation of the ventricular pressure signal can be achieved

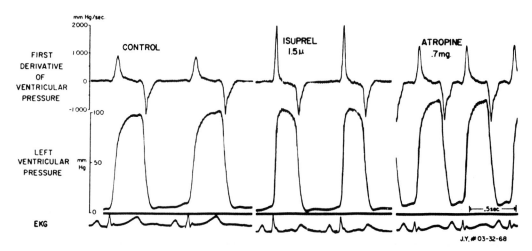

Fig. 20–1. Micromanometer recordings of left ventricular pressure and its first derivative, dP/dt, in a patient with normal left ventricular function. Isoproterenol markedly increases contractility with large increments in positive dP/dt. Atropine produces tachycardia, which results in a treppe effect and a rise in +dP/dt above control. (Reproduced, with permission, from Gleason WL, Braunwald E: Studies on the first derivative of the ventricular pressure pulse in man. J Clin Invest 41:80, 1962.)

by (1) analog techniques on-line (Figs. 20–1 and 20–2), using an RC differentiating circuit;[5,10] (2) computer digitization of the analog LV pressure tracing and subsequent differentiation of a polynominal best fit to the averaged LV isovolumic pressure;[17] or (3) computer digitization of the analog LV pressure tracing with subsequent Fourier analysis and differentiation.[18]

In addition to dP/dt, several other isovolumic indices have been introduced in an attempt to obtain a "pure" contractility index, completely independent of alterations in preload and afterload.[10,19–26] Of these indices, the maximum value of [(dP/dt)/P], where P is LV pressure, has been used by several groups over the past 20 years. On theoretic grounds, the quantity (dP/dt)/P has been related to the ve-

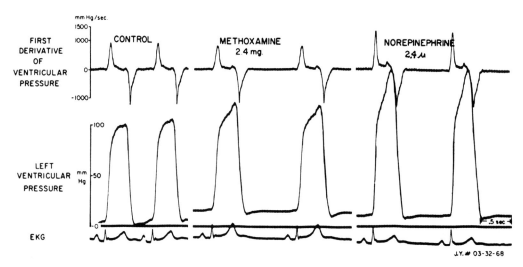

Fig. 20–2. Micromanometer recordings of left ventricular (LV) pressure and dP/dt, as in Figure 20–1. Methoxamine raises arterial and LV systolic pressure, but does not increase +dP/dt. In contrast, the combined α and β adrenergic effects of norepinephrine increase with LV systolic pressure and +dP/dt. (Reproduced, with permission, from Gleason WL and Braunwald E: Studies on the first derivative of the ventricular pressure pulse in man. J Clin Invest 41:80, 1962.)

locity of contractile element shortening, V_{CE}; the mathematical basis for this relation is given by several authors[20,21,23,27] and is not presented here in detail. A fundamental problem with the use of (dP/dt)/P as a measure of contractile element velocity is that the mathematics upon which this concept is based are highly model-dependent and require knowledge of the compliance of series and parallel elastic elements. From a *practical* standpoint, although (dP/dt)/P does directly reflect changes in contractility (e.g., it increases with isoproterenol or calcium infusion), it is sensitive to alterations in preload.[10] Thus, (dP/dt)/P falls during dextran infusion in animals and in response to increased venous return (passive straight leg raising) in man.[10] This preload sensitivity can be abolished if the P used in calculating (dP/dt)/P is "developed" LV pressure (total LV intraventricular pressure minus LVEDP), which corrects for shifts in preload.

The maximum value of (dP/dt)/P is sometimes called V_{PM}; as mentioned, it reflects changes in contractility directly, but is related inversely to changes in preload. Nevertheless, if an intervention produces an increase in V_{PM} at a time when LVEDP is unchanged or rising, an increase in contractility has almost certainly occurred.

Other isovolumic indices include (peak dP/dt)/IIT, where IIT = integrated isovolumic tension; (dP/dt)/CPIP, where CPIP = common developed isovolumic pressure; V_{max}, the extrapolated value of (dP/dt)/P versus P, when P = 0; (dP/dt)/P_D when developed LV pressure, P_D, equals 5, 10, or 40 mm Hg; and the fractional rate of change of power, which involves the second derivative of LV pressure. The reader is referred elsewhere for more information on these less commonly used isovolumic indices.[19,22,23,25,27]

While changes in dP/dt reflect acute changes in inotropy in a given individual, the usefulness of dP/dt is reduced when attempting to compare one individual with another, especially when there has been chronic LV pressure or volume overload. Thus, peak dP/dt is generally *increased* in patients with chronic aortic stenosis even though contractility is normal or

decreased in most of these patients. To account for chronic changes in LV geometry and mass that occur with chronic LV overload, some investigators have examined the rate of rise of systolic wall stress.[17] The peak value of dσ/dt may be used as a contractility index, as may the spectrum plot that relates dσ/dt to instantaneous σ (Fig. 20–3).

Pressure-Volume Analysis

Since the time of Frank and Starling, pressure-volume diagrams have been used to analyze ventricular function. The normally contracting left ventricle ejects blood under pressure, and the relationship of its pressure generation and ejection can be expressed in a plot of LV pressure against volume (Fig. 20–4). As can be seen in Figure 20–4, end-diastole is represented by point A, isovolumic contraction by line AB, aortic valve opening by point B, ejection by line BC, end ejection and aortic valve closure by point C, isovolumic relaxation by line CD, mitral valve opening by point D, and LV diastolic filling by line DA.

Stroke Work. The area ABCD enclosed within the PV diagram in Figure 20–4 is the external LV stroke work (SW), represented mathematically as ∫PdV. Although the calculation of LVSW is most accurate when derived by integrating the area within complete PV diagrams, a practical approximation can be obtained as:

$$\text{LVSW} = (\overline{\text{LVSP}} - \overline{\text{LVDP}})\text{SV}(0.0136) \quad (1)$$

where $\overline{\text{LVSP}}$ and $\overline{\text{LVDP}}$ are the mean LV systolic and diastolic pressures in mm Hg, SV is the LV total stroke volume in ml, and 0.0136 is a constant for converting mm Hg·ml into gm-m. $\overline{\text{LVSP}}$ and $\overline{\text{LVDP}}$ may be obtained from planimetry of direct pressure tracings, as shown in Figure 20–5. When the total LV stroke volume is the same as the forward stroke volume, SV may be calculated as cardiac output ÷ heart rate. In patients in whom LV total stroke volume differs from forward stroke volume (e.g., mitral or aortic regurgitation, ventricular septal defect), the PV diagram may

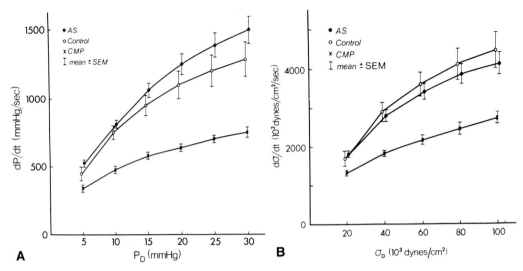

Fig. 20–3. Left ventricular (LV) isovolumic indexes of contractility. (A) Rate of pressure development (dP/dt) as a function of LV developed pressure (P_D). Mean values in control subjects (open circles), patients with aortic stenosis (AS, closed circles), and those with dilated cardiomyopathy (CMP, crosses) are shown. Brackets represent standard errors of the mean (SEM). (B) Rate of wall stress development (dσ/dt) as a function of LV developed stress (σ_D) for the same groups. There are no significant differences for patients with AS compared to controls, although patients with CMP clearly show depressed values for dP/dt and dσ/dt at all levels of P_D and σ_D. (Reproduced, with permission, from Fifer MA et al: Myocardial contractile function in aortic stenosis as determined from the rate of stress development during isovolumic systole. Am J Cardiol 44:1318, 1979.)

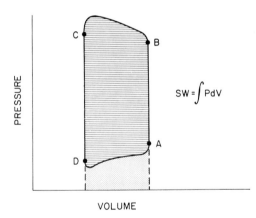

Fig. 20–4. Diagram of ventricular pressure (P) plotted against simultaneous ventricular volume (V) for a single cardiac contraction. For the left ventricle, point A represents end-diastole, segment AB is isovolumic contraction, point B is aortic valve opening, segment BC is LV ejection, point C is aortic valve closure and represents end-ejection, segment CD is isovolumic relaxation, point D is mitral valve opening, and segment DA is LV filling. LV stroke work (SW) is the cross-hatched area, while the stippled area is diastolic work done on the left ventricle by right ventricle and left atrium. See text for details.

differ substantially in configuration from that shown in Figure 20–4, and LVSW cannot be calculated from equation 1. Instead, planimetric integration of the entire PV plot is required.

If LV pressure tracings are not available, in the absence of major regurgitation SW can be approximated using aortic and pulmonary capillary wedge pressures as:

$$\text{LVSW} = (\overline{\text{AoSP}} - \overline{\text{PCW}})\text{SV}(0.0136) \quad (2)$$

where $\overline{\text{AoSP}}$ and $\overline{\text{PCW}}$ are the aortic systolic mean pressure (planimetered from the aortic pressure tracing, Fig. 20–5) and the mean pulmonary capillary wedge pressure. Because the mean systemic arterial pressure closely approximates $\overline{\text{AoSP}}$, a further approximation may be made by substituting mean arterial pressure ($\overline{\text{Ao}}$) for $\overline{\text{AoSP}}$.

LVSW is a reasonably good measure of LV systolic function in the absence of volume or pressure overload conditions, both of which may substantially increase calculated LVSW. The normal LVSW in adults is approximately 90 ± 30 gm·m (mean ± S.D.); in adult pa-

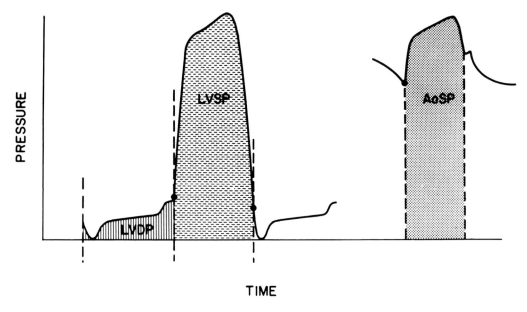

TIME

Fig. 20–5. Left ventricular (LV) and aortic (Ao) pressure tracings illustrate areas planimetered to measure LV mean systolic pressure (LVSP), mean diastolic pressure (LVDP), and aortic mean systolic pressure (AoSP). LVSP is the area contained under the LV pressure curve, bounded by perpendicular lines defining end-diastole and mitral valve opening; LVDP is the diastolic area similarly defined. AoSP is the area contained under the Ao pressure curve, bounded by perpendicular lines defining aortic valve opening and closure.

tients with dilated cardiomyopathy or heart failure from extensive prior myocardial infarction, LVSW is often less than 40 gm-m. Values less than 25 gm-m indicate severe LV systolic failure, and when LVSW is less than 20 gm·m, the prognosis is grave.

LVSW is a measure of total LV chamber function and can be considered to reflect myocardial contractility only when the ventricle is reasonably homogeneous in its composition, as in most patients with dilated cardiomyopathy. For patients with coronary artery disease and extensive myocardial infarction, LVSW may be depressed even though well perfused areas of the myocardium with normal contractility remain.

Ejection Phase Indices. LV systolic function can be assessed using only the volume data from the PV diagram. Thus, one of the most widely used indices of LV systolic performance is the *ejection fraction* (EF), which is defined as:

$$EF = (LVEDV - LVESV)/LVEDV \quad (3)$$

where LVEDV and LVESV are the LV end-diastolic and end-systolic volumes, respectively. In the cardiac catheterization laboratory, LVEF is most often derived from the LV angiogram, as discussed in Chapter 19. If the EF is divided by the ejection time (ET), measured from the aortic pressure tracing, the quotient is called *mean normalized systolic ejection rate (MNSER)*.

$$MNSER = \frac{(LVEDV - LVESV)}{(LVEDV)(ET)} \quad (4)$$

Finally, another ejection phase index of LV systolic function is velocity of circumferential fiber shortening, V_{CF}.[28,29] This is calculated as the rate of shortening of a theoretic LV myocardial fiber in a circumferential plane at the midpoint of the long axis of the ventricle. For convenience, mean V_{CF} is used most often, rather than instantaneous or peak V_{CF}. Mean V_{CF} is obtained as end-diastolic endocardial circumferential fiber length (πD_{ED}) minus end-systolic endocardial circumferential fiber length (πD_{ES}), divided by ET and normalized for end-diastolic circumferential fiber length:

$$V_{CF} = (\pi D_{ED} - \pi D_{ES})/\pi D_{ED}(ET)$$
$$= (D_{ED} - D_{ES})/D_{ED}(ET) \quad (5)$$

D_{ED} and D_{ES} are end-diastolic and end-systolic minor axis dimensions. Although V_{CF} can be calculated from angiographic data using the area-length method (D = 4 A/πL), it is most commonly calculated from values for D measured by M-mode echocardiography. Normal values for isovolumic and ejection phase indices are given in Table 20–2.

Ejection phase indices are obtained easily from LV angiography and can also be derived reliably from a variety of noninvasive techniques such as radionuclide ventriculography and echocardiography. The most widely used ejection phase index, the *ejection fraction*, is generally depressed when myocardial contractility is diminished. The ejection indices depend heavily, however, on preload and after-load and cannot be regarded as reliable indices of contractility in conditions associated with altered loading conditions. Thus, increases in preload cause the EF (and other ejection indices) to rise: consequently, left ventricular EF may be increased in patients with mitral or aortic regurgitation, severe anemia, or other causes of increased diastolic LV inflow and may mask underlying deterioration of myocardial contractility. Conversely, increases in afterload cause the EF to fall: consequently, left ventricular EF may be low in patients with severe aortic stenosis or other causes of increased resistance to systolic ejection and may falsely suggest underlying depression of myocardial contractility.

In actual practice, acute elevation of LV preload causes some increase in LV chamber size and aortic pressure, and these increases in afterload (systolic σ resisting shortening) tend to decrease the EF and other ejection indices, offsetting the rise in EF that a pure rise in preload would produce. Thus, Rankin and co-

Table 20–2. *Evaluation of Left Ventricular Systolic Performance: Normal Values for Some Isovolumic and Ejection Phase Indices*

Contractility Indices		Normal Values (mean ± S.D.)	References
Isovolumic Indices:			
Maximum dP/dt		1610 ± 290 mm Hg/sec	7
		1670 ± 320 mm Hg/sec	26
		1661 ± 323 mm Hg/sec	19
Maximum (dP/dt)/P)		44 ± 8.4 sec^{-1}	19
V_{PM} or peak $\left[\dfrac{dP/dt}{28P}\right]$		1.47 ± 0.19 ML/sec	26
dP/dt/DP at DP = 40 mm Hg		37.6 ± 12.2 sec^{-1}	19
Ejection Phase Indices:			
LVSW		81 ± 23 gm-m	6
LVSWI		53 ± 22 gm-m/M²	30 & 31, combined
		41 ± 12 gm-m/M²	32
EF	angio:	0.72 ± 0.08	33
MNSER	angio:	3.32 ± 0.84 EDV/sec	19
	echo:	2.29 ± 0.30 EDV/sec	34
Mean V_{CF}	angio:	1.83 ± 0.56 ED circ/sec	19
		1.50 ± 0.27 ED circ/sec	29
	echo:	1.09 ± 0.12 ED circ/sec	34

dP/dt = rate of rise of left ventricular (LV) pressure; DP = developed LV pressure; ML = muscle lengths; MNSER = mean normalized systolic ejection rate; ED = end-diastolic; V = volume; circ = circumference; EF = ejection fraction.

workers[34] produced changes in venous return by total body tilt in normal subjects: despite substantial changes in LV end-diastolic dimension and volume, there were no significant changes in EF, MNSER, or V_{CF}. Similarly, acute elevation of afterload by raising aortic pressure causes an increase in LVEDP, and the resultant rise in preload (end-diastolic fiber stretch) tends to increase the EF and other ejection indices, offsetting the fall in EF produced by a pure rise in afterload. These physiologic adjustments explain why the ejection indices are much more useful clinically than might be expected on the basis of studies in the isolated heart or muscle preparation.

An LV ejection fraction of less than 0.40 indicates depressed LV systolic pump function, and if there is no abnormal loading to account for it, an LVEF ≤ 0.40 can be taken to signify depressed myocardial contractility. An LVEF of <0.20 corresponds to severe depression of LV systolic performance and is usually associated with a poor prognosis. Interpretation of EF and other ejection indices is improved by consideration of the ventricular preload and afterload, and the latter are defined most precisely by end-diastolic and end-systolic wall stresses, respectively.

End-Systolic Pressure-Volume, and σ-Length Relations. Over the past 15 years, several groups have shown that the LV end-systolic pressure-volume, pressure-diameter, and σ-length relationships accurately reflect myocardial contractility, independent of changes in ventricular loading. This has been established in a series of studies in animals[35-43] and man.[44-50] The fundamental principle of end-systolic pressure-volume analysis is that at end-systole there is a single line relating LV chamber pressure to volume, unique for the level of contractility and independent of loading conditions. The LV end-systolic PV line can be generated by producing a series of PV loops (such as the one in Figure 20–4), over a range of loading conditions (Figs. 20–6 and 20–7). The line connecting the upper left hand corners of the individual PV diagrams is the end-systolic PV line, characterized by a slope and by an x-axis intercept, called V_0 (the extrapolated end-systolic volume when end-systolic pressure is zero). Current evidence indicates that an increase in contractility shifts the end-systolic PV line to the left with a steeper slope, and a depression in contractility is associated with a displacement of the line downward and to the right, with a reduced slope. While there is some uncertainty as to the meaning of V_0, it is agreed generally that an increase in slope of the end systolic PV line is a sensitive indicator of an increase in contractility. Unfortunately, the technique of end-systolic analysis may not be as useful in comparing one subject with another as in comparing values in one subject to those measured in the same subject after an intervention. The end-systolic PV lines for groups of patients with normal, intermediate, and depressed LV contractility are shown in Figure 20–8.

To measure the end-systolic PV line, one can use aortic dicrotic notch pressure as end-systolic LV pressure and minimum LV chamber volume as end-systolic volume. LV volume can be measured by angiography, using either direct LV injection or right-sided injection with image enhancement by digital subtraction angiography. Alternatively, LV volume can be measured by radionuclide techniques, ultrasonic techniques, or a specially designed impedance (conductance) catheter.[50-52]

The dP/dt_{MAX}–End-diastolic Volume Relationship. Little and co-workers[53,54] have examined the LV dP/dt_{MAX}-end diastolic volume relationship, and have proposed the slope of this relationship as an index of contractile state. They have shown that, on theoretic grounds, this relationship can be derived from the LV end-systolic pressure-volume relationship; both provide estimates of maximal myocardial elastance. This relationship is simpler to derive because both LV end-diastolic volume and dP/dt_{MAX} are more readily defined than either end-systolic pressure or volume. One does not need to be concerned about a lack of coincidence between end-systole and maximal elastance, as with the end-systolic pressure-volume relationship. The dP/dt_{MAX}-end diastolic volume relationship, however,

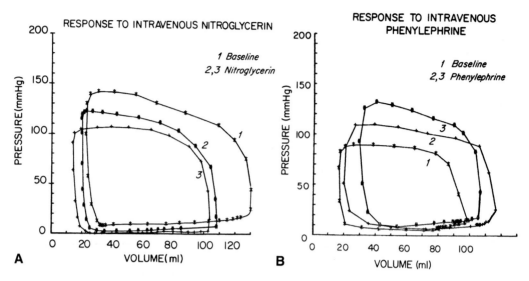

Fig. 20–6. Left ventricular (LV) pressure-volume plots constructed using radionuclide ventriculography to measure LV volume simultaneous with measurement of LV pressure during cardiac catheterization. (A) Three sequential plots measured during baseline and at two sequential doses of intravenous nitroglycerin to lower LV pressure. (B) Similar plots in a patient whose baseline LV systolic pressure was low: in this case phenylephrine was used in increasing doses to produce three levels of systolic loading. The upper left hand (end-systolic) corners of the three pressure-volume plots in each panel define a straight line, the LV end-systolic pressure-volume line. See text for discussion. (Reproduced, with permission, from McKay RG et al: Left ventricular pressure-volume diagrams and end-systolic pressure relations in human beings. J Am Coll Cardiol 3:301, 1984.)

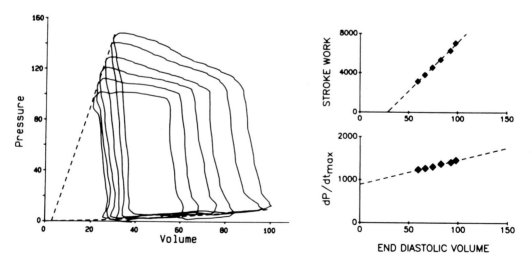

Fig. 20–7. The left panel shows LV pressure-volume loops obtained during rapid LV unloading achieved by IVC balloon occlusion in a patient undergoing cardiac catheterization. Volume was obtained using a conductance catheter technique. The right panels show relationships between stroke volume (upper right), LV dP/dt (lower right) and LV end-diastolic volume. (Reproduced, with permission, from Kass DA and Maughan WL: From E_{Max} to pressure-volume relations: A broader view. Circulation 77:1203–1212, 1988.)

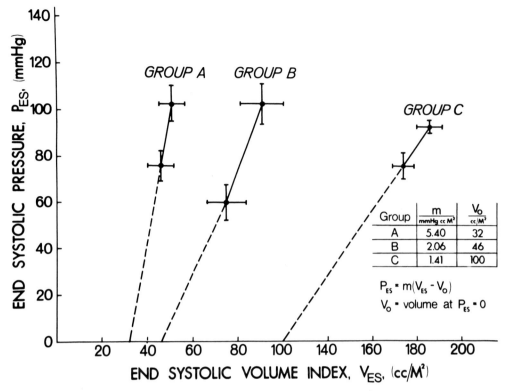

Fig. 20–8. Left ventricular end-systolic pressure (P_{ES}) plotted against end-systolic volume index (V_{ES}) at two levels of loading for each of 3 patient groups: Group A, patients with normal LV contractile function; Group B, patients with moderate depression of LV contractile performance; Group C, patients with marked depression of LV contractility. Depressed contractility shifts the $P_{ES} - V_{ES}$ relation to the right, with a reduced slope (m) and intercept (V_O) of the relation for each group. (Reproduced, with permission, from Grossman W, et al: Contractile state of the left ventricle in man as evaluated from end-systolic pressure relations. Circulation 45:845, 1977.)

has yet to be evaluated extensively in the clinical setting. Also, the end-systolic pressure-volume relationship can be estimated clinically using entirely noninvasive methods.[48,55] Nevertheless, the dP/dt$_{MAX}$-end-diastolic volume relationship represents an intriguing concept and may prove a valuable index of contractile state.

Stress-shortening Relations. Another approach to the assessment of LV systolic performance and myocardial contractility involves measuring the extent of cardiac muscle shortening and relating this shortening to the systolic wall stress (σ) resisting shortening.

If a ventricle is presented with progressively increasing resistance to ejection, σ rises while extent of myocardial shortening declines. Thus, a plot of systolic σ (horizontal axis) against myocardial shortening expressed as

EF, V_{CF}, or $\%\Delta D$ (vertical axis) yields a tight inverse relationship (Fig. 20–9). Data from studies of individual patients may then be compared with these normal values. In Figure 20–9, if the point relating end-systolic σ (σ_{ES}) and $\%\Delta D$ for a given patient lies within the confidence lines of the normal population, myocardial contractility is likely to be normal; however, if the σ_{ES}-$\%\Delta D$ point lies below the normal range, contractility is depressed even though $\%\Delta D$ may be normal. Figure 20–10 shows that the LV end-systolic wall stress–$\%\Delta D$ relationship is shifted upward by an increase in contractility resulting from a dobutamine infusion. One caution concerning the σ_{ES}-$\%\Delta D$ relationship is that it is preload-sensitive. That is, increases in preload will increase $\%\Delta D$ for any level of σ_{ES}. There is some evidence that when V_{CF} is substituted for

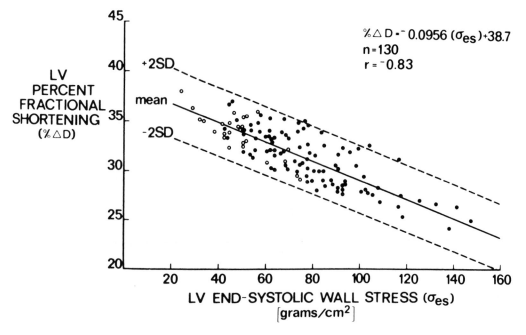

Fig. 20–9.   Relationship between LV end systolic wall stress (σ_{ES}) and % fractional shortening (%ΔD) measured by echo for 130 control points measured at rest (open circles) or during methoxamine infusion (closed circles). The inverse relationship defines normal LV myocardial contractility. (Reproduced, with permission, from Borow KM, et al: Left ventricular end-systolic stress-shortening and stress-length relations in humans. Am J Cardiol 50:1301, 1982.)

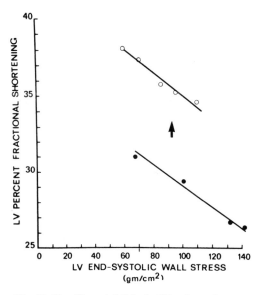

Fig. 20–10.   Upward shift in the LV end-systolic stress-shortening relation resulting from dobutamine infusion. See text. (Reproduced, with permission, from Borow KM, et al: Left ventricular end-systolic stress-shortening and stress-length relations in humans. Am J Cardiol 50:1301, 1982.)

%ΔD, the preload dependence of the stress-shortening relationship is attenuated or abolished.

Plots of systolic wall stress against LV ejection fraction have been analyzed for patients with a variety of conditions, including LV pressure overload (Fig. 20–11). In these plots, comprised of multiple individual data points (each point relating LV wall σ and EF for an individual patient) an inverse systolic σ-EF relationship is apparent for patients with chronic LV pressure-overload. This suggests that the depressed LVEF in some of these individuals is caused by excessive systolic σ; that is, the load resisting systolic shortening is abnormally high and is responsible for a reduced extent of shortening. This combination of high σ and low EF is sometimes referred to as "afterload mismatch"[56–58] and implies that hypertrophy has been inadequate to return systolic wall stress to its relatively low normal level. Patients in whom LVEF is diminished out of proportion to any increase in systolic wall stress can be assumed to have depressed myocardial contractility (Fig. 20–12).

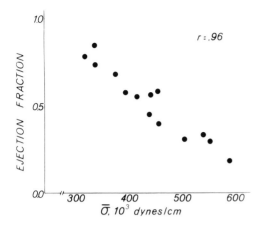

Fig. 20–11. Left ventricular (LV) ejection fraction plotted against mean systolic circumferential wall stress, $\bar{\sigma}$, for 14 patients with pure aortic stenosis (normal coronary arteries, no other valve disease) and varying degrees of LV decompensation. The inverse relationship is consistent with afterload excess as a principal cause of the decreased ejection fraction. (Reproduced, with permission, from Gunther S, Grossman W: Determinants of ventricular function in pressure-overload hypertrophy in man. Circulation 59:679, 1979.)

The advantage of σ-shortening analysis over PV diagram analysis is that wall σ takes into consideration changes in LV geometry and muscle mass that occur in response to chronic alterations in loading. Thus, a systolic pressure of 250 to 300 mm Hg imposed acutely on a normal left ventricular chamber would result in considerable reduction in LVEF, perhaps down to the 20 to 30% range. This change

occurs because, in the absence of any increase in LV wall thickness or decrease in chamber radius, systolic σ would more than double in response to such an acute pressure-overload, and this would lead to a major reduction in LVEF. If the increase in systolic pressure to 250 to 300 mm Hg occurs gradually, however, and is matched by the development of sufficient hypertrophy in the appropriate pattern, systolic wall σ remains normal and therefore fiber shortening and LVEF does not decrease. Thus, in the presence of significant hypertrophy and/or altered LV geometry, σ-shortening analysis may have considerable value.

DIASTOLIC FUNCTION

Left Ventricular Diastolic Distensibility: Pressure-Volume Relationship

As pointed out by Henderson in 1923: "In the heart, diastolic relaxation is a vital factor and not merely the passive stretching of a rubber bag. Being vital, it is variable."[59] Analysis of diastolic function today requires appreciation of the fact that diastolic compliance is variable and may change substantially in a given patient from one minute to the next. Diastolic function is summated physiologically in the relation between LV pressure and volume during diastole (Fig. 20–4, segment DA). Traditionally, an upward shift in this

Fig. 20–12. Plot of LV ejection fraction against systolic $\bar{\sigma}$, similar to Figure 20–11, but including patients with aortic stenosis (solid dots), dilated cardiomyopathy (crosses), and normal ventricular function (open squares). The regression line was constructed from the patients with normal LV function and those with aortic stenosis. See text for discussion. (Reprinted, with permission, from Gunther S, Grossman W: Determination of ventricular function in pressure overload hypertrophy in man. Circulation 5:679, 1979.)

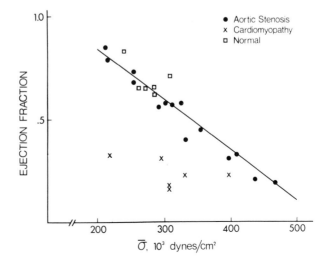

diastolic PV relation is regarded as indicating increased LV diastolic chamber *stiffness* and a downward shift indicates decreased stiffness or increased LV diastolic chamber *compliance*. In the terminology of physics and engineering, stiffness, and its opposite, compliance, relate a change in pressure (ΔP) to a change in volume (ΔV); therefore, some investigators have restricted these terms to refer to the *slope* of the diastolic PV relation. In this regard, as seen in segment DA of Figure 20–4, LV diastolic stiffness ($\Delta P/\Delta V$) is low early in diastole and rises steadily throughout diastolic filling.

Figure 20–13 shows theoretic LV diastolic PV plots for patients with normal, stiff, and compliant ventricular chambers. Several problems arise when stiffness and compliance are defined strictly in terms of the slope of the diastolic PV diagram, and these problems are illustrated in Figure 20–14. First, in some clinical conditions the LV diastolic PV plot may shift upward in a parallel fashion (e.g., during angina pectoris), without a noticeable change in slope. These patients have increased LV filling pressure, often with normal chamber volumes, and from a hydrodynamic point of view the LV chamber must be regarded as presenting increased resistance to diastolic filling. To say that LV diastolic stiffness and compliance are normal in such individuals because the upward shift has been a parallel one, without slope change, seems inappropriate. In some cases, patients may have a downward shift in the LV diastolic PV plot (e.g., following nitroprusside infusion in patients with heart failure) with an increase in the steepness of

the plot; again, to say that such patients exhibit increased LV diastolic stiffness seems inappropriate because they require a lower filling pressure to achieve the same diastolic chamber dimension and fiber stretch. Thus, the LV diastolic PV plot can show changes of two types: *displacement* or movement of the entire relationship upward, downward, or laterally, and *configuration change,* including change in curvature. In our studies, we have referred to upward or downward displacement changes as associated with a change in *ventricular distensibility.*[60] Thus, if the LV diastolic PV plot shifts upward, as is common during attacks of angina pectoris, we would say that the LV chamber has become *less distensible;* a higher diastolic pressure is required to fill or distend the chamber to its prior volume (Fig. 20–14). Similarly, a downward shift in the diastolic PV plot, as occurs commonly during nitroprusside infusion in patients with heart failure, would be said to indicate an increase in LV diastolic distensibility. The changes in curvature and/or configuration that may accompany these displacement changes are difficult to quantify and to interpret.[61]

Various formulae have been developed for analyzing the curvature of the LV diastolic PV plot.[62–67] These generally assume that the curvature is exponential, an assumption that is often but not always reasonable. Diastolic PV and P-segment length (SL) plots constructed from a series of *end*-diastolic points have been used in animal experiments to assess LV diastolic compliance,[66,68] and this technique is having its first application to clinical studies. When a series of end-diastolic PV or P-SL points are plotted, the relation is more strictly exponential, and application of mathematical models and analysis is more easily justified by the good agreement of measured data and mathematical predictions.

Factors that influence the position of the LV diastolic PV plot (that is, factors that influence LV diastolic *distensibility*) are listed in Table 20–3. Factors extrinsic to the LV chamber may influence the diastolic PV plot in striking fashion. Constrictive pericarditis and pericardial tamponade are associated with a striking up-

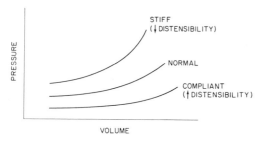

Fig. 20–13. Diagrammatic representation of ventricular diastolic pressure-volume relations for normal, stiff, and compliant ventricles. See text for discussion.

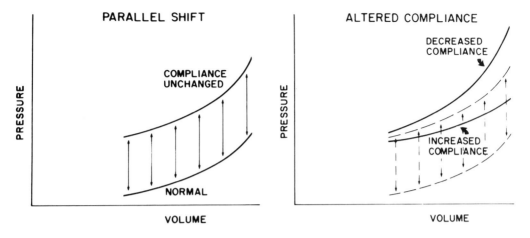

Fig. 20–14. Schematic illustration of the difference between diastolic distensibility and compliance. On the left, the ventricular diastolic pressure-volume relation has undergone a parallel upward shift. Distensibility is decreased (higher diastolic pressure required to fill the ventricle to the same chamber volume), although compliance, defined as the slope of the pressure-volume relation, is unchanged. On the right, superimposed on the parallel upward shift, are curves whose slopes are steeper (decreased compliance) or less steep (increased compliance) than either of the two parallel pressure-volume curves. This illustrates the importance of distinguishing distensibility from compliance because the curve labeled "increased compliance" nevertheless exhibits decreased diastolic distensibility in comparison to the normal pressure-volume relation. (Reproduced, with permission, from Grossman W: Relaxation and diastolic distensibility of the regionally ischemic left ventricle. In Grossman W, Lorell BH, eds.: Diastolic Relaxation of the Heart. Boston, Martinus Nijhoff Publishing, 1988, pp 193–203.)

Table 20–3. *Factors That Influence LV Diastolic Chamber Distensibility*

I. Factors extrinsic to the LV chamber
   A. Pericardial restraint
   B. Right ventricular loading
   C. Coronary vascular turgor (erectile effect)
   D. Extrinsic compression by tumor, pleural pressure, etc.

II. Factors intrinsic to LV chamber
   A. Passive elasticity of LV wall (stiffness or compliance when myocytes are completely relaxed)
     1. Thickness of LV wall
     2. Composition of LV wall (muscle, fibrosis, edema, amyloid, hemosiderin) including both endocardium and myocardium
     3. Temperature, osmolality
   B. Active elasticity of LV wall due to residual cross-bridge activation (cycling and/or latch state) through part or all of diastole:
     1. Slow relaxation affecting early diastole only
     2. Incomplete relaxation affecting early, mid- and end-diastolic distensibility
     3. Diastolic tone, contracture, or rigor
   C. Elastic recoil (diastolic suction)
   D. Viscoelasticity (stress relaxation, creep)

ward shift in the diastolic PV relation. In dogs with experimental tamponade, it has been shown that this upward shift is a *parallel* shift, without substantial change in curvature. When distended, the right ventricle can decrease LV diastolic distensibility by exerting an extrinsic pressure on the LV chamber in diastole through the shared interventricular septum, which may actually bulge into the LV chamber. Acute RV infarction causes dilatation of the RV chamber that, in the presence of an intact, previously unstressed pericardium, may lead to extrinsic compression of the LV in diastole with a hemodynamic pattern resembling cardiac tamponade.[69] The effect of increased RV loading on LV diastolic distensibility is an example of ventricular interaction, which is more prominent in the presence of an intact and relatively snug pericardium. In fact, in animal experiments it is difficult to demonstrate diastolic ventricular interaction once the pericardium has been opened wide.[67]

Coronary vascular turgor can influence LV diastolic chamber stiffness.[70] The LV wall has a rich blood supply, and engorgement of the capillaries and venules with blood makes the wall relatively stiff: for obvious reasons, this has been referred to as the erectile effect. While the erectile effect is probably not of much importance when coronary blood flow and pressure (the two components determining the degree of turgor) are in the physiologic range, a marked fall in coronary flow and pressure (as occurs distal to a coronary occlusion when collateral flow is poor or absent) is associated with a decrease in stiffness of the affected myocardium and an increase in LV diastolic distensibility.

Recent evidence[71] supports an important role for increased *coronary venous pressure* as a major determinant of coronary vascular turgor. Increases in right atrial pressure from 0 mm Hg to 15 mm Hg and 30 mm Hg led to substantial upward shifts in the LV end-diastolic PV relation that could not be attributed to right ventricular distension and a shift in the interventricular septum.

Extrinsic compression of the heart by tumor may cause decreased LV diastolic distensibility and may mimic cardiac tamponade. An example of this is presented in Chapter 35.

When an upward shift in the diastolic PV relation is present and the extrinsic factors listed in Table 20–3 cannot clearly explain the altered distensibility, a change in one of the intrinsic determinants of LV distensibility is likely to be present. Altered passive elasticity caused by amyloidosis, edema, or diffuse fibrosis may cause a restrictive cardiomyopathic pattern, with high LV diastolic pressure relative to volume in the presence of reasonably well-preserved systolic function. Clinically, heart failure may be present. Endomyocardial biopsy of RV or LV may be needed to establish the diagnosis (see Chapter 23).

Abnormal diastolic relaxation can cause the diastolic PV relation to shift upward strikingly. During angina pectoris, a 10 to 15 mm Hg rise in average LV diastolic pressure may occur with little or no change in diastolic volume; if this persists for a sufficient duration (≥10 to 20 minutes), pulmonary edema may occur. Such episodes of "flash pulmonary edema" in patients with essentially normal LV systolic function and normal LV chamber size gener-

ally indicate a large mass of ischemic myocardium[72] and suggest three-vessel or left main coronary obstruction. The decreased LV distensibility during ischemia may be prevented in many patients by a Ca^{++} channel blocking agent.[73] The mechanism of impaired myocardial relaxation during the ischemia of angina pectoris is not understood completely, but may be associated with diastolic Ca^{++} overload of the ischemic myocytes, in part due to ischemic dysfunction of the sarcoplasmic reticulum.[74] During the ischemia of acute coronary occlusion, an upward shift of the diastolic PV relation may occur if sufficient collateral blood flow is present to permit continued systolic contraction of the ischemic segment. If ischemia is sufficiently severe to cause complete akinesis of the affected myocardium, however, altered distensibility does not occur: "incomplete" relaxation can occur only in myocytes when there has been systolic cross-bridge activation. Also, the marked decrease in coronary vascular turgor distal to a coronary occlusion with poor or absent collaterals, together with local accumulation of H^+, contributes to an increase in regional distensibility, so that the net effect on the ventricular diastolic PV relation may be one of no change.

Impaired relaxation with decreased LV diastolic distensibility is also seen in patients with hypertrophic cardiomyopathy, and during angina pectoris in patients with aortic stenosis and normal coronary arteries.

Indices of LV Diastolic Relaxation Rate

There has been much attention to measures of LV diastolic relaxation during the isovolumic relaxation period and early diastolic filling. A listing of some of these indices and their normal values is given in Table 20–4. The time course of LV pressure decline following aortic valve closure is altered in conditions known to be associated with abnormalities of myocardial relaxation.

Isovolumic Pressure Decay. One of the simplest ways of quantifying the time course of LV pressure decline is to measure the maxi-

Table 20–4. *Evaluation of Left Ventricular Diastolic Performance: Normal Values for Some Indices of Relaxation and Filling*

	Normal Values	*Reference*
Peak $-dP/dt$	2660 ± 700 mm Hg/sec	7
	2922 ± 750 mm Hg/sec	89
	1864 ± 390 mm Hg/sec	90
	1825 ± 261 mm Hg/sec	91
T (logarithmic method, equation 7)	38 ± 7 msec	89
	33 ± 8 msec	90
	31 ± 3 msec	91
T (derivative method, equations 8 and 9)	55 ± 12 msec	91
	47 ± 10	92
P_B (derivative method, equations 8 and 9)	-25 ± 9 mm Hg	91
PFR	3.3 ± 0.6 EDV/sec	85
Time to PFR	136 ± 23 msec	85
Peak $-dh/dt$ (posterior wall)	8.4 ± 3.0 cm/sec	86
	8.2 ± 3.7 cm/sec	87

Peak $-dP/dt$ = maximum rate of LV isovolumic pressure decline; T = time constant of LV isovolumic relaxation, calculated assuming both zero pressure intercept (equation 7) and variable pressure (P_B) intercept (equations 8 and 9); PFR = LV peak filling rate, from radionuclide ventriculography, normalized to end-diastolic volumes (EDV)/sec; Peak $-dh/dt$ = maximum rate of posterior wall thinning, measured by echo.

mum rate of pressure fall, peak $-dP/dt$. Although peak $-dP/dt$ is altered by conditions that change myocardial relaxation, it is also altered by changes in loading conditions. For example, peak LV $-dP/dt$ increases (that is, rises in absolute value) when aortic pressure rises. Thus, an increase in LV $-dP/dt$ from -1500 mm Hg/sec to -1800 mm Hg/sec could be due to an increase in the rate of myocardial relaxation, a rise in aortic pressure, or both. An increase in peak $-dP/dt$ at a time when aortic pressure is unchanged or declining, however, signifies an improvement of LV relaxation. LV peak $-dP/dt$ is decreased during the myocardial ischemia of either angina pectoris or infarction, and is increased in response to beta adrenergic stimulation and the new bipyridine inotrope milrinone.[75] It is not increased by digitalis glycosides.

Time Constant of Relaxation. Because of the load dependency of peak $-dP/dt$, and the fact that it uses information from only 1 point on the LV pressure-time plot, other indices have been introduced that analyze the time course of LV isovolumic pressure fall more completely. In 1976, Weiss et al. introduced

the time constant T (or tau) of LV isovolumic pressure decline.[76] They pointed out that LV isovolumic pressure decline could be fit by the equation:

$$P = e^{At + B} \tag{6}$$

where P is LV isovolumic pressure, t is time after peak negative dP/dt, and A and B are constants. This can also be expressed as:

$$\ln P = At + B \tag{7}$$

A plot of ln LV pressure versus time allows calculation of the slope A, a negative number whose units are sec^{-1}. The time constant tau or T of isovolumic pressure fall is then defined as $-1/A$, expressed in milliseconds, and is the time that it takes P to decline $1/e$ of its value. Studies by the Johns Hopkins group have suggested that myocardial relaxation is normally complete by approximately 3.5 T after the onset of isovolumic relaxation. The normal value for T as calculated using a plot of LnP-versus-t is 25 to 40 msec in man. Thus, by 140 msec after the dicrotic notch, LV diastolic PV relations should be determined primarily by passive elastic properties of the myocardium. Because the normal LV diastolic filling period is >400 msec, it is unlikely, according to this concept, that late and end-diastolic PV relations are still influenced by the relaxation process. There is now considerable evidence, however, that even in the normal myocardium cross-bridge cycling persists to some extent throughout diastole. This resting myocardial activity or tone makes it difficult to know what significance to apply to the concept that relaxation is complete at 3.5 T. Nevertheless, it is important to emphasize that the relaxation process does progress with time through diastole, so that slowing of the process (prolongation of T) or shortening of the diastolic filling period (e.g., tachycardia) will result in a greater resistance to early and even late diastolic filling.

An approach to the measurement of T that has become more widely accepted uses a more general equation to describe LV isovolumic pressure decline:[77]

$$P = P_o e^{-t/T} + P_B \qquad (8)$$

In this formulation, if diastole were infinite in duration (t = ∞), P decays to a residual pressure P_B. In the initial formulation by Weiss et al.,[76] P always declines toward zero in long diastoles. The more general formula allows for 2 variables; tau or T (which equals $-1/A$) and P_B. Work by Carroll and coworkers,[78] as well other groups,[75] has shown that both P_B and T can vary with physiologic maneuvers (e.g., exercise, ischemia). The biologic meaning of P_B is uncertain, although there has been speculation that it may reflect the level of diastolic myocardial tone. A problem with both P_B and T is that there is experimental evidence that the speed of this relaxation process itself is altered by myofiber stretch that occurs after mitral valve opening.

When T is to be derived from the formulae that assume a variable pressure intercept (P_B), the calculation is often accomplished by taking the first derivative:[77]

$$P = P_o e^{-t/T} + P_B$$
$$\qquad (9)$$
$$dP/dt = -\frac{1}{T}(P - P_B)$$

Here, a plot of dP/dt vs (P − P_B) has the slope −1/T.

T may be prolonged from slow myocardial relaxation, but asynchrony of the relaxation process within the ventricular chamber will also result in a prolongation of T. In addition, T is probably not completely independent of loading conditions, although the influence of altered loading is relatively small.

Regional diastolic dysfunction may be difficult to assess solely by examination of a global parameter of LV diastolic function such as the time constant of relaxation. As has been pointed out by Pouleur,[79] the time course of LV isovolumic pressure decline underestimates the severity of regional impairment in the rate of relaxation. Thus, marked slowing of regional relaxation in an area of myocardial ischemia is partially masked by normal or enhanced rates of relaxation in adjacent normal regions of myocardium. Regional wall stress measurements are needed to assess regional rates of relaxation, and these can be made using knowledge of LV wall thickness and geometry.[80,81]

Peak Filling Rate. After mitral valve opening, ventricular filling usually proceeds briskly with an initial rapid filling phase, a middle slow filling phase, and a terminal increase in filling rate associated with atrial systole. The rapid filling phase may be characterized by a maximum or peak filling rate (PFR) and time to PFR. PFR is usually determined by plotting LV volume against time, fitting the initial portion of this plot after mitral valve opening to a third (or higher) order polynomial, and solving for the first derivative of this polynomial. LV volume for this calculation may be obtained from the LV cineangiogram, or from radionuclide techniques. As one might expect, PFR is preload-dependent: interventions that raise left atrial pressure increase PFR; interventions that reduce pulmonary venous return and left atrial pressure cause PFR to decrease.[82] An increase in PFR that occurs when LV filling pressure (pulmonary capillary wedge pressure, left atrial pressure, or LV diastolic pressure) is unchanged or falling can, however, reasonably be taken as an indication that LV relaxation has improved. Thus, PFR has been shown to decrease during angina pectoris[83] when LV filling pressure is increasing. Because the rise in LV filling pressure by itself would cause an increase in PFR, the fall in PFR that is actually observed most likely indicates slowed relaxation of the myocardium, consistent with the other findings in this condition (fall in peak negative dP/dt, prolongation of T) suggesting impaired relaxation of the ischemic myocardium. PFR is reduced in patients with coronary stenoses, even in the absence of overt ischemia, and improves after coronary angioplasty.[84] PFR is also reduced in patients with hypertrophic cardiomyopathy and improves after administration of a calcium-blocking agent.[85] PFR is usually normalized for end-diastolic volume (EDV) and expressed as EDV/sec. Thus, cardiac dilatation by itself tends to depress PFR, exaggerating its preload dependence.

Rate of Wall Thinning. Another index of diastolic function, similar in some ways to PFR, is the peak rate of diastolic LV wall thinning. This can be measured echocardiographically by plotting posterior or septal wall thickness against time, fitting the data to a polynomial, and taking the first derivative.[86-88] The posterior wall thickness, h, and its first derivative, dh/dt, reflect regional diastolic function of the posterior wall myocardium. An advantage of peak negative dh/dt as opposed to PFR is that peak negative dh/dt assesses regional myocardial function whereas PFR describes behavior for the whole ventricle and is insensitive when equal and opposite changes in diastolic function are occurring in different parts of the LV chamber. Peak negative dh/dt decreases during angina, even though LV filling pressure rises.[88]

Various other indices of diastolic myocardial relaxation have been proposed. Most are imperfect, as are the ones discussed above. Important information about diastolic relaxation and distensibility can, however, usually be gleaned from examination of the parameters discussed in this chapter, taken in the context of the clinical setting and other hemodynamic findings in an individual patient.

REFERENCES

1. Parmley WW, Chuck L: Length-dependent changes in myocardial contractile state. Am J Physiol 224:1194, 1973.
2. Lakatta EG: Starling's Law of the Heart is explained by an intimate interaction of muscle length and myofilament calcium activation. J Am Coll Cardiol 10:1157, 1987.
3. Lew WYW: Time-dependent increase in left ventricular contractility following acute volume loading in the dog. Circ Res 63:635, 1988.
4. Wiggers CJ: Studies on the cardiodynamic actions of drugs. I. The application of the optical methods of pressure registration in the study of cardiac stimulants and depressants. J Pharmacol Exp Ther 30:217, 1927.
5. Gleason WL, Braunwald E: Studies on the first derivative of the ventricular pressure pulse in man. J Clin Invest 41:80–91, 1962.
6. Grossman W, et al: Changes in inotropic state of the left ventricle during isometric exercise. Br Heart J 35:697, 1973.
7. McLaurin LP, Rolett EL, Grossman W: Impaired left ventricular relaxation during pacing induced ischemia. Am J Cardiol 32:751, 1973.
8. Feldman MD, et al: Depression of systolic and diastolic myocardial reserve during atrial pacing tachycardia in patients with dilated cardiomyopathy. J Clin Invest 82:1661, 1988.
9. Mason DT, Braunwald E: Studies on digitalis. IX. Effects of ouabain on the nonfailing human heart. J Clin Invest 42:1105, 1963.
10. Grossman W, et al: Alterations in preload and myocardial mechanics. Circ Res 31:83, 1972.
11. Brodie BR, Grossman W, Mann T, McLaurin LP: Effects of sodium nitroprusside on left ventricular diastolic pressure-volume relations. J Clin Invest 59:59, 1977.
12. Wallace AG, Skinner NS, Mitchell JH: Hemodynamic determinants of the maximal rate of rise of left ventricular pressure. Am J Physiol 205:30, 1963.
13. Zimpfer M, Vatner SF: Effects of acute increases in left ventricular preload on indices of myocardial function in conscious, unrestrained and intact, tranquilized baboons. J Clin Invest 67:430, 1981.
14. Broughton A, Korner PI: Steady-state effects of preload and afterload on isovolumic indices of contractility in autonomically blocked dogs. Cardiovasc Res 14:245, 1980.
15. Barnes GE, Horwitz LD, Bishop VS: Reliability of the maximum derivatives of left ventricular pressure and internal diameter as indices of the inotropic state of the depressed myocardium. Cardiovasc Res 13:652, 1979.
16. Gersh BJ, Hahn CEW, Prys-Roberts C: Physical criteria for measurement of left ventricular pressure and its first derivative. Cardiovasc Res 5:32, 1971.
17. Fifer MA, et al: Myocardial contractile function in aortic stenosis as determined from the rate of stress development during isovolumic systole. Am J Cardiol 44:1318, 1979.
18. Arentzen CE, et al: Force-frequency characteristics of the left ventricle in the conscious dog. Circ Res 42:64, 1978.
19. Peterson KL, et al: Comparison of isovolumic and ejection phase indices of myocardial performance in man. Circulation 49:1088, 1974.
20. Grossman W, et al: New technique for determining

instantaneous myocardial force-velocity relations in the intact heart. Circ Res 28:290, 1971.

21. Mirsky I, Pasternac A, Ellison RC: General index for the assessment of cardiac function. Am J Cardiol 30:483, 1972.

22. Falsetti HL, Mates RE, Green DG, Bunnel IL: V_{max} as an index of contractile state in man. Circulation 43:467, 1971.

23. Mason DT: Usefulness and limitations of the rate of rise of intraventricular pressure (dp/dt) in the evaluation of myocardial contractility in man. Am J Cardiol 23:516, 1969.

24. Mehmel H, Krayenbuehl HP, Rutishauser W: Peak measured velocity of shortening in the canine left ventricle. J Appl Physiol 29:637, 1970.

25. Stein PD, McBride GG, Sabbah NH: The fractional rate of change of ventricular power during isovolumic contraction. Derivation of haemodynamic terms and studies in dogs. Cardiovasc Res 9:456, 1975.

26. Krayenbuehl HP, et al: High-fidelity left ventricular pressure measurements for the assessment of cardiac contractility in man. Am J Cardiol 31:415, 1973.

27. Sonnennblick EH, Parmley WW, Urschel CW: The contractile state of the heart as expressed by force-velocity relations. Am J Cardiol 23:488, 1969.

28. Paraskos JA, et al: A non-invasive technique for the determination of velocity of circumferential fiber shortening in man. Circ Res 29:610, 1971.

29. Karliner JS, et al: Mean velocity of fiber shortening. A simplified measure of left ventricular myocardial contractility. Circulation 44:323, 1971.

30. Ross J Jr, et al: Left ventricular performance during muscular exercise in patients with and without cardiac dysfunction. Circulation 34:597, 1966.

31. Ross J Jr, Braunwald E: The study of left ventricular function in man by increasing resistance to ventricular ejection with angiotensin. Circulation 29:739, 1964.

32. McLaurin LP, et al: A new technique for the study of left ventricular pressure-volume relations in man. Circulation 48:56, 1973.

33. Wynne J, et al: Estimation of left ventricular volumes in man from biplane cineangiograms filmed in oblique projections. Am J Cardiol 41:726, 1978.

34. Rankin LS, Moos S, Grossman W: Alterations in preload and ejection phase indices of left ventricular performance. Circulation 51:910, 1975.

35. Suga H, Sagawa K, Shoukas AA: Load independence of the instantaneous pressure-volume ratio of the canine left ventricle and effects of epinephrine and heart rate on the ratio. Circ Res 32:314, 1973.

36. Weber KT, Janicki JS, Reeves RC, Hefner LL: Factors influencing left ventricular shortening in isolated canine heart. Am J Physiol 230:419, 1976.

37. Maughan WL, Sunagawa K, Burkhoff D, et al: Effect of heart rate on the canine end-systolic pressure-volume relationship. Circulation 72:654, 1985.

38. Kass DA, Yamazaki T, Burkhoff D, et al: Determination of left ventricular end-systolic pressure-volume relationships by the conductance (volume) catheter technique. Circulation 73:586, 1986.

39. Burkhoff D, Sugiura S, Yue DT, Sagawa K: Contractility-dependent curvilinearity of end-systolic pressure-volume relations. Am J Physiol 252:H1218, 1987.

40. McKay RG, Miller MJ, Ferguson JJ, et al: Assessment of left ventricular end-systolic pressure-volume relations with an impedance catheter and transient inferior vena cava occlusion: Use of this system in the evaluation of the cardiotonic effects of dobuta-

mine, milrinone, posicor and epinephrine. J Am Coll Cardiol 8:1152, 1986.

41. Mirsky I, Tajimi T, Peterson KL: The development of the entire end-systolic pressure-volume and ejection fraction-afterload relations: A new concept of systolic myocardial stiffness. Circulation 76:343, 1987.

42. Wisenbaugh T, Yu G, Evans J: The superiority of maximum fiber elastance over maximum stress-volume ratio as an index of contractile state. Circulation 72:648, 1985.

43. Sagawa K, Suga H, Shoukas AA, Bakalar KM: End-systolic pressure/volume ratio: A new index of ventricular contractility. Circulation 63:1223, 1981.

44. Grossman W, et al: Contractile state of the left ventricle in man as evaluated from end-systolic pressure-volume relations. Circulation 45:845, 1977.

45. McKay RG, Aroesty JM, Heller GV, et al: Assessment of the end-systolic pressure-volume relationship in human beings with the use of a time-varying elastance model. Circulation 74:97, 1986.

46. Aroney CN, Herrmann HC, Semigran M, et al: Linearity of the left ventricular end-systolic pressure-volume relation in patients with severe heart failure. J Am Coll Cardiol 14:127, 1989.

47. Starling MR, Walsh RA, Dell'Italia LJ, et al: The relationship of various measures of end-systole to left ventricular maximum time-varying elastance in man. Circulation 76:32, 1987.

48. Borow KM, Neumann A, Wynne J: Sensitivity of end-systolic pressure-dimension and pressure-volume relations to the inotropic state in humans. Circulation 65:988, 1982.

49. Konstam MA, Cohen SR, Salem DN, et al: Comparison of left and right ventricular end-systolic pressure-volume relations in congestive heart failure. J Am Coll Cardiol 5:1326, 1985.

50. Kass DA, Maughan WL: From 'Emax' to pressure-volume relations: A broader view. Circulation 77:1203, 1988.

51. Kass DA, Midei M, Graves W, et al: Use of a conductance (volume) catheter and transient inferior vena caval occlusion for rapid determination of pressure-volume relationships in man. Cathet Cardiovasc Diagn 15:192, 1988.

52. McKay RG, et al: Instantaneous measurement of left and right ventricular stroke volume and pressure-volume relationships with an impedance catheter. Circulation 69:703, 1984.

53. Little WC: The left ventricular dP/dt_{MAX}-end-diastolic volume relation in closed-chest dogs. Circ Res 56:808, 1985.

54. Little WC, Park RC, Freeman GL: Effects of regional ischemia and ventricular pacing on LV dP/dt_{MAX}-end diastolic volume relation. Am J Physiol 252:H993, 1987.

55. Marsh JD, Green LH, Wynne J, Cohn WF, Grossman W: Left ventricular end-systolic pressure-dimension and stress-length relations in normal human subjects. Am J Cardiol 44:1311, 1979.

56. Ross J Jr: Afterload mismatch and preload reserve: a conceptual framework for the analysis of ventricular function. Progr Cardiovasc Dis 18:255, 1976.

57. Gunther S, Grossman W: Determinants of ventricular function in pressure-overload hypertrophy in man. Circulation 59:679, 1979.

58. Grossman W: Cardiac hypertrophy: Useful adaptation or pathologic process? Am J Med 69:576, 1980.

59. Henderson Y: Volume changes of the heart. Physiol Rev 3:165, 1923.

60. Grossman W: Relaxation and diastolic distensibility of the regionally ischemic left ventricle. In Grossman W, Lorell BH, eds: Diastolic Relaxation of the Heart. Basic Research and Current Applications for Clinical Cardiology. Boston, Martinus Nijhoff Publishing, 1987, pp 193–203.

61. Glantz SA: Computing indices of diastolic stiffness has been counterproductive. Fed Proc 39:162, 1980.

62. Zile MR: Diastolic dysfunction: detection, consequences, and treatment. Part 1: Definition and determinants of diastolic function. Modern Concepts of Cardiovascular Disease 58:67, 1989.

63. McPherson DD, Skorton DJ, Kodiyalam S, et al: Finite element analysis of myocardial diastolic function using three-dimensional echocardiographic reconstructions: Application of a new method for study of acute ischemia in dogs. Circ Res 60:674, 1987.

64. Gaasch WH, et al: Left ventricular stress and compliance in man. With special reference to normalized ventricular function curves. Circulation 45:746, 1972.

65. Mirsky I: Assessment of diastolic function: suggested methods and future considerations. Circulation 69:836, 1984.

66. Rankin JS, et al: Viscoelastic properties of the diastolic left ventricle in the conscious dog. Circ Res 41:37, 1977.

67. Glantz SA, et al: The pericardium substantially affects the left ventricular diastolic pressure-volume relationship in the dog. Circ Res 42:433, 1978.

68. Momomura SI, Bradley AB, Grossman W: Left ventricular diastolic pressure-segment length relations and end-diastolic distensibility in dogs with coronary stenoses: an angina physiology model. Circ Res 55:203, 1984.

69. Lorell BH, et al: Right ventricular infarction. Clinical diagnosis and differentiation from cardiac tamponade and constriction. Am J Cardiol 43:465, 1979.

70. Vogel WM, et al: Acute alterations in left ventricular diastolic chamber stiffness. Role of the "erectile" effect of coronary arterial pressure and flow in normal and damaged hearts. Circ Res 51:465, 1982.

71. Watanabe J, Levine MJ, Bellotto F, et al: Effects of coronary venous pressure on left ventricular diastolic chamber distensibility. Circ Res (in press).

72. McKay RG, et al: The pacing thallium test reexamined: Correlation of pacing-induced hemodynamic changes with the amount of myocardium at risk. J Am Coll Cardiol 3:1469, 1984.

73. Lorell BH, Turi Z, Grossman W: Modification of left ventricular response to pacing tachycardia by nifedipine in patients with coronary artery disease. Am J Med 71:667, 1981.

74. Paulus WJ, Serizawa T, Grossman W: Altered left ventricular diastolic properties during pacing-induced ischemia in dogs with coronary stenosis. Potentiation by caffeine. Circ Res 50:218, 1982.

75. Monrad ES, et al: Improvements in indices of diastolic performance in patients with congestive heart failure treated with milrinone. Circulation 70:1030, 1984.

76. Weiss JL, Frederiksen JW, Weisfeldt ML: Hemodynamic determinants of the time-course of fall in canine left ventricular pressure. J Clin Invest 58:751, 1976.

77. Raff GL, Glantz SA: Volume loading slows left ventricular isovolumic relaxation rate. Circ Res 48:813, 1981.

78. Carroll JD, Hess OM, Hirzel HO, Krayenbuehl HP: Exercise-induced ischemia: The influence of altered relaxation on early diastolic pressure. Circulation 67:521, 1983.

79. Pouleur H, Rousseau M: Regional diastolic dysfunction in coronary artery disease: clinical and therapeutic implications. In Grossman W, Lorell BH, eds: Diastolic Relaxation of the Heart. Basic Research and Current Applications for Clinical Cardiology. Boston, Martinus Nijhoff Publishing, 1987, pp 245–254.

80. Pouleur H, Rousseau M, van Eyll C, et al: Impaired regional diastolic distensibility in coronary artery disease. Relations with dynamic left ventricular compliance. Am Heart J 112:721, 1986.

81. Pouleur H, Rousseau M, van Eyll C, Charlier AA: Assessment of regional left ventricular relaxation in patients with coronary artery disease: Importance of geometric factors and changes in wall thickness. Circulation 69:696, 1984.

82. Chong CY, Herrmann HC, Weyman AE, Fifer MA: Preload dependence of Doppler-derived indexes of left ventricular diastolic function in humans. J Am Coll Cardiol 10:800, 1987.

83. Aroesty JM, McKay RG, Heller GV, et al: Simultaneous assessment of left ventricular systolic and diastolic dysfunction during pacing-induced ischemia. Circulation 71:889, 1985.

84. Bonow RO, et al: Improved left ventricular diastolic filling in patients with coronary artery disease after percutaneous transluminal coronary angioplasty. Circulation 66:1159, 1982.

85. Bonow RO, et al: Effects of verapamil on left ventricular systolic function and diastolic filling in patients with hypertrophic cardiomyopathy. Circulation 64:787, 1981.

86. Mason SJ, et al: Exercise echocardiography: Detection of wall motion abnormalities during ischemia. Circulation 59:50, 1979.

87. St. John Sutton MG, Tajik AJ, Smith HC, Ritman EL: Angina in idiopathic hypertrophic subaortic stenosis. Circulation 61:561, 1980.

88. Bourdillon PD, et al: Increased regional myocardial stiffness of the left ventricle during pacing-induced angina in man. Circulation 76:316, 1983.

89. Pouleur H, et al: Force-velocity-length relations in hypertrophic cardiomyopathy: evidence of normal or depressed myocardial contractility. Am J Cardiol 52:813, 1983.

90. Hirota Y: A clinical study of left ventricular relaxation. Circulation 62:756, 1980.

91. Thompson DS, et al: Analysis of left ventricular pressure during isovolumic relaxation in coronary artery disease. Circulation 65:690, 1982.

92. Nonogi H, Hess OM, Bortone AS, et al: Left ventricular pressure-length relation during exercise-induced ischemia. J Am Coll Cardiol 13:1062, 1989.

Part VI

Special Catheter Techniques

21

Evaluation of Myocardial Blood Flow and Metabolism

ARLENE B. LEVINE and DONALD S. BAIM

Over the past three decades, numerous techniques have been developed to measure coronary blood flow in man. These methods have yielded valuable information about the regulation of coronary blood flow in clinical settings, and about coronary dynamics during and after various coronary interventions.

Presently, in most cases, decisions on therapy are based on the visual estimation of stenosis severity on the coronary angiogram, in conjunction with an assessment of regional myocardial wall motion. The marked intraobserver and interobserver variability in the visual estimation of stenosis severity is well known[1] (See Chapter 13). Even quantitative coronary angiography with computer-assisted determination of vessel cross-sectional area may not be helpful in the presence of angiographically inapparent diffuse coronary atherosclerosis. Finally, mechanical myocardial dysfunction does not necessarily imply metabolic inactivity and myocardial nonviability. It is thus evident that more information is needed to direct interventional approaches appropriately for optimal patient benefit.

REGULATION OF CORONARY BLOOD FLOW IN HUMANS

Coronary arterial flow may be expressed as the ratio between *transmyocardial perfusion pressure* (PP) and *coronary vascular resistance* (CVR). In patients with normal left ventricular filling pressures, average coronary driving pressure approximates mean aortic pressure (MAP), but the presence of elevated ventricular filling pressures causes MAP to overestimate the true perfusion pressure. One of two corrections may be in order. First, because the coronary sinus drains into the right atrium, perfusion pressure may be corrected for elevations in right atrial pressure (RAP) (i.e., PP = MAP − RAP).[3] Alternatively, because elevations in left ventricular filling pressure raise intramyocardial pressures and the measured zero flow pressure (P_{zf}) (Fig. 21–1),[4] perfusion pressure can be corrected by subtracting the pulmonary capillary wedge pressure (PCWP) (i.e., PP = MAP − PCWP), even though true P_{zf} cannot be measured clinically.

For the sake of simplicity, coronary vascular resistance may be considered as the sum of three distinct components, R_1, R_2, and R_3.[12] R_1 represents the resistance to flow in the larger epicardial coronary vessels, conduit vessels that function primarily as vascular capacitors and contribute only minimally to total coronary vascular resistance in the absence of fixed or dynamic epicardial stenoses. R_2 results from arteriolar smooth muscle tone, and

343

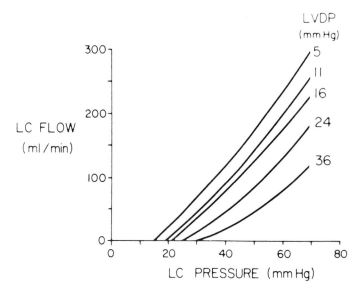

Fig. 21–1. Capacitance-free left circumflex coronary artery (LC) pressure-flow relationships at increasing preload in the dog heart. As left ventricular diastolic pressure (LVDP) increases from 5 to 36 mm Hg, the LC perfusion pressure at which flow ceases rises from 15 to 30 mm Hg. (From Aversano T, et al: Preload-induced alterations in capacitance-free diastolic pressure-flow relationships. Am J Physiol 246:H410, 1984, with permission.)

is normally the major component of coronary vascular resistance. R_3 results from external compression on intramural coronary vessels during ventricular contraction, which reduces systolic relative to enhanced diastolic coronary blood flow.

Changes in epicardial or arteriolar coronary resistances during physiologic or pharmacologic stimuli can be considered either "primary" or "secondary" vasomotive events (Fig. 21–2). *Primary* vasomotion signifies an alteration in myocardial vessel tone and perfusion with no change in myocardial oxygen demand. *Secondary* vasomotion refers to changes in vessel tone and blood flow in response to alterations in myocardial oxygen consumption.[5]

The myocardium relies almost exclusively on oxidative metabolism for its energy needs. Even at rest, transmyocardial oxygen extraction is near maximal, with resting coronary venous oxygen saturations the lowest in the body (typically as low as 25% to 35%).[6] Changes in myocardial oxygen demand can thus be met only by proportional alterations in myocardial blood flow, mediated by changes in local coronary arteriolar tone, R_2. These adjustments in coronary arteriolar resistance underlie the phenomenon of myocardial "autoregulation," the ability of the coronary circulation to maintain flow constant in the face of varying coronary perfusion pressure.[7]

"Coronary vasodilator reserve" or "flow reserve" refers to the ability of a coronary bed to increase coronary blood flow after release of a transient coronary occlusion or in response to various pharmacologic stimuli[8] that produce maximal reduction in the R_2 resistance. Flow reserve can be expressed as the ratio of *maximal* to *resting* coronary flow, and averages 4 to 7 in both experimental animals and man. This large vasodilator reserve explains why coronary "autoregulation" can maintain resting myocardial flow at normal levels despite the presence of increasingly severe coronary obstruction, though this maintenance of resting flow takes place at the expense of subsequent ability to increase flow in response to stress. Only at critical stenosis severity (>90% diameter reduction) does resting coronary flow fall, once all available coronary reserve has been exhausted.[9–10] This reciprocal relationship between stenosis and available flow reserve can thus be used to assess the effective physiologic severity of any given coronary lesion.

Measured coronary flow reserve is a function of the position of the pressure-flow relationship at maximal vasodilation, the coronary perfusion pressure, and basal coronary flow before maximal vasodilation (Fig. 21–3). Al-

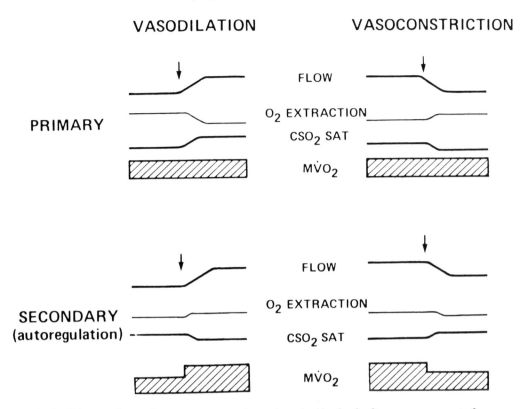

Fig. 21–2. Primary and secondary coronary vasomotion as determined by the simultaneous measurement of coronary blood flow (FLOW) and coronary venous oxygen saturation (CSO₂ SAT). Primary vasodilation causes a rise in flow at constant myocardial oxygen consumption (MVO₂), resulting in lower transmyocardial oxygen extraction. In contrast, in secondary coronary vasodilation, an increase in myocardial oxygen consumption obliges a secondary rise in coronary blood flow with either constant or reduced coronary sinus oxygen saturation. (From Baim DS, Rothman MT, and Harrison DC: Simultaneous measurement of coronary venous blood flow and oxygen saturation during transient alterations in myocardial oxygen supply and demand. Am J Cardiol 49:743, 1982, with permission.)

terations in intramyocardial pressures alter the maximally vasodilated pressure-flow relationship and affect flow reserve measurements. For any given pressure-flow relationship, maximally achievable coronary flow is a linear function of central aortic pressure, and flow reserve varies with perfusion pressure. Because coronary reserve flow represents the ratio of maximal over basal flow, it is affected by the level of basal coronary flow. Increases in resting flow thus tend to lower the apparent reserve ratio in the absence of any other alterations.

MYOCARDIAL METABOLISM

Myocardial metabolism links regional blood flow to mechanical function by means of the transport of oxygen, glucose, free fatty acids, lactate, amino acids, and ketones, which act as substrates for the generation of high-energy phosphates (ATP and creatine phosphate).[11] These high-energy phosphates are used to supply the energy requirements of the myocardium as determined by *tension development* during ventricular contraction, including the rate of force development and the frequency of force generation per unit time (which accounts for approximately 60% of energy utilization), *myocardial relaxation* (which accounts for approximately 15% of energy utilization), *electrical activity* (3 to 5%), and *basal cellular maintenance* and "wear and tear" (20% of energy utilization).[12] At higher workloads, myocardial contractile function clearly consumes an even greater fraction of

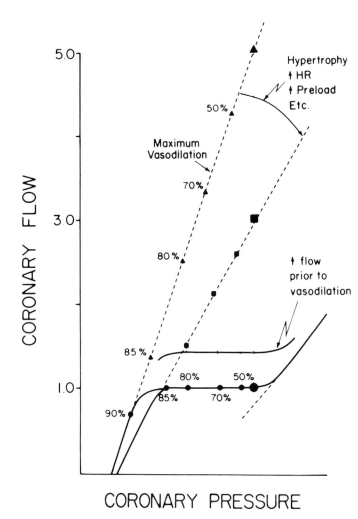

Fig. 21–3. Resting and maximally vasodilated coronary pressure-flow relationships. Coronary flow reserve, the ratio of maximally vasodilated over resting flow, can be seen to be a complex function of the actual position of the maximally vasodilated and resting flow curves. (From Klocke FJ: Measurements of coronary flow reserve: Defining pathophysiology versus making decisions about patient care. Circulation 76:1183, 1987, with permission.)

high-energy phosphate availability. Because myocardial cellular survival is the highest priority, outranking all other mechanical or electrical tasks, however, any compromise in substrate supply causes the myocardium to minimize its energy expenditure on mechanical work and use remaining high-energy substrates for the continued maintenance of cellular integrity. Clearly, neither the assessment of myocardial blood flow nor the measurement of myocardial mechanical function alone can provide reliable information about the residual myocardial viability.

Under normal aerobic conditions, several substrates are used simultaneously to meet myocardial energy needs: free fatty acids (65%), glucose (15%), lactate and pyruvate (12%), and amino acids (5%).[24,25] Under aerobic conditions, glycolysis plays only a minor role, with lactate extracted by the myocardium, converted into pyruvate, and oxidized by way of the Krebs cycle.[13]

In the fasting state, when serum fatty acids are high, myocardial glucose uptake is suppressed by fatty acid utilization. After an oral glucose load, however, or when a fall in myocardial blood flow and oxygen supply leads to a reduction and loss in mechanical function, glucose uptake is enhanced and fatty acid oxidation declines.[13] Glucose metabolism is initially aerobic, but as decreasing oxygen availability depletes high-energy phosphate stores, ADP, AMP, and other nucleosides accumulate. These ATP breakdown products enhance glycogenolysis and glycolysis to augment ATP production. This causes generation of pyruvate, which shifts the pyruvate-lactate equilibrium toward lactate formation, causing net transmyocardial lactate *production* rather than *extraction*. Under extreme conditions, increasing cytosolic lactate and hydrogen ion concentrations lead to further inhibition of residual glycolysis, and deprive the cell of even anaerobic ATP production, a sequence of biochemical events that may lead to complete cessation of energy production with irreversible cellular injury.

METHODS OF CORONARY FLOW MEASUREMENT

There are three basic approaches to the evaluation of myocardial blood flow and/or metabolism: measurement of *epicardial* coronary blood flow, assessment of *myocardial tissue perfusion* or metabolism, and measurement of *coronary venous flow*. The ideal coronary flow measurement technique would provide low risk for the patient; be simple, rapid, and reproducible to perform and absolute and linear over the physiologically relevant range of flows; and allow assessment of regional myocardial blood flow to the subendocardium as well as subepicardium. Such a method has yet to be devised, but the strengths and weaknesses of the currently available techniques are described below.

Epicardial Blood Flow Velocity

Doppler Velocity Probes. The Doppler flow meter is based on the principle that sound waves reflected from moving particles (e.g., red blood cells) undergo a shift in frequency which is linearly proportional to the particle velocity. A single piezoelectric crystal is mounted at or near the tip of a 3 Fr catheter, and placed subselectively into the coronary circulation over a 0.014″ guide wire (Millar Instruments, Houston, TX) (Fig. 21–4). The piezoelectric crystal is connected to the 20 MHz pulsed Doppler processor by means of two copper wires that run the length of the catheter

and allow the same transducer to both emit and receive the reflected soundwaves. The magnitude of the Doppler shift is then determined electronically, providing an output signal proportional to the instantaneous phasic blood flow velocity.[14,15]

The Doppler method has undergone extensive animal validation studies comparing it to timed venous coronary sinus collection, labeled microsphere, and electromagnetic flow probe techniques. Doppler measurements linearly reflect changes in flow over the entire physiologic range. They do not appear to be distorted significantly by the size of the transducing catheter,[16] but reproducible Doppler flow measurements do require careful and stable positioning of the Doppler catheter tip coaxially and centrally within the arterial lumen. The velocity probe should be placed beyond any major branches that arise proximal to the stenosis of interest. Care needs to be taken to avoid impairment of maximal coronary flow from guiding catheter obstruction, and to avoid mechanically induced epicardial coronary spasm intracoronary nitroglycerin should be administered before flow measurements. Nitroglycerin administration also minimizes potential variations in epicardial coronary diameter that might otherwise allow changes in volume flow not reflected in velocity changes. Intracoronary guide wire and catheter manipulations warrant the same level of systemic anticoagulation as is customary for coronary angioplasty procedures.

Although Doppler measurement of *absolute* coronary volume flow would require quantitative assessment of the arterial cross-sectional area, the Doppler technique is customarily used to measure relative changes in flow during the determination of the coronary reserve flow ratio. In the clinical setting, flow reserve is considered normal if it exceeds 3.5:1.[9] Maximal flow can be stimulated with *adenosine*, but the unpredictability of the dose required and associated bradyarrhythmias limit its clinical usefulness.[17] Intracoronary *papaverine* has been used widely and safely, although it may rarely cause QT interval prolongation and ventricular tachycardia.[18–19] The typical dose

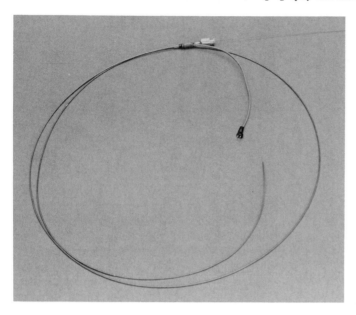

Fig. 21–4. 3 F Millar Mikro-tip disposable Doppler catheter with end-mounted 20 MHz crystal and central guide wire lumen (0.014″).

of intracoronary papaverine is 8 mg for the right coronary artery and 12 mg for the left coronary artery, producing a reproducible peak flow effect within 25 seconds that lasts for up to 2 minutes. It typically causes only a minimal decline in systemic arterial pressure with no appreciable change in heart rate, and is thus safe and useful in the assessment of coronary vascular reserve. Other vasodilator agents have been used: intravenous dipyridamole in adequate dosage does produce maximal coronary vasodilation,[20] but its long-lasting effects render repeated assessment of hyperemic responses impossible, and prolonged dipyridamole effect may exacerbate ischemia by causing coronary steal (dipyridamole's effect can be terminated by the administration of aminophylline). *Hyperosmolar ionic contrast media,* although easy and practical to use, do not produce maximal arteriolar vasodilation.

Doppler techniques have proven safe in the hands of experienced operators. Their high-frequency response allows measurement of phasic blood flow. The zero flow reference point is stable, so that repeated coronary flow measurements can be performed following sequential physiologic or pharmacologic stimuli. The *disadvantages* of the Doppler technique include the fact that it measures changes in blood flow velocity, not volumetric flow; that

it is of limited value in the setting of diffuse coronary artery disease with systolic and diastolic LV dysfunction,[21] that intracoronary catheter manipulation is required; and that although it allows determination of regional coronary flow, transmural perfusion cannot be assessed.

Coronary Videodensitometry. A variety of videodensitometric techniques have been developed for the measurement of coronary flow.[22–23] Biplane angiographic filming allows quantitative assessment of vessel cross-sectional area, with measurement of blood flow *velocity* obtained by monitoring radiographic contrast density as a function of time at two separate points within a given vessel segment. Blood flow is then calculated as the product of cross-sectional area and flow velocity (Fig. 21–5). Although this approach is applicable to large caliber coronary bypass grafts, application of this technique to the native coronary circulation has been seriously limited by small vessel caliber, complex three-dimensional anatomy and vessel arborizations, and the superimposed cyclic cardiac and respiratory background changes. Because each measurement takes several seconds, phasic flow cannot be assessed.

Similar videodensitometric principles have been applied to the measurement of bypass

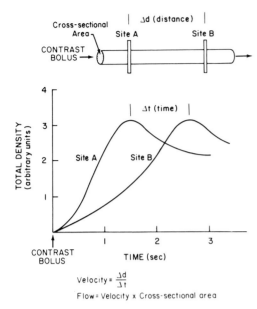

Fig. 21–5. Measurement of coronary graft flow by videodensitometry. Following injection of the radiographic contrast bolus, contrast density is measured as a function of time at two sites (A and B) along the vessel. The monitored sites should be in the same plane and along a straight portion of the artery with no interposing branches and have similar cross-sectional areas. Blood flow velocity is derived from the transit time (Δt). Volume flow is calculated as a product of velocity and cross-sectional area.

graft flow reserve by means of ultrafast computed tomography (CT). The improved image afforded by ultrafast CT allows intravenous or aortic root injection of radiographic contrast and is thus a more practical approach to the assessment of both bypass graft patency and flow reserve.[24]

Measurement of Myocardial Tissue Perfusion and Metabolism

Clearance Techniques. Clearance measurements of myocardial perfusion permit assessment of *blood flow per gram of myocardial tissue.* Clearance methods derive from the Fick principle, applying conservation of matter to either myocardial uptake (saturation) or washout (desaturation) of a tracer substance as reflected by systemic arterial and coronary venous tracer levels or precordial scintigraphy (Fig. 21–6).[25]

Individual clearance procedures vary with

respect to the indicators used, the method of administration, and the method of indicator analysis. Indicators should be physiologically inert, diffuse readily across the capillary endothelium to allow rapid myocardial tissue saturation and desaturation, be detectable by coronary sinus sampling or precordial scintigraphy, and have minimal recirculation. Several gases (nitrous oxide, hydrogen, helium, and xenon-133) have been used as indicators.

Measurements with nonradioactive gases are primarily applicable in patients with normal coronary anatomy in the absence of regional abnormalities of left ventricular perfusion or function. Radioactive Xe-133 is the tracer that has been used most frequently in research applications (Fig. 21–7). The inert gas is dissolved in saline and injected selectively into the coronary circulation at the time of coronary angiography. Precordial gamma irradiation emitted by the trapped radioisotope is recorded by a multicrystal scintillation camera, allowing visualization of isotope washout. The initial Xe-133 washout from each region of the myocardium is fitted to a computer-derived monoexponential equation, allowing the slope of the initial washout curve to be determined. Myocardial blood flow (F, in mL/100 gm/min) is then derived by the Kety formula:

$$F = kl/r$$

where k is the myocardial Xe-133 washout slope, l is the blood:myocardium partition coefficient for Xe-133, and r is the specific gravity of the myocardial tissue. Scintigraphically determined regional myocardial blood flow distribution can be correlated with the angiographically delineated coronary anatomy.[26]

The radioactive Xe-133 technique carries some risk to the patient because it requires intra-arterial injection. The temporal resolution of this technique is limited so that rapid flow changes cannot be detected accurately, and transmural myocardial perfusion differences cannot be assessed. Inasmuch as Xe-133 is 8 to 10 times more soluble in fat than in cardiac muscle, only a limited number of serial

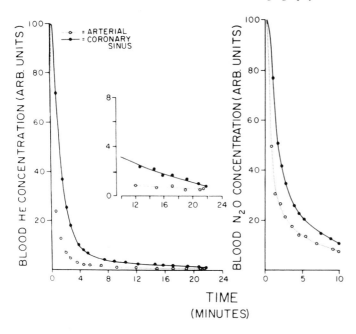

Fig. 21–6. Systemic arterial (open circles) and coronary sinus (closed circles) desaturation curves for helium (HE) and nitrous oxide (N_2O). Myocardial blood flow per 100 g N_2O (F/W) = 100 times the difference in coronary venous helium concentrations at two points in time (ΔC_v) divided by the area between the venous and arterial desaturation curves in that period of time $\int_0^t (C_v - C_a)$. (From Klocke FJ, et al: Average coronary blood flow per unit weight of left ventricle in patients with and without coronary artery disease. Circulation 50:547, 1974, with permission.)

measurements can be performed. This differential solubility may also affect Xe-133 washout curves, leading to underestimation of flow. Furthermore, it is not clear whether the partition coefficient of Xe-133 is affected by myocardial ischemia or myocardial fibrosis, and validation of Xe-133 measurements at high myocardial flows remains questionable, making it poorly suited to the assessment of myocardial flow reserve.

Myocardial Videodensitometry. A modification of the videodensitometric principles discussed previously involves assessment of regional myocardial perfusion through peak contrast density (C_{max}) and contrast arrival time (T_{arr}) within a *myocardial* region of interest.[27] Contrast is selectively power-injected into the coronary artery, and image acquisition is synchronized with the ECG signal. Sequential preinjection and postinjection images are obtained at fixed intervals after the R-wave and digitally stored. The precontrast mask image is subtracted from the contrast images, and the resulting subtraction images are analyzed subsequently to determine C_{max} and the corresponding T_{arr} for every pixel. A parameter (Q) related to coronary blood flow is calculated as:

$$Q = C_{max}/T_{arr}$$

with the flow ratio value (R_Q, for hyperemic flow divided by resting flow) calculated as:

$$R_Q = (C_{max}/T_{arr})_{hyper}/(C_{max}/T_{arr})_{rest}$$

With the use of potent coronary vasodilator agents such as papaverine and adenosine, appropriate reserve flow ratios have been measured.[28] Videodensitometric flow measurements are relatively safe, but require atrial pacing, ECG-gated power injection of coronary arteries, as well as specialized digital imaging equipment. They allow regional flow assessment but provide no information regarding transmural flow distribution. Rapid flow changes cannot be assessed, and any patient motion may distort the results.

Adaptation of these videodensitometric principles to ultrafast computed tomography[24] offers the prospect of achieving a relatively noninvasive approach to the measurement of both regional and transmural flow distribution in the resting and hyperemic state, with theoretic spatial resolution as fine as 1 mm^2.

Positron Emission Tomography. Positron emission tomography (PET) can be used to assess regional and transmural myocardial perfusion, flow reserve, or myocardial metabolism, depending on the tracer and the techniques used. PET depends on the use of tracers

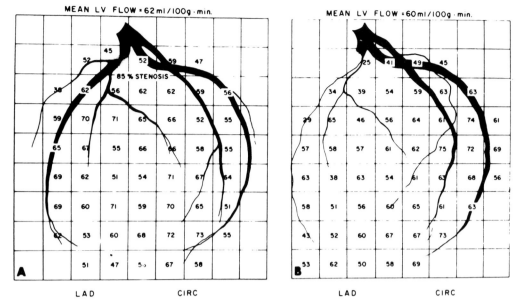

Fig. 21–7. Xe-133 precordial scintigram in the LAO projection following selective tracer injection into the left coronary artery. A. Despite the presence of an 85% stenosis in a proximal LAD, resting myocardial perfusion rates were similar throughout the left ventricle. B. Three months after an anterior myocardial infarction, the same patient has a 100% proximal LAD occlusion. Regional myocardial flows distal to the occlusion are lower when compared to the remainder of the ventricle. (From Cannon PJ, Weiss MB, Sciacca RR: Myocardial blood flow in coronary artery disease: studies at rest and during stress with inert gas washout techniques. Prog Cardiovasc Dis 20:95, 1977, with permission.)

that emit positrons (particles whose mass equals that of the electrons but whose electrical charge is positive). Released positrons travel through tissue until they lose kinetic energy and combine with electrons. The resulting mass annihilation releases energy in the form of two photons, which leave the annihilation site in opposite directions. This "annihilation event" is recorded as simultaneously sensing of 511 keV photons by two separate scintillation detectors positioned 180 degrees apart (coincidence detection). Typically, one or more circular arrays of these detectors surround the patient, to allow data collection from all angles simultaneously and reconstruction of high spatial resolution tomographic myocardial slices.[29]

In a variation of the microsphere technique used in animals, quantitative measurements of myocardial perfusion (expressed in units of ml/min/gram) can be obtained by PET scanning after injecting C-11 labeled albumin microspheres into the left ventricle and performing simultaneous arterial reference sampling. The invasive nature of this approach limits the clinical applicability of this microsphere technique in man.[29]

N-13 ammonia, H_2O-15, and Rb-82 have also been used in noninvasive PET assessment of myocardial blood flow. Although the ammonium ion can substitute for potassium in the Na-K ATP-ase transport system, N-13 ammonia enters myocytes primarily by way of lipophilic diffusion of its nonionic species across the sarcolemmal membranes. The N-13 ionic species is then trapped intracellularly, providing a long tissue half-life for N-13 ammonium to permit noninvasive quantitation of myocardial flow.[29] Rb-82 is an alternative radionuclide tracer for assessment of myocardial blood flow, which acts as a potassium analog. Its short 76-second physical half-life allows studies to be repeated at short intervals, approximately every 10 to 15 minutes.[30]

The extraction of N-13 ammonia and Rb-82 is inversely related to flow, and myocardial uptake depends on both perfusion and active metabolism, limiting the clinical utility of these two tracers. Although Rb-82 can be eluted from an inexpensive self-contained generator, the other positron-emitting radionuclides require expensive on-site cyclotrons for their production. Transmural myocardial perfusion can be assessed by this technique but resolution is limited to 8 to 12 mm, and cardiac, respiratory, or patient motion artifacts interfere with this technique.[29]

Importantly, PET scanning may supply unique and essential information on the viability of dysfunctional myocardium, differentiating between ischemic and necrotic tissue by positron emission imaging with F-18 2-deoxyglucose (FDG). In the fasting state, with suppression of normal myocardial glucose uptake, FDG is taken up selectively by ischemic myocardial tissue, which is forced to rely on anaerobic glycolysis. Following oral glucose loading, both normal and ischemic (but not necrotic) myocardium take up the tracer. Importantly, mismatches between PET flow and metabolic imaging may point to areas of myocardial ischemia, stunning, or hibernation, which may be salvaged by revascularization.[29,31]

Coronary Venous Flow

Coronary Sinus Thermodilution and Oximetry. The measurement of coronary venous flow is widely available and inexpensive, and requires only right-heart cardiac catheterization.

Unlike coronary *arterial* flow, coronary venous flow occurs predominantly during *systole*. Approximately two thirds of left anterior descending coronary artery flow drains into the great cardiac vein, the continuation of the anterior intraventricular vein as it reaches the atrioventricular groove. The great cardiac vein becomes the coronary sinus per se at the valve of Vieussens and the oblique vein of Marshall (a left atrial venous remnant of the embryonic left-sided superior vena cava, Fig. 21–8). The remaining portion of LAD venous drainage enters the coronary sinus along with blood from the circumflex territory, by way of the left marginal vein and circumflex venous

branches. Only a small percentage of left circumflex venous effluent reaches the great cardiac vein. Great cardiac vein flow thus represents primarily LAD venous outflow, whereas coronary sinus flow represents a mixture of both left anterior descending and left circumflex coronary artery outflow, with 80 to 85% of total left coronary inflow drained by this route.[32,33]

Measurement of coronary venous flow is based on the thermodilution principle, with the assumption that the heat lost by blood equals the heat gained by a cold indicator solution (Fig. 21–9). Room temperature fluid (5% dextrose or normal saline) is injected upstream in the coronary sinus for 20 to 30 seconds at a rate of 35 to 55 mL/min (using a 200 cc Harvard pump or angiographic power injector to ensure turbulent mixing with venous blood). Coronary venous flow is then computed according to the following formula:[33,34]

$$Q = F \times C \times (T_m - T_i)/(T_b - T_m)$$

Where Q is coronary venous flow, F is the rate of injection of the thermodilution indicator, C is the ratio of the specific heats of blood and the injectate (equaling 1.08 for 5% dextrose and 1.19 for normal saline): and T_m, T_i, and T_b are the temperatures of the mixture, the injectate, and blood respectively.

The clinical utility of available coronary sinus catheters (Wilton Webster, Altadena, California; Baim Electro-catheter, Rahway, New Jersey) is enhanced by incorporation of various features (Fig. 21–10): the presence of two sampling thermistors allows simultaneous selective measurement of LAD and more proximal coronary sinus flow by a catheter whose tip is positioned at the great cardiac vein. The presence of pacing electrodes facilitates the measurement of blood flow changes in response to coronary sinus pacing. Reflectance oximetry allows the continuous measurement of great cardiac vein oxygen saturation and permits on-line determination of regional myocardial oxygen consumption ($M\dot{V}O_2$)[5]:

$$M\dot{V}O_2 = Q \times (A_{O_2} - CS_{O_2})$$

where Q equals coronary venous flow, A_{O_2} is

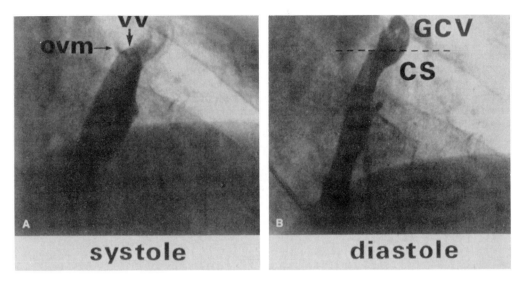

Fig. 21–8. Human coronary venogram in the RAO projection. The catheter tip is at the junction of the coronary sinus (CS) and the great cardiac vein (GCV). A. During ventricular systole, unopacified, venous blood from the great cardiac vein silhouettes the valve of Vieussens (VV) at the CS-GCV junction. The oblique vein of Marshall (OVM), the remnant of the embryonic left-sided superior vena cava lies adjacent to the valve of Vieussens and is filled by contrast. B. During ventricular diastole, contrast refluxes beyond the valve of Vieussens to fill the great cardiac vein. Several small marginal veins are similarly seen to fill in retrograde fashion. (From Bradley AB, Baim DS: Measurement of coronary blood flow in man: methods and implication for clinical practice. Cardiovasc Clinics 14(3):67, 1984, with permission.)

arterial, and CS_{O_2} is coronary sinus oxygen saturation.

The coronary sinus is located slightly behind the tricuspid annulus. Coronary sinus cannulation has traditionally been performed from a left brachial approach because a catheter with a single curve easily enters the ostium of the coronary sinus from the left arm in the majority of patients. A right brachial or femoral venous approach is feasible using a reverse loop technique. Our preferred approach is percutaneous placement from the right internal jugular vein. This allows excellent catheter control by virtue of the proximity of the coronary sinus ostium. The catheter tip is initially pointed laterally towards the right atrial border. The catheter is then rotated counterclockwise and advanced slightly until it just enters the right ventricle. After slight additional counterclockwise rotation, the catheter is then withdrawn slowly until an atrial pressure tracing is restored. Gentle readvancement of the catheter from this position leads to cannulation of the coronary sinus. Should the right ventricle be re-entered, the same maneuver is repeated with accentuation of counterclockwise rotation.

Successful coronary sinus entry is confirmed by the maintenance of a right atrial pressure trace as the catheter is smoothly advanced across the right heart border. If resistance is encountered during catheter advancement, this usually signifies impingement upon venous branches or the valve of Vieussens. If slight catheter repositioning fails to correct the situation, the anatomic obstacle can usually be crossed with a 0.018-inch soft-tipped angioplasty guide wire, allowing advancement of the catheter over this wire to reach the desired sampling site in the great cardiac vein. The coronary sinus is a thin-walled venous structure that can be easily perforated with the application of force, so that care should be taken to ascertain continued intravascular position.

Reproducible coronary venous flow measurements require a stable position of the catheter to avoid variable inclusion of blood entering from venous tributaries adjacent to the sampling site. The proximal (coronary sinus) thermistor needs to be positioned at least 2 to 3 cm from the sinus ostium to avoid contamination of the temperature profile by right atrial

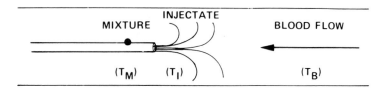

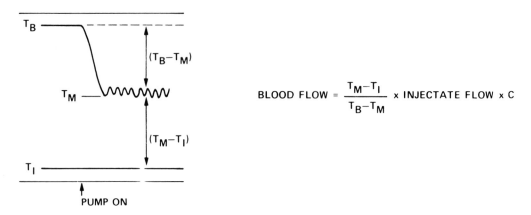

$$\text{BLOOD FLOW} = \frac{T_M - T_I}{T_B - T_M} \times \text{INJECTATE FLOW} \times C$$

Fig. 21–9. Schematic diagram of the thermodilution technique. The thermal indicator (injectate) at temperature T_I is infused at fixed rate, typically 50 cc/min. The ensuing turbulence causes mixing of the injectate with coronary venous blood at temperature T_B resulting in a mixture at temperature T_M. The temperatures monitored by the catheter tip (T_B and T_M) and injectate (T_I) thermistors are recorded continuously on a uniform temperature scale. Because the heat lost by blood is gained by the injectate, coronary venous flow can be calculated using the respective measured temperatures, the rate of indicator injection, and a constant derived from the specific heats of blood and injectate. (From Bradley AB, Baim DS: Measurement of coronary blood flow in man: methods and implications for clinical practice. Cardiovasc Clinics 14(3):67, 1984, with permission.)

admixture. Typically, the most stable position for the catheter tip is near the point where the anterior intraventricular vein meets the great cardiac vein. This position also provides the most selective measurement of LAD territory outflow (Fig. 21–11).

Coronary venous flow measurements are easy to perform, inexpensive, and can be done at low risk to the patient. The approach allows insights into regional (LAD) myocardial flow and metabolic changes. Serial measurements can be performed to detect transient changes in flow and oxygen extraction.[35]

The technique has several limitations. It does not allow assessment of phasic or very rapid changes in coronary flow. Transmural myocardial perfusion also cannot be assessed. Regionality of flow measurements is confined to the LAD territory. The technique is extremely sensitive to alterations in catheter positioning and is insufficiently validated for

flow measurements in severe coronary artery disease. There is, furthermore, a tendency to significantly underestimate coronary flow reserve. Rarely, coronary sinus thrombosis has been reported to occur as a result of right atrial and coronary sinus instrumentation, particularly in the setting of heart failure.[36]

MEASUREMENT OF MYOCARDIAL PERFUSION IN CLINICAL SITUATIONS

Coronary Artery Disease. An accurate assessment of the physiologic significance of coronary obstructions is essential for proper decision-making regarding medical therapy and percutaneous or surgical revascularization. Although marked intra- and interobserver variability has hampered the clinician's visual interpretation of the coronary angiogram, quantitative coronary angiography allows a

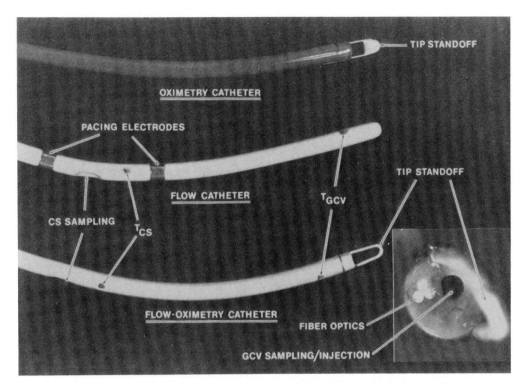

Fig. 21–10. Coronary venous oximetry, thermodilution flow, and combined flow oximetry catheters (top to bottom). The flow and flow oximetry catheters have the following features in common: two lumina for indicator injection or sampling at the great cardiac vein (see insert) and coronary sinus sites and two great cardiac vein (T_{GCV}) and coronary sinus (T_{CS}) thermistors for regional flow determinations. The flow catheter additionally has two pacing electrodes. The oximetry and flow oximetry catheters have fiberoptic bundles for the continuous measurement of great cardiac vein oxygen saturation. (From Baim DS, Rothman MT, Harrison DC: Simultaneous measurement of coronary venous flow and oxygen saturation during transient alterations in myocardial oxygen supply and demand. Am J Cardiol 49:743, 1982, with permission.)

more objective assessment of percent diameter and area stenosis, as well as of absolute luminal cross-sectional area. The utility of this quantitative approach, however, is compromised by the effects of stenosis geometry (stenosis entrance and exit angle, length) and of diffuse coronary disease on the physiologic effect of coronary lesions.[37,38] Proper assessment of coronary obstructive disease should, therefore, take into account both geometric-anatomic and physiologic considerations. Because normal resting coronary flow is preserved until the development of critical occlusions, measurement of coronary flow reserve may be necessary to ascertain the physiologic significance of some lesions.

Studies employing Xe-133 clearance methods as well as thermodilution techniques in

instances of single vessel coronary artery disease have found resting coronary flows that match those of normal control subjects. Abnormalities in coronary flow were found only in the context of pacing tachycardia, during which patients with coronary artery disease had a blunted increment in coronary flow associated with angina and electrocardiographic changes, suggesting exhaustion of coronary reserve in the ischemic territory.[39] Other investigators have used Xe-133 and helium clearance methods to show reduction in left ventricular perfusion per unit weight in patients with multivessel coronary artery disease at rest, possibly representing a reduction in regional metabolic demand.[26,40]

In patients with single vessel coronary artery disease, there is a good agreement between

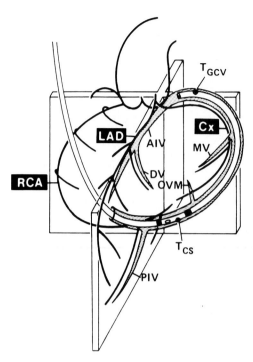

Fig. 21–11. Schematic diagram of the cannulated coronary venous system in relation to the coronary artery anatomy: diagonal vein (DV), anterior intraventricular vein (AIV), marginal vein (MV), oblique vein of Marshall (OVM), posterior intraventricular vein (PIV), and the right, left anterior descending, and circumflex coronary arteries (RCA, LAD, CX respectively). (From Baim DS, Rothman MT, Harrison DC: Simultaneous measurement of coronary venous flow and oxygen saturation during transient alterations in myocardial oxygen supply and demand. Am J Cardiol 49:743, 1982, with permission.)

quantitatively determined stenosis severity and Doppler-measured coronary flow reserve (Fig. 21–12). Lesions obstructing luminal area by no more than 70% showed normal coronary flow reserve (defined as greater than 3.5), whereas coronary flow reserve was compromised (i.e., less than 3.5), for all obstructions reducing luminal area by more than 80%. There was significant overlap in flow reserve values for 70 to 80% lesions.[9] Regional flow reserve measurements by digtal subtraction cineangiography have shown similar impairment for minimal coronary luminal cross-sectional areas less than 2 mm[2].[41]

In contrast to the findings in single vessel coronary artery disease, measurements in patients with multivessel disease have shown poor correlation between the quantitatively determined stenosis severity and flow reserve. Percent stenosis tends to underestimate the physiologic significance of a lesion on flow reserve compared to measurements of absolute lesion cross-sectional area. The inability of percent stenosis to predict abnormalities of flow reserve reflects primarily the fact that diffuse luminal infringement is not reflected.[42]

It should be noted that these studies were done in a highly selected patient population without previous infarction, left ventricular hypertrophy, left ventricular dysfunction, multivessel disease, or evident coronary collateralization, any of which might independently affect flow reserve. Thus, flow reserve measurements are of value primarily in assessing patients with discrete single-vessel coronary disease and normal ventricular function.

Imaging by positron emission tomography has shed new light on the management of patients with severe coronary artery disease. N-13 ammonia flow studies followed by F-18 deoxyglucose imaging can distinguish myocardial scar from severely ischemic but viable myocardium. Matched flow and metabolic defects reflect scar tissue, whereas a mismatch in flow and metabolic activity, characterized by reduced myocardial perfusion with persistent F-18 deoxyglucose uptake, reflects viable myocardium that may recover mechanical function after revascularization. PET is more sensitive than thallium-201 scanning because it has demonstrated continued tissue viability in over 50% of fixed defects found during thallium scintigraphy.[2]

Coronary Artery Spasm. Coronary sinus measurement of myocardial blood flow and oxygen saturation during spontaneous or pharmacologically induced coronary artery spasm demonstrate that episodes of ischemia at rest are not preceded by changes in the hemodynamic determinants of myocardial oxygen consumption. Rather, a primary reduction in flow precedes the conventional signs of myocardial ischemia (diminished systolic function, electrocardiographic changes, or angina).[43] Interestingly, these measurement techniques also documented a rebound overshoot in coronary

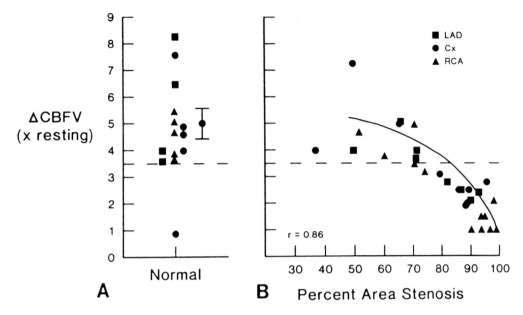

Fig. 21–12. Coronary flow reserved (ΔCBFV) expressed as multiples of resting flow (A) in normal vessels and (B) in the presence of increasingly severe percent area stenosis. Normal flow reserve was greater than 3.5, and remained so until area stenoses exceeded 70 to 80%. (From Marcus ML, et al: Assessing the physiologic significance of coronary obstructions in patients: importance of diffuse undetected atherosclerosis. Prog Cardiovasc Dis 31:39, 1988, with permission.)

flow on resolution of spasm, coincident with a fall in coronary arteriovenous oxygen extraction, a pattern consistent with reactive hyperemia in response to spasm-induced ischemia.[44]

Coronary flow measurements in patients with documented coronary artery spasm may show impairment of coronary flow reserve in the absence of epicardial stenosis or concurrent spasm, conceivably caused by persistent abnormalities of arteriolar vasomotor tone or to diffuse atherosclerosis. This observation may account in part for the occurrence of exercise-induced ischemia in subgroups of patients with coronary spasm.[45]

Other Chest Pain Syndromes. Twenty to thirty percent of patients referred for diagnostic cardiac catheterization experience angina-like symptoms in the absence of myocardial hypertrophy, fixed obstructive coronary artery disease, or inducible focal epicardial spasm.[46] Investigations using both the argon clearance method and coronary sinus thermodilution have identified a group of patients with "Syndrome X" who have normal resting myocar-

dial blood flow but impaired vasodilatory capacity in response to exercise or to intravenous dipyridamole.[47] Such patients may actually show a fall in coronary flow after the administration of intravenous ergonovine, despite a rise in myocardial oxygen consumption. Cold pressor testing and intravenous ergonovine administration may similarly impair the vasodilatory response to pacing tachycardia. Coronary flow reserve measurement is essential in documenting this disorder in arteriolar vasoregulation and establishing the diagnosis in these patients (Fig. 21–13).[48]

Heart Failure and Cardiac Transplantation. Xe-133 clearance techniques have demonstrated myocardial perfusion per unit weight that is decreased at rest in patients with congestive heart failure.[49]

Heart failure resulting in elevated ventricular filling pressures may cause a rightward shift of the maximally vasodilated pressure-flow relationship, resulting in an impairment of flow reserve.[4,21] Although there is limited use for flow measurements in heart failure, the measurement of coronary flow reserve may

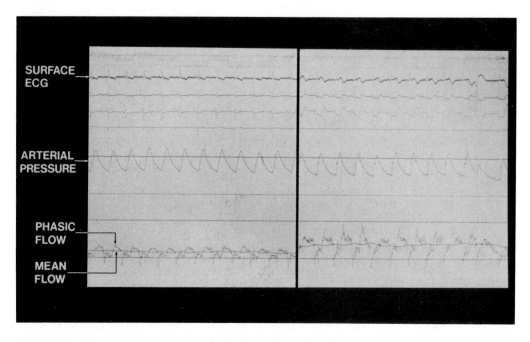

Fig. 21–13. Left panel: Phasic and mean LAD Doppler flow signal in a 65-year-old woman with exertional angina but normal coronary anatomy and left ventricular function. Right panel: After administration of 12 mg of intracoronary papaverine, there was no appreciable change in heart rate or blood pressure. Doppler velocity flow increased only by a factor of 2, and the patient experienced her typical angina associated with marked electrocardiographic changes, consistent with impaired vasodilatory reserve and pharmacologically induced coronary steal.

find clinical application in the care of patients after orthotopic cardiac transplantation. Accelerated coronary atherosclerosis, presumably caused by immune-mediated vascular injury, may not be detectable by standard coronary angiography. In the absence of graft rejection or acquired left ventricular hypertrophy, coronary vasodilator reserve has been found to be normal (3.8 to 7.3). Coronary reserve, however, is severely eroded as proliferative vascular injury supervenes.[50]

Coronary sinus thermodilution techniques have been used to assess the effect of therapeutic agents on the balance of myocardial oxygen supply and demand in patients with heart failure. Thus, the rise in ventricular contractility induced by dobutamine increases myocardial oxygen demand ($M\dot{V}O_2$) and obligates a "secondary" rise in coronary blood flow. In contrast, the vasodilatory phosphodiesterase inhibitors amrinone and milrinone have both been found to *reduce* myocardial oxygen demand slightly in patients with heart failure by decreasing left ventricular wall stress, although their direct arteriolar vasodilator properties lead to a small "primary" rise in coronary blood flow associated with a simultaneous fall in transmyocardial oxygen extraction.[51]

Myocardial Hypertrophy. Patients with hypertrophied ventricles frequently exhibit signs of myocardial ischemia including exertional angina and ST segment depression on the resting or exercise electrocardiograms, even in the absence of angiographically detectable coronary artery stenoses. While Xe-133 clearance techniques have shown elevated resting coronary flow, perfusion *per unit weight* was found to be decreased, possibly reflecting diminished resting myocardial wall stress in these hypertrophied ventricles.[49] Both thermodilution techniques and Doppler flow measurements have also shown that *coronary flow reserve* is markedly impaired in patients with left ventricular hypertrophy, whether it was caused by aortic stenosis, aortic regurgitation, supravalvular aortic stenosis, systemic hypertension, or primary hypertrophic cardiomyopathy.[52-54] Inadequate growth of the microvascular bed as myocardial mass increases may result in a fall in the capillary to myocyte surface area ratio, leading to a mismatch between myocardial mass and flow.[55] Further erosion of available reserve capacity would cause a rightward shift of the maximally dilated pressure-flow relationship in the presence of high intramyocardial pressures, and elevation in resting coronary flow would contribute to a fall in measured flow reserve. This reduction of coronary flow reserve may explain stress-induced myocardial ischemia in patients with hypertrophy despite normal-appearing epicardial coronary arteries.

Importantly, this known impairment of flow reserve with hypertrophy alone complicates interpretation of flow reserve in patients with coronary artery disease and ventricular hypertrophy.

Coronary Artery Bypass Surgery and Percutaneous Transluminal Angioplasty. Electromagnetic and Doppler flow probes have been used commonly during coronary artery bypass surgery to assess the adequacy of bypass graft flow. Bypass grafts anastomosed to nonstenotic distal coronary vessels that perfuse normal myocardium have normal coronary flow reserve.[56] In such patients, coronary flow reserve can then be used clinically to follow the functional adequacy of the graft by means of either Doppler technology or newer ultrafast CT methods.

To date, flow measurements have not been used routinely to assess the immediate or long-term adequacy of percutaneous revascularization procedures. Thermodilution methods have permitted the observation of post-occlu-

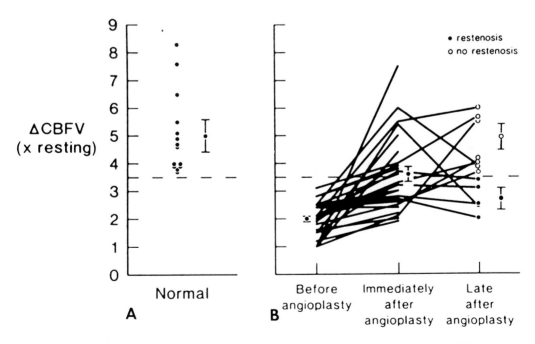

Fig. 21–14. A. Change in coronary blood flow velocity (ΔCBFV) following papaverine in 14 patients without coronary artery disease. B. Change in coronary blood flow velocity or flow reserve in 31 patients before angioplasty, immediately after successful angioplasty, and 7.5 months after angioplasty. Flow reserve before angioplasty was abnormal. In approximately half of the patients, flow reserve continued to remain below normal levels immediately after successful angioplasty. In the absence of restenosis, coronary flow reserve normalized at late follow-up. (From Wilson RF, Johnson MR, Marcus ML, Aylard PE, Skorton DJ, Collins S, White CW: The effect of coronary angioplasty on coronary flow reserve. Circulation 77:873, 1988, with permission.)

sion reactive hyperemia during PTCA, and numerous investigators have demonstrated that reduction in luminal stenosis severity restores coronary reserve capacity and the magnitude of reactive hyperemia.[57,58]

Interestingly, several investigators have found that flow reserve does not return to normal immediately after angioplasty despite apparent angiographic success. Flow reserve does normalize within several weeks to months with continued vessel patency (Fig. 21–14).[59] Abnormal coronary flow reserve immediately after angioplasty may be caused by an elevation in resting coronary blood flow velocity, altered coronary microcirculatory responsiveness from prolonged ischemia and low distal perfusion pressures, or the continued mechanically obstructive effects of vessel dissection as a result of PTCA. Unfortunately, these abnormal flow reserve measurements after PTCA limit their applicability in assessing immediate postangioplasty results.

In summary, although the techniques for measurement of coronary blood flow and metabolism have played a pivotal role in understanding the physiology of the human coronary circulation, they have only recently begun to find application in clinical practice. Coronary sinus thermodilution measurements remain a low-risk practical approach for monitoring both coronary flow and myocardial oxygen consumption in the cardiac catheterization laboratory. Methods of assessing coronary flow reserve (intracoronary Doppler flow measurements and digital subtraction angiography) have gained increasing acceptance in the evaluation and assessment of fixed coronary obstructive disease, coronary spasm, chest pain syndromes, post-transplant management, and follow-up of bypass surgery and angioplasty. Because a growing interventional armamentarium mandates increased physiologic understanding, measurements of flow reserve and metabolism are expected to help significantly in clinical decision making.

REFERENCES

1. Marcus ML, et al: Visual estimates of percent diameter coronary stenosis: ''A battered gold standard.'' J Am Coll Cardiol 2:882, 1988.
2. Schelbert HR, Buxton D: Insights into coronary artery disease gained from metabolic imaging. Circulation 78:496, 1988.
3. Klocke FJ: Coronary blood flow in man. Prog Cardiovasc Dis 19:117, 1976.
4. Aversano T, Klocke FJ, Mates RE, Canty JM: Preload-induced alterations in capacitance-free diastolic pressure-flow relationships. Am J Physiol 246:H410, 1984.
5. Baim DS, Rothman MT, Harrison DC: Simultaneous measurement of coronary venous blood flow and oxygen saturation during transient alterations in myocardial oxygen supply and demand. Am J Cardiol 49:743, 1982.
6. Weber KT, Janicki JS: The metabolic demand and oxygen supply of the heart: physiologic and clinical considerations. Am J Cardiol 44:722, 1979.
7. Bache RJ, Dymek DJ: Local and regional regulation of coronary vascular tone. Prog Cardiovasc Dis 24:191, 1981.
8. Kirkeeide RL, Gould KL, Parsel L: Assessment of coronary stenoses by myocardial perfusion imaging during pharmacologic coronary vasodilation. VII. Validation of coronary flow reserve as a single integrated functional measure of stenosis severity reflecting all its geometric dimensions. J Am Coll Cardiol 7:103, 1986.
9. Wilson RF, Marcus ML, White CW: Prediction of the physiologic significance or coronary arterial lesions by quantitative lesion geometry in patients with limited coronary artery disease. Circulation 75:723–732, 1987.
10. Zijlstra F, Fioretti P, Reiber JH, Serruys PW: Which cineangiographically assessed anatomic variable correlates best with functional measurements of stenosis severity? A comparison of quantitative analysis of the coronary cineangiogram with measured coronary flow reserve and exercise/redistribution thallium-201 scintigraphy. J Am Coll Cardiol 12:686, 1988.
11. Opie LH: Metabolism of the heart in health and disease, Part I. Am Heart J 76:685, 1968. Part II 77:100, 1969. Part III 77:383, 1969.
12. Scheuer J, Penpargkul S: Myocardial metabolism. In Willerson S, Sanders C (ed): Clinical Cardiology. New York, Stratton, 1977.
13. Krasnow N, et al: Myocardial lactate and metabolism. J Clin Invest 41:2075, 1962.
14. Hartley CJ, Cole JS: An ultrasonic pulsed Doppler system for measuring blood flow in small vessels. J Appl Physiol 37:626, 1974.
15. Sibley DH, Millar HD, Hartley CJ, Whitlow PL: Subselective measurement of coronary blood flow velocity using a steerable Doppler catheter. J Am Coll Cardiol 8:1332, 1986.
16. Marcus ML, Wilson RF, White CW: Methods of measurement of myocardial blood flow in patients: a critical review. Circulation 76:245, 1987.
17. Zijlstra F, Juilliere Y, Serruys PW, Roelandt JRTC: Value and limitations of intracoronary adenosine for the assessment of coronary flow reserve. Cath Cardiovasc Diag 15:76, 1988.
18. Zijlstra F, Serruys PW, Hugenholtz PG: Papaverine: The ideal coronary vasodilator for investigating coronary flow reserve? A study of timing, magnitude, reproducibility, and safety of the coronary hyperemic

response after intracoronary papaverine. Cath Cardiovasc Diag 12:298, 1986.

19. Wilson RF, White CW: Serious ventricular dysrhythmias after intracoronary papaverine. Am J Cardiol 62:1301, 1988.

20. Rossen JD, Simonetti I, Marcus ML, Winniford MD: Coronary dilation with standard dose dipyridamole and dipyridamole combined with handgrip. Circulation 79:566, 1989.

21. Klocke FJ: Measurement of coronary flow reserve: defining pathophysiology versus making decisions about patient care. Circulation 76:1183, 1987.

22. Rutishauser W, et al: Evaluation of roentgen cinedensitometry for flow measurements in models and in intact circulation. Circulation 36:951, 1967.

23. Smith HC, Strum RE, Wood EH: Videodensitometric system for measurement of vessel blood flow, particularly in the coronary arteries, in man. Am J Cardiol 32:144, 1973.

24. Marcus ML, Stanford W, Hajduczok ZD, Weiss RM: Ultrafast computed tomography in the diagnosis of cardiac disease. Am J Cardiol 64:54E, 1989.

25. Bassingthwaighte JP: Physiology and theory of tracer washout techniques for the estimation of myocardial blood flow: flow estimation from tracer washout. Prog Cardiovasc Dis 20:165, 1977.

26. Cannon PJ, Weiss MB, Sciacca RR: Myocardial blood flow in coronary artery disease: studies at rest and during stress with inert gas washout techniques. Prog Cardiovasc Dis 29:95, 1977.

27. Vogel R, et al: Application of digital technique to selective coronary arteriography: use of myocardial contrast appearance time to measure coronary flow reserve. Am Heart J 107:153, 1984.

28. Cusma JT, et al: Digital subtraction angiographic imaging of coronary flow reserve. Circulation 75:461, 1987.

29. Schelbert HR: Current status and prospects of new radionuclides and radiopharmaceuticals for cardiovascular nuclear medicine. Semin Nuc Med 17:145, 1987.

30. Wilson RA, et al: Rubidium-82 myocardial uptake and extraction after transient ischemia: PET characteristics. J Comput Assist Tomogr 11:60, 1987.

31. Schelbert HR: Myocardial ischemia and clinical applications of positron emission tomography. Am J Cardiol 64:46E, 1989.

32. Nakazawa HK, Roberts DL, Klocke FJ: Quantitation of anterior descending vs circumflex venous drainage the canine great cardiac vein and coronary sinus. Am J Physiol 234:H163, 1978.

33. Ganz W, et al: Measurement of coronary sinus blood flow by continuous thermodilution in man. Circulation 44:181, 1971.

34. Baim DS, Rothman MT, Harrison DC: Improved catheter for regional coronary sinus flow and metabolic studies. Am J Cardiol 46:997, 1980.

35. Pepine CJ, et al: In vivo validation of a thermodilution method to determine regional left ventricular blood flow in patients with coronary disease. Circulation 58:795, 1978.

36. Guindi MM, Walley VM: Coronary sinus thrombosis: a potential complication of right heart catheterization. Can J Surg 30:66, 1987.

37. Demer L, Gould KL, Kirkeeide R: Assessing stenosis severity: coronary flow reserve, collateral function, quantitative coronary arteriography, positron imaging, and digital subtraction angiography. A review and analysis. Prog Cardiovasc Dis 30:307, 1988.

38. Marcus ML, et al: Assessing the physiologic significance of coronary obstructions in patients: Importance of diffuse undetected atherosclerosis. Prog Cardiovasc Dis 31:39, 1988.

39. Fuchs RM, et al: Coronary flow limitation during development of ischemia. Effect of atrial pacing in patients with left anterior descending coronary artery disease. Am J Cardiol 48:1029, 1981.

40. Klocke FJ, et al: Average coronary blood flow per unit weight of left ventricle in patients with and without coronary artery disease. Circulation 509:547, 1974.

41. Zijlstra F, van Ommeren J, Reiber JH, Serruys PW: Does the quantitative assessment of coronary artery dimensions predict the physiologic significance of a coronary stenosis? Circulation 75:1154, 1987.

42. McPherson DD, et al: Delineation of the extent of coronary atherosclerosis by high-frequency epicardial echocardiography. N Engl J Med 316:304, 1987.

43. Chierchia S, et al: Sequence of events in angina at rest: primary reduction in coronary flow. Circulation 61:759, 1980.

44. Ricci DR, et al: Reduction of coronary blood flow during coronary artery spasm occurring spontaneously and after provocation by ergonovine maleate. Circulation 57:392, 1978.

45. Legrand V, Mancini GB, Bates ER, Vogel RA: Evidence of abnormal vasodilator reserve in coronary spasm. Am J Cardiol 57:481, 1986.

46. Ockene IS, et al: Unexplained chest pain in patients with normal coronary arteriograms. N Engl J Med 303:1249, 1980.

47. Bortone AS, et al: Abnormal coronary vasomotion during exercise in patients with normal coronary arteries and reduced coronary flow reserve. Circulation 79:516, 1989.

48. Cannon RO, et al: Angina caused by reduced vasodilator reserve of the small coronary arteries. J Am Coll Cardiol 1:1359, 1983.

49. Weiss MB, et al: Myocardial blood flow in congestive and hypertrophic cardiomyopathy: relationship to peak wall stress and mean velocity of circumferential fiber shortening. Circulation 54:484, 1976.

50. McGinn AL, et al: Coronary vasodilator reserve after human orthotopic cardiac transplantation. Circulation 78:1200, 1988.

51. Monrad ES, et al: Milrinone, dobutamine, and nitroprusside: comparative effects on hemodynamics and myocardial energetics in patients with severe congestive heart failure. Circulation 73:III–168, 1986.

52. Marcus ML, et al: Decreased coronary reserve—a mechanism for angina pectoris in patients with aortic stenosis and normal coronary arteries. N Engl J Med 307:1362–1366, 1982.

53. Pichard AD, et al: Coronary vascular reserve in left ventricular hypertrophy secondary to chronic aortic regurgitation. Am J Cardiol 51:315, 1983.

54. Cannon RO, et al: Myocardial ischemia in patients with hypertrophic cardiomyopathy: contribution of inadequate vasodilator reserve and elevated left ventricular filling pressures. Circulation 71:234, 1985.

55. Dellsperger KC, Marcus ML: The effects of pressure-induced cardiac hypertrophy on the functional capacity of the coronary circulation. Am J Hypertens 1:200, 1988.

56. Wilson RF, Marcus ML, White CW: Effects of coronary bypass surgery and angioplasty on coronary blood flow and flow reserve. Prog Cardiovasc Dis 31:95, 1988.

57. Rothman MT, et al: Coronary hemodynamics during percutaneous transluminal coronary angioplasty. Am J Cardiol 49:1615, 1982.

58. Serruys PW, et al: Left ventricular performance, regional blood flow, wall motion, and lactate metabolism during transluminal angioplasty. Circulation 70:25, 1984.

59. Zijlstra F, et al: Assessment of intermediate and long-term functional results of percutaneous transluminal coronary angioplasty. Circulation 78:15, 1988.

22

Intracardiac Electrophysiology

JOHN P. DiMARCO

The development of catheter techniques for intracardiac recording and stimulation has greatly enhanced our knowledge of the mechanisms responsible for cardiac arrhythmias in man. Since the first description of the clinical use of His bundle recordings in 1969,[1] cardiac electrophysiologists have described methods for assessing sinus node function, atrioventricular (AV) conduction, and the mechanisms of atrial and ventricular tachyarrhythmias.[2,3] Although many questions remain unanswered, stimulation techniques have also been used in serial fashion to predict the future clinical efficacy of pharmacologic and nonpharmacologic modes of antiarrhythmic therapy. This chapter attempts to provide a general introduction to the techniques of clinical electrophysiology.

EQUIPMENT

Like all other catheterization procedures, intracardiac electrophysiologic studies must be performed in an environment that ensures patient safety and comfort during the procedure. The room should be large enough for a patient litter, fluoroscopy unit, instrument table, a physiologic recorder, and stimulators. An emergency cart that carries a monitor-defibrillator, supplies to allow manually assisted ventilation, and emergency drug stocks should be accessible for immediate use. A second back-up defibrillator is strongly recommended. Wall outlets for oxygen and suction should be conveniently located. Although portable fluoroscopy equipment is adequate for many procedures, multiplane fluoroscopy is required if left or right ventricular catheter mapping is to be performed. All electrical devices should be adequately grounded with individual leakage currents of less than 10 microamps and connected to circuits that have immediate emergency backup in case of power failure or interruption.

Intracardiac electrograms are displayed on a multichannel oscilloscope-recorder. An instrument for these studies should permit simultaneous display of at least three or four surface ECG leads and a minimum of five intracardiac channels. Amplifiers for the intracardiac channels are usually filtered below 30 and above 500 or 1000 Hz for standard procedures and should be free of significant line noise at a sensitivity of at least 0.05 mV/cm, preferably at 0.02 mV/cm. Additional amplifiers for hemodynamic measurements are convenient. Some types of recording (e.g., sinus node electrograms) require different filter settings, and one or more specialized amplifiers may be required. Although bipolar recordings are used for most purposes, unipolar recordings may occasionally be of interest and may be recorded using an indifferent electrode placed above the heart in the superior vena cava or other major vein. Each channel should have a standard calibration signal. Electrical signals are either recorded directly onto recording paper or stored on optical or magnetic media for subsequent retrieval and analysis. The printer should be capable of producing high-quality tracings at paper speeds up to 200 mm/sec. Intracardiac stimulation may be performed using one of several commercial devices. The stimulator selected should be capable of delivering a minimum of 3 extrastimuli after either an externally-sensed event or a drive train of delivered stimuli. The impulses delivered should be of a constant current. Most laboratories use a stimulus width of 1 to 2 msec and a current intensity set at 2 to 5 times diastolic threshold. The ability to deliver longer pulse widths (up to 10 msec) or higher currents (up to 40 ma) may be useful if special techniques such as transesophageal pacing are to be performed.

CATHETERIZATION TECHNIQUES

Diagnostic electrophysiologic procedures usually require insertion of between two and five multipolar, 6 or 7 Fr electrode catheters into the heart (Fig. 22–1). The catheters themselves are made of woven Dacron and have three or more platinum ring electrodes positioned along their length. A preformed curve at the tip of the catheter facilitates placement. We use quadripolar catheters with an inter-electrode spacing of 0.5 or 1.0 cm with the distal ring at the tip of the catheter for routine studies. This permits bipolar stimulation and recording from each catheter. Other electrode configurations may be useful for selected purposes. Each electrode is then connected to a switch box, which directs signals from the recording poles to the oscilloscope-recorder and transmits impulses from the stimulator. Because these cables are sensitive to interference from stray electrical signals, shielding of connections from patient to amplifiers is recommended.

The patient is brought to the laboratory in a fasting state. If possible, prior antiarrhythmic therapy will have been discontinued and the drugs allowed to wash out for 5 half-lives. Oral or intravenous benzodiazepines may be used to allay anxiety when necessary. Both groins are prepared and draped, and the skin overlying the femoral vessels is anesthetized with 0.5 or 1% lidocaine. Excessive amounts of lidocaine should be avoided because significant amounts may be absorbed systemically

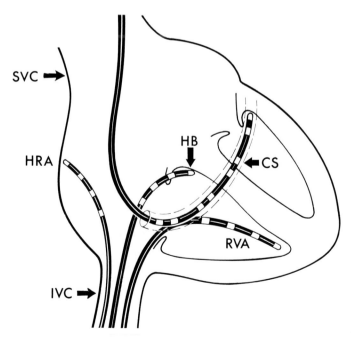

Fig. 22–1. Diagram of standard catheter positions for electrophysiologic studies. Quadripolar catheters to the high right atrium (HRA), the right ventricular apex (RVA), and the bundle of His (HB) are usually inserted via the femoral veins and inferior vena cava (IVC). Left atrial recording and stimulation are usually performed with a catheter in the coronary sinus (CS). The coronary sinus catheter may have 3 to 5 pairs of electrodes spaced near its tip to facilitate localization of left-sided accessory pathways. (SVC, superior vena cava.)

and potentially affect the results obtained.[4] The femoral artery is palpated about 1 to 2 cm below the iliac crease, using the anatomic guideline described in Chapter 5. A small skin incision is made with a scalpel blade, and the subcutaneous tissue is dilated with a hemostat. A guide wire is then inserted into the common femoral vein using the Seldinger technique (see Chapter 5). An appropriately sized introducing sheath is then passed over the guide wire, and the electrode catheter is passed through the sheath to the inferior vena cava. A second catheter may be inserted using the same procedure on the opposite groin. When three or more electrode catheters are required for the study, second sheaths may usually be inserted into the right and/or left femoral vein for the third and fourth catheters. A puncture is made about 1 cm proximal to the previous insertion site, and a second sheath is inserted over a guide wire. If a catheter has already been advanced through the first sheath, the possibility of puncturing the thin walls of the initial sheath during the second puncture is minimized. Some electrophysiologists prefer to insert 2 or 3 guide wires through a single sheath, then remove the first sheath and use these guide wires for subsequent sheaths. This obviates the need for a second puncture but may slightly increase the possibility of venous damage and cause friction between catheters to make positioning more difficult.

Once the catheters have been inserted, they are advanced to the heart under fluoroscopic guidance. The catheters usually employed in these studies are somewhat more rigid than those used for most other catheterization procedures, and care must be taken to avoid vessel or cardiac perforation. One catheter is usually positioned high in the right atrium near its junction with the superior vena cava (Fig. 22–1). This places the catheter just adjacent to the sinus node. A second catheter is positioned in the right ventricular apex (Fig. 22–1). The distal and proximal poles of these catheters are used for right atrial and right ventricular stimulation and recording, respectively.

The bundle of His lies in the high membra-nous septum, and a local electrogram containing the His bundle potential may be recorded with the electrodes positioned just across the tricuspid valve. In practice, the catheter should be advanced into the right ventricular cavity and electrical activity from its tip displayed on the oscilloscope for monitoring. The catheter is then slowly withdrawn until the characteristic bi- or triphasic His bundle potential is recognized before the onset of ventricular depolarization (Fig. 22–2). Small movements of the catheter or by the patient may cause the His bundle potential signal to be lost or even

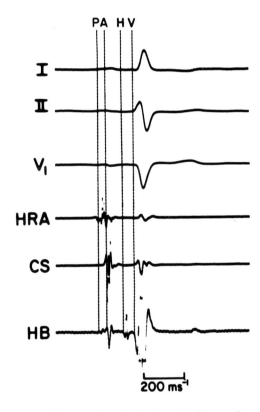

Fig. 22–2. Normal conduction intervals. Three surface electrocardiographic leads (I, II, and V_1) are displayed simultaneously. In addition, a high right atrial (HRA) electrogram, a coronary sinus (CS) electrogram, and a His bundle (HB) electrogram are also displayed. The PA interval is measured from the onset of the P wave on the surface ECG to the first rapid atrial deflection on the His bundle electrogram. AV nodal conduction time is approximated as the interval from onset of septal atrial activation to the onset of the His potential (AH interval). His-Purkinje conduction time is measured as the HV interval, where V is the first point of ventricular activity on either the surface ECG or ventricular electrogram.

cause the catheter to flip back into the atrium, and it is occasionally necessary to reposition this catheter one or more times during the procedure. His bundle recording may also be performed using a superior approach (catheter advanced from brachial, cephalic, or internal jugular vein) by making a figure six-shaped loop with the catheter across the tricuspid valve, but this technique is considerably more difficult and yields a less stable recording than the transfemoral approach. In rare cases, His bundle recording may be performed using a catheter positioned either just above or just below the noncoronary cusp of the aortic valve.

Most electrophysiologic studies for assessment of AV conduction, sinus node function, or ventricular tachycardia do not require left atrial recording. Analysis of atrial activation patterns and responses to left atrial stimulation may, however, be critical for the evaluation of supraventricular arrhythmias or pre-excitation patterns. Left atrial activity is most commonly recorded using a catheter placed in the coronary sinus. The ostium of the coronary sinus lies in the floor of the right atrium near the tricuspid valve ring. Although coronary sinus catheterization by way of a femoral approach is possible, it is technically easier to perform from either a subclavian or an internal jugular site. In some patients, a medial left antecubital vein also allows suitable access. Occasionally, a catheter may be placed in the left atrium through a patent foramen ovale or a transseptal puncture from a transfemoral approach. Use of catheters with multiple (3 to 5) pairs of electrodes along their distal portion facilitates mapping of left atrial activation sequence in patients with supraventricular tachycardias.

BASELINE INTERVALS

As illustrated in Figure 22–2, a number of standard measurements may be made from the initial recordings obtained. The PA interval is measured from the onset of the P wave on the ECG to the first rapid atrial deflection on the His bundle electrogram. We have not found

measurement of the PA interval a clinically valuable exercise. It has not been possible to record AV nodal activation directly with a catheter. Therefore, AV nodal conduction time has been approximated as the interval from onset of septal atrial activation to the onset of the His bundle potential (AH interval). His-Purkinje conduction time is measured as the interval from the onset of the His bundle potential to the first point of ventricular activity on either the surface ECG leads or on the ventricular electrogram (HV or HQ interval). The normal ranges for these intervals in our laboratory are given in Table 22–1.

Sinus Node Function

Sinus node dysfunction may be diagnosed when marked sinus bradycardia or inappropriate tachycardia is recorded during routine ambulatory electrocardiography. These findings may appear only intermittently, however, and correlation with previously experienced symptoms may not be available. In patients with intermittent symptoms and inconclusive findings during ambulatory monitoring, firm conclusions about the need for implantation of a permanent pacemaker may be difficult. For this reason, a number of tests of sinus node function have been used clinically. Those most commonly used are an assessment of the response of the sinus node to overdrive stimulation (sinus node recovery time) and the direct or indirect measurement of sinoatrial conduction times.[5]

Table 22–1. *Normal Electrophysiologic Parameters*

Intervals	
PA	25–50 msec
AH	60–140 msec
HV	30–55 msec
His duration	10–25 msec
Effective refractory periods	
Atrium	200–270 msec
AV node	280–450 msec
Ventricle	200–270 msec
Corrected Sinus Node	
recovery time	<525 msec
Sinoatrial conduction	
Time (Total)	100–210 msec

Sinus Node Recovery Time. If cardiac tissue with intrinsic automaticity is repetitively depolarized by impulses conducted from another source, its intrinsic automaticity will be suppressed transiently after the external drive is discontinued. This phenomenon has been termed overdrive suppression, and the response of the sinus node to overdrive stimulation has been used as a measure of sinus node automaticity.[6]

In practice, a pacing catheter is positioned in the high right atrium and, beginning at a cycle length just below the intrinsic sinus cycle length, 30- to 60-second trains of pacing are delivered. The delay between the last stimulus to the onset of atrial activity originating near the high right atrial catheter is termed the *sinus node recovery time* (SNRT) (Fig. 22–3).

For the SNRT to reflect the effects of overdrive suppression on the sinus node accurately, each stimulus must conduct into the sinus node and depolarize it. In addition, the magnitude of overdrive suppression may vary with different rates of pacing in an individual subject. Maximum sensitivity is therefore achieved if pacing at each cycle length is repeated twice and if multiple cycle lengths are tested, ranging from just below the patient's sinus cycle length down to 300 msec.

The sinus node recovery time depends on the intrinsic sinus cycle length, and most authors report a corrected sinus node recovery time (CSNRT) calculated by subtracting the basic sinus cycle length (SCL) from the recovery time (CSNRT = SNRT − SCL). The upper limit of normal for a measured CSNRT in our laboratory is 525 msec. As mentioned above, this test assumes that the last atrial stimulus has penetrated the sinus node and depolarized it. This may not always be true. In such cases, unexplained pauses after the first intrinsic beat may occur. When such secondary pauses are greater than 525 msec above the intrinsic sinus cycle length, they should be considered markers of abnormal sinus node recovery.

Sinoatrial Conduction. In some patients, intrinsic sinus node automaticity is normal, but conduction of the impulse to the atrium is blocked or delayed, leading to apparent sinus arrest. Both direct and indirect methods for assessing sinoatrial conduction have been described.

Two indirect methods for measuring sinoatrial conduction times have been used. The Strauss method measures the delay in atrial recovery after a single atrial premature depolarization introduced during sinus rhythm.[7] Single atrial premature stimuli (A_2) are delivered during stable sinus rhythm (A_1-A_1) beginning with the initial coupling interval just below the sinus cycle length (A_1-A_1). Four

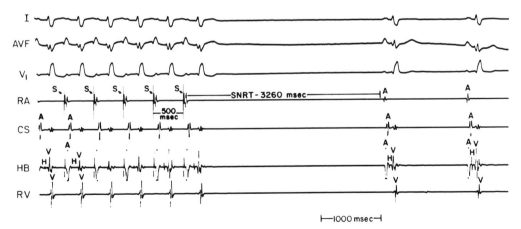

Fig. 22–3. Abnormal sinus node recovery time in a patient with recurrent syncope. The end of a train of right atrial stimuli at a cycle length of 500 msec is shown. A 3260 msec pause follows the termination of pacing. The intrinsic sinus cycle length was 1140 msec, giving a markedly abnormal corrected SNRT of 2120 msec. (RA, right atrium; CS, coronary sinus; HB, His bundle; RV, right ventricle; S, stimulus artifact; SNRT, sinus node recovery time.)

zones of response may be identified as the extrastimulus is made progressively more premature. In zone 1, the premature beat (A_2) depolarizes the atrium, but the sinus node itself has already depolarized. Thus, the impulse exiting from the sinus node collides with the stimulated impulse, and the interval from the premature beat to the next sinus beat (A_2-A_3) is fully compensatory, i.e., (A_1-A_2) + (A_2-A_3) = 2 (A_1-A_1). If the extra stimulus is moved earlier, the impulse penetrates the sinus node and resets it. The A_2-A_3 return cycle is therefore composed of three periods: the time for penetration into the node, the reset interval, and the time for conduction out of the node. The reset interval should be the same as the basic cycle length, (A_1-A_1). Therefore, (A_2-A_3) − (A_1-A_1) = conduction time (in) + conduction time (out). In practice, either total sinoatrial conduction times [SACT$_{TOTAL}$ = (A_2-A_3) − (A_1-A_1)] or, if one assumes equal antegrade and retrograde conduction, unidirectional sinoatrial conduction times

$$SACT_{A \text{ or } R} = \frac{(A_2\text{-}A_3) - (A_1\text{-}A_1)}{2}$$

are reported. As the A_1-A_2 interval is further shortened, A_2-A_3 shortens to less than A_1-A_1. This shortening is caused by either interpolation (zone 3) or re-entry (zone 4). The most reliable and reproducible values for sinoatrial conduction time are obtained with A_1-A_2 intervals in the latter half of zone 2.

A second method for estimating sinoatrial conduction has been proposed by Narula et al.[8] The atrium is paced at a rate slightly above the intrinsic sinus rate for eight consecutive beats, pacing is stopped, and the interval from the last paced beat to the next sinus beat is measured. The basic cycle length is then subtracted from this interval, and the mean of several such determinations is used as an estimate of SACT$_{TOTAL}$.

A direct method for estimating sinoatrial conduction has also been proposed.[9] An electrode catheter is placed at the junction of the superior vena cava and the high right atrium adjacent to the expected location of the sinus node. With appropriate gain (0.05 mV/cm) and filtering (0.1 to 50 Hz), a low-amplitude deflection can be seen to precede both the P wave and the local atrial electrogram. This deflection is thought to represent the sinus node electrogram, and the time from its first deflection to the onset of atrial activation has been used as a direct measure of sinoatrial conduction. Values obtained with this method are in general agreement with those obtained by the indirect methods described earlier. The upper limit of normal for a directly or indirectly measured total SACT in our laboratory is 210 msec.

The clinical value of electrophysiologic testing in patients with suspected sinus node dysfunction has been disappointing. Although an abnormal SNRT is a relatively specific marker for patients with significant sinus node dysfunction, it is frequently normal in patients with a clear history of symptoms associated with sinus bradyarrhythmias. Autonomic nervous system influences on sinus nodal function, which are difficult to reproduce during the study, may account for some of these inconsistencies. Measurement of sinoatrial conduction times has also not proven particularly valuable as a test to screen patients for suspected sinus node dysfunction. At present, ambulatory monitoring remains the most reliable guide to therapy in patients with disorders of sinus node function, and the tests outlined are used chiefly to confirm or clarify other clinical findings.

AV Conduction

The specialized AV conduction system consists of the AV node, the common bundle of His, the bundle branches, and the distal Purkinje fiber network. In most cases, the mechanism responsible for a prolongation in AV conduction can be deduced from standard electrocardiographic criteria. Analysis of AV conduction intervals as outlined previously may also be of value. In certain situations, however, it may be useful to assess the responses of the AV conduction system to both incremental atrial stimulation and atrial extra-stimuli.

Atrial pacing is usually performed from the right atrium, but coronary sinus pacing may also be used. Pacing is started at a cycle length just below the sinus cycle length, and the cycle length is decreased by 20 to 50 msec every 30 to 60 seconds. Periodic pauses between runs should be allowed to avoid reflex changes due to prolonged rapid heart rates. The onset of AV nodal Wenckebach and the point at which 2:1 AV nodal block develops should be noted. In resting adults, the development of AV nodal Wenckebach at a cycle length of greater than 500 msec or less than 300 msec is considered abnormal. It must be remembered that drugs, age, and autonomic tone all have profound effects on AV nodal conduction, and these factors must be considered in interpreting the data, both in absolute terms and when serial comparisons are made.

During incremental atrial pacing, the HV interval usually remains constant. The development of block within or below the bundle of His during atrial pacing, particularly at a pacing cycle length of >400 msec, is an abnormal finding.[10] Rate-related bundle branch block may also be observed during incremental atrial pacing, and its demonstration may be of value for the interpretation of previously observed wide complex beats or tachycardias of uncertain origin.

The clinical value of isolated His bundle recording is usually limited, because moderate prolongation of the HV interval is common. In asymptomatic patients with bundle branch block, HV intervals of under 80 to 100 msec have not been associated with a high rate of progression to complete heart block.[11] As illustrated in Figure 22–4, however, His bundle recording may be helpful in explaining atypical electrocardiographic patterns of AV block.

The effective, relative, and functional refractory periods of the AV conduction system may be measured using the atrial extrastimulus method. A stimulation train of eight atrial beats (A_1) at a constant cycle length is followed by a single premature stimulus (A_2). The drive train is repeated after a 2- to 6-second pause, and the extrastimulus is introduced at progressive decrements of 10 or 20 msec. The effective refractory period (ERP) of the AV node is defined as the longest A_1-A_2 interval that captures the atrium but fails to conduct to the bundle of His. The relative refractory period is the longest atrial premature interval that results in a measurable increase in the AH interval over that measured during the drive train. The functional refractory period is the shortest interval between His bundle depolarizations (H_1-H_2) that results from any A_1-A_2.

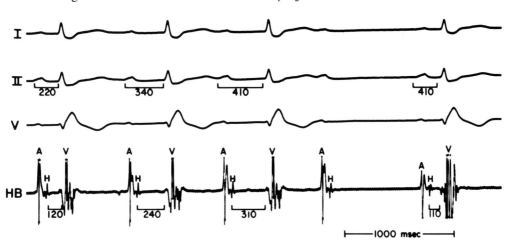

Fig. 22–4. Infra-Hisian Wenckebach block. The tracings were obtained in a 31-year-old man with Wenckebach type second-degree AV block on his ECG and a history of syncope. Intracardiac recordings documented that the site of conduction delay was below the bundle of His (HB) despite the Wenckebach periodicity. Note that all of the progressive conduction delay occurs within the HV interval.

The response of the AV node to premature stimuli usually yields a relatively smooth curve when A_2-H_2 intervals are plotted against A_1-A_2 intervals. In some patients, however, the curve may be discontinuous (Fig. 22–5), and longitudinal dissociation of conduction due to dual pathways in the AV node has been postulated as the underlying mechanism.[12] This phenomenon can be demonstrated in many patients with paroxysmal supraventricular tachycardia (SVT) caused by AV nodal re-entry but can also be observed in some patients without a clinical history of episodic SVT.

PROGRAMMED ELECTRICAL STIMULATION

Many chronic cardiac tachyarrhythmias are caused by the re-entry of impulses over fixed circuits within the heart. Re-entrant arrhythmias may be either monomorphic, when only a single circuit is involved, or polymorphic, when multiple circuits are involved simultaneously. Re-entry depends on dissociation of conduction and refractory properties of contiguous tissue enabling unidirectional block to occur in one limb of the circuit and slow conduction in the opposite limb. If conduction in the initially blocked circuit recovers after an appropriate interval, it will conduct an impulse that has completed the circuit in retrograde fashion. If the tissue proximal to the region of initial block has recovered excitability, a re-entrant beat is initiated. Premature stimulation, by decreasing the time allowed for tissues to recover, is able to induce re-entrant arrhythmias by enhancing the inhomogeneity of conduction and refractory properties of adjacent tissues.

A number of factors influence the results of programmed cardiac stimulation (Table 22–2). These factors may all interact in a fashion that has not been totally characterized. As a result, it is often difficult to compare results obtained in different laboratories that use different stimulation protocols. At present, there is no general agreement on the techniques that afford optimal sensitivity without sacrificing specificity. The protocol we use currently for programmed stimulation is outlined below.

Atrial Stimulation. Single (S_2) and double (S_2-S_3) atrial extrastimuli are introduced during sinus rhythm and after eight beats of atrial pacing (S_1) at cycle lengths of 600 and 400 msec. A pause of 2 to 6 seconds is allowed to occur between successive drive trains. The initial S_1-S_2 interval is set to put S_2 in late diastole, and the interval is decreased in 10 or 20 msec decrements until S_2 no longer captures. This defines the atrial effective refractory period (ERP) for that cycle length. The S_1-S_2 interval is then set at 50 msec above the atrial ERP, and the S_2-S_3 interval is set equal to that S_1-S_2 interval. S_2-S_3 is then decreased in 10 msec decrements until S_3 is refractory.

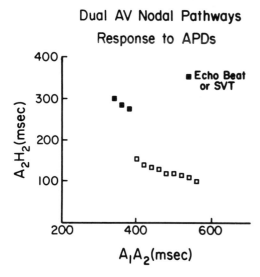

Dual AV Nodal Pathways
Response to APDs

■ Echo Beat
  or SVT

Fig. 22–5. AV conduction in a patient with dual AV nodal pathways. The A_2-H_2 intervals are plotted against the A_1-A_2 intervals. The sudden increase in A_2-H_2 signifies a shift in conduction to the slow pathway as the refractory period of the faster pathway is reached.

Table 22–2. *Factors Affecting Results of Programmed Stimulation*

Site of stimulation
Amplitude and duration of stimuli
Number of extrastimuli
Coupling intervals for extrastimuli
Cycle lengths of drive trains
Rate and duration of burst pacing
Definition of a positive response
Use of provocative stimuli
Population studied

S_1-S_2 is then shortened by 10 msec until S_3 captures. The sequence is repeated until S_2 no longer captures. In patients with supraventricular arrhythmias, atrial premature stimulation is repeated from the left atrium using the same protocol. Finally, bursts of atrial pacing at rates up to 300 beats per minute may be used to assess the point at which AV conduction delay occurs and the effects of conduction delay on arrhythmia initiation. When indicated, triple extrastimuli or bursts of rapid atrial pacing at rates up to 800 per minute may be used to induce atrial flutter or atrial fibrillation.

Ventricular Stimulation. Retrograde conduction is assessed during short trains of fixed-rate ventricular pacing and single extrastimuli, and the cycle length, coupling interval, and site at which VA block occurs should be noted. Single, double, and triple ventricular extrastimuli are delivered to the right ventricular apex during both sinus rhythm and ventricular pacing at cycle lengths of 600 and 400 msec. The coupling intervals are varied in a similar manner to the sequence described above. Use of only coupling intervals longer than or equal to 180 msec helps prevent induction of nonspecific polymorphic arrhythmias.[13] If no arrhythmia is initiated with right ventricular apical stimulation, stimulation is repeated from a second right ventricular site, usually the outflow tract. Some other laboratories prefer to stimulate with double extrastimuli at two right ventricular sites before proceeding to triple extrastimuli at either site. A number of other additional steps are used by others or in selected patients. These include repetition of each coupling interval before proceeding, the use of abrupt cycle length change (400 to 600 msec) after the seventh or eighth beat of the drive,[14] use of 3 or more drive cycle lengths, isoproterenol infusions, and left ventricular stimulation.

Supraventricular Arrhythmias

Programmed atrial and ventricular stimulation is frequently useful in patients with a history of supraventricular arrhythmias. These studies can be used to define the mechanism responsible for the arrhythmia, to localize any extranodal pathways that might be involved, to assess risk of more serious arrhythmias in patients with Wolff-Parkinson-White syndrome, to measure the effects of drug therapy, and to provide a guide for attempts to interrupt a pathway required for arrhythmia propagation, either surgically or with catheter techniques.[12,15–16]

Paroxysmal Supraventricular Tachycardia

Five electrophysiologic mechanisms account for the majority of cases of paroxysmal supraventricular tachycardia (PSVT) that occur clinically. Four of these are due to re-entry. Patients with these latter types manifest characteristic patterns of responses to atrial and ventricular stimulation (Table 22–3). The electrophysiologic study should determine the mode(s) of stimulation required to initiate and terminate the tachycardia, the requirements of atria or ventricles for tachycardia initiation and continuation, the atrial activation sequence during PSVT, and the effects of atrial and ventricular stimulation during tachycardia. In addition, it is often helpful to evaluate the effects of drugs or physical maneuvers on the tachycardia.

Re-entry within the AV node is the most common cause for recurrent PSVT. The tachycardia circuit involves antegrade conduction over a "slow" antegrade AV nodal pathway and retrograde conduction over a "fast" pathway. This "fast" pathway may be either true nodal tissue or perinodal fibers. With atrial premature stimulation, a discontinuous AV nodal conduction curve can often be demonstrated (Fig. 22–5). Initiation of AV nodal re-entrant SVT usually occurs after atrial or, less commonly, ventricular premature beats that produce a critical AV nodal conduction delay or during atrial pacing that results in 2-degree AV block. As the antegrade refractory period of the fast pathway is reached, the AH interval is abruptly prolonged because the slow pathway is then used for antegrade conduction. If PSVT is initiated, or if an echo beat occurs, retrograde septal atrial activation often occurs

Table 22–3. *Characteristics of Common Forms of Supraventricular Tachycardia*

Arrhythmia	Mode of Initiation	Requirement for Atrium/Ventricle	P Wave Morphology, Position	Atrial Activation Sequence	Notes
AV nodal re-entry	APD, VPD, AP	Neither	Retrograde, usually obscured by QRS	Caudocephalad, AVJ earliest	Discontinuous AV nodal conduction curve common
AV re-entry in patients with WPW or CBT	APD, VPD, AP, VP	Both	Variable, usually after QRS	Depends on AP location	Smooth AV nodal conduction, ipsilateral BBB increases CL
Intra-atrial re-entry	APD, AP	Atrium	Variable, PR related to rate	Depends on location	AV block common
Sinoatrial re-entry	APD	Atrium	Normal, PR related to rate	Identical to sinus	AV block may occur
Automatic atrial tachycardia	Spontaneous	Atrium	Variable, PR related to rate	Depends on location	AV block may occur

Abbreviations: AP = atrial pacing; APD = atrial premature depolarizations; AV = atrioventricular; AVJ = atrioventricular junction; CBT = concealed bypass tract; SVT = supraventricular tachycardia; VP = ventricular pacing; VPD = ventricular premature depolarizations; WPW = Wolff-Parkinson-White syndrome.

simultaneously with ventricular activation. The septal atrial deflection on the His bundle electrogram is then obscured by ventricular activity, but left and right atrial activation indicates a normal retrograde activation pattern. Because the re-entry circuit is located within the AV node, AV dissociation may occur and be demonstrated with premature stimulation during tachycardia.

The second most common form of recurrent SVT involves antegrade conduction over the AV node and retrograde conduction over an extranodal pathway (orthodromic AV reciprocating tachycardia). This arrhythmia mechanism may be documented in patients with manifest pre-excitation (Wolff-Parkinson-White syndrome) and in patients whose accessory pathways conduct only in retrograde fashion (concealed bypass tracts). PSVT initiation may occur when an atrial extrastimulus encounters antegrade block in the accessory pathway and causes prolonged AV conduction through the normal pathway. An example is shown in Figure 22–6. Initiation may also occur when a ventricular extrastimulus blocks

retrogradely in the His-Purkinje system and conducts over the accessory pathway only. Atrial activation during SVT depends on the location of the accessory pathway, and a precise location may be determined if atrial activity is recorded from multiple sites (Fig. 22–7). If eccentric activation is not seen and the first retrograde activity is recorded at the AV junction, it is useful to confirm the presence of a septal bypass tract by advancing atrial activation during PSVT with a premature ventricular stimulus introduced at the time of antegrade His bundle activation. In PSVT due to AV re-entry, ventricular activation is required before the accessory pathway can be entered; thus atrial activity of necessity follows ventricular activity, and the development of bundle branch block ipsilateral to the pathway increases the tachycardia cycle length. Contralateral bundle branch block does not affect cycle length. Both atria and ventricles are required for the arrhythmia circuit, and AV dissociation should not occur.

Sinus node re-entry and intra-atrial re-entry are the two other common re-entrant forms of

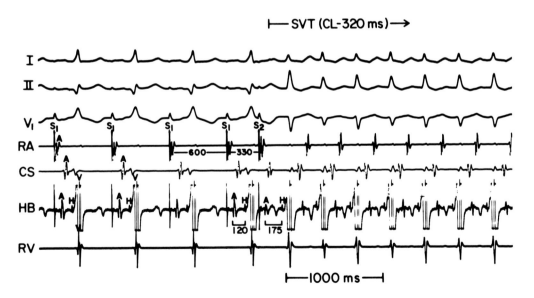

Fig. 22–6. Initiation of AV reciprocating tachycardia in a patient with Wolff-Parkinson-White syndrome. After eight atrially paced beats at a cycle length of 600 msec, a single atrial premature stimulus (S₂) is introduced. Antegrade block is produced in the accessory pathway, and the change in QRS morphology indicates that AV conduction is by way of the normal pathway. The impulse then can engage the left-sided pathway in the retrograde conduction, and the re-entrant circuit is completed. (SVT, supraventricular tachycardia; CL, cycle length; RA, right atrium; CS, coronary sinus; HB, His bundle; RV, right ventricle.)

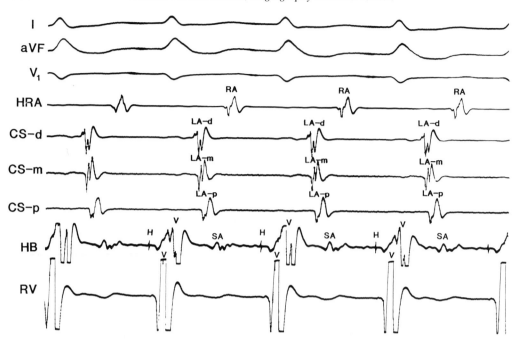

Fig. 22–7. Atrial activation sequence in supraventricular tachycardia (SVT) caused by a concealed bypass tract. The tracings are high speed (150 mm/sec) recordings made during SVT. Note that the first retrograde atrial activity recorded after ventricular depolarization is from the left atrium (LA) as recorded on the distal coronary sinus (CS-d) catheter. High right atrial (HRA) and septal right atrial (SA) activations are recorded later. (HB, His bundle; RV, right ventricle.)

PSVT. Both are independent of AV nodal conduction delay and may continue in the presence of AV block. PSVT may also be caused by increased automaticity in an ectopic atrial focus, by re-entry over multiple accessory pathways, and by a variety of patterns in patients with atypical variants of pre-excitation. Discussion of the electrophysiologic characteristics of these latter arrhythmias is beyond the scope of this chapter.

The indications for electrophysiologic study in patients with recurrent PSVT have broadened as new surgical and catheter approaches that offer the promise of correction of the substrate underlying the arrhythmia have become available. Such nonpharmacologic therapies must be guided by information obtained at electrophysiologic study. At present, electrophysiologic studies for selecting and guiding therapy are indicated whenever the symptoms from arrhythmia are severe so that the risk from any recurrence is high or whenever nonpharmacologic therapy is considered.

Atrial Flutter and Fibrillation

Intracardiac recording and programmed stimulation are of less value in other atrial arrhythmias. Atrial flutter may be diagnosed by recording discrete atrial depolarizations with a constant cycle length ranging between 240 and 180 msec. Bursts of rapid atrial pacing, usually at rates between 320 and 420 beats per minute, terminate flutter in about two thirds of patients if atrial capture can be achieved, particularly if the patient has been pretreated with an antiarrhythmic drug.[17,18] It is frequently difficult to confirm atrial capture at these rapid pacing rates using only a surface ECG, and we have preferred to monitor a local electrogram from the recording poles of an endocardial catheter during each attempt at termination. The initial pacing cycle length is set just shorter than the flutter cycle length, and 5- to 15-second bursts of pacing are delivered. If the first attempt is unsuccessful, shorter cycle lengths are tried until 1:1 atrial capture is no longer possible. The primary advantages of atrial pacing over transthoracic cardioversion are the avoidance of anesthesia and the ability to institute pacing if sinus node dysfunction is present. We have noted that it may be necessary to try pacing from several different sites within the atrium before successful termination of the arrhythmia can be achieved.

Atrial fibrillation and some cases of atrial flutter cannot be terminated with burst pacing, and the value of serial drug testing by repeated attempts to initiate arrhythmia in these patients has not been proven. For these reasons, electrophysiologic studies in patients with paroxysmal atrial flutter or paroxysmal atrial fibrillation as their only rhythm disturbance are only occasionally useful.

Accessory Pathways

In patients with pre-excitation, it is necessary to measure the effective refractory period of the accessory pathway for both antegrade and retrograde conduction and to localize the pathway. The effective refractory period of the pathway may be defined as the shortest coupling interval after which an extrastimulus cannot be conducted over the pathway. During atrial decremental extrastimulation in patients with pre-excitation, the QRS may become more and more bizarre as the contribution of conduction over the accessory pathway to ventricular activation becomes more pronounced. Once the effective refractory period of the pathway is reached, either no AV conduction occurs or, if the ERP of the pathway is relatively long, the PR length and the QRS normalize as conduction is shifted to the normal AV conduction system. It is also advisable to initiate atrial fibrillation in these patients because the shortest RR interval measured during atrial fibrillation approximates the true antegrade ERP of the accessory pathway and correlates with the risk of future occurrence of a life-threatening arrhythmia.[19]

The location of the accessory pathway can be determined best by atrial activation mapping during either SVT or ventricular stimulation. The earliest site of atrial activation found correlates with the location of the accessory pathway. Atrial stimulation from this site should also result in the shortest possible stimulus-to-ventricle activation time and usually shows the greatest degree of pre-excitation at any given pacing cycle length. Multiple accessory pathways may be present, but are often difficult to identify at electrophysiologic study. Careful attention should be paid to changes in antegrade or retrograde activation patterns to detect changes that might indicate a second pathway. It is necessary to record activation at multiple sites along the coronary sinus and around the tricuspid ring to evaluate this possibility. Serial electrophysiologic measurements are often used to characterize the effects of drugs on the pathways involved in PSVT. Many drug effects on either the AV node or accessory pathways can be reversed by catecholamine administration,[20] and data obtained by serial comparisons may not always predict clinical response. These responses, however, may be useful as rough estimates of the magnitude and direction of drug effect.

Ventricular Arrhythmias

The successful use of electrophysiologic studies in patients with supraventricular arrhythmias led several groups of investigators to use a similar approach in patients with recurrent ventricular tachycardia and ventricular fibrillation.[21-24] Many questions about the optimal methods for evaluating such patients remain unanswered, however, and the role of such studies in these patients has not been completely defined.

The ventricular stimulation protocol used in our laboratory has been outlined. Like any other stimulation protocol, it attempts to reach a compromise between sensitivity and specificity. Sensitivity is increased if more extrastimuli are used,[25-27] if several sites are stimulated,[28,29] if stimulus intensity is increased, and if either nonsustained or polymorphic runs of ventricular tachycardia or ventricular fibrillation are accepted as positive responses.[30,31] Any attempts to increase sensitivity through the use of more aggressive stimulation protocols, however, have resulted in decreased specificity, i.e., when the stimulation protocol is used in patients without a history of prior arrhythmia, "positive" responses are obtained. In addition, an aggressive stimulation protocol may make suppression of the arrhythmia at subsequent testing difficult or impossible, thereby limiting the value of electrophysiologic testing for evaluating therapy.[32]

The definition of a positive response is also difficult because there is not a clearly defined separation in response to a reasonably sensitive stimulation protocol between populations with and without previous arrhythmias. All investigators would agree that sustained, monomorphic ventricular tachycardia that is morphologically identical to a clinically documented arrhythmia is a positive response. Unfortunately, a 12-lead ECG during tachycardia with the patient off antiarrhythmic drug therapy is available in only a small number of patients, and such a correlation cannot always be made. It has been our practice to define the reproducible initiation of >30 sec of any ventricular tachycardia in response to 1, 2, or 3 extrastimuli as a positive response. It is important to try to reproduce the clinically documented arrhythmia in all patients with a history of sustained ventricular tachycardia. Therefore, we recommend that the stimulation protocol always be carried out, either to its conclusion or to initiation of a sustained arrhythmia. When these definitions are used, a ventricular arrhythmia can be reproducibly initiated with our protocol in over 95% of patients with coronary artery disease and a history of ventricular tachycardia and in about 60 to 75% of patients with that diagnosis who present with out-of-hospital cardiac arrest. Lower percentages of successful initiation are observed in other forms of heart disease.

For serial electrophysiologic studies to be a valid method for guiding antiarrhythmic therapy, it is necessary that the results be reproducible from study to study. It is clear that there are often day-to-day and even same-day differences in the point during the stimulation protocol at which sustained arrhythmia is initiated. Minor changes in the number of extrastimuli required for initiation should not be considered significant because they can be caused by a spontaneous variability in response.[33,34] Many patients also have more than one type of tachycardia, and therefore changes in cycle length and morphology between studies should be interpreted conservatively.

Initial Study. In preparation for the patient's initial electrophysiologic study, antiarrhythmic therapy should be discontinued, and the patient should be observed in a monitored setting until plasma drug concentrations are undetectable. Sinus node function and AV conduction should be assessed routinely, and several recording catheters should be used to exclude PSVT with aberrancy as the mechanism for any arrhythmia. Programmed ventricular stimulation is then performed according to the protocol outlined. If a sustained ventricular arrhythmia is initiated, the patient's ability to tolerate the arrhythmia should be evaluated immediately. Some laboratories routinely record intra-arterial pressure during these studies, but we have not found this necessary except during prolonged mapping procedures. If the arrhythmia is poorly tolerated, attempts should be made to terminate it with bursts of rapid ventricular pacing beginning at a cycle length just below that of the tachycardia (Fig. 22–8). In well-tolerated tachycardias, single or double extrastimuli may produce termination with less risk of acceleration. If syncope or severe chest pain develops or if the tachycardia either cannot be terminated with drugs or pacing or accelerates when pacing is attempted, direct current countershock should be used. We have found it helpful to monitor response to countershock by watching the intraventricular electrogram as opposed to a surface ECG lead because its signal is not distorted by muscle activity caused by the countershock or seizure activity. It is also helpful to use self-adhesive defibrillator pads because they provide a more stable ECG and facilitate shock delivery.

Electrophysiologic studies may be carried out in serial fashion to evaluate the effects of antiarrhythmic drugs or surgical procedures. During a drug trial, programmed ventricular

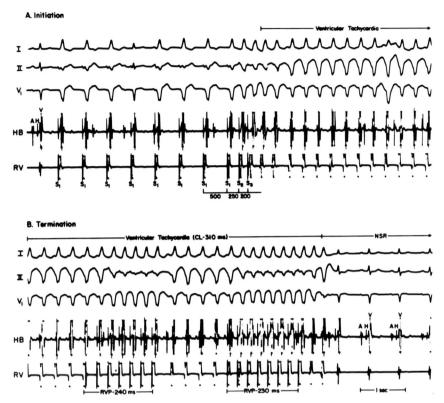

Fig. 22–8. Electrophysiologic study in a patient with recurrent ventricular tachycardia. A. Sustained ventricular tachycardia is initiated by double extrastimuli (S_2-S_3) after eight paced beats at a cycle length of 500 msec. B. Two bursts of rapid ventricular pacing (RVP) are delivered. The first fails to terminate the arrhythmia, but the second at a shorter cycle length is effective and sinus rhythm is restored. Note that the His bundle (HB) electrogram shows an absent His potential and AV dissociation during tachycardia.

stimulation using the original protocol is repeated. Although many laboratories advocate stimulation at multiple sites during each drug trial, it has been our practice to use only the site from which ventricular tachycardia was initiated at the initial study. Suppression of the ability to induce an arrhythmia has correlated well with subsequent protection from recurrent arrhythmias by any form of therapy in our experience[35] and in that of others.[36–38] Unfortunately, many patients do not respond completely to any drug tested and, for this reason, criteria for partially beneficial responses would be desirable. Proposed criteria have included an increase in the stimulation intensity required for arrhythmia induction, prolongation of tachycardia cycle length, and changes in duration or morphology. All of these criteria have some limitations, however, and should

be used cautiously because firm data about their validity are lacking.

Catheter Mapping. The concept that sustained ventricular tachycardia (VT) is due to re-entry in a small area of the ventricle has led to a number of innovative nonpharmacologic approaches to its control. If patients are able to tolerate their arrhythmia, an electrode catheter can be inserted retrogradely into the left ventricle, and bipolar recordings can be made from multiple sites. The mapping scheme originally proposed by the investigators at the University of Pennsylvania is most widely used (Fig. 22–9).[39] In this manner, activation sequence maps of the left ventricle during tachycardia can be generated and the site of earliest activity identified. In patients with coronary artery disease, these areas have usually been found within the border zones of ventricular

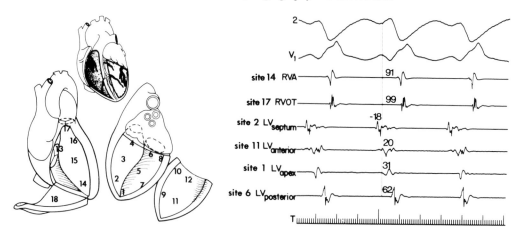

Fig. 22–9. Catheter mapping of ventricular tachycardia. The left panel shows a schematic diagram of standard recording positions used during catheter mapping. The right panel shows selected local electrograms recorded during ventricular tachycardia. Activation at site 2 precedes the onset of the QRS (dotted line) and identifies the site or region of tachycardia origin. LV-left ventricle, RVA-right ventricular apex, RVOT-right ventricular outflow tract. (Reproduced by permission from Josephson ME, et al: Role of catheter mapping in the preoperative evaluation of ventricular tachycardia. Am J Cardiol 49:207, 1982.)

aneurysms or scars resulting from previous myocardial infarction. Although preoperative catheter mapping is often valuable, more precise information is gained during intraoperative endocardial mapping and serial stimulation during cardiopulmonary bypass can be used to guide the extent of resection or the need for cryoablation. This is of particular value because many patients manifest more than one morphologically distinct tachycardia during intraoperative stimulation.[40,41] Patients are restudied as soon as they are stable postoperatively, and suppression of the ability to induce arrhythmia may be seen in a high percentage of patients. Further refinement of these techniques may improve the prognosis for many patients who cannot be optimally managed with drug therapy alone or for those with other indications (e.g., valve dysfunction, critical coronary stenoses) for cardiac surgery.

Device Therapy. During the last decade, the use of implantable devices for the management of arrhythmias has become increasingly important. Because most chronic arrhythmias are due to re-entry, they are often susceptible to interruption by pacing. Pacemakers have been devised that can sense a tachycardia and then, according to a preset algorithm, deliver a series of pacing interventions to terminate the ar-

rhythmia. Sensing criteria commonly used include cycle length, abrupt change in cycle length at arrhythmia onset, and duration of arrhythmia. Pacing modes usually include short bursts of pacing that are adjusted to the cycle length of the tachycardia. If the arrhythmia is not terminated by the initial pacing attempt, the algorithm adjusts the cycle length or duration of the next burst. In some algorithms, the unit recalls the pacing intervention that was last effective and begins with it at the next episode.

Although antitachycardia pacing is often effective under controlled conditions in the laboratory, there is a risk of accelerating or disorganizing the arrhythmia in virtually all patients.[42] For this reason, permanent antitachycardia pacing alone is useful primarily in patients with atrial as opposed to ventricular arrhythmias. Patients with pre-excitation in whom the initiation of atrial fibrillation could be dangerous would also not be good candidates for an antitachycardia pacemaker. The incorporation of antitachycardia pacing into a device that also has the capacity of back-up defibrillation is an exciting technology that is now reaching clinical application.

The automatic implantable cardioverter defibrillator (AICD) was introduced into clinical practice in 1980. The original device had only a limited function, to charge and deliver a shock whenever it sensed ventricular fibrillation. Subsequently, many improvements in these devices have been made, and AICD therapy is now recognized as a critical option in arrhythmia management.[43,44] The basic components of an AICD are an electronic module, capacitors, and an energy source encased in titanium. Bipolar pacing leads that permit rate counting and, in some devices, pacing, are implanted in the heart. Two other leads are used for morphology sensing, if desired, and defibrillation. Either a transvenous electrode-LV epicardial patch combination or two epicardial patches may be used. Other types of lead systems that might permit implantation without thoracotomy or allow delivery of sequential shocks are currently undergoing testing. No matter what combination of leads are chosen, the ends to be inserted into the AICD are tunneled subcutaneously to the abdomen, where a pocket for the generator has been created.

The rate-counting leads may be either endocardial or epicardial. After positioning of these leads, R-wave amplitude (> 5 mV) and the duration of the local electrogram (< 110 msec) are measured to ensure accurate rate determination. The defibrillating leads are then implanted and the adequacy of their electrograms assessed as above. The leads are then connected to an external cardioverter-defibrillator that can deliver shocks of from 1 to 40 J. Ventricular fibrillation is induced by delivering AC current and the defibrillation threshold determined. There should be at least a 10 J margin of safety between the defibrillation threshold and the amount of energy the device will deliver. If the defibrillation threshold is high, either the types of leads, their orientation, or their polarity should be changed until a satisfactory defibrillation threshold is achieved. A follow-up study to confirm the stability of the device is usually performed just before hospital discharge.

Devices that combine antitachycardia pacing with back-up defibrillation, have electrogram storage for events, reanalyze the pa-

tient's arrhythmia just before shock delivery, and incorporate advanced algorithms for arrhythmia recognition are undergoing clinical trials. By greatly improving flexibility, these devices will make such therapy applicable to many additional patients.

Catheter Ablation. Catheter ablation of the AV conduction system was originally developed as a means of controlling ventricular rates in patients with drug-refractory supraventricular arrhythmias.[16] Inducing AV block and inserting an adaptive rate pacemaker can often improve symptoms in such patients dramatically.[45,46]

Figure 22–10 illustrates the setup for AV junctional ablation. A temporary pacing wire is positioned in the right ventricular apex and a previously unused 6 or 7 Fr electrode catheter is positioned across the tricuspid valve. The catheter is manipulated so that a large unipolar His bundle deflection is recorded from one of the electrodes. This pole is then connected to the cathodal output of a standard defibrillator. A large adhesive electrode placed on the patient's back over the left scapula is used as the anode. Once the intracardiac electrode is in a satisfactory position, the patient is anesthetized using a short-acting barbiturate, and a 200 or 300 J cathodal shock is delivered. This usually results in complete heart block. After this first shock, it usually becomes difficult to record a high quality His bundle deflection. The catheter position is then visually confirmed and a second shock of the same energy is delivered to the same region. Heart rate is supported by the temporary pacemaker, which should be set at a high output because the pacing threshold may rise transiently after each catheter shock. The patient is then observed in the laboratory for 30 to 45 minutes because some patients may resume AV conduction during this time. If AV block persists, the patient requires permanent pacemaker insertion, either immediately or within 24 hours.

The expected success rate for His bundle ablation should be greater than 80% in experienced centers.[45] Some patients will have a return of AV conduction within the first weeks after ablation. A second procedure is usually

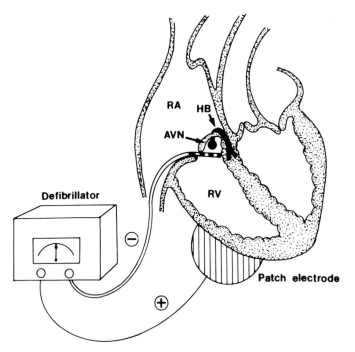

RA   HB

AVN

Defibrillator

RV

⊖

Patch electrode

⊕

Fig. 22–10. Schematic diagram of an AV junctional ablation. A new electrode catheter has been positioned across the tricuspid valve and the pole yielding the largest His deflection has been connected as the cathode to a standard defibrillator. The patch electrode placed over the left scapula serves as the anode. A transvenous pacing electrode will also be inserted to provide demand pacing if the post-ablation escape rhythm is not well tolerated. AVN-AV node, HB-His bundle, RA-right atrium, RV-right ventricle. (Reproduced by permission from Morady F: Interventional electrophysiology: Catheter ablation techniques. *In* Management of Cardiac Arrhythmias, The Nonpharmacologic Approach. Platia, E, ed. Philadelphia, J.B. Lippincott Co., 1987, pp 364–376.)

successful even though the His bundle electrogram may be fractionated and of low amplitude.

Modifications of the basic technique described above have been proposed. Radiofrequency energy eliminates the need for anesthesia but produces smaller lesions, and highly precise catheter positioning is required. The delivery of shocks more proximally in the AV nodal region may achieve modification rather than ablation of AV nodal conduction. This may be particularly useful in patients with AV nodal re-entry.[47] Catheter ablation techniques for right-sided and posteroseptal pathways have also been described.[48] Catheter shocks should not be delivered within the coronary sinus itself because there is a substantial risk of rupture and hemorrhage. Catheter ablation in patients with ventricular tachycardia has achieved only a modest rate of success and should rarely be used.

COMPLICATIONS OF ELECTROPHYSIOLOGIC STUDIES

One of the purposes of an electrophysiologic study is to reproduce a patient's clinical ar-

rhythmia. In many cases, these arrhythmias cause hemodynamic deterioration which, if not terminated promptly, might result in death. For this reason, it is critically important to evaluate every patient carefully before study for factors that might complicate any attempt at resuscitation. We try to screen out patients with unstable ischemia, uncompensated heart failure, severe, uncorrected valvular lesions, metabolic abnormalities, or drug toxicity in whom provocation of an arrhythmia might lead to irreversible collapse. By taking these precautions, we have been able to perform studies safely even in patients with advanced heart disease. If these precautions are taken, the complications of the electrophysiologic studies should be similar to those of any other catheterization procedure.

Deaths during electrophysiologic studies should be extremely rare. Only one death occurred among 1000 consecutive patients reported by Horowitz et al.[49] Cardioversion or defibrillation is, however, required in many patients who develop unstable arrhythmias. Other reported complications in that series included vascular injury (0.4%), thrombophlebitis (0.6%) or pulmonary embolism (0.3%),

arterial embolism (0.1%), and cardiac perforation (0.2%). A higher prevalence of thromboembolic complications is seen if patients are
followed long-term.[50] For this reason, we prefer to use intravenous heparin during the case,
except when a coronary sinus catheter is used,
and prescribe subcutaneous heparin while the
patient is hospitalized after the study. Drug
reactions including proarrhythmia may also be
seen whenever medications are given during
the study.

REFERENCES

1. Scherlag BJ, et al: Catheter technique for recording His bundle activity in man. Circulation 39:13, 1969.
2. Fisher JD: The role of electrophysiologic testing in the diagnosis and treatment of patients with known and suspected bradycardias and tachycardias. Prog Cardiovasc Dis 24:25, 1981.
3. Michelson EL, Dreifus LS: Present status of clinical electrophysiologic studies: Introduction—What studies are necessary. PACE 7:421, 1984.
4. Nattel S, Rinkenberger RL, Lehrman LL, Zipes DP: Therapeutic blood lidocaine concentration after local anesthesia for cardiac electrophysiologic studies. N Engl J Med 301:418, 1979.
5. Strauss HC, et al: Current diagnosis and therapeutic maneuvers in patients with sinus node disease. *In* Rappaport E (ed.): Cardiology Update—1983. New York, Elsevier, 1983, pp 193–218.
6. Mandell W, Hayakawa H, Danzig R, Marcus HS: Evaluation of sinoatrial function in man by overdrive suppression. Circulation 44:59, 1971.
7. Strauss HC, Saroff AL, Bigger JT Jr, Giardina EGV: Premature atrial stimulation as a key to the understanding of sinoatrial conduction in man. Circulation 47:86, 1973.
8. Narula OS, et al: A new method for measurement of sinoatrial conduction time. Circulation 58:706, 1978.
9. Reiffel JA, et al: The human sinus node electrogram. A transvenous catheter technique and a comparison of directly measured and indirectly estimated sinoatrial conduction time in adults. Circulation 62:1324, 1980.
10. Dhingra RC, et al: Significance of block distal to the His bundle induced by atrial pacing in patients with chronic bifascicular block. Circulation 60:1455, 1979.
11. McAnulty JH, et al: Natural history of "high-risk" bundle branch block. N Engl J Med 307:137, 1982.
12. Denes P, et al: Demonstration of dual A-V nodal pathways in patients with paroxysmal supraventricular tachycardia. Circulation 48:549, 1973.
13. Morady F, DiCarlo LA, Baerman JM, deBuitleir M: Comparison of coupling intervals that induce clinical and nonclinical forms of ventricular tachycardia during programmed stimulation. Am J Cardiol 57:1269, 1986.
14. Denker S, et al: Facilitation of ventricular tachycardia induction with abrupt changes in ventricular cycle length. Am J Cardiol 53:508, 1984.
15. Gallagher JJ, et al: Wolff-Parkinson-White syndrome. The problem, evaluation and surgical correction. Circulation 51:767, 1975.
16. Gallagher JJ, et al: Catheter technique for closed-chest ablation of the atrioventricular conduction system. N Engl J Med 306:194, 1982.
17. Della Bella P, et al: Facilitating influence of disopyramide on atrial flutter termination by overdrive pacing. Am J Cardiol 61:1046, 1988.
18. Greenberg ML, Kelly TA, Lerman BB, DiMarco JP: Atrial pacing for conversion of atrial flutter. Am J Cardiol 58:95, 1986.
19. Klein GJ, et al: Ventricular fibrillation in the Wolff-Parkinson-White syndrome. N Engl J Med 301:1080, 1979.
20. Niazi I, et al: Treatment of atrioventricular node reentrant tachycardia with encainide: reversal of drug effect with isoproterenol. J Am Coll Cardiol 13:904, 1989.
21. Horowitz LN, et al: Recurrent sustained ventricular tachycardia. 3. Role of the electrophysiologic study in selection of antiarrhythmic therapy. Circulation 58:987, 1978.
22. Mason JW, Winkle RA: Accuracy of the ventricular tachycardia-induction study for predicting long-term efficacy and inefficacy of antiarrhythmic drugs. N Engl J Med 303:1073, 1980.
23. Ruskin JN, DiMarco JP, Garan H: Out-of-hospital cardiac arrest. Electrophysiologic observations and selection of long-term antiarrhythmic therapy. N Engl J Med 303:607, 1980.
24. Josephson ME, Horowitz LN, Spielman SR, Greenspan AM: Electrophysiologic and hemodynamic studies in patients resuscitated from cardiac arrest. Am J Cardiol 46:948, 1980.
25. Mann DE, et al: Induction of clinical ventricular tachycardia using programmed stimulation: Value of third and fourth extrastimuli. Am J Cardiol 52:501, 1983.
26. Brugada P, Abdollah H, Heddle B, Wellens HJJ: Results of a ventricular stimulation protocol using a maximum of 4 premature stimuli in patients without documented or suspected ventricular arrhythmias. Am J Cardiol 52:1214, 1983.
27. Buxton AE, et al: Role of triple extrastimuli during electrophysiologic study of patients with documented sustained ventricular tachyarrhythmias. Circulation 69:532, 1984.
28. Doherty JU, et al: Programmed ventricular stimulation at a second right ventricular site: an analysis of 100 patients with special reference to sensitivity, specificity and characteristics of patients with induced ventricular tachycardia. Am J Cardiol 52:1184, 1983.
29. Morady F, Hess D, Scheinman MM: Electrophysiologic drug testing in patients with malignant ventricular arrhythmias: importance of stimulation at more than one ventricular site. Am J Cardiol 50:1055, 1982.
30. Swerdlow CD, Winkel RA, Mason JW: Prognostic significance of the number of induced ventricular complexes during assessment of therapy for ventricular arrhythmias. Circulation 68:400, 1983.
31. Brugada P, Green M, Abdollah H, Wellens HJJ: Significance of ventricular arrhythmias initiated by pro-

grammed ventricular stimulation: The importance of the type of arrhythmia induced and the number of premature stimuli required. Circulation 69:87, 1984.

32. Swerdlow CD, et al: Decreased incidence of antiarrhythmic drug efficacy at electrophysiologic study associated with the use of a third extrastimulus. Am Heart J 104:1004, 1982.

33. Cooper MJ, et al: Comparison of immediate versus day-to-day variability of ventricular tachycardia induction by programmed stimulation. J Am Coll Cardiol 13:599, 1989.

34. Kudenchuk PF, et al: Reproducibility of arrhythmia induction with intracardiac electrophysiologic testing in patients with clinical sustained ventricular tachyarrhythmias. J Am Coll Cardiol 7:819, 1986.

35. Zhu J, Haines DE, Lerman BB, DiMarco JP: Predictors of efficacy of amiodarone and characteristics of recurrence of arrhythmia in patients with sustained ventricular tachycardia and coronary artery disease. Circulation 76:802, 1987.

36. Swerdlow CD, Winkle RA, Mason JW: Determinants of survival in patients with ventricular tachyarrhythmias. N Engl J Med 208:1346, 1983.

37. Waller TJ, et al: Reduction in sudden death and total mortality by antiarrhythmic therapy evaluated by electrophysiologic drug testing: criteria of efficacy in patients with sustained ventricular tachyarrhythmias. J Am Coll Cardiol 10:83, 1987.

38. Rae AP, et al: Antiarrhythmic drug efficacy for ventricular tachyarrhythmias associated with coronary artery disease as assessed by electrophysiologic studies. Am J Cardiol 55:1494, 1985.

39. Josephson ME, et al: Role of catheter mapping in the preoperative evaluation of ventricular tachycardia. Am J Cardiol 49:207, 1982.

40. Miller JM, Kienzle MG, Harken AH, Josephson ME: Subendocardial resection for ventricular tachycardia:

predictors of surgical success. Circulation 70:624, 1984.

41. Wilber DJ, et al: Incidence and determinants of multiple morphologically distinct tachycardias. J Am Coll Cardiol 10:583, 1987.

42. Fisher JD, Kim SG, Waspe LE, Matos JA: Mechanisms for the success and failure of pacing for termination of ventricular tachycardia: Clinical and hypothetical considerations. PACE 6:1095, 1983.

43. Winkle RA, et al: Long-term outcome with the automatic implantable cardioverter-defibrillator. J Am Coll Cardiol 13:1353, 1989.

44. Kelly PA, et al: The automatic implantable cardioverter-defibrillator: efficacy, complications and survival in patients with malignant ventricular arrhythmias. J Am Coll Cardiol 11:1278, 1988.

45. Evans GT Jr, et al: The Percutaneous Cardiac Mapping and Ablation Registry: final summary of results. PACE 11:1621, 1988.

46. Morady F: Interventional electrophysiology: Catheter ablation techniques. *In* Management of Cardiac Arrhythmias, The Nonpharmacologic Approach. Platia, E, ed. Philadelphia, J.B. Lippincott Co., 1987, pp 364–386.

47. Epstein LM, et al: Percutaneous catheter modification of the atrioventricular node: A potential cure for atrioventricular nodal reentrant tachycardia. Circulation 80:757, 1989.

48. Morady F, et al: Long-term results of catheter ablation of a posteroseptal accessory atrioventricular connection in 48 patients. Circulation 79:1160, 1989.

49. Horowitz LN, et al: Risks and complications of clinical cardiac electrophysiologic studies: A prospective analysis of 1000 consecutive patients. J Am Coll Cardiol 9:1261, 1987.

50. DiMarco JP, Garan H, Ruskin JN: Complications in patients undergoing electrophysiologic procedures. Ann Intern Med 97:490, 1982.

23

Endomyocardial Biopsy

MARC J. LEVINE and DONALD S. BAIM*

As a result of recent improvements in catheter design and pathologic interpretation, transvascular endomyocardial biopsy has become an important component in the invasive evaluation of patients with known or suspected primary myocardial dysfunction.[1] Because significant controversy remains about the definition, frequency, natural history, and optimal treatment of many of these myocardial disorders, however, use of the endomyocardial biopsy in the routine evaluation of patients with myocardial disease varies from center to center. This chapter will focus on the currently available techniques for endomyocardial biopsy and the disease states in which myocardial histology appears most valuable, rather than on a precise listing of current indications for this procedure.

BIOPSY DEVICES

Cardiac biopsy in the 1950s was initially performed by means of limited thoracotomy. Subsequent attempts at transthoracic needle biopsy were frustrated by a nearly 10% incidence of major complications, including pneumothorax, tamponade, and coronary laceration.[2,3] Over the past several decades, these techniques have been replaced by a series of biopsy catheter systems (or bioptomes) that permit

*Some of the material in this chapter was developed in the previous edition in conjunction with Dr. Robert E. Fowles.

rapid and safe transvascular endomyocardial biopsy. There are two basic types of bioptomes: (1) stiff devices that are maneuvered independently through the vasculature, and (2) floppy devices that are positioned with the aid of a long sheath or introducing catheter.

Independent Bioptomes

The Konno Bioptome. In 1962, Sakakibara and Konno developed a biopsy catheter capable of transvascular introduction and procurement of endomyocardial biopsy samples from either the left or the right ventricular chamber.[4] The original device consisted of a 100-cm catheter shaft with two sharpened cups (diameter either 2.5 or 3.5 mm) at its tip. These cups could be opened or closed under the control of a single wire activated by a sliding assembly attached to the proximal end of the catheter. Because of the large size of the catheter head, it was usually introduced by means of cutdown on the saphenous or basilic vein or the femoral or brachial artery, maneuvered into the desired ventricle under fluoroscopic guidance, and applied to the endocardial surface with its jaws closed. The catheter was then withdrawn slightly, opened, readvanced into contact with the endocardium, reclosed, and withdrawn. While the Konno bioptome is still in limited use, the stiffness of its shaft complicates intravascular and intracardiac manipulation and has led to a variety of other devices based on the same theme.

The Kawai Bioptome

Developed by Kawai and Kitaura in 1977, this device has a highly flexible tip that can be deflected up to 40 degrees in one direction and up to 10 degrees in the opposite direction by rotation of a knob on the operating handle[5,6] (Fig. 23–1). This allows easy maneuvering through the vasculature and across the aortic or tricuspid valve for the right or left ventricular biopsy. Because of its extremely flexible tip, a stylet must be advanced into the catheter shaft before excision of an endomyocardial sample.

The Stanford (Caves-Schulz) Bioptome.

This device, developed as a modification of the Konno bioptome, was designed specifically for right ventricular biopsy by way of the right internal jugular vein[7,8] (Fig. 23–2) and has wide application in the United States. It consists of a somewhat flexible coil shaft fabricated from stainless steel and coated by clear plastic tubing (Sholten Surgical Supply, Palo Alto, CA). The tip of the catheter has two hemispheric cutting jaws with a combined diameter of 3.0 mm (9 Fr); one jaw is opened

and closed by a stainless steel wire running through the center of the bioptome shaft, and the other jaw is stationary. The control wire is attached to a ratcheting surgical mosquito clamp by means of a pair of adjustable nuts that allow the operator to set the force applied during opening and closing of the surgical clamp. These nuts should be adjusted so that the two biopsy jaws close just as the two halves of the ratchet mechanism make contact. The distal end of the catheter is equipped with a curve that forms an angle between 45 and 90 degrees (depending on whether the clamp is closed to its first or second click) with the shaft and lies in the same orientation as the handle of the clamp. With adequate care and cleaning, each instrument can be used for more than 50 procedures without the need for sharpening or service.

The biopsy procedure involves percutaneous entry of the right internal jugular vein. This is performed with the patient lying supine without a pillow and with his or her head turned far to the left. With the patient in this position, the operator should be able to identify the sternal notch, the sternal and clavicular heads of the right sternocleidomastoid muscle, and the top of the clavicle (Fig. 23–3). These

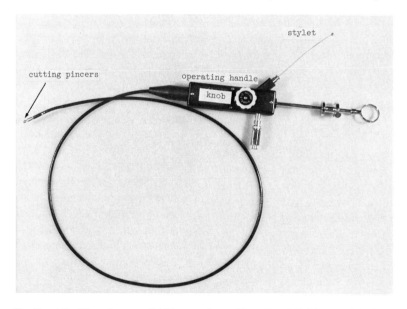

Fig. 23–1. The Kawai flexible endomyocardial biopsy catheter. (From Kawai C, Matsumori A, Kawamura K: Myocardial biopsy. Ann Rev Med 31:139, 1980. with permission.)

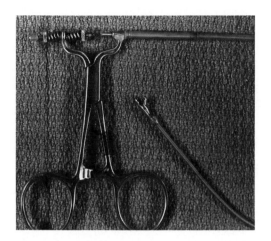

Fig. 23–2. Stanford (Caves-Schulz) bioptome. The surgical clamp drives the control wire by way of its connection through the two adjustable nuts, thereby controlling the position of the single mobile jaw.

anatomic features can be defined more easily if the patient is asked to lift his or her head just off the table. With a 25-gauge needle, a small intradermal bleb of 1% xylocaine is injected into the center of the triangle formed by the two muscle heads and the clavicle, at a point approximately two fingerbreadths above the top of the clavicle. A skin nick is created with the tip of a No. 11 blade and enlarged with a small mosquito clamp. A 6-ml non-Luer syringe is filled with 2 ml of xylocaine and attached to a 22-gauge, 1.5-inch needle. This needle is advanced through the skin nick at an angle 30 to 40 degrees from vertical, and 20 to 30 degrees right of the sagittal plane. Continuous suction is applied until the vein is entered, usually at a depth of 1 to 2.5 cm below the skin, using the steep angle of entry described above. If desired, small boluses of xylocaine can be injected into the soft tissues along the way, but the total volume injected should be kept under 1 ml to avoid compression of the vein within the carotid sheath. If the vein is not found, the needle should be withdrawn to the skin under continued suction, and puncture should be attempted with a slightly more lateral angulation; if this fails, a more medial angulation may be tried, but this increases the risk of

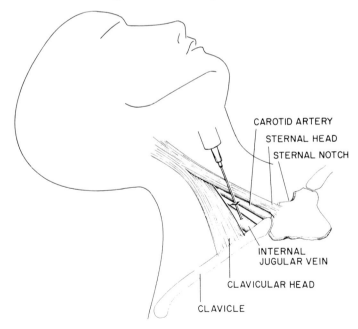

Fig. 23–3. Regional anatomy for right internal jugular vein puncture. With the patient's head rotated to the left, the sternal notch, clavicle, and the sternal and clavicular heads of the sternocleidomastoid muscle are identified. A skin nick is made between the two heads of the muscle, two fingerbreadths above the top of the clavicle, and the needle is inserted at an angle of 30 to 40 degrees from vertical and 20 to 30 degrees right of sagittal. This approach leads to reliable puncture of the internal jugular vein, and aims the needle away from the more medially located carotid artery.

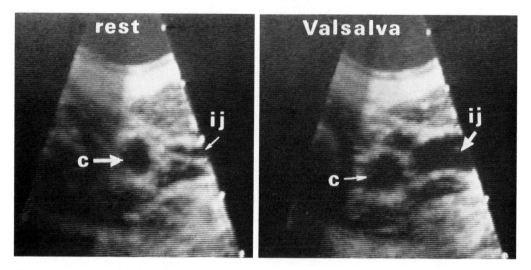

Fig. 23–4. Two-dimensional echo of the carotid artery (c) and the internal jugular vein (ij) at rest (left) and during a Valsalva maneuver (right), showing the marked enlargement in jugular venous caliber with increased distending pressure.

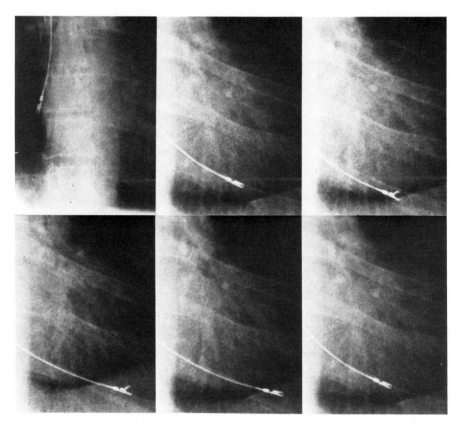

Fig. 23–5. Cineangiographic frames obtained during right ventricular endomyocardial biopsy using the Stanford bioptome: From left to right, the bioptome is shown against the lateral right atrial wall, against the ventricular septum, withdrawn slightly with jaws opened, reapplied to the septum with subsequent closure of the jaws, and withdrawn with sample.

carotid puncture. In patients with normal or low right atrial pressure, jugular venous puncture may be facilitated by elevation of the legs, the Trendelenburg position, or a Valsalva maneuver (Fig. 23–4). Once the vein is entered, we usually leave the "test" needle in place and perform a parallel puncture using a 2¾-inch 18-gauge thin-wall needle (UMI, Universal Medical Instruments, Ballston Spa, NY), through which a 40 cm J guide wire is then advanced into the right atrium. The "test" needle is now removed, and a 9 Fr sheath with a side-arm and backbleed-valve (Cordis Corp., Miami, FL) is then advanced over the guide wire and attached to a continuous intravenous drip adjusted to a moderate flow rate.

With the clamp closed on its first click, the bioptome is advanced into the sheath until its tip lies against the lateral right atrial wall in its lower third (Fig. 23–5). The catheter is then rotated counterclockwise into an anteromedial orientation and advanced across the tricuspid valve. As the valve is crossed, counterclockwise rotation is continued until the handle clamp is pointed nearly straight posteriorly, thus directing the tip of the bioptome at the interventricular septum. The bioptome should then appear on fluoroscopy to have its tip across the spine and below the upper margins of the left hemidiaphragm, in contact with the ventricular myocardium (recognized by the lack of further advancement, the occurrence of premature ventricular contractions, and the transmission of ventricular impulses to the operator's hand). This maneuver must be performed with both finesse and assurance. The bioptome is stiff and perforates the heart if advanced too vigorously in the wrong orientation (Fig. 23–6). If there is any doubt about its final position in the right ventricle and against the septum, this can be evaluated further by fluoroscopy in the 30-degree right anterior oblique and 60-degree left anterior oblique views. On occasion these views have disclosed unintentional positioning of the bioptome in the coronary sinus (i.e., in the A-V groove in the RAO projection) or in an infradiaphragmatic vein (i.e., under the heart and beyond the left heart border in the LAO projection). If the bioptome is not in the correct position, it must be withdrawn into the atrium and repositioned appropriately before sampling. In some patients, correct positioning may be facilitated by closing the handle clamp to its second click, thus increasing the curve of the bioptome to 90 degrees. Two-dimensional echocardiography has been reported as a useful alternative or adjunct to fluoroscopy for guiding endocardial biopsy.[9]

Once the biopsy catheter is in the desired position against the septal endocardium, it is

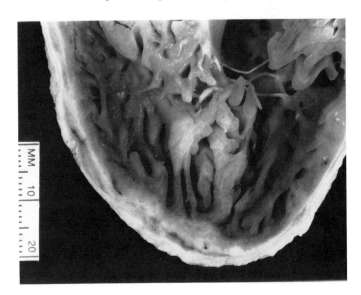

Fig. 23–6. Postmortem specimen shows the heavy trabeculation of the interior surface of the right ventricle and the thinness of the right ventricular free wall.

withdrawn about 1 cm, the jaws are opened, and the catheter is gently readvanced into contact with the endocardium (Fig. 23–5). The jaws are closed and the catheter is gently withdrawn with its enclosed sample. Although there is frequently a slight "tug" on the catheter as the sample is removed from the wall, forceful tugging with multiple premature ventricular contractions and inward retraction of the ventricular wall suggests that the jaws may have trapped a sample that includes the pericardium, in which case the jaws should be opened and the bioptome withdrawn without the sample.

A special 7 Fr pediatric Stanford bioptome is also available, and may be used from the subclavian vein in adults with difficult jugular venous access. Use of any rigid bioptome from the subclavian vein is more difficult than use from the right internal jugular vein, however, and the possibility of using one of the long-sheath techniques from an alternate site should be considered.

Long-sheath Devices

The King's Bioptome. The King's bioptome is a modification of the stainless steel Olympus bronchoscopic biopsy forceps (Olympus Corporation of America, Lake Success, NY), which is widely used in Europe[10,11] (Fig. 23–7). Its double opening scissor-action jaws are controlled by an inner drive wire attached to a proximal control handle. A compression spring on the control handle keeps the jaws in their closed position unless the handle's thumb ring is pushed in. The flexible forceps shaft and closed jaws have an outer diameter of 1.8 mm, allowing the catheter to be introduced into the desired ventricle through a radiopaque 6 or 7 Fr sheath which has been previously placed within the desired chamber. The sample is retrieved as described for the Stanford bioptome.

Disposable 50- and 104-cm versions of the King's type bioptome are now available (Cordis Corp., Miama, FL and Mansfield Scientific, Inc., Mansfield, MA), which can be used for biopsy of either the left or right ventricle.

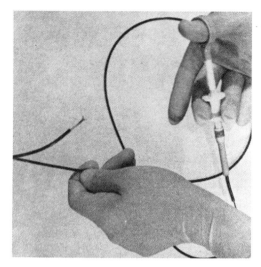

Fig. 23–7. The Olympus bioptome positioned through a modified Stanford biopsy sheath. (From Anderson JL, Marshall HW: The femoral venous approach to endomyocardial biopsy: comparison with internal jugular and transarterial approaches. Am J Cardiol 53:833, 1984, with permission.)

The longer bioptome is introduced through a 7 or 8 Fr, 98-cm curved Teflon introducing sheath (equipped with a back-bleed valve and side-arm flush mechanism) which has been previously positioned within the desired chamber over a conventional cardiac catheter. Once the tip of the sheath is in position, the conventional catheter is withdrawn and the bioptome is introduced. The shorter bioptome is employed for right ventricular biopsy using a 45-cm length sheath inserted by way of the right internal jugular vein. A similar system has been used to permit transseptal catheterization and endomyocardial biopsy of the left ventricle in children.[12]

The Stanford Left Ventricular Bioptome. The original Stanford bioptome has been modified for left ventricular biopsy by doubling its length to 100 cm and reducing its outer diameter to 6 Fr.[8] With this reduction in shaft diameter, the catheter is no longer capable of independent movement through the vasculature and must be positioned with the aid of a 90-cm curved Teflon sheath, which is itself introduced into the left ventricle over a conventional 100 cm 6.7 Fr pigtail catheter (Stanford Biopsy Set, Cook Inc., Bloomington,

IN). The tip of the sheath is positioned below the mitral apparatus and away from the posterobasal segment, which is more easily perforated than other areas of the left ventricle. The pigtail catheter is then removed, the sheath flushed, and the bioptome introduced.

The Stanford left ventricular sheath has been modified by Anderson to permit biopsy of the right ventricular septum by way of the percutaneous femoral venous approach.[13] The Teflon sheath is heated over a forming wire to create an 8-cm distal semicircular curve with 70-degree posterior angulation of the final 3 cm (Fig. 23–7). When this sheath is placed in the right ventricle over the 6.7 Fr pigtail catheter (itself heated to form a distal Cournand-like curve), it rests against the septum to allow safe biopsy of that structure without risk of free wall perforation (Fig. 23–8). Commercially developed guiding sheaths (Cordis Corp., Miami, FL), preformed with the desired distal curves,[14] are also available for use with either reusable or disposable transfemoral bioptomes. Sheathless uréthane-coated disposable bioptomes are also available for use by the internal jugular approach. It may be wise to consider use of disposable biopsy equipment, in view of widespread concern over acquired immunodeficiency syndrome (AIDS) and other blood-borne infectious diseases.

COMPLICATIONS

Transvascular endomyocardial biopsy of either the left or right ventricle can be performed safely using any of the techniques described. A worldwide survey of more than 6000 cases showed a procedure-related mortality of only 0.05%.[15]

The main hazard of endomyocardial biopsy (using any of the biopsy techniques) is cardiac perforation, which occurs in 0.3 to 0.5% of cases and can lead rapidly to tamponade and circulatory collapse.[1,15] This risk can be minimized by careful attention to catheter position, suitable caution during catheter advancement, and continuous monitoring of the patient. Biopsy passes associated with chest pain or those producing samples that float in 10% formalin (suggesting the presence of epicardial fat) are of particular concern and should prompt monitoring of the blood pressure, right atrial pressure, and the fluoroscopic appearance of the heart border for at least 10 minutes following the final biopsy sample. Frank cardiac perforation is usually heralded by sudden bradycardia and hypotension, associated with loss of the normal fluoroscopic motion of the right atrial and left ventricular heart borders. If the diagnosis of perforation with hemopericardium is in question in a hemodynamically stable patient, it may be de-

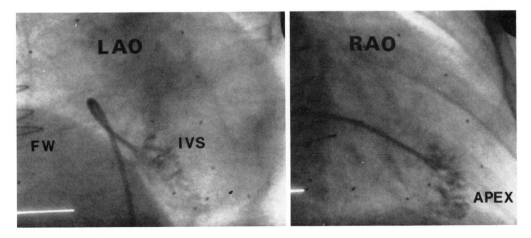

Fig. 23–8. Contrast injection in the left anterior oblique (left) and right anterior oblique projections demonstrates correct position of the long sheath against the apical-septal wall. FW = free wall of right ventricle; IVS = interventricular septum.

sirable to confirm the presence of pericardial effusion by means of a portable echocardiogram in the cardiac catheterization laboratory, but the operator must be prepared to perform pericardiocentesis without hesitation if hemodynamic compromise develops. In most cases, simple aspiration or temporary catheter drainage of the pericardial space allows nonoperative management of biopsy-induced cardiac perforation in a patient with normal coagulation parameters. *We avoid right ventricular biopsy in any patient with a prothrombin time greater than 17 seconds, any patient who is heparinized, or any patient with a clinical coagulopathy.* On the other hand, left ventricular biopsies are generally performed *with* systemic anticoagulation (heparin 5000 u), which is *not* reversed with protamine at the end of the procedure to minimize the risk of thrombus formation at the biopsy site. Left ventricular biopsy should not be done in patients with recent myocardial infarction, since local wall thinning or weakness may increase the risk of perforation. Coronary artery to right ventricular fistula has been reported as a newly recognized complication of endomyocardial biopsy,[16-18] although the clinical significance of this lesion appears to be negligible.

An additional hazard of cardiac biopsy is embolization. With continuous flushing of the entry sheath, right-sided thromboembolism during cardiac biopsy is rare. Air embolization has been described, however, as the result of the smaller size of the bioptome shaft relative to its head. This allows aspiration of air through any sheath lacking a suitable valve when the bioptome is used in a patient with a low central venous pressure. The possibility of paradoxical air or thromboembolism constitutes a relative contraindication for right ventricular biopsy in patients with significant right-to-left intracardiac shunting. Of course, thromboembolism poses a greater potential problem during left ventricular biopsy, in which cerebral embolization has been reported despite careful technique, systemic angiocoagulation, and avoidance of patients with mural thrombi.[6] Finally, a number of less serious complications of endomyocardial biopsy have been described, including transient arrhythmias and transient or permanent bundle branch block. Because these complications are invariably evident before the patient leaves the catheterization laboratory, we are currently performing serial right ventricular biopsies (in cardiac transplant or myocarditis patients) on an outpatient basis.

TISSUE PROCESSING

The operator must take responsibility for obtaining an adequate tissue sample and performing the initial preparations that permit subsequent pathologic evaluation. It is usually recommended that 3 to 5 separate specimens be obtained from either the right or the left ventricle to minimize sampling errors. Most myocardial diseases affect both ventricles, so that either chamber may be sampled, depending on operator experience and preference. Selective left ventricular involvement may be present in certain diseases (endomyocardial fibrosis, scleroderma, left heart radiation, and cardiac fibroelastosis of infants and newborns). Left ventricular biopsy should be performed in these conditions or in patients in whom right ventricular biopsy has been unsuccessful or nondiagnostic. In the remaining patients, we generally prefer right rather than left ventricular biopsy because of greater ease, speed, and less likelihood of morbidity.

The safest and most elegant techniques of endomyocardial biopsy are useless without expert pathologic interpretation. The availability of a cardiac pathologist who is fully trained in the evaluation of biopsy-obtained tissue is mandatory in any biopsy program. Artifacts such as crushing or contraction bands are frequently present in endomyocardial biopsy specimens and may be overinterpreted by an inexperienced pathologist or one used to evaluating only postmortem specimens. The operator may assist the pathologist by appropriate handling of the tissue in the catheterization laboratory. Biopsy specimens should be removed gently from the jaws of the bioptome with a fine needle and placed on moistened filter paper to be transferred immediately to the appropriate fixative—10% formalin for light microscopy, or 2.5% buffered glutaraldehyde for electron microscopy. Frozen specimens may be prepared in the catheterization laboratory by placing samples in a suitable fluid embedding medium and immersing them in liquid nitrogen or a dry ice-isopentate mixture to allow immediate interpretation (as in the case of transplant rejection) or subsequent immunologic staining. Special sample preparation or staining may be indicated for the evaluation of specific disease states (see below).

FINDINGS IN SPECIFIC DISEASE STATES

Transplant Rejection

Endomyocardial biopsy has been the cornerstone of monitoring of antirejection therapy in patients with heart or heart-lung transplants.[19] It allows the detection of early rejection before the clinical findings of advanced cardiac damage (arrhythmias, third heart sound, congestive heart failure) become manifest, and confirms the adequacy of pulsed immunosuppressive therapy to control each acute rejection episode. Because immunologic transplant rejection is a diffuse process, sampling errors are rare. The light-microscopic histologic features of rejection include interstitial edema, inflammatory infiltration, and immunoglobulin deposition. More severe rejection is marked by myocytolysis and even interstitial hemorrhage.

Adriamycin Cardiotoxicity

Doxorubricin hydrochloride (Adriamycin) is a potent anthracycline antibiotic that is active against many tumors, but whose usefulness is limited by its tendency to cause irreversible dose-related cardiotoxicity. One approach to safe clinical use has been to limit the total cumulative dose to 500 mg/sq m, but this constitutes an unnecessary limitation in patients who can tolerate substantially higher doses without cardiotoxicity and who depend on the drug for tumor control. On the other hand, patients with pre-existing heart disease, prior radiotherapy or cyclophosphamide administration, or who are over age 70, may develop cardiac toxicity at substantially lower doses. Because overt impairment of cardiac function is a relatively late finding in adriamycin toxicity, noninvasive testing may fail to disclose whether additional doses of adriamycin can be given safely. Bristow and coworkers have demonstrated, however, that a progressive series of histologic changes (including electron microscopic evidence of myofibrillar loss and cytoplasmic vacuolization) takes place during the development of adriamycin cardiotoxicity.[20] The extent of these changes can predict whether a patient is likely to develop clinical cardiotoxicity during the subsequent chemotherapy cycle, permitting maximal yet safe dosing with adriamycin while substantially decreasing the incidence of morbidity and mortality from adriamycin cardiotoxicity.

Dilated Cardiomyopathy

Approximately 10,000 cases of dilated cardiomyopathy—primary myocardial failure in the absence of underlying coronary, valvular, or pericardial disease—occur in the United States each year.[21-23] Most patients present with well-established cardiac damage, and the majority of patients with dilated cardiomyopathy display only the monotonous findings of myocyte hypertrophy, interstitial and replacement fibrosis, and endocardial thickening,[24] underlying the fact that idiopathic dilated cardiomyopathy itself has no diagnostic morphologic features.[25-26] These findings do not necessarily aid in establishing etiology, long-term prognosis, or appropriate specific therapy. Accordingly, some authorities have suggested that endomyocardial biopsy is of little value in patients with dilated cardiomyopathy.[1,27-29] In a review of the utility of cardiac biopsy in patients with heart disease of unknown cause,[1] Mason and O'Connell concluded that fewer than 5% of patients had biopsy diagnosis of a myocardial disorder for which specific therapy existed. They noted, however, that this figure underestimates the overall usefulness of cardiac biopsy, which includes negative results or biopsies that reveal a specific but untreatable disorder. Dilated cardiomyopathy carries a substantial 5-year mortality, so that our approach for any young or middle-aged patient with dilated cardiomyopathy includes an invasive evaluation with endomyocardial biopsy.

Myocarditis

The clinical recognition of myocarditis remains difficult, its relation to dilated cardiomyopathy uncertain, and its current therapy largely unsatisfactory.[30] Epidemiologic studies suggest that approximately 5% of a coxsackie B virus-infected population show some evidence of cardiac involvement.[21–23] In most cases, these abnormalities do not come to medical attention and subside with the resolution of the acute viral infection. In some patients, however, cardiac inflammation associated with viral, protozoal, metazoal, or bacterial infections may persist, leading to ongoing symptoms of heart failure, chest pain, or arrhythmias. Interestingly, previous studies have demonstrated that fewer than 25% of patients with clinically suspected acute myocarditis have positive biopsies.[31–33] One group has suggested that the yield may be increased by prebiopsy screening with a gallium 67 scan.[34]

In some studies, 15 to 30% of patients with established dilated cardiomyopathy, unexplained chest pain, or ventricular arrhythmias have had biopsy evidence of inflammatory myocarditis despite the absence of clinical findings such as fever, leukocytosis, or an elevated erythrocyte sedimentation rate.[33,35,36]

In a recent study of endomyocardial biopsy in patients with heart failure and dilated cardiomyopathy,[37] 8 of 61 patients (13%) demonstrated myocardial lymphocytic infiltration. Most pathologists would concur with this diagnosis in a patient who has foci of round-cell infiltration in proximity to areas of myocyte damage.[38] In practice, however, several major problems[39] still surround the biopsy diagnosis of myocarditis:

1. Tissue sampling may be inadequate.[40]
2. Idiopathic dilated cardiomyopathy has no specific histologic features.
3. There has been a high degree of interobserver variability in the interpretation of biopsy samples.

"Myocarditis" is both a specific and a general term.[41] *Specifically,* it refers to a combination of inflammation and nonischemic myocyte damage. Although many factors may cause this histologic picture, the most recent criteria[42] for the diagnosis of myocarditis (the "Dallas Criteria") were developed by a group of eight pathologists in conjunction with the American College of Cardiology. These authors defined myocarditis as a process characterized by an infiltrate of the myocardium with necrosis and/or degeneration of adjacent myocytes not typical of the ischemic damage associated with coronary artery disease. Their system relies solely on morphology and sets forth histopathologic criteria for the diagnosis of myocarditis, whereby patients are assigned to one of three categories:

1. *Active myocarditis* (with or without fibrosis)
2. *Borderline myocarditis* (inflammatory infiltrate but no myocyte necrosis)
3. *No myocarditis.*

Based on this classification scheme, Chow and co-workers[43] demonstrated myocarditis in 4 of 90 patients who underwent endomyocardial biopsy after presenting with unexplained congestive heart failure. Although controlled trials are still in progress, up to 60% of patients with inflammatory myocarditis improve when treated with a regimen of prednisone and azothioprine, according to some reports.[8,21] On the other hand, patients may also improve spontaneously, and death from sepsis and opportunistic infections has been reported in immunosuppressive-treated patients. Conclusive proof of the efficacy of immunosuppressive therapy can be established only by a large-scale randomized trial, and the results of such a trial will be pivotal in establishing the ultimate role of cardiac biopsy in the diagnosis and treatment of myocarditis.

To this end, the Myocarditis Treatment Trial,[1] an international study of the efficacy of immunosuppression in myocarditis, was begun in 1988, sponsored by the National Heart, Lung, and Blood Institute. Patients with suspected myocarditis undergo endomyocardial biopsy, and the histologic findings are reviewed by a member of the trial's pathology panel. If myocarditis is present histologically, and if the patient has a left ventricular ejection fraction less than 0.45, the patient can be randomized to one of two treatment arms: (1) *immunosuppression* with cyclosporine and a small prednisone dose, or (2) *conventional therapy* for congestive heart failure, without immunosuppression. Maximum treadmill exercise time is used as an adjunct to monitor effects of therapy. Assigned therapy is maintained for 6 months. After an additional 6 months, at 1 year after diagnosis, final assessment of the patient's cardiac functional status is performed.

Through September 1, 1988, 1378 biopsies had been performed at 23 centers in the trial to rule out myocarditis.[1] Myocarditis was detected in 139 patients (10%).

With the exception of patients with inflammatory myocarditis, endomyocardial biopsy in most patients with dilated cardiomyopathy shows simply the nonspecific findings described previously. Occasionally, however, specific findings allow the diagnosis of disorders such as hemochromatosis,[44,45] sarcoidosis,[46,47] and recently, Lyme carditis,[48] for which specific therapy may exist. Other disorders, such as postpartum or alcoholic cardiomyopathy,[49] lack both distinctive histologic features and specific therapy and cannot be separated from idiopathic myocardial failure.

Restrictive versus Constrictive Disease

Heart failure caused by impaired diastolic functioning of a normal-sized or mildly dilated left ventricle is an uncommon but important clinical entity. In some cases, this may be due to pericardial constriction or hypertrophic myopathy, in which instance endomyocardial biopsy would offer no further information. On the other hand, diastolic dysfunction may also be caused by one of a series of diseases that can be readily diagnosed with endomyocardial biopsy, thus sparing the patient from inappropriate medical or surgical therapy.[50] These disorders include primary amyloidosis,[51] Loeffler's endomyocardial fibrosis, carcinoidosis, Fabry's disease,[52] and the glycogen storage diseases.[22,23]

One potential new area where cardiac biopsy may prove useful is acquired immunodeficiency syndrome (AIDS). Several recent autopsy studies in patients with AIDS have shown that serious clinical cardiac abnormalities were common and associated with myocarditis.[52,53] What role endomyocardial biopsy will have in this syndrome depends on specific etiologies and the development of new therapy.

FUTURE DIRECTIONS

Based on the increased ease and safety of endomyocardial biopsy, the increased awareness of inflammatory myocarditis, and the proliferation of cardiac pathologists trained to evaluate endomyocardial biopsy samples, endomyocardial biopsy is playing an increasing role in the invasive evaluation of patients with primary myocardial disorders. As further knowledge is gained about the natural history and therapy of the various myocardial disorders, the use of endomyocardial biopsy should continue to expand.

REFERENCES

1. Mason JW, O'Connell JB: Clinical merit of endomyocardial biopsy. Circulation 79:971, 1989.
2. Shugoll GI: Percutaneous myocardial and pericardial biopsy with the Menghini needle. Am Heart J 85:35, 1973.
3. Shirey EK, Hawk WA, Mukerji D, Effler DB: Percutaneous myocardial biopsy of the left ventricle: Experience in 198 patients. Circulation 46:112, 1972.
4. Sakakibara S, Konno S: Endomyocardial biopsy. Jpn Heart J 3:537, 1962.
5. Kawai C, Kitaura Y: New endomyocardial biopsy catheter for the left ventricle. Am J Cardiol 40:63, 1977.

6. Kawai C, Matsumori A, Kawamura K: Myocardial biopsy. Ann Rev Med 31:139, 1980.
7. Caves PK, Stinson EB, Dong E Jr: New instrument for transvenous cardiac biopsy. Am J Cardiol 33:264, 1974.
8. Mason JW: Techniques for right and left ventricular endomyocardial biopsy. Am J Cardiol 41:887, 1978.
9. Miller LW, Labovitz AJ, McBride LA, Pennington DG, Kanter K: Echocardiography-guided endomyocardial biopsy. A 5-year experience. Circulation 78(suppl III):III-99–III-102, 1988.
10. Richardson PJ: King's endomyocardial bioptome. Lancet 1:660, 1974.
11. Brooksby IAB, et al: Left ventricular endomyocardial biopsy. Lancet 2:1222, 1974.
12. Rios B, Nihill MR, Mullins CE: Left ventricular endomyocardial biopsy in children with the transseptal long sheath technique. Cathet Cardiovasc Diagn 10:417, 1984.
13. Anderson JL, Marshall HW: The femoral venous approach to endomyocardial biopsy: Comparison with internal jugular and transarterial approaches. Am J Cardiol 53:833, 1984.
14. Anastasiou-Nana MI et al: Validation of a new femoral venous method of endomyocardial biopsy. Comparison with internal jugular approach. J Interven Cardiol 1:263, 1988.
15. Sekiguchi M, Take M: World survey of catheter biopsy of the heart. In Sekiguchi M, Olsen EGJ (eds): Cardiomyopathy. Clinical, Pathological, and Theoretical Aspects. Baltimore, University Park Press, 1980, pp. 217–225.
16. Henzlova MJ et al: Coronary artery to right ventricle fistula in heart transplant recipients: a complication of endomyocardial biopsy. J Am Coll Cardiol 14:258, 1989.
17. Fitchett DH, Forbes C, Guerraty AJ: Repeated endomyocardial biopsy causing coronary arterial-right ventricular fistula after cardiac transplantation. Am J Cardiol 62:829, 1988.
18. Sandhu JS et al: Coronary artery fistula in the heart transplant patient. A potential complication of endomyocardial biopsy. Circulation 79:350, 1989.
19. Billingham ME, Mason JW: The role of endomyocardial biopsy in the management of acute rejection in cardiac allografts. In Fenoglio JJ Jr (ed.): Endomyocardial Biopsy: Techniques and Applications. Boca Raton, FL, CRC Press, 1982, pp. 57–64.
20. Bristow MR, Mason JW, Billingham ME, Daniels JR: Doxorubicin cardiotoxicity: Evaluation of phonocardiography, endomyocardial biopsy, and cardiac catheterization. Ann Intern Med 88:168, 1978.
21. Kereiakes DJ, Parmley WW: Myocarditis and cardiomyopathy. Am Heart J 108:1318, 1984.
22. Abelmann WH: Classification and natural history of primary myocardial disease. Prog Cardiovasc Dis 27:73, 1984.
23. Johnson RA, Palacios I: Dilated cardiomyopathies of the adult. N Engl J Med 307:1051, 1119, 1982.
24. Unverferth DV, et al: Human myocardial histologic characteristics in congestive heart failure. Circulation 68:1194, 1983.
25. Rose AG, Beck W: Dilated (congestive) cardiomyopathy: A syndrome of severe cardiac dysfunction

with remarkably few morphological features of myocardial damage. Histopathology 9:367, 1985.
26. Yonesaka S, Becker AE: Dilated cardiomyopathy: diagnostic accuracy of endomyocardial biopsy. Br Heart J 58:156, 1987.
27. MacKay EH, Littler WA, Sleight P: Critical assessment of diagnostic value of endomyocardial biopsy. Br Heart J 40:69, 1978.
28. Ferrans VJ, Roberts WC: Myocardial biopsy: A useful diagnostic procedure or only a research tool? Am J Cardiol 41:965, 1978.
29. Mason JW: Endomyocardial biopsy: Balance of success and failure. Circulation 71:185, 1985.
30. Wenger NK: Myocarditis: Unresolved diagnostic and therapeutic issues. Current Opinion in Cardiology 4:406, 1989.
31. Mason JW, Billingham ME, Ricci DR: Treatment of acute inflammatory myocarditis assisted by endomyocardial biopsy. Am J Cardiol 45:1037, 1980.
32. Aretz HT, Chapman C, Fallon JJ: Morphologic and immunologic findings in patients with clinically suspected acute myocarditis (abstract). Circulation 68 (Supp III):27, 1983.
33. Parrillo JE, et al: The results of transvenous endomyocardial biopsy can frequently be used to diagnose myocardial diseases in patients with idiopathic heart failure. Circulation 69:93, 1984.
34. O'Connell JB, Robinson JA, Henkin RE, Gunnar RM: Immunosuppressive therapy in patients with congestive cardiomyopathy and myocardial uptake of gallium-67. Circulation 64:780, 1981.
35. Nippoldt TB, et al: Right ventricular endomyocardial biopsy—Clinicopathologic correlates in 100 consecutive patients. Mayo Clin Proc 57:407, 1982.
36. Zee-Chung C, et al: High incidence of myocarditis by endomyocardial biopsy in patients with idiopathic congestive cardiomyopathy. J Am Coll Cardiol 3:63, 1984.
37. Popma JJ, Cigarroa RG, Buja MB, Hillis LD: Diagnostic and prognostic utility of right sided catheterization and endomyocardial biopsy in idiopathic dilated cardiomyopathy. Am J Cardiol 63:955, 1989.
38. Fenoglio JJ, et al: Diagnosis and classification of myocarditis by endomyocardial biopsy. N Engl J Med 308:12, 1983.
39. Lie JT: Myocarditis and endomyocardial biopsy in unexplained heart failure: A diagnosis in search of a disease. Ann Intern Med 109:525, 1988.
40. Hauck AJ, Kearney OL, Edwards WD: Evaluation of postmortem endomyocardial biopsy specimens from 38 patients with lymphocytic myocarditis: Implications for role of sampling error. Mayo Clin Proc 64:1235, 1989.
41. Marboe CC, Fenoglio JJ: Biopsy diagnosis of myocarditis. Cardiovasc Clin 18:137, 1988.
42. Aretz HT et al: Myocarditis—A histopathologic definition and classification. Am J Cardiovasc Pathol 1:3, 1986.
43. Chow LC, Dittrich HC, Shabetai R: Endomyocardial biopsy in patients with unexplained congestive heart failure. Ann Intern Med 109:535, 1988.
44. Short EM, Winkle RA, Billingham ME: Myocardial involvement in idiopathic hemochromatosis: Morphologic and clinical improvement following venesection. Am J Med 70:1275, 1981.

45. Olson LJ, et al: Endomyocardial biopsy in hemochromatosis: clinicopathologic correlates in six cases. J Am Coll Cardiol 13:116, 1989.
46. Silverman KJ, Hutchins GM, Bulkley BH: Cardiac sarcoid: A clinicopathologic study of 84 unselected patients with systemic sarcoidosis. Circulation 58:1204, 1978.
47. Lorell B, Alderman EL, Mason JW: Cardiac sarcoidosis: Diagnosis by transvenous endomyocardial biopsy and treatment with corticosteroids. Am J Cardiol 42:143, 1978.
48. Reznick JW et al: Lyme carditis. Electrophysiologic and histopathologic study. Am J Med 81:923, 1986.
49. Rubin E: Alcoholic myopathy in heart and skeletal muscle. N Engl J Med 301:28, 1979.
50. Schoenfeld MH, Supple EW, Dec GW, et al: Restrictive cardiomyopathy versus constrictive pericarditis: Role of endomyocardial biopsy in avoiding unnecessary thoracotomy. Circulation 75:1012, 1987.
51. Schroeder JS, Billingham ME, Rider AK: Cardiac amyloidosis: Diagnosis by transvenous endomyocardial biopsy. Am J Med 59:269, 1975.
52. Colucci WS, et al: Hypertrophic obstructive cardiomyopathy due to Fabry's disease. N Engl J Med 307:926, 1982.
53. Reilly JM, et al: Frequency of myocarditis, left ventricular dysfunction and ventricular tachycardia in the acquired immune deficiency syndrome. Am J Cardiol 62:789, 1988.

24

Temporary and Permanent Pacemakers

STAFFORD I. COHEN

D
r. Paul Zoll made the first serious attempt to accelerate an excessively
slow heart rate in man with external
cardiac stimulation applied to the chest wall.[1]
Although effective in controlling heart action,
the electric shock and skeletal muscle stimulation caused discomfort. The transvenous
method of pacing followed and was painless,[2]
and implantable permanent cardiac pacing
proved to be the first reliable long term-method
of managing Stokes-Adams attacks.[3] Most of
the early workers in the permanent pacemaker
field were thoracic surgeons who placed epimyocardial leads directly on the exposed heart.
The technically simpler permanent transvenous pacemaker technique aroused the interest of general surgeons and cardiologists
with surgical skills.

The evolution of cardiac pacemaker therapy
has required collaboration among cardiac
physiologists, biomedical engineers, and the
pacemaker industry. Pacemaker technology
has advanced so rapidly that it confounds some
implanters and is not understood by many physicians and cardiologists who are primarily
committed to patient care. A pacemaker certification requirement has been proposed and
is administered by the North American Society
for Pacing and Electrophysiology. Competency ensures that there are proper indications
for implanting a pacemaker and that the selected device is well suited to the patient's
special need.[4]

Technologic advance in the design of pacemaker electrodes and generators now permits
several options in the selection of a temporary
or permanent pacemaker system. There is single-chamber right atrial or right ventricular
pacing. There is also dual chamber pacemaker
technology, which not only maintains a satisfactory heart rate but does so by simulating
physiologic cardiac excitation. Rate-responsive pacemakers have recently become available. The Intersociety Commission for Heart
Disease Resources established a *three-letter
code* for characterizing antibradycardia pacemaker capability.[5] *The first letter signifies the
chamber paced, the second letter the chamber
sensed, and the third letter the response of the
pacemaker to sensed intrinsic cardiac activity.*
Fourth and fifth letters have recently been
added to identify programmability and antitachycardia characteristics.[5,6] (Table 24–1)

TEMPORARY PACEMAKER

Indications. Table 24–2 lists the indications
for temporary pacemaker placement, and Figure 24–1 represents an example of one of these
indications. Pacemakers were first used to
manage high-grade atrioventricular (A-V)
block or so-called Stokes-Adams attacks. The
indications for pacemaker placement have expanded to include acute or anticipated bradyarrhythmias from any electrophysiologic
mechanism. Although pacemakers are also

396

Table 24–1. *ICHD Five-Position Code of Pacemaker Mode and Function*

Position of letter	I	II	III	IV	V
Letter designates	Chamber(s) paced	Chamber(s) sensed	Modes of response(s)	Programmable functions	Special anti-tachyarrhythmia functions
Letters used	V—ventricle	V—ventricle	T—triggered	P—programmable rate and/or output	B—bursts
	A—atrium	A—atrium	I—inhibited	M—multi-programmable	N—normal rate competition
	D—double	D—double	D—double	C—communicating	S—scanning
		O—none	O—none	R—rate modulation	E—external
			R—reverse	O—none	

used to treat or prevent tachyarrhythmias, this chapter will not review antitachycardia principles or devices.

The management of a bradyarrhythmia crisis is usually pharmacologic or mechanical. Atropine, isoproterenol, and epinephrine are generally available and are often effective. The simple act of a chest thump or forceful slap can excite an asystolic heart to contract. Rhythmic chest thumping can sustain life until other methods are substituted.

Electrical methods to accelerate heart rate can be applied if the underlying cause of bradyarrhythmia is not rapidly reversed, if the life-threatening bradyarrhythmia is likely to recur, or if the excessively slow heart rate persists.

External electrical stimulation can be applied swiftly, and a recent modification of this historic technique, using prolongation of stimulus duration and large-diameter pacing pads, permits effective cardiac pacing without pain in most conscious patients.[7,8] When there is an absolute emergency such as a cardiac arrest requiring cardiopulmonary resuscitation, a transthoracic pacing wire can be placed quickly through an intracardiac needle positioned from a subxyphoid approach. The desperate circumstance of a stubborn asystolic heart justifies potential injury to a coronary artery as the needle passes through the myocardial wall. If the patient survives, a temporary transvenous pacer must be substituted

Table 24–2. *Indications for Placement of a Temporary Pacemaker*

Symptomatic bradycardia
Sinus node dysfunction	arrest
	bradycardia
	S-A block
A-V node dysfunction	second degree block
	third degree block
His-Purkinje dysfunction	Mobitz II block
	trifascicular block
	bifascicular and Wenckebach block
	right and left bundle branch block

Prophylactic pacemaker placement
   Right heart catheterization in presence of LBBB
   Electrical cardioversion in presence of known sick slow sinus
   Acute anterior myocardial infarction with new onset bifascicular block (example, Fig. 24–1)

Tachyarrhythmia control
   Convert atrial tachycardia and flutter
   Overdrive suppress ventricular ectopy/tachycardia
   Accelerate rate in setting of torsade de pointes with long Q-T interval

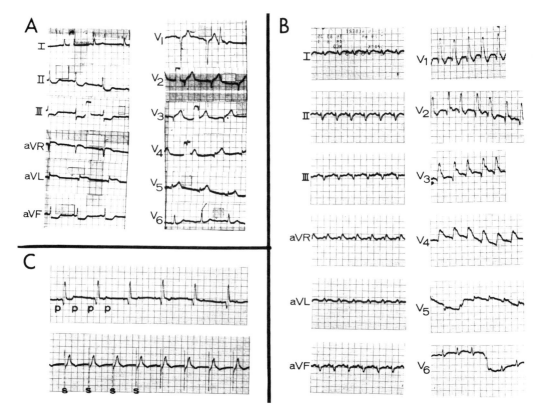

Fig. 24–1. Prophylactic temporary pacemaker during acute myocardial infarction. A. Presenting ECG in emergency ward of a patient with crushing chest pain. Poor R wave progression V_1–V_4, ST depression leads II, III, aVF, ST elevation aVL and V_4. B. Several hours later, there is a pattern of acute anterior infarction and new onset of right bundle branch block with left axis deviation. A temporary pacemaker is placed because of the likelihood of high grade A-V block. C. High grade heart block: Top, monitor strip reveals 2:1 heart block. Bottom, temporary unipolar pacer is required. S = pacemaker stimulus.

for the transthoracic pacemaker. The placement of a temporary transvenous pacemaker requires preparation and care. Ideally, the procedure is performed on a relatively stable patient.

Temporary pacemakers are indicated whenever there is symptomatic bradycardia from any cause that is not quickly reversed and is expected to continue to recur. Symptoms of bradyarrhythmia usually relate to cerebral insufficiency and consist of frank syncope, dizziness, or light-headed spells. It should be noted that some patients with syncope and a witnessed unconscious state later insist that they were fully alert. Other manifestations of bradycardia include fatigue and heart failure.

Procedure for Temporary Pacemaker Placement. Temporary pacing requires that a catheter be introduced into a vein and advanced to the right atrium or ventricle. There are several options for venous access. The choice should depend on the expected duration of the bradyarrhythmia, anatomic considerations, and the anticipated need and timing of a permanent pacemaker. The venous access sites commonly used are internal jugular, external jugular, subclavian, brachial, median basilic, and femoral veins. Hynes et al.[9] reviewed the clinical course of more than 1000 consecutive temporary pacer placements at the Mayo Clinic. Overall pacemaker-related morbidity occurred in 14%, and the internal jugular and subclavian routes were associated with low complication rates. Percutaneous transvenous introducer techniques can be used to enter each of the major venous routes. Cutdown techniques are often applied to the median basilic, brachial, or external jugular veins. Considerations regarding selection of a venous approach are presented in Table 24–3. Whatever the venous site, placement must be done under aseptic conditions such as those prevailing in a catheterization laboratory or operating room.

The operator must select from several catheter models and several guidance systems available to help direct the catheter from the venous introduction site to the right ventricle. There are three guidance systems: (1) fluoroscopic surveillance, (2) catheter-tip electrogram, and (3) cardiac monitor or electrocardiogram rhythm strip during pacemaker stimulation. Most temporary pacing catheters are bipolar, come in a variety of diameter sizes, and have a range of relative flexibility. Some have an inflatable balloon tip, which allows venous flow to direct the catheter tip to the right ventricle.

Fluoroscopy is clearly the best method for assisting the operator to direct the pacing catheter through the venous system and right atrium to a final position in the right ventricle. The availability and location of fluoroscopic equipment and the severity of the arrhythmia dictate the approach and physical location of the pacemaker procedure. Some hospitals have a procedure room within or adjacent to a critical care unit, or there may be radiolucent patient beds and a portable fluoroscope machine, which permit pacemaker placement in any intensive care room. Patients with a failing permanent pacemaker or a Swan-Ganz catheter should have a temporary pacemaker placed under fluoroscopic guidance to avoid entangling or knotting the catheters within the heart.[10] Fluoroscopy is also suggested when the pacemaker is inserted into the femoral vein or when tricuspid regurgitation, a dilated right atrium, and cardiogenic shock or a low flow state is present.

Placement can also be achieved by monitoring the electrogram derived from the pacing catheter's distal electrode.[11] The terminal pin of the distal electrode is connected to the central lead of a standard patient ECG cable after the limb leads have been attached. The ECG lead selector is placed in the V position, and the electrogram is monitored as the pacing catheter is advanced. The pattern of intrinsic atrial excitation is recognized when the catheter tip is within the right atrial cavity. Further advancement of the catheter results in a ventricular intracavity electrogram pattern. When the ventricular pacing and sensing thresholds are satisfactory, a chest roentgenogram should be obtained to confirm the catheter's position and orientation. Catheter placement with electrogram guidance should be used only in an environment under strict surveillance for electrical safety. Ventricular fibrillation can occur

Table 24–3. *Special Considerations when Selecting Vein Access for Temporary Pacing*

Vein	Consider
Internal jugular	Can patient lie flat? Avoid air embolism
Subclavian	Avoid preferred side of permanent pacer placement Avoid air embolism
External jugular	Can patient lie flat? Avoid preferred side of permanent pacer placement
Femoral	Avoid if edema, phlebitis, or varicosities of leg Avoid if ambulation important Not possible if past IVC ligation, clip, or umbrella Requires fluoroscopy
Median basilic	Long tortuous course Prone to spasm High displacement rate

if there is inadequate grounding of equipment, electrical leaks, or improperly functioning wall receptacles. A temporary pacing catheter in the right ventricle is a low resistance pathway from the external environment to the heart. Very low 60-cycle electric current can produce ventricular fibrillation when applied directly to the heart. Also, it is obvious that there must be sustained cardiac excitation to record intracavitary electrical activity; therefore, electrogram guidance is not useful during asystolic cardiac arrest.

The last technique for guiding the pacing catheter to the right ventricle is use of combined sensing and pacing during continuous electrocardiographic monitoring. This approach is necessary when fluoroscopy is unavailable, when the electrograms are not of diagnostic quality, or when the heart is asystolic. After the pacing catheter is introduced into and advanced within the venous system, the bipolar pacemaker's electrode terminal pins are attached with a standard cable to an external pacemaker-generator. If the patient has intrinsic cardiac activity with reasonable rate and rhythm, the pacemaker's sensing circuit is adjusted to its lowest threshold; the energy output and rate are also adjusted to their lowest level. If the intrinsic heart rate is too slow, the pacemaker's rate is set at 60 to 70/min., and the energy output increased to 3.0 volts or 6.0 milliamperes (mA). The pacing catheter is again advanced. If the pacemaker-generator indicates sensing of intrinsic cardiac activity, the paced rate is adjusted to a faster rate. The energy output is increased. The cardiac monitor is observed for excitation of the atria or ventricles. If the former occurs, the generator settings are returned to their original position, and the catheter is withdrawn slightly and readvanced with rotation to enter the right ventricle. If the pacing catheter is balloon-tipped, the balloon must be deflated each time the catheter is withdrawn. Fragile chordae tendinae have been known to be torn as an inflated balloon is forcefully withdrawn against chordal resistance. After manipulation, the catheter should advance across the tricuspid valve and result in ventricular excitation when the rate and energy settings are properly adjusted. Entry into the right ventricle is usually heralded by ectopy; therefore, the electrocardiographic monitor should be observed carefully during catheter manipulation. If the initial indication for a pacemaker was asystolic arrest, the pacemaker-generator is activated for pacing as the catheter is advanced. Low thresholds for stimulation are desirable. Although a pacing threshold of less than 1.0 mA is ideal, thresholds between 1.0 and 2.0 mA are common.

After satisfactory positioning, the catheter must be secured to prevent inadvertent withdrawal by the patient or medical personnel. The pacing catheter should be secured to the skin by a lock stitch and then arranged with an accessory loop so that a "tug" on the proximal catheter will cause the circumference of the loop to contract rather than the catheter to be withdrawn from the vein. Antibiotic or iodinated ointment should be applied over the insertion site before the wound is dressed. A chest roentgenogram is then obtained to document the catheter position. The introduction site should be examined at intervals, and the pacing system should be checked for malfunctions, most of which will be discussed in the section of this chapter on permanent pacing.

Need for Temporary Physiologic Pacing. A variety of pathologic cardiac conditions have been identified that need the normal sequence of atrial and ventricular activation to maintain a satisfactory cardiac output and blood pressure. Aortic stenosis, mitral stenosis, and obstructive myopathies should alert the operator to the theoretic or actual need of a physiologic pacing system. Other cardiac states that may require physiologic pacing include myocardial infarction, the immediate postoperative period following heart surgery, and left ventricular hypertrophy from any cause. Except in mitral stenosis, there is usually a noncompliant left ventricle in need of the "priming" action of atrial systole.

Atrial pacing alone maintains physiologic chamber activation in the presence of intact A-V conduction. The anatomy of the right atrium does not easily permit a conventional temporary pacing catheter to remain in contact with the atrial wall. On occasion, a catheter can be effectively positioned at the atrial inflow, looped against the lateral wall, or advanced from the femoral vein directly to the atrial appendage. Because of unreliable atrial pacing with conventional catheters, models have been specifically designed for the purpose.

A catheter is relatively secure against displacement while in the coronary sinus or veins.[12] Some catheters have been adapted specifically for coronary sinus pacing by positioning the electrode rings several centimeters proximal to the tip. Other temporary atrial pacing catheters include a preformed J-shaped distal end for placement in the atrial appendage, or those that must be positioned in the right atrium through a strategically placed introducer catheter. The end of the atrial pacing catheter may assume a ring-like form with each of the oppositely charged semicircles making contact with opposing sides of the atrial wall.[13] The ends of another atrial catheter design have two electrode prongs, which flare in opposite directions to contact opposing walls of the atrium (Atri-pace I, Mansfield Scientific, Mansfield, MA), and this catheter is discussed in Chapter 18.

Dual-chamber temporary pacing is beneficial when there is A-V heart block and need for preservation of physiologic chamber activation. Separate pacing catheters may be required. There are pacing catheters designed for dual chamber pacing, however. Some have multipolar electrodes situated along the atrial and ventricular course of the catheter. Other designs need an introducer through which a single catheter with two sets of flared prongs or two catheters can be passed.

Temporary pacemakers can remain in position for days to weeks. The longer the catheters remain, the greater the risk of infection. Therefore, a permanent pacing system should be placed as soon as the clinical status permits. If placement of a permanent pacemaker is an obvious long-term therapeutic consideration, the preferred veins should be reserved for the permanent pacemaker, and the temporary pacer should be introduced through another approach. In addition, the patient should not have skin electrodes for cardiac monitoring placed near the preferred sites of permanent pacemaker placement. The skin should be free of excoriations and allergic reaction to adhesives, which could predispose to infection. Anticoagulants and antiplatelet agents should be avoided or adjusted if permanent pacer placement is imminent.

In addition to infection, an important potential complication of a temporary pacemaker is cardiac perforation (Fig. 24–2). This complication is more likely when the pacemaker is placed without fluoroscopic guidance, when stiff pacing catheters are used, and when there is recent right ventricular infarction where the ventricular myocardium is necrotic

PERMANENT PACEMAKER

Preoperative Evaluation. Guidelines for permanent cardiac pacemaker implantation have been developed by a task force of cardiologists and surgeons representing the American Heart Association and the American College of Cardiology.[14] The guidelines include three patient categories: those with unqualified need, qualified need, and doubtful need. The categories are listed in Table 24–4.

There are many approaches to permanent pacer implantation.[15–19] The suggestions that follow are personalized and relate to my own experience. Permanent pacemaker implantation is performed under local anesthesia. The patient is awake, and patients who are expected to cooperate need not be sedated. Confused patients or those with a high level of anxiety during the preoperative evaluation should be sedated just before pacemaker implantation. Triazolam, diazepam, lorazepam, haloperidol, midazolam, and thoridazine work well in most patients.

If there is a history of angina pectoris or heart failure, the status of each patient should be carefully reviewed. Additional nitrate or diuretic therapy might be required to enhance comfort and to reduce risk during the opera-

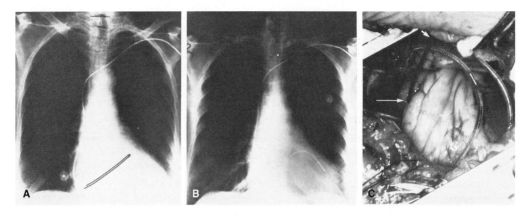

Fig. 24–2. Cardiac perforation by temporary pacemaker catheter. A. Temporary pacer catheter inserted from left arm to right ventricular outflow tract. Course of catheter in the right ventricle has been outlined. It is pointing towards the left shoulder. B. Repeat roentgenogram following intermittent failure of capture and rising threshold for pacing. There is myocardial perforation by the catheter which is turning down along the lateral border towards the ventricular apex. C. An epimyocardial permanent pacer system is being placed. Viewing the left ventricular apex, two epicardial leads are curving about the lateral heart border to their fixation position on the diaphragmatic surface. The perforated temporary pacer exits from the base of the right ventricle (large arrow) and is directed superiorly. The small arrow points to the tip electrode. The temporary pacer was withdrawn under direct vision without bleeding from the site of perforation.

tion. If there is unstable angina and an unreliable intrinsic mechanism to support adequate heart rate, a temporary pacemaker is preferable to isoproterenol or atropine for rate control during placement of a permanent pacer. The history of allergy should specify local anesthetics, sedatives, analgesics, adhesive tape, antibiotics, x-ray contrast medium, and iodine. Each of these agents might be used in the course of a pacemaker implantation.

The cardiovascular examination should emphasize issues relevant to pacer placement. Physical findings of tricuspid regurgitation prepare the operator to use a fixation ventricular electrode. The preliminary assessment should include an estimate of the need for physiologic pacing. If the patient's condition permits, the physical examination should include a determination of blood pressure in the supine, sitting, and standing positions. The finding of varicose veins suggests the possibility of orthostatic hypotension. Knowledge of orthostatic hypotension could be crucial to selecting a physiologic pacing system, especially if sole ventricular excitation also causes relative hypotension. Significant mitral stenosis or aortic stenosis prepares the operator to use a physiologic pacing system. If there is a systolic murmur and carotid pulse contour,

both characteristic of IHSS, an echocardiogram should be obtained to confirm the diagnosis and the probable need for a physiological pacing system.

The areas of venous access should be examined carefully. The presence or absence of external jugular, internal jugular, and cephalic veins should be noted. A large distended vein might result from partial venous obstruction, as might a prominent plexus of veins over the shoulder area. The thickness and integrity of the skin overlying potential sites for placing the pacemaker bear close examination. Abrasions and excoriations are potential sources of infection and should be avoided. The clavicles and overlying skin should be inspected carefully; if the clavicle is prominent and the skin thin, the catheter should be placed in the cephalic vein or subclavian vein. A neck placement might eventually result in necrosis of the skin overlying the clavicular portion of the pacing catheter. In addition, the breasts of female patients are examined carefully for pathologic conditions. If there is a suspicious lump, the pacemaker should be placed from the contralateral approach.

Laboratory data are checked for potential problems: there should be correction of abnormal levels of glucose, hematocrit, potas-

Table 24–4. *Indications for Implantation of Permanent Cardiac Pacemakers*

Group I. Conditions under which implantation of a cardiac pacemaker is generally considered acceptable or necessary, provided that the conditions are chronic or recurrent and not from transient causes such as acute myocardial infarction, drug toxicity, or electrolyte imbalance. In cases of chronic or recurrent rhythm disturbance a single episode of a symptom such as syncope or seizure is adequate to establish medical necessity.

1. Acquired complete AV heart block with symptoms (e.g., syncope, seizures, congestive heart failure, dizziness, confusion, or limited exercise tolerance).

2. Congenital complete heart block with severe bradycardia (in relation to age), or significant physiologic deficits or significant symptoms due to the bradycardia.

3. Second degree AV heart block of Mobitz Type II with symptoms attributable to intermittent complete heart block.

4. Second degree AV heart block of Mobitz Type I with significant symptoms caused by hemodynamic instability associated with the heart block.

5. Sinus bradycardia associated with major symptoms or substantial sinus bradycardia (heart rate less than 50) associated with dizziness or confusion. The correlation between symptoms and bradycardia must be documented, or the symptoms must be clearly attributable to the bradycardia rather than some other cause.

6. In a few selected patients, sinus bradycardia of lesser severity (heart rate 50–59) with dizziness or confusion. The correlation between symptoms and bradycardia must be documented, or the symptoms must be clearly attributable to the bradycardia rather than some other cause.

7. Sinus bradycardia that is the consequence of long-term necessary drug treatment for which there is no acceptable alternative, when accompanied by significant symptoms. The correlation between symptoms and bradycardia must be documented, or the symptoms must be clearly attributable to the bradycardia rather than some other cause.

8. Sinus node dysfunction with or without tachyarrhythmias or AV conduction block—i.e., the bradycardia-tachycardia syndrome, sinoatrial block, sinus arrest—when accompanied by significant symptoms.

9. Sinus node dysfunction with or without symptoms when there are potentially life-threatening ventricular arrhythmias or tachycardia secondary to the bradycardia.

10. Symptomatic bradycardia associated with supraventricular tachycardia.

11. The occasional patient with hypersensitive carotid sinus syndrome with syncope due to bradycardia and unresponsive to prophylactic medical measures.

Group II. Conditions under which implantation of a cardiac pacemaker may be found acceptable or necessary, provided that the medical history and prognosis of the patient involved can be documented and there is evidence that the pacemaker implantation will assist in the overall management of the patient. As with Group I, the conditions must be present chronically or recurrently and not due to such transient causes as acute myocardial infarction, drug toxicity, or electrolyte imbalance.

1. Acquired complete AV heart block without symptoms.

2. Congenital complete heart block with less severe bradycardia (in relation to age).

3. Bifascicular or trifascicular block accompanied by syncope attributed to transient complete heart block after other plausible causes of syncope have been reasonably excluded.

4. Prophylactic pacemaker use following recovery from acute myocardial infarction during which there was temporary complete (third-degree) and/or Mobitz Type II second-degree AV block.

5. Asymptomatic second-degree AV block of Mobitz Type II.

6. Very substantial sinus bradycardia (heart rate less than 45) that is a consequence of long-term necessary drug treatment for which there is no acceptable alternative, when not accompanied by significant symptoms.

7. In patients with recurrent and refractory ventricular tachycardia, "overdrive pacing" (pacing above the basal rate) to prevent ventricular tachycardia.

Table 24–4. *Indications for Implantation of Permanent Cardiac Pacemakers* **Continued**

Group III. Conditions that, although used by some physicians as bases for permanent pacemaker implantation, are considered unsupported by adequate evidence of benefit and therefore should not generally be considered appropriate uses for pacemakers in the absence of indications cited in the above two groups.

1. Syncope of undetermined cause.
2. Sinus bradycardia without significant symptoms.
3. Sinoatrial block or sinus arrest without significant symptoms.
4. Prolonged R-R intervals with atrial fibrillation (without third degree AV block) or with other causes of transient ventricular pause.
5. Bradycardia during sleep.
6. Right bundle branch block with left axis deviation (and other forms of fascicular or bundle branch block) without syncope or other symptoms of intermittent AV block.
7. Asymptomatic second-degree AV block of Mobitz Type I.

Note: This table is based upon recommendations in references 5 and 14.

sium, gas exchange, clotting parameters, and toxic levels of drugs such as digitalis. The chest roentgenogram is carefully reviewed for evidence of pneumonia or other pathologic conditions. Is there evidence of infection such as fever or unexplained high white blood count?

The preoperative orders might include the considerations in Table 24–5. Operative consent includes a description of the patient's rhythm disturbance, the best pacemaker modality for correction, and the technical requirements for pacemaker placement. The benefits and risks of the operation are detailed, as well as other therapeutic options and the risks of not having the operation. Operative risks include the possibility of death, infection, arrhythmias, including bradyarrhythmias and catheter-induced tachyarrythmias; the possible need for cardioversion in the event of a tachyarrhythmia; perforation of the heart and its consequences; displacement of the electrode with pacemaker failure; the possible need for

a reoperation; a discussion of secondary approaches for venous access in the event of failure of the initial approach; and the long-term need for antibiotic prophylaxis because of the implantation of a foreign body.

Permanent Pacemaker Procedure. The pacemaker implantation is usually performed in an operating room or cardiac catheterization laboratory. At some institutions, satisfactory results and lack of complications accompany pacemaker placement in either locale.[20] The patient is made as comfortable as possible on the x-ray table, with his or her head and shoulders elevated slightly. If left heart failure is present, the shoulders are elevated higher and nasal oxygen is administered. The patient's hands are restrained loosely at the sides of the table to prevent inadvertent movement and possible contamination of the operative field. If there is restlessness, confusion, or a general inability to cooperate, the legs are restrained and a binder is placed across the knees.

There are highly visible cardiac monitors to

Table 24–5. *Pre- and Postoperative Orders for Permanent Pacemaker Placement*

Preoperative	*Postoperative*
• Coagulation blood screen	• Bed rest for 24 hours with graded increase in subsequent activity
• Chest roentgenogram	• Portable chest roentgenogram—same day
• Surgical skin scrubs to the chest and neck 24 hours before procedure	• EKG—same day
• Functioning intravenous or heparin lock	• Cardiac monitor until ambulating
• Consent for operation	• Analgesia
• Transportation by stretcher with portable cardiac monitor	• Chest roentgenograms P-A and lateral before discharge

display and record the electrocardiographic events during the pacemaker implantation. An audio "beep" capability to signal each heartbeat is helpful. A control 12-lead ECG recording is taken at the start of the operation as a reference in the event of change during the course of the procedure. Our laboratory monitors ECG leads II and V_1. A defibrillator is in a state of readiness within the room, and an emergency drug cart is in the vicinity. An external transcutaneous pacemaker capability is recommended in the event of unexpected asystole before permanent placement of the pacing catheter. A sterile drape covers the fluoroscopic tube.

The operative field is shaved; the neck veins are marked; and the entire field, including the axilla, chest, and neck, is cleansed with surgical skin scrubs. An elevated bar is positioned at the level of the neck and parallel to the shoulders so that when sterile drapes are properly positioned across the bar, the patient's face is screened from the sterile field.

The skin is infiltrated with a local anesthetic in preparation for the incision. Only enough lidocaine to achieve a state of satisfactory anesthesia is administered because lidocaine is absorbed systemically to levels that can suppress subsidiary intrinsic pacemaker activity. If the cephalic vein is sought, its course is constant in the deltopectoral groove.[21] A small artery frequently crosses the vein; it must be anticipated and may require division. The diameter of the cephalic vein is often small. As it courses in a superior and medial direction towards the subclavian vein, the cephalic vein becomes larger. At times, some pectoralis muscle must be dissected from the clavicle to expose a large segment of the vein. A length of vein is isolated and cleansed of fat and adventitia. The distal end of the vein segment can be ligated, and a loose silk should be placed on the proximal end to control bleeding. Suction should be available in the event of brisk arterial or venous bleeding.

A subcutaneous "pocket" must be prepared for the pacemaker-generator before or after the pacing catheter is placed in the vein. The subcutaneous space is created by sharp or blunt dissection in the fascial plane just above the pectoralis muscle. Adequate local anesthesia is required, because this is usually the most uncomfortable part of the operation. An antibiotic-soaked radiopaque sponge is placed within the pocket, and the size of the created space should correspond to the size of the pacemaker generator.

The vein should be incised near its ligated end with a blade or a fine sharp-tipped scissors. A vein introducer will facilitate the entrance of the pacing catheter. Bathing the vein and the electrode tip in lidocaine may prevent venospasm. If the cephalic vein is thick-walled but too small to accept the pacing catheter, a vein dilator or small snap may be introduced to stretch the vein to a larger diameter. When the tip of the pacing catheter cannot completely enter the vein, a curved snap can gently tease the edges over the catheter tip's largest diameter.

A variety of pacing catheters are suitable for the uncomplicated or the problem patient. There are thin leads for small veins, screw-in active fixation electrodes that minimize the risks of dislodgement, and tined-tip leads that acquire excellent fixation, so good, in fact, that in time removal by traction may be impossible despite some innovative techniques[22]—a vexing problem if there is an infected pacer system.

The permanent pacing catheter is very flexible and very "floppy." The catheter is guided through the venous system and right heart chambers by a stiffening wire stylet that is placed in a central channel extending throughout the catheter and stopping at the tip electrode of the catheter. The stylet can be shaped into any desired curve or combination of curves by the operator. A single gentle curve of the distal 2 inches is usually all that is required.

The pacing catheter enters the cephalic vein with a straight or curved stylet in place, and the catheter is advanced several inches into the vein without rotation. The stylet is then withdrawn 1 to 2 inches to give the catheter a more flexible tip, and the catheter is now advanced further to negotiate curves en route to the subclavian vein. Further advance should be with fluoroscopic assistance. Difficulty may be encountered in entering the subclavian vein. The pacing catheter may turn back toward the axilla or enter the subclavian vein pointing laterally toward the arm rather than medially toward the heart. The stylet should be withdrawn and a single curve or variety of curves fashioned until the catheter takes the correct route. Experience and skill are necessary in manipulating the stylet and catheter. One hand slowly advances or withdraws the pacing catheter at the point of entry to the vein. The thumb and index finger of the other hand turn the stylet while the body of the catheter is held firmly between the palm and the remaining fingers (Fig. 24–3).

The pacing catheter is guided into the subclavian vein and superior vena cava. If the catheter cannot be advanced along the proper route, it must be withdrawn and a venogram performed from the cephalic vein to demonstrate the true route or the stenosis-thrombosis that is preventing passage. If the cephalic approach fails, there are two options. The skin incision can be extended medially to prepare for the placement of a subclavian introducer, or the sterile drapes can be readjusted to expose the neck where external and internal jugular veins are accessible.

The gentle curve of the stylet permits smooth passage of the catheter from the subclavian vein to the superior vena cava and helps direct passage from the right atrium to the ventricle. When the tricuspid valve is difficult to traverse, success may be achieved by looping the tip of the catheter against the lateral atrial wall and then rotating the loop medially against the atrial septum with the catheter tip just above the tricuspid valve. Gentle withdrawal of the catheter straightens the loop and directs the tip inferiorly past the tricuspid valve.

Difficulty in crossing the tricuspid valve can be expected when there is a large right atrium or tricuspid regurgitation. In the latter condition, the regurgitant jet may reject the catheter from the ventricle back to the atrium. Entry of the catheter into the ventricle often results

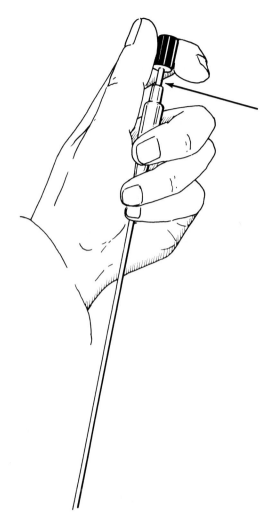

Fig. 24–3. Stylet and pacing catheter. See text for explanation. For illustrative purposes, the diameter of the stylet guide wire (arrow) is exaggerated and the hand is not gloved.

in ventricular ectopy, ventricular couplets, and occasional nonsustained or sustained ventricular tachycardia. The pacing catheter should be permanently positioned at a distance from any arrhythmogenic areas. The operator observes the fluoroscopic image during catheter manipulations; thus laboratory personnel must observe the heart rhythm on the cardiac monitor. If ectopy is excessive, intravenous lidocaine can be safely administered if there is no danger of suppressing a subsidiary pacemaker or if there is a temporary pacer in place.

Because entry into an inferior branch of the

coronary vein can occasionally mimic a right ventricular position, some operators routinely pass the catheter to the pulmonary artery to be certain of a right ventricular position. The ideal catheter placement is on the diaphragmatic surface or "floor" of the right ventricle anywhere between its midpoint and its apex. The "floor" of the proximal ventricle is a second choice. The least desirable option is in the midventricle or apex with the catheter tip pointing toward the outflow tract (Fig. 24–4).

When the pacing catheter has been advanced to the right ventricle, the stylet is rotated to direct the tip inferiorly. The stylet is then withdrawn about 2 inches, and the catheter is advanced toward the cardiac apex. When the catheter tip is advanced to the endocardial wall of the ventricle or to a trabeculated muscle bridge, the operator feels some resistance, and a buckling is seen in the unstiffened distal part of the catheter. A slight forward movement of the catheter tip could indicate a "wedging" of the tip under a trabeculum. If the pacing catheter tip fails to follow the desired intraventricular route, or will not "wedge," the curved stylet is exchanged for a straight stylet while the pacing catheter remains in the right ventricle. The straight stylet usually directs the catheter tip to the diaphragmatic surface of the ventricle.

Once the pacing catheter has a satisfactory intracardiac position by fluoroscopic appearance, other studies and maneuvers are undertaken to test adequate position and fixation. A ventricular catheter with fixation or "wedging" of the tip can be slowly withdrawn until the atrial curve straightens and a slight "tug" is felt during diastole similar to that of a fish nibble on a hand-held fishing line. This maneuver is helpful only when the catheter moves freely within the vein. If there is venous spasm or an excessively tortuous route from the cephalic vein to the ventricle, the "tug" test should not be used. If the catheter tip is not "wedged," the mere reduction of the atrial arc of the pacing catheter will usually displace the tip electrode from its position. Conversely, if the atrial curve is straightened without movement of the tip, the electrode is most likely in a "wedged" position.

Respiratory maneuvers are also helpful in determining proper placement, stability, and arc of a pacing catheter. During deep inspiration, the diaphragm moves downward, the mediastinum elongates, and the heart moves inferiorly. When the tip and atrial curve of the pacing catheter are observed fluoroscopically during deep inspiration, the tip should not move but the arc of the atrial curve should reduce and move away from the lateral wall (Fig. 24–5). During deep inspiration, the site where the catheter enters the vein must be sat-

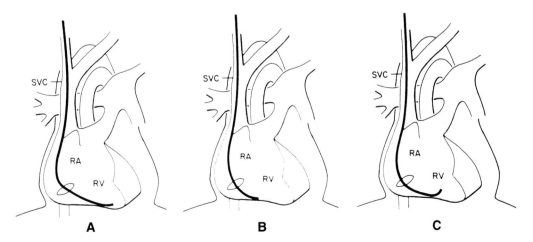

Fig. 24–4. Common catheter positions for right ventricular pacing (see text). A. Most desirable position. B. Acceptable position. C. Acceptable but least desirable position. SVC = superior vena cava; RA = right atrium; RV = right ventricle.

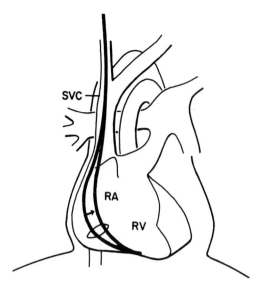

Fig. 24–5. Catheter motion during respiration. The catheter's arc decreases during inspiration (arrow) as the heart descends during diaphragmatic excursion; however, the pacing tip does not move.

urated with a sponge soaked in saline to prevent air embolism. As this maneuver is being performed to determine stability of the catheter, a judgment can be made regarding the proper amount of atrial curve, or catheter slack, required in the system (Fig. 24–6). During ventricular systole there is often a desirable gentle upward bowing in the catheter segment

between the tricuspid valve and the tip electrode. If there is excess catheter in the right atrium, the catheter often hugs the lateral wall and projects more inferiorly into the atrium than is usually the case. In this circumstance, the catheter segment from the tricuspid valve to the electrode tip has an exaggerated upward bowing during systole (Fig. 24–6). Some patients have an exaggerated mediastinal excursion during inspiration, which requires that an excessive amount of right atrial catheter curvature be retained to prevent tip dislodgement during cough, stretch, or exercise.

Perforation is the major risk of an excessive arc in the right atrial portion of the catheter, since a pacemaker catheter that hugs the right atrial wall can direct excessive force toward the tip electrode and perforate the ventricle (Fig. 24–7).

Another determinant of a satisfactory placement of a ventricular pacing catheter is the intracardiac electrogram. The electrogram is helpful in documenting constant contact between the electrode and the endocardial wall. An electrogram is displayed by attaching the central V lead terminal of the patient's ECG cable to the distal electrode terminal pin of the pacemaker catheter with a sterile connecting cable. A variety of intraventricular patterns may be displayed, the most typical of which

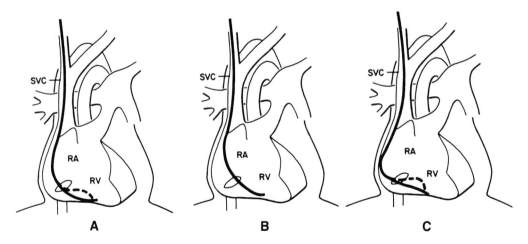

Fig. 24–6. Adjusting the arc of the catheter. A. The catheter has a gentle arc through the atrium to the ventricle. There is a slight upward bow during ventricular systole (dotted line). B. The catheter is too straight. Displacement of the tip is likely. Adjustment is required. C. The catheter has too much slack (arc). It is hugging the wall of the atrium and has an exaggerated upward bow (dotted line) during systole. Adjustment is required.

is a negative complex with a current of injury (Fig. 24–8). ST segment elevation should persist when the catheter's loop is reduced to relieve pressure at the interface between the tip electrode and the endocardial wall. The current of injury should also remain unchanged during respiratory maneuvers. Loss of ST elevation could indicate withdrawal of the electrode from good contact with the endocardial surface, and an atypical electrogram pattern could suggest ventricular perforation, especially if the electrode tip had advanced to the lateral border of the heart on the fluoroscopic image as in Figure 24–7.

The electrical properties of the pacemaker system represent the most crucial test of an acceptable pacing catheter position. A pacemaker system analyzer is used to test the electrical properties of the catheter and the generator. The electrical properties are measured in terms of voltage, current, and resistance. The electrical threshold for stimulating the heart is an important measurement. Historically, the early pacemakers had a stimulus duration of 2.0 msec. Most modern pacemakers have multiprogrammable stimulus durations with a nominal factory setting of 0.5 msec. Our laboratory continues to threshold-test at 2.0 msec as well as the nominal stimulus duration at 0.5 msec. At a 2.0 msec duration of

stimulus, we accept a threshold measurement for ventricular pacing of 1.0 mA current, 500 to 600 ohms resistance, and 0.5 volts. During electrical testing of the pacing threshold, a subcutaneous needle placed in the lower margin of the skin incision is used for the grounding (anode) electrode of a monopolar system. Other workers use a metal disk placed within the subcutaneous pocket. If a threshold determination is unacceptable, the connecting cable, grounding needle, analyzer system, and all electrical connections must be checked. If each is in good order and the threshold remains poor, the pacing catheter must be repositioned. The pacing threshold can be rigorously stressed by setting the energy level slightly above threshold while the patient takes several deep breaths. Failure to maintain continuous pacing during respiratory maneuvers suggests poor contact between the tip electrode and the endocardium.

A low pacing threshold at the time of pacemaker implantation is essential because it usually increases sharply during the first few weeks before returning to a lower level. As fibrosis develops about the electrode's tip, the threshold again gradually rises to two or three times the original value before stabilizing. Sensing thresholds are also affected by this process. A steroid elution tip may reduce the

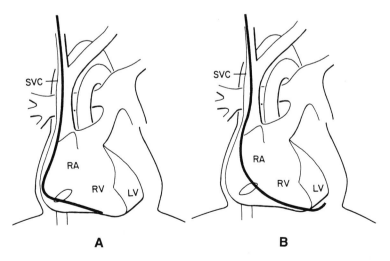

Fig. 24–7. Cardiac perforation by pacing catheter. A. Catheter positioned near apex of the right ventricle with abundant slack and an excessive arc to the catheter segment in right atrium. B. The catheter tip has perforated the myocardial wall and is overlying the left ventricle between the epicardium and pericardium.

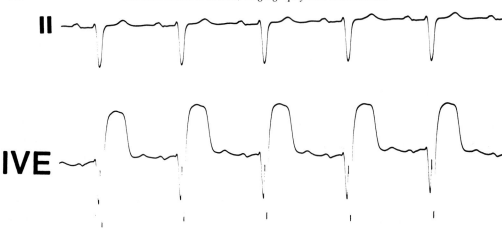

Fig. 24–8. Intraventricular electrogram (IVE) recorded from the tip of a permanent pacemaker catheter being positioned in the right ventricle. Two-channel simultaneous recording of ECG lead II (top) and IVE (bottom) reveals R:S ratio of less than one with current of injury.

inflammatory reaction and subsequent fibrosis at the electrode-myocardial interface.[23,24] Because a slowing of pacemaker rate is one indicator of the approaching end of battery life, there should be a large margin of safety between the energy level that indicates the impending end of battery life and the energy level required to pace the heart continuously. Most generators have a 5.0 volt discharge or 10 mA current (assuming a 500-ohm resistance). The rate-slowing warning that signals the near-end of battery life usually occurs when the voltage drops to approximately 3.5 to 2.3 volts, or a current of 7.0 to 4.6 mA. If the threshold for cardiac stimulation is greater than 7.0 mA, there is no warning before failure of effective pacing. Therefore, only optimal thresholds should be accepted at the time of permanent pacer implantation.

Several helpful physical and electrophysiologic observations may be made during ventricular pacing. Standard cuff blood pressure determinations are recorded during sinus or intrinsic rhythm and ventricular pacing. If there is a marked reduction in blood pressure during the transition from sinus rhythm to ventricular paced rhythm, a physiologic pacing system may be required.[25,26]

During ventricular pacing, the dual channel oscilloscope recorder is scrutinized for evidence of atrial activity. P waves may follow each pacemaker-induced complex indicating retrograde V-A conduction, during which time the heart is at a hemodynamic disadvantage, or the P waves may be independent and totally dissociated from the paced ventricular beats. The dual-channel ECG oscilloscope/recorder is also scrutinized for the pattern of the paced beats. If the pacing catheter is situated on the "floor" of the right ventricle, simultaneous leads II and V_1 display a pattern of left bundle branch block with left axis deviation. An anteroposterior fluoroscopic field could show a pacing catheter in apparently acceptable position even though this was not the case. Examples include the catheter in an inferior branch of the coronary sinus, perforating the free right ventricular wall or septum, and overlying or being within the left ventricle. Pacing in each circumstance initiates left ventricular excitation and late excitation of the right ventricle, which yield an ECG pattern of right bundle branch block. Echocardiography may be helpful in determining a faulty electrode position, which results in right bundle branch block.[27]

After the pacing catheter is well positioned and has satisfactory electrical properties for stimulating the ventricle, the fluoroscopic image is directed to the left diaphragm, and 5.0 volts of energy, or an equivalent of the maximum energy of the selected permanent pacemaker, are used to stimulate the right ventricle. The fluoroscopic image and patient are observed for evidence of extracardiac stimulation, such as contraction of the diaphragm or chest wall, in synchrony with pacemaker-induced cardiac stimulation. If this occurs, the catheter must be repositioned.

Competition between pacemaker stimuli and intrinsic spontaneous cardiac excitation is prevented by the pacemaker's ability to sense the latter. The pacemaker-generator can easily sense an endocardial electrogram with at least a 3.0 millivolt (mv) maximum signal and a 1 mv per msec rate of rise (slew rate).[28] A marginal sensing threshold is sufficient cause to reposition the pacing catheter unless the pacer generator can be reprogrammed to low-threshold sensing capability. Some pacer systems have late sensing failure because the elevated ST segment current of injury is being sensed rather than an R or S wave. Sensing fails when the injury current diminishes. Sensing failure may also occur because of decay in either the maximal signal or slew rate as the tip electrode is enveloped in fibrous tissue.

After the electrical properties are fully tested and found adequate, a gentle tie secures the catheter within the vein. The pacing catheter is also fixed to the pectoralis muscle or its overlying fascia with a butterfly or similar plastic anchoring apparatus. A tie should not be placed directly on the body of a polyurethane pacing catheter because of the risk of material fracture.

The pacemaker is then reprogrammed to the patient's needs while still within its sterile packaging. Before implantation, the pacemaker unit is tested with the system analyzer to ensure against a rare component failure between the last factory review and placement. The pacing generator is then attached to the pacing catheter. After removal of the antibiotic-soaked irrigating sponges, both the catheter and the pacemaker-generators are arranged in the subcutaneous pocket with the catheter on the underside of the pacemaker-generator. If the pacing system is unipolar and the generator has a noninsulated and an insulated surface, the noninsulated side of the generator (anode) should be positioned against the undersurface of the skin to minimize the likelihood of pectoralis muscle stimulation from the pacemaker's electrical field. Once the pacemaker-generator is positioned, the implantation site should be carefully scrutinized. Local muscle stimulation, if present, might be eliminated by placing an insulating cover about the pacemaker-generator.

The system should be reviewed fluoroscopically before skin closure. The catheter should not have changed orientation or position. Radiopaque sponges should not be in the pacemaker pocket, and there should be no sharp angulations in the extravascular catheter segment. The wound is then closed in layers and dressed. A strip chart recording should be made to document proper permanent pacemaker function. The patient is then discharged from the procedure room with a portable monitor.

The post-pacemaker orders depend on hospital custom and personal preference. There are advocates of abbreviated hospitalization or ambulatory initial pacemaker implantation.[29,30] Because pacemaker failure is highest in the first few days, there should be close surveillance during this period. The patient can be observed on either an inpatient or outpatient basis. Typical postoperative orders are listed in Table 24–5.

Postoperative Evaluation. A daily postoperative evaluation of patient and pacemaker is performed at the bedside. The cardiac monitor is observed for failure of pacing or sensing. Postimplantation Holter monitor studies reveal a high frequency of malfunctions in dual-chamber (42%) and single-chamber (27%) pacemakers.[31] If the pacemaker is inhibited by a fast intrinsic rate, a magnet placed over the pacemaker-generator will activate its asynchronous fixed-rate mode and demonstrate the pacemaker's ability to stimulate the ventricle. During paced rhythm, the chest wall and costal margin are observed for extracardiac stimulation of the pectoralis or the diaphragm. The wound is examined for evidence of infection or bleeding.

The examiner should be attentive to the

presence of a new pericardial friction rub or a pacemaker click during cardiac auscultation. These findings could result from cardiac perforation. Signs of cardiac tamponade, such as distended neck veins and pulsus paradoxus, should be sought. The examiner should also palpate the pulse while observing the cardiac monitor. If the pulse amplitude becomes weak during paced beats that are not preceded by P waves, the heart may be demonstrating a strong dependence on the atrial contribution to ventricular filling, which was not present or was not appreciated at the time of pacemaker implantation.

Chart and laboratory data are scrutinized carefully. The temperature chart is reviewed for fever, the hematocrit should be stable, and the postoperative electrocardiogram should maintain a left bundle branch block pattern during ventricular pacing.

The positions of the generator and the pacing catheter on a chest roentgenogram should resemble those seen on fluoroscopy during the implantation procedure. The immediate postoperative chest x ray can identify early problems or serve as a reference to identify a later malfunction. Selected illustrated examples include intracardiac displacement of the electrode (Fig 24–9), generator "flip-over" with the ground plate against pectoralis muscle (Fig. 24–10A), migration of the electrode pin out of the connector block (Fig. 24–10B), electrode coiling and twisting because of the patient's frequent manual flipping of the generator within its loose subcutaneous pocket. This phenomenon is termed "twiddler's syndrome"[33] (Fig. 24–10C) and electrode fracture (Fig. 24–11).

Physiologic (Dual-Chamber and Rate-Responsive) Permanent Pacing. Preservation of the normal A-V sequence to maintain optimal cardiac performance is required in a variety of conditions, most of which are associated with a noncompliant "stiff" left

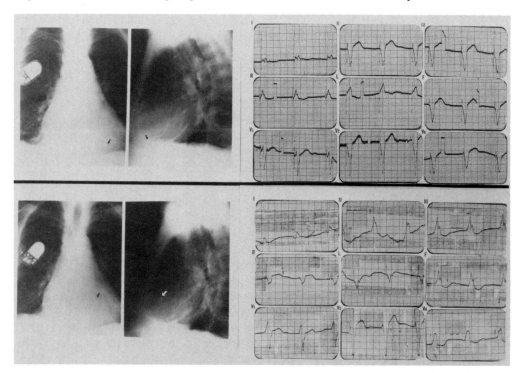

Fig. 24–9. The electrode is properly positioned in the right ventricular apex. The paced electrocardiogram reveals the expected left bundle branch block pattern with superior oriented forces. One month later, the electrode tip has displaced towards the right ventricular outflow tract with a corresponding shift of electrocardiographic forces from superior to inferior.

Fig. 24–10. A. This patient complained of muscle contractions "twitching" in the area of the pacemaker generator. Comparative x ray analysis revealed that the generator had flipped over with the ground plate pressed against pectoralis muscle (A-2) rather than against subcutaneous tissues of the skin's underside (A-1). The symptoms can be relieved by returning the pacer to its proper position or reprogramming the pacer to a lower stimulus energy. Reoperation is rarely required. B. This patient had intermittent failure of ventricular capture 6 months after placement of a dual-chamber pacemaker. On close scrutiny, the x ray revealed that the ventricular electrode pin had migrated out of the connector block because of a loose set screw. Note the relation of the ventricular electrode pin to its connector block (arrow) in contrast to the atrial electrode pin which is completely through its connector block. C. This patient unconsciously twirled the pacemaker generator within its subcutaneous pacemaker pocket. As a result, the electrode twisted around itself. Extreme twirling may result in withdrawal of the pacemaker tip from its position of fixation.

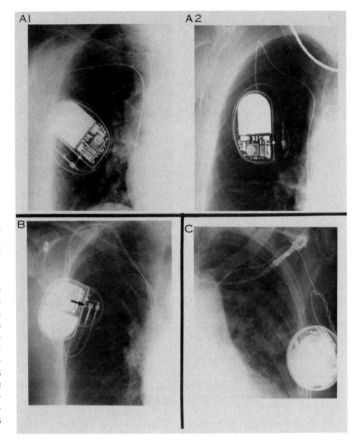

ventricle or V-A conduction. Recent or old myocardial infarction and significant mitral or aortic stenosis are classic examples of conditions in which there is left ventricular dependence on atrial transport. Other conditions associated with such a dependence include hypertrophic, obstructive, hypertensive, and ischemic cardiomyopathies. Doppler echocardiographic studies have characterized patients who will receive significant hemodynamic benefit from dual-chamber pacing as those with a stroke volume of less than 50 ml in VVI mode, V-A conduction, and a percent atrial contribution of more than 38%.[32] Sick sinus syndrome without A-V conduction abnormality is also a relatively common indication for A-V sequential pacemaker placement. Such patients might fare better with physiologic pacing. Patients with rare conditions such as recurrent carotid sinus, vasovagal, and glossopharyngeal (swallowing) syncope might also

receive consideration for a dual-chamber physiologic pacing system because it is better able to counter the vasodepressor effects of the vagal reflex.

Technical advances in atrial lead design have made permanent atrial and dual-chambered pacing practical. If the cephalic vein is used for the ventricular lead, the atrial lead is most often introduced by way of a jugular vein. Other options for the atrial lead include the cephalic vein if it is large or the subclavian vein. The use of a percutaneous subclavian vein introducer is currently very popular because it is rapid and relatively safe, and permits introduction of a single or dual catheter.[34,35] In one study, however, the introducer method of vein access contributed significantly to the complication rate because of hemothorax and pneumothorax.[36]

Although the right atrium does not have many trabeculations in its free wall, the atrial

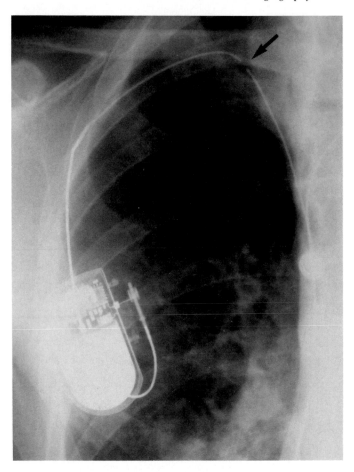

Fig. 24–11. This patient with complete heart block had a sudden decline in pulse rate. The pacer system was old and the electrode had a previous extravascular fracture which had been repaired. An intravascular fracture (arrow) was evident in the portion within the subclavian vein. An entirely new pacing system was then placed on the opposite side.

appendage is richly endowed with trabeculae. Atrial leads with a distal end curved in the shape of the letter J permit the tip electrode to be positioned in the atrial appendage, where fixation can be accomplished with a tine or screw-in tip. The screw-in lead can also be secured to the atrial free wall, a necessity in patients who have had open-heart surgery and lost their right atrial appendage.

A pacing catheter properly positioned in the right atrial appendage has a distinctive fluoroscopic appearance. During atrial systole, the loop moves medially and the tip moves laterally (Fig. 24–12). When placing the atrial pacing catheter in the appendage, the tip must be anterior and the J loop posterior. It is difficult to determine on the standard A-P fluoroscopic projection if the tip electrode is properly oriented anteriorly or improperly oriented posteriorly. Clockwise rotation of a properly oriented electrode forces the loop medially toward the septum and directs the tip laterally as in the systolic frame of Figure 24–12. The amount of free catheter in the right atrium is crucial because an excessive length of atrial catheter can result in its loop projecting through the tricuspid valve and causing ventricular ectopy. In contrast, insufficient catheter slack in the right atrium can result in displacement during deep inspiratory effort or stretching of the upper body.

The atrial catheter is tested for electrical properties of stimulation, resistance, and sensing. The atrial electrogram has a low amplitude, which explains why failure to sense is the most common problem of atrial pacing systems. The phrenic nerve overlies the right atrium and is susceptible to stimulation through the thin atrial wall. Therefore, the catheter must be tested with a 5.0 volt stimulus before accepting a final position.

Potential problems with dual-chamber pac-

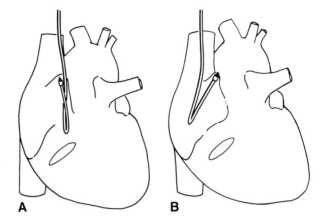

Fig. 24–12. Motion of pacing catheter in the right atrial appendage. A. During atrial systole the catheter tip appears to move in a lateral direction and the loop moves in a medial direction. B. During atrial diastole the catheter tip moves medially and the loop laterally.

A **B**

ing include a greater chance of malfunction because of the system's complexity. Retrograde P waves may trigger ventricular excitation in the DDD mode. Dual-pacemaker catheters double the risk of catheter failure and increase the chance of venous thrombosis in the upper body. All modern dual-chamber pacemakers are multiprogrammable; thus, a malfunctioning atrial component can be eliminated by programming to DVI mode in the frequent case of failure of atrial sensing, or VVI mode in the case of failure of atrial pacing or the patient converting from normal sinus rhythm to atrial fibrillation. Approximately 35% of DDD pacemakers have been reprogrammed to an alternative mode within 4 years of implantation.[37]

Programming a pacemaker between a physiologic mode (VAT) and sole ventricular pacing (VVI) has permitted hemodynamic and subjective comparisons in the same patient. In general, there is a significant improvement in hemodynamic state, exercise tolerance, and subjective state of well-being during physiologic pacing.[38] Physiologic pacing can be achieved by either atrial pacing in the presence of an intact A-V node[39] or DDD pacing in the presence of a pathologic A-V node. If there is fixed atrial fibrillation or no perceived advantage to physiologic pacing, a conventional ventricular pacemaker should be placed.

Heart rate modulation and the normal sequence of atrioventricular activation are two important determinants of an optimal cardiac output. Dual-chamber pacing was initially termed "physiologic pacing" because the heart's normal sequence of chamber activation was preserved. True physiologic pacing, however, requires the type of rate modulation provided by an intact, normally functioning sino-atrial node when impacted by a variety of stimuli such as physical activity, emotional stress, and body temperature. During a restful or sleep state, there is withdrawal of stimuli with concurrent slowing of heart rate.

Cardiac output can be increased in some patients, more from accelerated heart rate than by atrioventricular synchrony. In patients with atrial fibrillation, who comprise approximately 10% of the permanent pacemaker population, rate modulation is an important mechanism for regulating cardiac output.

Since the advent of VAT (ventricular paced, atrial triggered) and DDD mode pacing systems, there has been a capacity of providing both the capacity of AV-synchrony and rate response if the sinoatrial node is competent. Many hearts, however, have a chronotropically incompetent sinus node that does not provide a "physiologic" range of rate response.[40] Physical exercise results in an accelerated rate of muscular contraction and respirations, an increased body temperature, and a slight shift of pH toward acidic. The heart's response to exercise or emotionally augmented catecholamines is to accelerate rate, shorten A-V conduction time, increase inotropic force, and shorten ventricular excitation time.

Although there were early attempts at rate-adaptive pacing linked to phenomena other than atrial rate,[41] since 1985 rate responsive ventricular pacing linked to muscular activity has been widely accepted and ideally suited to patients with atrial fibrillation and a slow ventricular response (Fig. 24–13), or patients with sinus rhythm and little dependence on the atrial contribution to ventricular filling. Rate-responsive atrial pacing would be beneficial in the circumstance of a chronotropically incompetent sinus node with intact A-V conduction. Rate-responsive DDD pacing was approved for general use in late 1989 and is beneficial to the patient with a chronotropically incompetent sinus node with impaired A-V conduction.

We are on the threshold of a new era in pacemaker technology. A variety of phenomena related to heart rate modulation are being used as sensors to govern the rate of pacemaker discharge. The majority of systems are in the experimental stages; a few are in their infancy. Table 24–6 lists the sensors that have been incorporated into rate-responsive permanent pacer systems. Some systems being contemplated will use combinations of sensors to ensure "physiologic" rate responses during variable states of emotion as well as varied states of physical activity.[42]

Although activity rate-responsive pacemakers have gained wide acceptance and there is a heightened level of general interest in rate-responsive pacers, we must not consider our time-tested technology obsolete. It is estimated that most patients with pacemakers will not

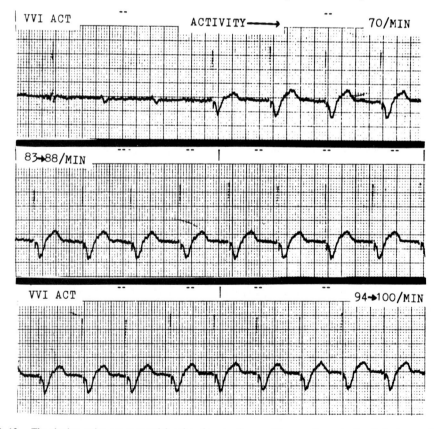

Fig. 24–13. The rhythm strips are sequential rather than continuous. Top panel: onset of activity in a patient with atrial fibrillation results in continuous ventricular pacing at a rate of 70/min. Middle panel: With continued activity, ventricular paced rhythm continues to accelerate from 83 to 88/min. Bottom panel: continued physical activity accelerates ventricular pacing to the programmed upper limit of 100/min.

Table 24–6. *Sensors for Pacemaker Rate Modulation*

Sensor	Reference
Skeletal muscle contraction	45–48
Temperature of central venous blood	49–52
Stroke volume or pre-ejection interval (dV/dT)	53
Respiration rate or respiratory minute volume	54–56
pH venous blood	57,58
Right ventricular pressure (dP/dT)	59
Evoked ventricular depolarization gradient or ventricular evoked potential	60
Oxygen saturation	58,61
Q-T interval or stimulus-T interval	62–64

use rate enhancement features more than 10 to 20% of the time.[43,44]

ACKNOWLEDGMENT

For many years, I have observed Dr. Howard A. Frank's skilled surgical approach to pacemaker implantation. Many of his techniques are described in this chapter.

REFERENCES

1. Zoll PM: Resuscitation of the heart in ventricular standstill by external electrical stimulation. N Engl J Med 247:768, 1952.
2. Furman S, Schweidel JB: An intracardiac pacemaker for Stokes-Adams seizures. N Engl J Med 261:943, 1959.
3. Elmquist R, Senning A: An implantable pacemaker for the heart. Proceedings of the Second International Conference on Medical Electronics. Paris, June 24, 1979.
4. Parsonett V: The proliferation of cardiac pacing; medical technology and socioeconomic dilemmas. Circulation 65:841, 1982.
5. Parsonnet V, Furman S, Smyth N, Bilitch M: Inter-Society Commission for Heart Disease Resources (ICHD): Optimal resources for implantable cardiac pacemakers. Pacemaker Study Group. Circulation 68:227A, 1983.
6. Ludmer PL, Goldschlager N: Cardiac pacing in the 1980s. N Engl J Med 311:1671, 1984.
7. Zoll PM, et al: External non-invasive temporary cardiac pacing: clinical trials. Circulation 71:937, 1985.
8. Zoll PM: Noninvasive temporary cardiac pacing. J Electrophysiology 1:156, 1987.
9. Hynes JK, Holmes DR Jr, Harrison CE: Five-year experience with temporary pacemaker therapy in the coronary care unit. Mayo Clin Proc 58:122, 1983.
10. Boal BH, Keller BD, Ascheim RS, Kaltman AJ:

Complications of intracardiac electrical pacing—knotting together of temporary and permanent electrodes. N Engl J Med 280:650, 1969.
11. Bing OHL, McDowell JW, Hantman J, Messer JV: Pacemaker placement by electrocardiographic monitoring. N Engl J Med 287:651, 1972.
12. Kramer DH, Moss AJ: Permanent atrial pacing from the coronary vein. Circulation 42:427, 1970.
13. Berens SC, Kolin A, MacAlpin RN, Lenz MW: New stable temporary atrial loop. Am J Cardiol 34:325, 1974.
14. Guidelines for permanent cardiac pacemaker implantation May 1984, Joint American College of Cardiology/American Heart Association Task Force on Assessment of Cardiovascular Procedures (Subcommittee on Pacemaker Implantation). J Am Coll Cardiol 4:434, 1984, and Circulation 70:331A, 1984.
15. Parsonnet V: Technique for implantation and replacement of permanent pacemakers. In Modern Techniques in Cardiac/Thoracic Surgery. New York; Futura, 1979, Chapter 12.
16. Meere C, Lesperance J: Surgical techniques in cardiac pacing. In Thalen HJ, Meere C. editors: Fundamentals of Cardiac Pacing. Hague/Boston/London, Martinus Nijhoff, 1979, pp. 127–169.
17. Smyth NPD: Techniques of pacemaker implantation: atrial and ventricular, thoracotomy and transvenous. Prog Cardiovasc Dis 23:435, 1981.
18. Martinis AJ: Pacemaker insertion. In Dillard DH, Miller DW: Atlas of Cardiac Surgery. New York, Macmillan, 1983, pp. 156–163.
19. Mond HG: The Cardiac Pacemaker: Function and Malfunction. New York, Grune and Stratton, 1983, pp. 191–232.
20. Miller GB, Leman RB, Kratz JM, Gillette PC: Comparison of lead dislodgement and pocket infection rates after pacemaker implantation in the operating room versus the catheterization laboratory. Am Heart J 115:1048, 1988.
21. Brinker JA: The cephalic vein revisited (editorial). Intelligence reports in cardiac pacing and electrophysiology. Health Scan Inc 7:1, 1988.
22. Goode LB, Clark JM, Fontaine JM, et al: Explanation of chronic pacemaker leads. Pace 12:677, 1989.
23. Mond H, Stokes K, Helland J, et al: The porous titanium steroid eluting electrode: A double blind study assessing the stimulation threshold effect of steroid. Pace 11:214, 1988.
24. Radovsky AS, Van Vleet JF: Effects of dexamethasone elution on tissue reaction around stimulation electrodes of endocardial pacing leads in dogs. Am Heart J 117:1288, 1989.
25. Cohen SI, Frank H: Preservation of active atrial transport. An important clinical consideration in cardiac pacing. Chest 81:51, 1982.
26. Ogawa S, et al: Hemodynamic consequences of atrioventricular and ventriculoatrial pacing. Pace 1:8, 1978.
27. Shettigar UR, Loungani RR, Smith RN: Inadvertent permanent ventricular pacing from the coronary vein: An electrocardiographic, roentgenographic and echocardiographic assessment. Clin Cardiol 12:267, 1989.
28. Furman S, Hurzler P, Decaprio V: The ventricular endocardial electrogram and pacemaker sensing. J Thorac Cardiovasc Surg 73:258, 1977.

29. Hayes DK, Vlietstra RE, Trusty J, et al: A shorter hospital stay after cardiac pacemaker implantation. Mayo Clin Proc 63:236, 1988.
30. Bellott PH: Ambulatory pacemaker procedures (editorial). Mayo Clinic Proc 63:301, 1988.
31. Janosik OL, Redd RM, Buckingham TA, et al: Utility of ambulatory electrocardiography in detecting pacemaker dysfunction in the early post implantation period. Am J Cardiol 60:1030, 1987.
32. Pearson AC, Janosik OL, Redd RM, et al: Hemodynamic benefit of atrioventricular synchrony: Prediction from baseline Doppler-echocardiographic variables. J Am Coll Cardiol 13:1613, 1989.
33. Tegtmyer CJ, Deignan JM: The cardiac pacemaker: A different twist. Am J Roentgenol 126:1017, 1976.
34. Friesen A, et al: Percutaneous insertion of a permanent transvenous pacemaker electrode throughout the subclavian vein. Can J Surg 20:131, 1977.
35. Janss B: Two leads in one introducer technique for A-V sequential implantations. Pace 5:217, 1982.
36. Parsonnet V, Bernstein AD, Lindsay B: Pacemaker implantation complication rates: An analysis of some contributing factors. J Am Coll Cardiol 13:917, 1989.
37. Kelmentowicz P, Oseroff O, Andrews C, Furman S: (Abs) An analysis of DDD pacing mode survival. The first five years. Pace 10:699, 1987.
38. Kruse I, Arman K, Conradson TB, Ryden L: A comparison of the acute and long-term hemodynamic effects of ventricular inhibited and atrial synchronous ventricular inhibited pacing. Circulation 65:846, 1982.
39. Bernstein SB, Van Natta BE, Ellestad MH. Experiences with right atrial pacing. Am J Cardiol 61:113, 1988.
40. Rickards AF: Rate responsive pacing. In Barold S (ed): Modern Cardiac Pacing. Futura Publishing Co., 1985, pp 199–809.
41. Nathan D, Center S, Wu CY, Keller W: An implantable synchronous pacer for the longer term correction of complete heart block. Am J Cardiol 2:362, 1963.
42. Paul V, Garratt C, Camm AJ: Combination of sensors to provide optimal pacing rate response. Clin Cardiol 12:400, 1989.
43. Parsonett V, Bernstein AD: Adaptive rate pacing. In Braunwald E (ed): Heart Disease Update, volume 5. W.B. Saunders Company 1989, pp 79–110.
44. Pipilis A, Sulke N, Henderson R, et al: How often do nondependent patients achieve rate response? NASPE Abstracts. Pace 12(Part I):655, 1989.
45. Humem DP, Kostuk WJ, Andklein GJ: Activity sensing rate responsive pacing. Improvement in myocardial performance with exercise. Pace 8:52, 1985.
46. Maura PJ, Gessman LJ, Lai T, et al: Chronotropic response of an activity detecting pacemaker compared with the normal sinus node. Pace 10:78, 1987.
47. Benditt DG, Mianulli M, Fetter J, et al: Single chamber cardiac pacing with activity initiated chronic response: evaluation by cardiopulmonary exercise testing. Circulation 75:184, 1987.
48. Stangl K, Wirtzfeld D, Lochshmidt O, Basler B, Mittnacht A: Physical movement sensitive pacing: comparison of two "activity" triggered pacing systems. Pace 12:102, 1989.
49. Griffin JC, Jutzy KR, Claude JP, Knutti JW: General body temperature as a guide to optimal heart rate. Pace 6:498, 1983.
50. Sellers T: A multicenter experience with a temperature based rate modulated pacemaker (Kelvin 500). Pace 11:486, 1988.
51. Boal B: A study of patients with modulated pacemakers which use blood temperature to determine rate followed for more than one year (Kelvin 500). Pace 11:795, 1988.
52. Alt E, Volker R, Högl B, Macarter D: The first clinical results with a new temperature-controlled rate responsive pacemaker. Comparison of Activitrax and Nova MR pacemakers with VV1/AA1 pacing. Circulation 78(suppl III):III-116, 1988.
53. Chirife R: Physiological principles of a new method of rate responsive pacing using the pre-ejection interval. Pace 11:1545, 1988.
54. Rossi, Plicchi G, Canoucci G, Ragnoni G, Aina F: Respiratory rate as a determinant of optimal pacing rate. Pace 6:502, 1983.
55. Mond HG, Kertes PJ: Rate responsive cardiac pacing. Sidney, Australia, Teletronics and Cordis Pacing Systems 1988, p 45.
56. Lau CP, Ward DE, Camm AJ: Rate responsive pacing with a pacemaker that detects respiratory rate (BioRate): Clinical advantages and complications. Clin Cardiol 11:318, 1988.
57. Camilli L, Alciol L, Shapland E, Obino S: Results, problems and perspectives with the autoregulating pacemaker. Pace 6:488, 1983.
58. McElroy PA, Janicki J, Weber KT: Physiologic correlates of the heart rate response to upright isotonic exercise: Relevance to rate responsive pacemakers. J Am Coll Cardiol 2:94, 1988.
59. Stangl K, Munteanu J, Wirtzfeld A: Right atrial pressure, right ventricular pressure and dP/dT: new pacemakers for regulative rate responsive pacemakers. Pace 10:1230, 1987.
60. Callighan F, Camerl O, Tarjan P: The ventricular depolarization gradient: exercise performance of a closed-loop rate responsive pacemaker. Pace 10:1212, 1987.
61. Wirtzfield A, Goedel-Meinen L, Bock T, et al: Central venous oxygen saturation for the control of automatic rate responsive pacing. Pace 5:829, 1982.
62. Donoldson RM, Richards AF: Rate responsive pacing using the evoked Q-T principle: A physiological alternative to atrial synchronous pacemakers. Pace 6:1344, 1983.
63. Anders Hedman: Rate responsive cardiac pacing by sensing of the evoked Q-T interval. Kongl Carolinska Medico Chirurgiaska Institutet Stockholm 1989.
64. Baig MW, Wilson J, Boute W, et al: Improved pattern of rate responsiveness with dynamic slope setting for the QT sensing pacemaker. Pace 12:311, 1989.

25

Intra-Aortic Balloon Counterpulsation and Other Forms of Cardiopulmonary Support

JULIAN M. AROESTY

Despite the recent development of new devices capable of percutaneous insertion and near-total cardiopulmonary support outside the operating room, the intra-aortic balloon pump (IABP) remains the most commonly used mechanical cardiac support device. While both insertion and removal of the intra-aortic balloon pump initially required the services of a vascular surgeon,[1,2] the development of the percutaneous insertion technique in 1980[3] has virtually eliminated this problem.

The intra-aortic balloon catheter has a flexible polyurethane bladder which is positioned within the descending thoracic aorta. This bladder is inflated with a low-density gas (such as CO_2 or helium) immediately after aortic valve closure, causing an increase in aortic diastolic pressure. As the aortic valve opens in early systole, the gas-control system deflates the balloon rapidly, producing a sharp fall in systolic aortic pressure and a decrease in resistance to left ventricular ejection. The gas-control console uses the electrocardiogram to trigger each balloon cycle, with fine adjustment of inflate and deflate times to optimize hemodynamic effect as reflected by the arterial pulse pressure tracing. Because balloon ex-

pansion occurs during diastole, and deflation during systole, the entire process is most appropriately called *counterpulsation*. This has major physiologic advantages, including a decrease in myocardial oxygen consumption and an increase in diastolic coronary perfusion pressure, along with improved left ventricular ejection.

CONSTRUCTION

Intra-aortic balloon catheters are available from four manufacturers (Aries, Datascope, Kontron, and Mansfield) in a variety of shaft sizes (9.5 to 12 Fr) and balloon volumes (30 to 50 ml). All manufacturers now use *helium* as the inflation gas because its low viscosity permits the use of smaller balloon shafts and more rapid pumping rates. Unlike CO_2, helium has low solubility in blood. This requires reliable mechanisms within the console that detect and react to balloon leak or rupture to minimize the risk of serious gas embolism.

Surgically Implanted Catheters

Surgical implantation requires direct exposure of the common femoral artery, with the attachment of a woven graft through which the balloon is advanced to the thoracic aorta. This approach has been almost completely supplanted by the percutaneous technique, which has comparable success and complication rates, but can be accomplished much more quickly in a coronary care unit or cardiac catheterization laboratory.[4]

Percutaneous Catheters

Double-lumen balloon catheters are available from all manufacturers and include a central lumen that allows advancement of the catheter over a previously placed guide wire, and subsequent monitoring of central aortic pressure. *Single*-lumen intra-aortic balloon catheters give up those advantages in exchange for a smaller shaft and smaller deflated balloon profile, which may be advantageous in patients with advanced atherosclerotic peripheral vascular disease or small stature.

The inflated balloon diameter should be 10 to 20% smaller than the diameter of the aorta. A balloon that is too large for the corresponding aorta will damage the intima, while one that is too small tends to produce ineffective counterpulsation. Most adults require a 40 ml balloon. For patients with very small or very large stature, 30 and 50 ml balloons are available[5] (Table 25–1).

INDICATIONS AND CONTRAINDICATIONS

Counterpulsation is most often used in medically refractory unstable angina,[6] cardiogenic shock,[7–9] or hemodynamic instability at the time of cardiac surgery,[10] coronary angioplasty, or balloon valvuloplasty. Less well established indications include the limitation of infarct size in patients with uncomplicated acute myocardial infarction,[11] support of patients with advanced heart disease or recent infarction who require general anesthesia during noncardiac surgical procedures,[12] and the treatment of intractable ventricular tachycardia.[13]

Counterpulsation is *contraindicated* in the presence of aortic regurgitation or a large arteriovenous shunt (e.g., patent ductus arteriosus) because either condition may be worsened by the elevation of aortic diastolic pressure during counterpulsation. Other contraindications to intra-aortic balloon counterpulsation include the presence of severe arterial insufficiency of the lower limbs, an atherosclerotic or dissecting abdominal aortic aneurysm, a marked bleeding diathesis, uncontrolled sepsis, and documented cholesterol embolism to abdomen or legs. Marked irregularity of the cardiac rhythm is not a contraindication, although it makes timing of balloon inflation more difficult. Percutaneous placement through prior Dacron aortofemoral grafts is possible, but should be avoided if there is another alternative.[14]

TECHNIQUE FOR INSERTION

Planning

If counterpulsation is planned before elective coronary arteriography, the possibility of intra-aortic balloon placement should be discussed with the patient and informed consent obtained. Because patients with unstable angina and those with critical left main or multivessel coronary obstructions may require counterpulsation following coronary angiography, one should be aware of the anatomy of the distal aorta, iliac arteries, and femoral arteries during performance of the diagnostic coronary angiogram. This does not necessarily require power injection through a special catheter. A large amount of information can be obtained from observation of the course taken by guide wire and catheter and/or small hand injections under fluoroscopic imaging if excessive tortuosity or significant arterial obstruction is encountered. Even in the absence of arterial obstruction, peripheral angiography may occasionally help to avoid complications by recognizing potential problems caused by unusual anatomy or tortuosity (Fig. 25–1).

Table 25–1. *Percutaneous Intra-aortic Balloons*

Manufacturer*	Balloon Catheter Size (Fr)	Volume of Balloon cc	Size of Introducer Internal	Size of Introducer External
Datascope				
Single lumen	4.5	2.5	Presently	
(Pediatric)	5.5	5.0	available for	
	5.5	7.0	surgical	
	7.0	12.0	insertion	
	7.0	20.0	only	
Single lumen	8.5	40.0	10.0	11.5
(Adult)	9.5	40.0	10.0	11.5
Double lumen	9.5	40.0	10.0	
(Adult)	10.5	40.0	11.4	13.2
	10.5	50.0	11.5	13.2
				11.0
Kontron	9.5	40.0	11.8	12.5
Double lumen	10.5	40.0	12.6	13.7
Mansfield				
Single lumen	9.5	30.0	10.5	12.0
Double lumen	9.5	40.0	11.0	12.0
	10.0	40.0	11.0	13.0
Aries				
Single lumen	9.0	30.0	(9.0)†	11.0
	9.0	40.0	(9.0)†	11.0
	9.0	50.0	(9.0)†	11.0
Double lumen	11.0	30.0	(11.0)†	12.5
	11.0	40.0	(11.0)†	12.5
	11.0	50.0	(11.0)†	12.5

*Manufacturers' Addresses: Datascope, Paramus, NJ 07653-0005; Kontron, Everett, MA 02149; Mansfield, Mansfield, MA 02048; Aries, Woburn, MA 01801.

†This system uses a peel-away sheath that is removed after insertion. The arterial puncture is sealed subsequently with a tapered plug.

Evaluation

If feasible, a complete blood count, prothrombin time, partial thromboplastic time, bleeding time, and platelet count should be obtained within 24 hours of the planned insertion to ensure that there is no serious bleeding problem. A careful history should be obtained, with specific questioning regarding symptoms of limb ischemia. The strength of bilateral femoral, popliteal, dorsalis pedis, and posterior tibial pulses should be recorded. The abdomen, pelvis, and both legs should be auscultated for the presence of bruits. If there is evidence of possible arterial insufficiency, *noninvasive* evaluation of limb circulation (Doppler pressures, pulse volume recording, etc.) is helpful in initial evaluation as well as

follow-up. Periodic evaluation of percutaneous intra-aortic balloon patients by a vascular surgeon and nurse before insertion, throughout the course of counterpulsation, and after removal of the balloon catheter may be helpful in the prevention and early recognition of vascular complications.

Puncture Technique

Before intra-aortic balloon insertion, both groins should be scrubbed and draped so that the opposite groin may be used if the initial site is unsuitable. Because the balloon catheter is a foreign body that may remain in the vasculature for several days, meticulous attention

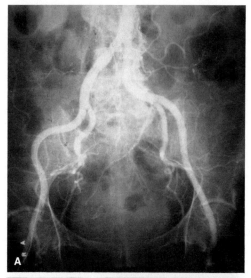

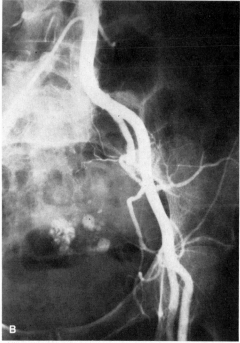

Fig. 25–1. A, Angiography in a 62-year-old woman reveals an unobstructed aorta, iliac and femoral system with marked tortuosity more prominent on the right side. Insertion by way of the left femoral artery would be preferable. B, Left iliac arteriography in a 65-year-old woman without arterial obstruction but with a very proximal femoral artery bifurcation on the left side. Puncture at the usual site 2 cm below the inguinal ligament would enter a femoral branch with probable limb ischemia. Note the relationship between femoral artery and the head of the femur. The artery usually crosses the femoral head at its medial half.

should be paid to sterile technique, even during emergency placement.

The most common complications of intra-aortic balloon placement are related to puncture at an improper site or forceful advancement of a guide wire which is not within the true lumen of the artery. Puncture should take place in the segment of the *common* femoral artery, which is distal to the inguinal ligament but proximal to the point at which the femoral artery bifurcates into its superficial and deep branches (see Chap. 5). Puncture proximal to this segment might not allow control of bleeding at the time of balloon catheter removal, increasing the risk of developing a false aneurysm or large hematoma. If the puncture is too distal rather than too proximal, the intra-aortic balloon catheter will be inserted into a relatively small artery (either the superficial or profunda branch of the femoral artery) with greater risk of obstruction to flow, immediate limb ischemia, or thrombosis-induced late ischemia.

For a right-handed operator, right groin insertion is somewhat easier. Enough time should be spent palpating the femoral artery to define accurately its location and course. If the patient is in cardiogenic shock, the femoral artery may not be palpable, but successful puncture can often be performed using fluoroscopy with the knowledge that the femoral artery overlies the medial half to medial third of the femoral head (Fig. 25–1).

Advancement of the Guide Wire

Advancement of the guide wire *should be painless* and should proceed without any sensation of resistance. If resistance, pain, or kinking of the guide wire is observed by fluoroscopy, it must not be forced. A movable core guide wire with a smaller J tip, a Wholey wire or a steerable guide wire may succeed when a standard guide wire cannot be advanced. In such instances, advancement of the large intra-aortic balloon introduction sheath may be difficult, and it would be wise to insert a 5 or 6 Fr catheter over the guide wire, followed by careful hand injections of non-ionic or diluted contrast material to define the arterial anatomy and preferable insertion site.

If passage of the guide wire to the descending thoracic aorta has been uneventful, an 8F dilator is inserted to predilate the artery. The tip of the guide wire is kept above the diaphragm while the 8F dilator is then removed and discarded. Firm pressure is applied over the puncture sight to prevent bleeding and the exposed guide wire is wiped clean with a wet sponge. The incision in the skin and fascia is enlarged to permit easy passage of the balloon sheath or catheter. To prevent kinking of the guide wire, firm pressure must be maintained over the femoral artery puncture site with the left hand as the dilator/sheath apparatus is inserted with a rotating motion, holding the dilator close to the skin. Once the dilator section is within the femoral artery, the sheath can be advanced from the distal or hub end of the assembly to prevent the sheath from sliding over the dilator.

Intra-aortic Balloon Insertion

Before the operator handles the balloon catheter, powder should be washed off sterile gloves because powder may alter the nonthrombogenic properties of the balloon surface. Most manufacturers now supply the balloons in a prefolded configuration to avoid direct manipulation before passage through the sheath. Each balloon should be prepared according to the specific instructions of the manufacturer because details differ for each brand (Datascope, Kontron, Mansfield, Aries) as well as each type (noncentral lumen, guide wire directed central lumen) of catheter.

The central lumen of the balloon catheter should be irrigated with heparinized solution before the balloon is advanced over a guide wire that has already been passed to the aortic knob. I prefer this to introduction of the sheath over the shorter (60 cm) 0.035 guide wire, with subsequent introduction of the balloon catheter after readvancing a 145 cm J tip guide wire to the aortic knob, especially if advancement of the initial guide wire was difficult.

If an introducing sheath is used, it can be "pinched" to reduce bleeding as the balloon is first passed. The balloon catheter should then fit within the sheath snugly enough that there is little bleeding. Once the balloon is within the sheath, the tip of the guide wire should be maintained in the aorta at a position near the level of the left subclavian artery. The wrapped balloon should advance over the guide wire without resistance until its radiopaque tip marker is within the descending thoracic aorta just below the origin of the left subclavian artery, usually at about the level of the carina or left mainstem bronchus. The guide wire is then removed and discarded, so that the central lumen of the balloon catheter can be aspirated vigorously and then irrigated cautiously with heparinized solution. Special care must be taken to avoid inadvertent injection of air bubbles or thrombi because the tip of the catheter lies at the aortic arch. The cuff on the balloon shaft is advanced to the hub of the introduction sheath to seal the sheath and prevent back-bleeding.

An alternative to percutaneous insertion through the sheath has been used in some patients in our institution. After the artery is predilated with a dilator 0.5 Fr smaller than the balloon catheter (i.e., 9 Fr for a 9.5 Fr balloon), the intra-aortic balloon itself is inserted directly, taking care to avoid injuring the artery or the catheter. Although the folded balloon has a slightly larger diameter than the balloon shaft, advancement of the balloon over a guide wire to its proper position in the descending thoracic aorta has not thus far resulted in marked bleeding around the balloon shaft at the puncture site. This modified technique may permit the use of a balloon in arteries that are otherwise too small or narrowed by atherosclerosis because the balloon shaft is roughly 1.5 Fr (0.5 mm) smaller than the outer diameter of the associated sheath. An alternative strategy involves partial or total withdrawal or peeling away of the sheath *after* balloon placement, but this would seem much more likely to produce significant bleeding around the balloon shaft at the puncture site.

The central lumen is attached to a heparinized transducer and continuous infusion system through a three-way stopcock. The infusion system is pressurized to 300 mmHg and provides a continuous flow of 3 ml/hr without distorting recorded arterial pressure.[15] Because air could pass through this apparatus and be released into the central aorta, *all* air must be purged from the system. Heparin is added to the flush solution at a concentration of 10 IU/ml (5000 IU heparin in a 500 ml bag of flush solution).

Because an embolus from the tip of the intra-aortic balloon catheter might enter the cerebral or coronary circulation, the central lumen must be flushed with extreme care. It should be flushed only with the continuous infusion system (which runs at 1.5 ml per second while its valve is held open) only while counterpulsation is temporarily interrupted. Except during initial insertion, the central lumen should *never* be flushed manually with a syringe, and it should not be used for drawing blood samples. If the central lumen pressure trace becomes damped and the cause is not related to a loose connection in the system, aspiration of the central lumen should be attempted. If there is marked resistance to aspiration of blood, *DO NOT FLUSH*. The lumen should then be considered occluded, and the central aortic pressure line should be capped and discontinued.

INITIATION OF COUNTERPULSATION

The balloon is attached to the appropriate connector for the Datascope, Kontron, Mansfield, or Aries console. Following a purge with helium inflation gas, the balloon is *half-filled* and counterpulsation is begun at 1:2 setting (every other beat) so that preliminary timing adjustments can be made (see subsequent text).

Fluoroscopy is used to identify the position of the proximal portion of the balloon. It ensures that the balloon is fully unwrapped and inflating without twist or kink, and that the distal portion of the balloon has fully exited the introduction sheath. If it is necessary to adjust the position of the balloon, it may be moved *within* the sheath but must never be

adjusted by advancing the sheath itself because the latter maneuver may produce arterial damage at the distal end of the introduction sheath as it advances within the artery without the protection of a snug fitting introduction catheter.

If the half-filled balloon is operating satisfactorily, the balloon should then be filled to its full volume using fluoroscopy to verify that the balloon position is appropriate and the filled balloon assumes a uniform symmetric cylindrical shape. The seal and the balloon shaft are sewn to the skin, betadine ointment is applied to the entrance site, a mark is placed across the balloon shaft and the skin to identify balloon migration, and a sterile dressing is applied. Aqueous heparin, 5000 IU, is administered intravenously followed by continuous intravenous heparin or dextran. A supine chest roentgenogram is obtained to confirm the presence of satisfactory balloon position.

COUNTERPULSATION TIMING

If balloon timing is not adjusted properly, left ventricular systolic emptying may take place during balloon inflation with disastrous consequences in critically ill patients. Timing is adjusted with the console set at 1:2 pumping (i.e., counterpulsation of every other beat) so that arterial pressure tracings with and without counterpulsation can be compared. Use of the aortic pressure tracing from the balloon lumen is preferable to monitoring the radial artery tracing because of the delay and change in arterial contour as the pulse wave moves from the central aorta to the periphery.

Inflation

While observing a high-fidelity central aortic pressure trace of good waveform, the operator should slowly move the inflation knob toward the right (later inflation) until the dicrotic notch is visible, and then back slightly to the left until inflation fuses with the central aortic dicrotic notch to form a "V." This position also produces maximal height of the augmented diastolic pressure (Fig. 25–2A).

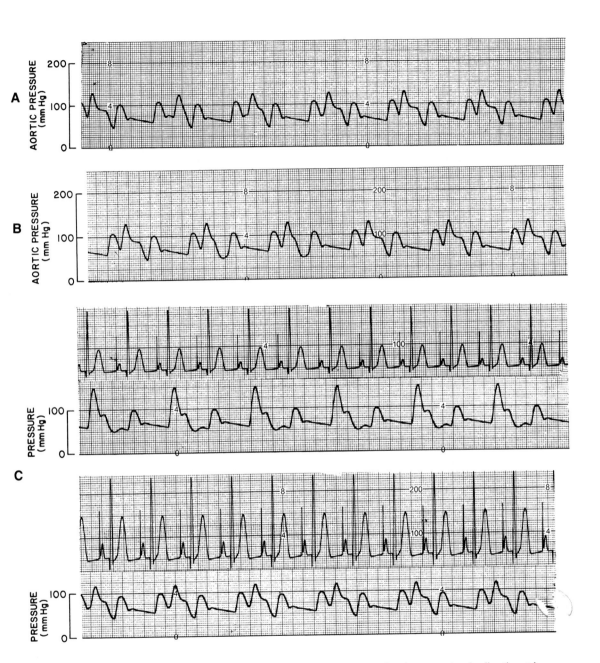

Fig. 25–2. A, The timing of balloon inflation is adjusted until it occurs late in diastole, uncovering the dicrotic notch. Subsequently, inflation timing is moved earlier in the cardiac cycle until the dicrotic notch on the central aortic tracing just disappears (beat #4). The augmented pressure will rise as inflation timing is moved earlier. B, Deflation knob is moved toward the right (later in the cardiac cycle) until the end diastolic dip is 10 to 15 mmHg below the patient's unassisted diastolic pressure. This will produce a maximal lowering of the patient's unassisted systolic pressure. C, The balloon console is triggering on an atrial pacing artifact. This is corrected by changing the console to a mode that will discriminate between a pacing spike and an R wave.

Deflation

Deflation should take place just before the opening of the aortic valve. Starting at the left (earlier deflation), the deflation knob is then moved slowly to the right until there is maximum reduction in the aortic systolic pressure of the beat following balloon deflation, usually associated with a dip in end-diastolic pressure 10 to 15 mmHg below the diastolic pressure of a nonaugmented beat (Fig. 25–2B).

If there is a marked irregularity of cardiac rhythm (e.g., atrial fibrillation with marked variation in cycle length), balloon timing is best adjusted so that deflation occurs on the peak of the R wave to avoid left ventricular ejection against an inflated balloon during occasional shorter cycles.

Atrial pacing may also produce difficulty with balloon timing if the balloon console misinterprets the atrial pacing spike as the peak of the R wave. This error can be corrected by setting the timing by the arterial pressure wave, choosing an ECG lead that magnifies the difference between QRS and atrial pacing spike, or by setting the console to a mode that discriminates between the pacing spike and the R wave by sensing both the height and duration of the signal (Fig. 25–2C).

BALLOON PRESSURE WAVEFORM

The balloon waveform (with the gas control system) ordinarily has a rectangular appearance with a sharp positive overshoot artifact just before the peak inflation pressure, and a negative deflation artifact at the end of deflation (Fig. 25–3A). Loss of these inflation and deflation artifacts produces a rectangular pressure wave with a blunted or somewhat rounded top. This pattern may be seen in the presence of a balloon that is too large for the aorta, a kink in the balloon catheter or connecting tubing, or a balloon that is not fully unwrapped (Fig. 25–3B). Correction of these problems should result in the prompt return of the proper waveform with clearly visible inflation and deflation artifacts.

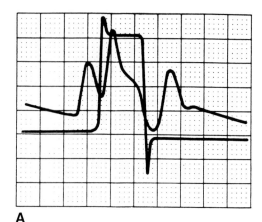

A

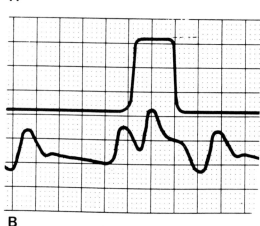

B

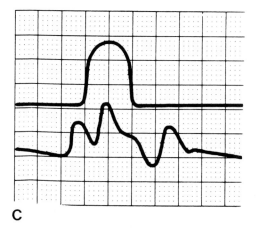

C

Fig. 25–3. A, Balloon pressure waveform superimposed on the arterial pressure wave. Note the overshoot at the peak of balloon inflation and the negative deflation artifact at the end of balloon emptying. B, Loss of the positive and negative artifacts, indicative of a balloon that is not filling completely because of incomplete unwrapping or a kink in the tubing. C, Rounding of the balloon pressure, which occurs when the balloon is too large for the aorta.

MANAGEMENT DURING COUNTERPULSATION

During counterpulsation, there should be daily evaluation for evidence of sepsis, thrombocytopenia, blood loss, hemolysis-induced anemia, vascular obstruction caused by the balloon, thrombus, embolus, or dissection. Thrombocytopenia is almost invariable, but the platelet count rarely falls below 50,000 to 100,000/ml. Platelet transfusions should be considered only if there is serious bleeding, but are rarely necessary. Following balloon removal, the platelet count returns to normal rapidly.[16]

Aortic dissection is rare, but can be present even in the presence of apparent successful balloon pump function. It is usually accompanied by significant pain in the back, limbs, or pelvis, and must be treated promptly by removal of the balloon and vascular evaluation.

Local sepsis can be minimized by good aseptic insertion technique, daily changes of dressings with application of povidone-iodine (Betadine) ointment to the insertion site, and careful technique in changing bottles of flush solution. However, disseminated sepsis is an emergency that may require balloon removal for control. Prophylactic antibiotics are not given routinely, but should be used if there is any compromise in sterile technique during insertion.

After balloon insertion, patients must be kept at bed rest. Hip flexion or elevation of the head of the bed beyond 30 degrees must be avoided, but the entire bed may be tilted head-up or head-down to treat pulmonary edema or hypotension. A loose bandage that attaches the involved ankle to the bed helps to maintain appropriate leg position during periods of sleep, confusion, or discomfort.

If cardiac angiography is necessary *after* balloon insertion, it can be performed by the Sones technique during continuous counterpulsation.[17] The opposite femoral artery can also be used safely as long as the balloon is turned off briefly while the coronary catheter traverses the area of the balloon and special care is exercised to avoid damage to the balloon by the tip of the catheter. We have performed several hundred catheter exchanges in this way without any recognized balloon damage.[18]

BALLOON REMOVAL

Before removal of an intra-aortic balloon catheter, the patient is weaned from 1:1 mode to 1:2, 1:4, and finally 1:8. Sufficient time should elapse between each stage to ensure that the patient will tolerate a progressive decrease in the level of counterpulsation without clinical deterioration. At 1:8 pumping, anticoagulation should be discontinued so that the balloon can be turned off and removed.

A 50 ml syringe is attached to the balloon inflation lumen by means of a stopcock and used to create a vacuum. The balloon is withdrawn to, but not into, the insertion sheath, because the latter maneuver may tear or even embolize a portion of the balloon membrane. After the skin ties are cut, the sheath and balloon are withdrawn as a single unit. A small spurt of blood should be allowed to escape while the artery is compressed, first distal and then proximal to the insertion site, to help flush out any adherent thrombus. The site is then compressed firmly by hand or with a mechanical compression device (Compressar, Intromedix, Portland, OR) for 30 to 60 minutes. Distal limb circulation should be checked during and after compression. The patient is kept at bed rest, and hip flexion is not allowed on the involved side for 24 hours.

COMPLICATIONS

In almost all reported series, percutaneous balloon insertion and counterpulsation can be accomplished with a 90% success rate. There is a wide variance in reported complication rates, at least partly related to differences in the patient population. The average rate of serious complications is 10 to 20%, mostly due to iliofemoral thrombosis, and is similar to that observed in several large *surgical* intra-aortic balloon series.[4,16,19–33] The wire-guided technique should produce fewer dangerous arterial lacerations, although the number of local thromboses may be increased by the obstructing effect of the introducing sheath.

A study of 206 consecutive patients between 1980 and 1982 compared 105 intra-aortic balloons introduced by percutaneous technique with 101 implanted surgically. Vascular complications were reported in 42 of 206 or 20% of patients, half of whom required vascular surgical repair for management. Multivariate analysis demonstrated that pre-existing peripheral vascular disease (history of claudication, presence of femoral bruit, or absence of foot pulses) and the use of the percutaneous approach increased the risk of major complications. In patients with prior peripheral vascular disease, the risk of major vascular complication was 31% with percutaneous technique versus 16% for surgical implantation. In patients without peripheral vascular disease, the risk of a major vascular complication was four times higher in women (15%) than in men (3.5%). Age, duration of counterpulsation, and indication for insertion were not significant risk factors. Specific complications included vascular injury/perforation, thrombosis, emboli, aortic dissection, limb ischemia, infection, renal failure, cerebrovascular accident, mesenteric infarction, balloon rupture, and death.[33]

A review of 733 patients by Kantrowitz[34] revealed an increased vascular complication rate in women and diabetic or hypertensive patients, but showed no relationship to the duration of counterpulsation. Infectious complications were fewer when insertion was performed in the operating room as compared to the coronary care unit (12% vs. 26%) and the occurrence of bacteremia increased significantly with the duration of counterpulsation. It should be noted that many of these insertions were performed using the surgical technique on patients with cardiogenic shock.[34]

An analysis of 103 patients who underwent insertion of percutaneous intra-aortic balloon catheters at our institution[35] showed that limb ischemia occurred in over 40% of patients and required balloon removal in just under 30%.

Limb ischemia was related to the presence of diabetes, peripheral vascular disease, female gender, and the presence of a postinsertion ankle-brachial pressure index less than 0.8. There was no association between the development of limb ischemia and age, body surface area, 10.5 F versus 12 Fr balloon size, or adequacy of anticoagulation.[35] The newer 9.5 Fr balloon and the sheathless insertion technique described above were not included in this series.

Of the 7333 patients undergoing percutaneous left heart catheterization procedures at the Beth Israel Hospital between 1980 and 1987, only 1% required operative repair of catheterization-related vascular complications, but the incidence of operative repair after transfemoral intra-aortic balloon placement was 11.5%.[36] Most patients developing limb ischemia following balloon placement, however, do *not* need surgical repair because limb ischemia often resolves once the intra-aortic balloon catheter has been removed.

HEMODYNAMIC EFFECTS OF COUNTERPULSATION

The hemodynamic effects of counterpulsation depend in part on the underlying problem for which it is used. When it is instituted relatively early in the course of cardiogenic shock in dogs, counterpulsation produces a 19 to 25% reduction in peak LV wall stress with a concomitant increase in coronary blood flow.[37] Studies have been performed on relatively small numbers of patients, who are often not comparable from one to another investigation. Seventy percent of patients in cardiogenic shock studied 14 hours after IABP insertion showed no change or a fall in coronary blood flow with counterpulsation and no significant change in myocardial lactate extraction,[38] yet a comparable group of patients studied 4 to 6 hours after initiation of counterpulsation showed an 18% decrease in LV systolic pressure and a 38% increase in cardiac index. Coronary sinus studies in these patients documented a 34% increase in coronary blood flow and a change from 6% lactate production to

15% extraction[39] or an improvement in lactate production toward normal.[40] With multiple ECG leads in a dog model or in man, counterpulsation produced a marked decrease in the extent and severity of myocardial ischemia (as determined by the sum of ST segment elevation in multiple electrocardiographic leads) if it was applied within 3 hours of coronary occlusion. In addition, IABP reversed the increased myocardial ischemia induced by isoproterenol infusion.[41]

In addition to the suggested benefits on coronary blood flow described above, almost all investigators have demonstrated a favorable effect of counterpulsation on LV performance: cardiac index and mean arterial pressure increase and left ventricular filling pressures decrease substantially[7,9,39,40,42,43] (Fig. 25–4). Although the intra-aortic balloon usually produces an initial improvement in hemodynamics, there is often recurrent deterioration in hemodynamics after 3 to 4 days unless corrective surgery is performed.

Patients with medically refractory unstable angina may be improved by counterpulsation, and this condition is the most common indication for intra-aortic balloon placement in our institution. Such patients may show only a small decrease in peak systolic pressure and in left ventricular filling pressure (Fig. 25–5), with unchanged left ventricular volumes and ejection fraction during counterpulsation,[44] and no clear improvement in regional coronary flow to the ischemic area.[45] Yet the addition of intra-aortic balloon pumping to a maximal medical program produces marked improvement in anginal status in the great majority of patients.[6] This benefit is underscored when it becomes necessary to discontinue counterpulsation transiently to refill the balloon with helium; unstable patients may manifest clinical deterioration within 1 or 2 minutes without counterpulsation (Fig. 25–5).

The variable effect of counterpulsation on coronary blood flow is probably related to the type of patient studied (i.e., cardiogenic shock versus unstable angina). Normally perfused myocardium may demonstrate a *decrease* in

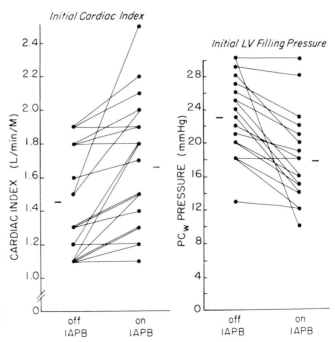

Fig. 25–4. Hemodynamic effects of intra-aortic balloon pump (IABP) in cardiogenic shock. Although cardiogenic shock patients sustained an initial improvement in cardiac index and left ventricular filling pressure (PCW), the largest changes were noted in patients with a mechanical defect (ventricular septal defect or mitral regurgitation).

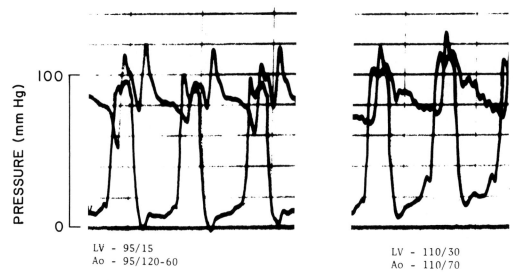

LV - 95/15
Ao - 95/120-60

LV - 110/30
Ao - 110/70

Fig. 25–5. One minute after temporary discontinuation of counterpulsation in a patient with three-vessel coronary artery disease, left main coronary artery stenosis, and severe unstable angina, there is a prompt increase in left ventricular systolic and end-diastolic pressure with rapid return of ischemic pain.

regional coronary flow because of a decrease in loading conditions, while ischemic myocardium (a region with maximal vasodilatation and therefore susceptible to marked changes in regional coronary blood flow with changes in perfusion pressure) may show an *increase* in regional blood flow.

An example of the effectiveness of intra-aortic balloon counterpulsation in cardiogenic shock due to mitral regurgitation is shown in Figures 25–6 and 25–7. These tracings were recorded in a 45-year-old woman who presented in cardiogenic shock with pulmonary edema from acute ruptured chordae and massive mitral regurgitation. As seen in Figure 25–6, counterpulsation reduced left ventricular diastolic pressure and the V wave in the pulmonary capillary wedge tracing. Figure 25–7 shows pressures during a pullback of the left heart catheter from the left ventricle to the aorta during balloon counterpulsation. Careful inspection of the tracings and their relation to the simultaneous ECG shows that the major pressure wave in the aorta is occurring during diastole and represents a 30 mmHg effect of counterpulsation. Thus, despite a left ventricular systolic pressure of 60 to 70 mmHg, the patient's condition stabilized, permitting successful mitral valve surgery.

OTHER FORMS OF CARDIOPULMONARY SUPPORT

The intra-aortic balloon pump has been useful mainly in the treatment of patients with medically refractory ischemic coronary heart disease. Although it has also been helpful in the management of cardiogenic shock, its usefulness has been most prominent in shock accompanied by reparable mechanical defects (acute severe mitral regurgitation or ventricular septal defect), or in patients with cardiogenic shock caused by reversible myocardial ischemia. Several newer forms of cardiopulmonary support are much more potent in supporting failing systemic hemodynamics. These cardiopulmonary support devices can support patients in full cardiopulmonary arrest, but may be less effective in reversing myocardial ischemia in the presence of a completely occluded coronary artery, because they work almost exclusively by decreasing cardiac work and myocardial oxygen consumption, elevating diastolic pressure only slightly.

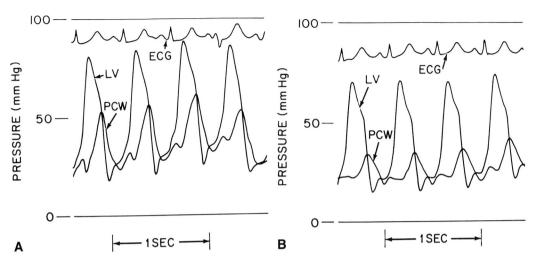

Fig. 25–6. Left ventricular (LV) and pulmonary capillary wedge (PCW) tracings A, without and B, with intra-aortic balloon counterpulsation in a 45-year-old woman in cardiogenic shock from ruptured chordae of the mitral valve. See text.

Bard CPS System

The Bard percutaneous cardiopulmonary support (CPS) system is analogous to the heart-lung machine used during open heart surgery, except that cannulation is performed percutaneously by way of the femoral artery and vein. The patient's venous blood is withdrawn from the right atrium and pumped mechanically through a semipermeable membrane oxygenator and then back into the arterial system through the femoral arterial cannula.

Design. The basic design of the system is illustrated schematically in Figure 25–8. Venous blood collected from the right atrium and vena cavae is passed through the Bio-medicus pump, a heat exchanger, and a membrane oxygenator, after which it is pumped back into the

aorta by way of the percutaneously introduced arterial cannula.

Because the venous and arterial cannulae are currently size 20 Fr (6.7 mm), iliofemoral and aortic angiography should be performed before insertion of the CPS system. Access is achieved in both the femoral artery and ipsilateral femoral vein using an .038 inch J guide wire and standard 8 Fr angioplasty sheath. The J guide wire is then replaced with a specially stiffened "heavy duty" 0.038 J tip guide wire. Following removal of the long 8 Fr dilator, the vessel is dilated with serial 12 Fr and then 14 Fr dilators. The 20 Fr arterial cannula is inserted to the desired position within the aorta. The dilator and guide wire are removed and the cannula tubing is clamped.

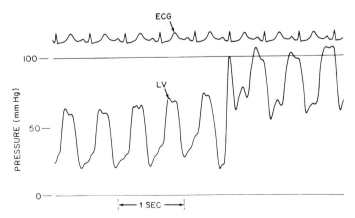

Fig. 25–7. Same patient as in Figure 25–6. Tracings during catheter pullback from left ventricle (LV) to central aorta during intra-aortic balloon counterpulsation. See text.

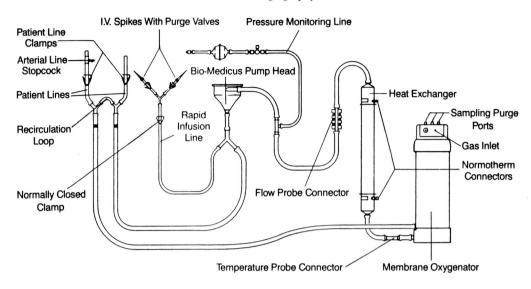

Fig. 25–8. The Bard cardiopulmonary support system uses a Bio-medicus pump to pass venous blood through a heat exchanger and membrane oxygenator and into the arterial system. The extra lines are available to provide pressure monitoring, a recirculation loop, and a purging circuit.

A similar entry technique is used for the femoral vein, placing a stiffened heavy duty .038 J tip guide wire in the SVC. In similar fashion, the 8F long dilator is removed and a 12 Fr followed by a 14 Fr dilator is passed into the venous system over the heavy duty guide wire. With the guide wire tip maintained in the superior vena cava, the 20 Fr venous cannula is advanced to the right atrium just above its juncture with the inferior vena cava. The dilator and guide wire are removed and a clamp is applied to the cannula tubing.

Starting 3 hours before insertion of the pump, low molecular weight dextran is infused at 50 cc per hour. Once access to the venous and arterial system has been achieved, heparinization is instituted using a high dose protocol (300 units per kg of body weight).

While the cannulae are being inserted, the CPS perfusion circuit is primed with crystalloid solution. Cardiopulmonary bypass is initiated at 2 L per minute and then increased progressively as needed to 2.5, 3.0, 3.5, 4.0, or 5.0 L per minute.

Bypass is initiated once the CPS catheters have been fixed securely. The venous line clamps are opened followed by gradual opening of the arterial line clamps. The motor speed on the console is increased gradually until a maximal blood flow is demonstrated, after which the motor speed is reduced to the slowest level that will continue to provide the desired blood flow. Oxygenation gas flow is adjusted in a 1:1 proportion with the blood flow rate. Activated clotting time determinations are used to adjust anticoagulation.

Management During Pumping. Blood flow may be increased to counterbalance any marked fall in resistance. The venous oxygen saturation should be maintained at approximately 70% while the arterial pCO$_2$ should be maintained at approximately 40 mmHg. At higher pumping levels, suction in the venous cannula may produce collapse of the vena cava resulting in reduction in blood flow. This can be corrected by reducing the speed of the pump or adding volume. Because of the high volume of blood withdrawal through the venous cannulae, any attempt to achieve central venous access during pumping carries the risk of air embolism. Therefore, central venous access should not be attempted while the pump is running.

Discontinuation of Pumping. If the pump has been inserted to perform high-risk angioplasty, the patient can be weaned from cardiopulmonary support gradually over 10 to 15 minutes. The cannulae are clamped but left in place for 30 minutes to permit rapid reinstitution of cardiopulmonary bypass should abrupt closure occur. When CPS blood flow reaches its minimum level (0.5 liters per minute), the arterial (red) clamp is closed while the pump continues operating at 2000 rpm, and volume can be infused as needed using the rapid infusion line. Subsequently, the blue clamp is closed slowly on the venous cannula, and the recirculation loop is opened to prevent thrombus formation because of stasis in the CPS arterial and venous cannulae. At this point, the oxygen ventilating gas can be turned off. If recurrent support is required, the recirculation line can be closed quickly, oxygen flow resumed, and pumping reinstituted.

The arterial and venous cannulae are removed and hemostasis is obtained using a mechanical clamp.

Results. The CPS system uses a nonpulsatile flow mechanism, producing a reduction in aortic systolic pressure and an increased aortic diastolic pressure. The pulmonary artery diastolic or pulmonary capillary wedge pressure often drops dramatically during pumping, falling as low as 0 to 5 mmHg. If hypotension occurs at a time when the systemic flow is satisfactory, volume infusion is required. If hypotension persists and systemic vascular resistance is significantly reduced, phenylephrine infusion may be helpful.

As the flow rates are tapered in preparation for removal of the pump, a 250 to 500 ml volume infusion is often necessary to restore a satisfactory pulmonary artery diastolic pressure.

A mechanical clamp is applied to the femoral puncture site and released slowly once the PTT has decreased to 70 seconds. Eight to 16 hours of mechanical clamp application are required to achieve good hemostasis.

Noninvasive studies at the femoral puncture sites are undertaken between 2 and 4 weeks after discharge to determine whether or not an AV fistula or pseudoaneurysm has occurred.

The CPS system has been used to perform high-risk angioplasty in patients with poor LV function or a large amount of myocardium at risk.[46–49] Because abrupt closure in a high-risk angioplasty patient might produce rapid hemodynamic deterioration, the cannulae need to remain in position for several extra hours. The 20 Fr catheters permit a flow rate of 6 liters per minute; newer 18 Fr catheters have been introduced that simplify the percutaneous approach but permit a maximum flow rate of only 5 liters per minute, although this level should still be sufficient to provide good systemic cardiopulmonary support.

If it is to be used for treatment of cardiac arrest, the CPS support seems to be of little value unless the event occurs when the patient is immediately accessible to the catheterization laboratory. The delay in mobilizing equipment was greater than 15 minutes in two thirds of patients and greater than 30 minutes in one third, resulting in brain death in many of the patients studied, with few long term survivors.[50,51] On the other hand, cardiogenic shock complicating acute myocardial infarction was successfully treated by CPS plus percutaneous coronary angioplasty (PTCA) with 6 of 7 patients remaining asymptomatic for 8 months.[52]

The failure of the CPS system to provide increased myocardial perfusion distal to a total occlusion is a potential limitation of the technique. Despite the presence of excellent systemic flows and extreme reduction in myocardial oxygen demand, an occluded coronary artery may continue to produce significant myocardial ischemia unless an autoperfusion catheter can be advanced across the occlusion. Thus, even in the presence of effective CPS support, acute coronary occlusion after PTCA, which cannot be stabilized by repeat dilatation, should be treated with coronary bypass surgery to prevent a large myocardial infarction. Thus, the availability of CPS does not change the requirement for rapid coronary artery bypass graft surgery (CABG) in the event of abrupt and uncorrectable coronary occlusion following PTCA.

Complications. While CPS can be applied for an upper limit of 6 to 7 hours presently, hemolysis, platelet clumping, and cell fragmentation with embolization are more likely to occur at the longer durations.[53] This may produce a syndrome characterized by an abnormal bleeding tendency, increased capillary permeability, plasma loss, and vasoconstriction. Fortunately, only an hour of CPS is required for supported coronary angioplasty, and 2 or 3 hours are usually sufficient for patients with cardiac arrest in the catheterization laboratory setting.

Hemopump (Nimbus, Johnson & Johnson)

Rather than being a full cardiopulmonary support device, the Hemopump (Fig. 25–9) is an investigational temporary left ventricular assist device using a single 21 Fr coaxial catheter inserted into the LV cavity by means of direct surgical exposure of the femoral artery. A smaller, 14 Fr catheter using femoral puncture technique is in development.

Design. The Hemopump left ventricular assist device is much less complicated than the full cardiopulmonary support system described above. A flexible silicone cannula is placed across the aortic valve into the left ventricular cavity. A rotating turbine fits snugly within the cannula and imparts both a rotational and longitudinal velocity to the blood. To eliminate the rotational motion of the blood as it exits the catheter, static vanes are mounted downstream from the rapidly rotating turbine pump. Power to the pump is provided by means of a magnetically coupled sheath/drive cable, providing a system that is entirely closed with no contact between blood and the drive motor. The pump can be driven at speeds up to 25,000 revolutions per minute to provide pumping rates up to 3.5 L per minute in a continuous nonpulsatile manner. Forty percent dextrose in water is used to lubricate the 9 Fr sheath which contains the drive cable for the pump, as well as the pump itself. This sheath is also a conduit for the 40% dextrose purge which is used to lubricate the drive cable. Only the portion of the catheter within the left ventricle and in the central aorta is 21 Fr in size; the remainder of the system, extending from the aortic arch and exiting the femoral artery, is only 9 Fr in di-

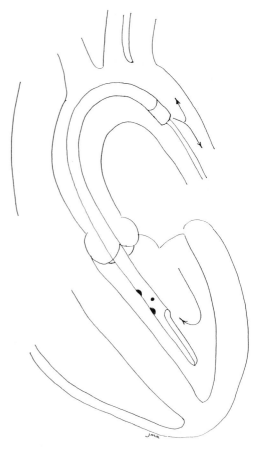

Fig. 25–9. The Hemopump system has a centrifugal screw pump at the proximal portion of the soft 21 F cannula which draws blood from the left ventricle and ejects it into the central aorta just beyond the pump. Note the smaller 9F sheath and coupling drive extending from the 21F cannula to the external drive, which is maintained outside the body. This arrangement produces much less vascular compromise than the cardiopulmonary support system, which requires a large catheter in both the femoral artery and femoral vein.

ameter. There are several lumens within this 9 Fr sheath. The four outer lumens carry the purge flow down the sheath to the pump's interior bearing cavity. The total purge flow is approximately 300 cc per day of 40% dextrose in water. Of this amount, approximately 200 cc per day passes through the pump's blood seal and is injected into the body and 100 cc per day flows retrograde through the sheath bore, providing lubrication to the cable and motor bearings, after which it is collected in an external bag. The control console weighs

25 lb, is easily portable, and may be run from 30 to 60 minutes on its battery system.

Two rechargeable lead acid batteries are used for battery backup. If longer battery power is required, the batteries can be used one at a time. Removal of both batteries simultaneously will cause the console to shut down. The electrical drive motor, which provides the rapid rotation of the flexible drive cable, must be external to the body because it requires bulky aluminum fins for cooling.

Technique of Catheter Insertion. Until a percutaneous system has been fully developed, catheter insertion requires surgical isolation of the femoral artery with anastomosis of a 12 mm graft. The pump housing is placed within the descending aortic arch and the inflow cannula is positioned across the aortic valve into the left ventricle.

Indications and Contraindications. Present indications for the still-investigational Hemopump system include reversible cardiogenic shock (e.g., acute myocardial infarction, acute rejection of transplanted heart) or inability to wean the patient from cardiopulmonary bypass postoperatively. Several contraindications to the use of this device include the presence of a prosthetic aortic valve, aortic aneurysm, aortic dissection, severe aortic or peripheral vascular disease, significant aortic stenosis, or the presence of a left ventricular thrombus. Before insertion of the cannula, peripheral angioplasty may be required to permit passage of the 7 mm diameter, 21 Fr catheter.

Management During Pumping. Before insertion, arterial blood gas analysis, CBC with platelet and differential counts, liver function tests, fibrinogen, fibrin split products, partial thromboplastin time, prothrombin time, and activated clotting time measurements are obtained. A pulmonary artery catheter, arterial catheter, and intravenous line should be in place and a baseline echocardiogram is obtained. Prophylactic antibiotics are administered. Care must be taken to avoid damage to the surface of the cannula to maintain its resistance to thrombus formation. After insertion of the pump, anticoagulation is achieved using intravenous heparin. The pump rotation speed

is increased progressively until a satisfactory pumping level has been achieved. A chest X ray is obtained to monitor cannula position. During the use of the Hemopump, the patient should be monitored closely for signs of complications, including coagulation abnormalities, sepsis, arrhythmias, embolization of LV thrombus either systemically or within the 21F pump cannula, decreased peripheral circulation, and cannula migration. The purge delivery set should be changed every 2 to 3 days. Soft restraints are used to prevent marked flexion of the cannulated leg and the head of the bed is kept below 30 degrees to prevent cannula migration. A daily chest x ray should be obtained to check cannula placement.

Discontinuation of Pumping. To evaluate the patient's ability to undergo weaning from the Hemopump support system, a trial of reduced-speed pumping is performed every 24 hours. During this trial, the patient is observed for signs of adequate perfusion, evidence of decreased respiratory support required to maintain appropriate arterial blood gases, and evidence of improving baseline values of arterial pulse, right heart pressures, and cardiac output. If these trials indicate that the weaning is appropriate, the pump rate is decreased gradually with repeat ECG and hemodynamic measurements at hourly intervals. If the patient tolerates each step well, continuing weaning can be performed at 4-hour intervals.

Preliminary Results. In animals, the system has been run for up to 2 weeks without any significant alteration in plasma hemoglobin, platelets, fibrinogen, bilirubin, or creatinine.[54] Because the Hemopump system produces nonpulsatile perfusion, coronary flow occurs throughout the cardiac cycle. In studies in dogs with mid-LAD occlusion, it produced marked left ventricular systolic unloading with maintained aortic pressure. In the ischemic LAD territory, wall motion improved markedly as compared to both baseline and intra-aortic balloon counterpulsation, and LAD flow decreased 26%.[55–57]

This device has been used successfully in patients with severe rejection of a cardiac allograft, deterioration following emergency coronary surgery, and cardiogenic shock caused by acute myocardial infarction.[58]

Despite the presence of a large cannula extending across the aortic valve into the left ventricle, angiography can be performed during Hemopump operation from either the brachial or femoral route.

REFERENCES

1. Moulopoulos SD, Topaz S, Kolff WJ: Diastolic balloon pumping (with carbon dioxide) in the aorta—A mechanical assistance to the failing circulation. Am Heart J 63:669, 1962.
2. Kantrowitz A, et al: Initial clinical experience with intraaortic balloon pumping in cardiogenic shock. JAMA 203:113, 1968.
3. Bregman D, Casarella WJ: Percutaneous intraaortic balloon pumping: Initial clinical experience. Ann Thorac Surg 29:153, 1980.
4. Goldberg MJ, et al: Intraaortic balloon insertion: A randomized study comparing percutaneous and surgical techniques. J Am Coll Cardiol 9:515, 1987.
5. Weber KT, Janicki JS: Intraaortic balloon counterpulsation: A review of physiological principles, clinical results, and device safety. Ann Thorac Surg 17:602, 1974.
6. Weintraub RM, et al: Medically refractory unstable angina pectoris: Long-term follow-up of patients undergoing intraaortic balloon counterpulsation and operation. Am J Cardiol 43:877, 1979.
7. Aroesty JM: Cardiogenic shock. In Donoso E, Cohen S (eds): Critical Cardiac Care. New York, Stratton Intercontinental Medical Book Corp, 1979, pp 51–64.
8. Gold HK, et al: Intraaortic balloon pumping for ventricular septal defect or mitral regurgitation complicating acute myocardial infarction. Circulation 47:1191, 1973.
9. Dunkman WB, et al: Clinical and hemodynamic results of intraaortic balloon pumping and surgery for cardiogenic shock. Circulation 46:465, 1972.
10. Sturm et al: Treatment of postoperative low output syndrome with intraaortic balloon pumping: Experience with 419 patients. Am J Cardiol 45:1033, 1980.
11. Leinbach RC, et al: Early intraaortic balloon pumping for anterior myocardial infarction without shock. Circulation 58:204, 1978.
12. Cohen S, Weintraub RM: A new application of counterpulsation; safer laparotomy after recent myocardial infarction. Arch Surg 110:116, 1975.
13. Hanson EC, et al: Control of post infarction ventricular irritability with intraaortic balloon pump. Circulation 62 (suppl I):130, 1978.
14. Shahian DM, Jewell ER: Intraaortic balloon pump placement through dacron aortofemoral grafts. J Vasc Surg 7:795, 1988.
15. Gardner RM, Bond EL, Clark JS: Safety and efficency of continuous flush systems for arterial and pulmonary artery catheters. Ann Thorac Surg 23:534, 1977.
16. McCabe JC, Abel RM, Subramanian VA, Gay WA: Complications of intra-aortic balloon insertion and counterpulsation. Circulation 57:769, 1978.
17. Leinbach RC, et al: Selective coronary and left ventricular cineangiography during intraaortic balloon pumping for cardiogenic shock. Circulation 45:845, 1972.
18. Aroesty JM, Schlossman D, Weintraub RM, Paulin S: Transfemoral selective coronary artery catheterization during intra-aortic balloon by-pass pumping. Radiology 111:307, 1974.
19. Isner JM, et al: Complications of the intraaortic counterpulsation device: Clinical and morphological observations in 45 necropsy patients. Am J Cardiol 45:260, 1980.
20. Goldberg MJ, et al: Intraaortic balloon pump insertion: A randomized study comparing percutaneous and surgical techniques. J Am Coll Cardiol 9:515, 1987.
21. Vignola PA, Swaye PS, Gosselin AJ: Guidelines for effective and safe percutaneous intraaortic balloon pump insertion and removal. Am J Cardiol 48:660, 1981.
22. Leinbach RC, et al: Percutaneous wire-guided balloon pumping. Am J Cardiol 49:1707, 1982.
23. Hauser AM, et al: Percutaneous intraaortic balloon counterpulsation. Clinical effectiveness and hazards. Chest 82:422, 1982.
24. Shahian D, Neptune WB, Ellis LH, Maggs PR: Intraaortic balloon pump morbidity: a comparative analysis of risk factors between percutaneous and surgical techniques. Ann Thorac Surg 36:644, 1983.
25. Alcan K, et al: Comparison of wire-guided percutaneous insertion and conventional surgical insertion of intra-aortic balloon pumps in 151 patients. Am J Med 75:24, 1983.
26. Todd G, Bregman D, Voorhees A, Reemstma K: Vascular complications associated with percutaneous intra-aortic balloon pumping. Arch Surg 118:963, 1983.
27. McEnany MT, et al: Clinical experience with intraaortic balloon pump support in 728 patients. Circulation 57, 58(Suppl I):124, 1978.
28. Weintraub RM, Thurer RL: The intraaortic balloon pump—A ten-year experience. Heart Transpl 3:8, 1983.
29. Bregman D, et al: Percutaneous intraaortic balloon insertion. Am J Cardiol 48:261, 1980.
30. Subramanian VA, et al: Preliminary clinical experience with percutaneous intraaortic balloon pumping. Circulation 62 (Suppl 1):123, 1980.
31. Singh AK, et al: Percutaneous vs. surgical placement of intra-aortic balloon assist. Cathet Cardiovasc Diagn 8:519, 1982.
32. Vignola PA, Swaye PS, Gosselin AJ: Percutaneous intra-aortic balloon pumping: new problems and dilemmas. Cathet Cardiovasc Diagn 9:117, 1983.
33. Gottlieb SO, et al: Identification of patients at high risk for complications of intraaortic balloon counterpulsation: A multivariate risk factor analysis. Am J Cardiol 53:1135, 1984.
34. Kantrowitz A, et al: Intraaortic balloon pumping 1967–1982: Analysis of complications in 733 patients. Am J Cardiol 57:976, 1986.
35. Alderman J, et al: Incidence and management of limb

ischemia with percutaneous wire guided intraaortic balloon catheters. J Am Coll Cardiol 9:524, 1987.

36. Skillman J, Kim D, Baim D: Vascular complications of percutaneous femoral interventions. Arch Surg 123:1207, 1988.

37. Braunwald E, Covell JW, Maroko PR, Ross J Jr: Effects of drugs and of counterpulsation on myocardial oxygen consumption. Circulation 39 and 40 (Suppl 4):220, 1970.

38. Leinbach RC, et al: Effects of intraaortic balloon pumping on coronary flow and metabolism in man. Circulation 43 and 44 (Suppl 1):77, 1971.

39. Mueller H, et al: The effects of intraaortic counterpulsation on cardiac performance and metabolism in shock associated with acute myocardial infarction. J Clin Invest 50:1885, 1971.

40. Mueller H, et al: Effect of isoproterenol, 1-norepinephrine, and intraaortic counterpulsation on hemodynamics and myocardial metabolism in shock following myocardial infarction. Circulation 45:335, 1972.

41. Maroko PR, et al: Effects of intraaortic balloon counterpulsation on the severity of myocardial ischemic injury following acute coronary occlusion. Circulation 45:1150, 1972.

42. Dilley RB, Ross J Jr, Bernstein EF: Serial hemodynamics during intraaortic balloon counterpulsation for cardiogenic shock. Circulation 47 and 48 (Suppl 3):99, 1973.

43. Bardet J, et al: Clinical and hemodynamic results of intraaortic balloon counterpulsation and surgery for cardiogenic shock. Am Heart J 93:280, 1977.

44. Aroesty JM, Weintraub RM, Paulin S, O'Grady GP: Medically refractory unstable angina pectoris II. Hemodynamic and angiographic effects of intraaortic balloon counterpulsation. Am J Cardiol 43:883, 1979.

45. Williams DO, Korr KS, Dewirtz H, Most AS: The effect of intraaortic balloon counterpulsation on regional myocardial blood flow and oxygen consumption in the presence of coronary artery stenosis in patients with unstable angina. Circulation 66:593, 1982.

46. Shawl FA, et al: Cardiopulmonary bypass supported coronary angioplasty in inoperable patients. J Am Coll Cardiol 13:53A, 1989.

47. Shawl FA, et al: Percutaneous cardiopulmonary bypass support in high risk patients undergoing percutaneous transluminal coronary angioplasty. Am J Cardiol 64:1258, 1989.

48. Tommaso CI: Management of high-risk coronary angioplasty. Am J Cardiol 64:33E, 1989.

49. Vogel RA, Tommaso CL, Gundry SR: Initial experience with coronary angioplasty and aortic valvuloplasty using elective semipercutaneous cardiopulmonary support. Am J Cardiol 62:811, 1988.

50. Heartz R, et al: Portable bypass does not improve survival in cardiac arrest patients. J Am Coll Cardiol 13:121A, 1989.

51. Overlie PA, et al: Emergency use of portable cardiopulmonary bypass in patients with cardiac arrest. J Am Coll Cardiol 13:160A, 1989.

52. Shawl FA, et al: Emergency percutaneous cardiopulmonary (bypass) support in cardiogenic shock. J Am Coll Cardiol 13:160A, 1989.

53. Kirkland J: In Braunwald E, ed, Heart Disease, 3rd edition. W.B. Saunders Co, Philadelphia, 1988, pp 1670–1.

54. Wampler WK, et al: In vivo evaluation of a peripheral vascular access axial flow blood pump. Trans Am Soc Artif Intern Organs Trans 34:450, 1988.

55. Mehrige ME, et al: Effect of the Hemopump left ventricular assist device on myocardial perfusion: reduction of ischemia during coronary occlusion. Circulation 78:II–580, 1988.

56. Mehrige ME, et al: Effect of the Hemopump left ventricular assist device on regional myocardial perfusion and function. Reduction of ischemia during coronary occlusion. Circulation 80:III–158, 1989.

57. Smalling RW, et al: Improved hemodynamic and left ventricular unloading during acute ischemia using the Hemopump left ventricular assist device compared to intraaortic balloon counterpulsation. J Am Coll Cardiol 13:160A, 1989.

58. Frazier OH, et al: First human use of the Hemopump, a catheter-mounted ventricular assist device. J Am Coll Cardiol 13:121A, 1989.

Part VII

Interventional Techniques

26

Coronary Angioplasty

DONALD S. BAIM*

Transluminal angioplasty—enlargement of the lumen of a stenotic vessel using an intravascular catheter—was conceived and initially reported by Dotter and Judkins in 1964.[1] In their technique, a guide wire was advanced through an atherosclerotic arterial stenosis, allowing the subsequent advancement of serially larger rigid dilators until an improvement in luminal caliber was evident. Although this technique was clearly effective in peripheral arteries, the need to insert large-caliber rigid dilators through an arterial puncture and the high shear forces that this approach applied to the atherosclerotic plaque limited its clinical application.

In 1974, Gruentzig modified this technique, replacing the rigid dilator with an inflatable nonelastomeric balloon mounted on a comparatively smaller catheter shaft.[2] This device could be introduced percutaneously with minimal trauma, advanced easily across a vascular stenosis, and then inflated with sufficient force to enlarge the stenotic lumen. In 1977, following a series of experiments in animals, cadavers, peripheral arteries, and the coronary arteries of patients undergoing bypass surgery, Gruentzig and co-workers extended the technique of percutaneous balloon angioplasty to the coronary arteries in conscious humans.[3] Subsequent further improvements in equipment and technique have resulted in the dramatic growth of percutaneous transluminal coronary angioplasty (PTCA) over 13 years, with performance of an estimated 200,000 procedures during 1988, compared to only 1,000 procedures in 1980[5] (Fig. 26–1). Roughly 60% of the patients who undergo diagnostic cardiac catheterization for coronary artery disease are referred for revascularization. With current techniques and indications,[6] up to half of the revascularization is performed by balloon dilatation rather than bypass surgery.[4] As equipment and technique continue to improve, and as new technologies increase safety, predictability, and durability, the use of coronary angioplasty is likely to increase even further. Each new application, however, warrants a clear and objective demonstration that angioplasty is to be preferred over the traditional alternatives of medical therapy or bypass surgery for the particular anatomic and clinical indication.

EQUIPMENT

A coronary angioplasty system consists of three components: (1) a guiding catheter, which provides stable access to the coronary ostium and allows advancement of the dilatation equipment; (2) a nonelastomeric balloon dilatation catheter filled with liquid contrast medium; and (3) a leading guide wire (Fig. 26–2). Technologic advances lead to major changes in specific equipment each year, but

---

*David P. Faxon, M.D., was a contributor to this chapter in the previous (3rd) edition.

441

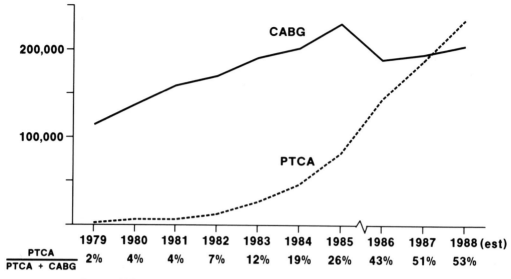

Fig. 26–1. Growth in the number of coronary angioplasty procedures between 1979 and 1988. Compared to the relatively stable number of bypass procedures (CABG), there has been a rapid and progressive growth in the number of coronary angioplasty (PTCA) procedures during this time period, and in PTCA as a fraction of all revascularization (PTCA + CABG).

one recent summary of available angioplasty components outlines many of the current products.[7]

Guiding Catheters. Guiding catheters remain a crucial component in PTCA. The typical catheter has an outer diameter of 8 or 9 Fr (2.7 or 3 mm), a nontapered tip, and a Teflon-lined lumen with a diameter of 0.071 to 0.092 inches (1.7 to 2.3 mm). Smaller (7 Fr) guiding catheters have just been introduced, although their restricted inner diameter (0.064 inches or 1.5 mm) makes them best

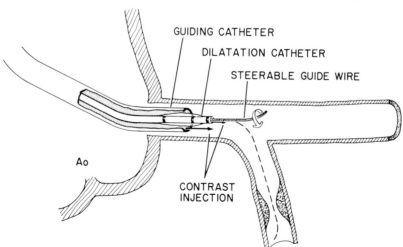

Fig. 26–2. Schematic diagram showing the three components used in coronary angioplasty: guiding catheter positioned in ostium of coronary artery, dilatation catheter positioned in left main artery ready to be advanced over the guide wire, and soft-tip, shapeable guide wire that can be steered to enter the desired vessel and advanced gently across the target stenosis.

suited for use with fixed-wire dilatation catheters, which have a slim enough shaft diameter to allow contrast injection through the guiding catheter lumen with the dilatation catheter in place. Current guiding catheters are available in shapes similar to conventional Judkins and Amplatz curves, as well as a woven Dacron configuration (Stertzer guiding catheter, USCI) designed to be used from the brachial approach. To function adequately, the guiding catheter must be able to selectively engage the ostium of the involved vessel without occluding arterial inflow. Although this is routinely possible in the left coronary artery, ostial damping was a vexing problem in the right coronary artery until the introduction of a Judkin's type catheter equipped with side holes to allow ongoing perfusion despite wedged engagement of the right coronary ostium. The guiding catheter is also used to deliver small boluses of contrast medium into the involved vessel to visualize vascular side branches and the target lesion for angioplasty. A second important function of the guiding catheter, however, is to provide adequate support for advancement of the dilatation catheter across the target stenosis. This support derives from the intrinsic stiffness of the guiding catheter material, buttressing of the catheter against the opposite aortic wall, and/or deep engagement of the guiding catheter into the coronary ostium. In the patient with a short left main coronary artery, correct choice of the shape and size of the guiding catheter may also facilitate direction of the dilatation system to the left anterior descending or circumflex coronary artery, as required. A slightly shorter catheter (i.e., a JL 3.5 rather than a JL 4) or an out-of-plane catheter with a preformed anterior deflection of the tip (or counterclockwise rotation and slight advancement of a standard catheter) helps to orient the dilatation system toward the left anterior descending. A slightly longer catheter (i.e., JL 4.5), a preformed catheter with a posterior out-of-plane tip orientation, or a left Amplatz catheter will help to direct the system toward the circumflex artery. On the other hand, steerable guide wires have made vessel selection quite easy and have re-duced the need for overzealous manipulation of the guiding catheter which may lead to dissection of the coronary ostium. Even so, we prefer guiding catheters with a soft, relatively atraumatic tip to minimize the risk of ostial injury.

Dilatation Catheters. The dilatation catheters for coronary angioplasty have undergone radical evolution since 1977. Whereas the original Gruentzig catheters were designed with a short segment of guide wire permanently affixed to the catheter tip, virtually all dilatation catheters since 1982 have used an independently movable and/or steerable guide wire extending the entire length of the dilatation catheter, as described by Simpson and co-workers (Fig. 26–2). The dilatation catheter must have a central lumen of sufficient caliber to allow free movement of the guide wire. Some operators also use this lumen to allow measurement of distal coronary arterial pressure from the tip of the dilatation catheter,[9] or the injection of small boluses of contrast material to visualize the distal coronary arterial lumen. A second important feature of the dilatation catheter is its "profile," defined as the diameter of the smallest opening through which the deflated balloon can be passed. Compared to the 0.060 inch (1.5 mm) profile of the original Gruentzig design, current over-the-wire dilatation catheters have profiles of less than 0.040 inch (1.0 mm). Specially designed "fixed wire" devices consist of a balloon mounted directly on a steerable wire core, allowing profiles as small as 0.020 inch (0.5 mm).[10,11] A third feature is the ability of the balloon to bend so as to permit advancement through tortuous vascular segments, without loss of the shaft stiffness required to force it through the stenosis. The final important characteristic of the dilatation catheter is its ability to inflate to a precisely defined diameter despite application of pressures as high as 10 atm (150 psi). Specialized balloons can retain their defined diameter up to a rupture pressure of 20 atm (300 psi), to allow dilatation of calcific or fibrotic stenoses without overdistending the adjacent normal vessel. Dilatation catheters that meet these design specifications are currently available with inflated diameters of 2.0, 2.5, 3.0, 3.5, and 4.0 mm, to match the size of coronary artery in which the stenosis is located.

Guide Wires. The original movable guide wire system designed by Simpson employed a standard 0.018-inch Teflon coated wire, which moved freely through the dilatation catheter. It could be directed past branches by removal from the dilatation catheter, reshaping of its tip, and reintroduction.[8] In contrast, the guide wires used in modern angioplasty are specifically designed devices that combine tip softness, radiographic visibility, and precise torque control, so that the guide wire can be steered past vascular side branches and through tortuous stenotic segments. These features are now obtainable in guide wires with diameters ranging from 0.014 to 0.018 inch (0.3 to 0.5 mm). Exchange length (300 cm) angioplasty wires are also available which allow serial advancement of different sized dilatation catheters (i.e., use of an initial low profile balloon to cross and partially dilate a severe stenosis, followed by a full-sized balloon to complete the dilatation) without the risk of subintimal passage of the second guide wire and balloon catheter as it crosses the partially dilated segment.[12] The movable guide wire concept and the current highly sophisticated steerable guide wires have simplified, shortened, and improved the success rate of coronary angioplasty. Even with these sophisticated devices, however, it is important to heed the advice of Dotter and Judkins that "the guide wire is passed across the atheromatous block more by the application of judgement than of force."[1]

PROCEDURE

Although the angioplasty procedure bears a superficial resemblance to diagnostic cardiac catheterization (in that catheters are introduced under local anesthesia), the procedure is a great deal more complicated and entails significantly greater risk,[13] including that of abrupt vessel closure (the development of complete coronary occlusion during attempted PTCA of a stenotic vessel), frequently necessitating emergency bypass surgery. Angioplasty should thus be attempted only by experienced personnel in a setting where full cardiac surgical and anesthetic support is available.[6] The patient is prepared as for cardiac surgery with an antiseptic soap shower, crossmatching of blood, and proscription of oral intake after midnight on the evening prior to the procedure. In our current regimen, calcium channel blockers and anti-platelet therapy (aspirin 325 mg/day and dipyridamole 200 mg/day) are begun 24 hours before angioplasty and continued for 6 months after the procedure, to prevent vessel spasm and to diminish platelet adhesion to the disrupted endothelium at the PTCA site. Although controlled trials have failed to show that aspirin decreases the incidence of subsequent *restenosis,* it clearly reduces the rate of acute complications.[14] Intravenous heparin (10,000 to 15,000 units) is administered during the procedure, adjusted to maintain an ACT (activated clotting time) of 250 to 300 seconds. Most centers have discontinued the routine use of low molecular weight dextran due to lack of experimental efficacy and side effects including increased blood loss, volume overload, and allergic reactions.

Angioplasty may be done by either the femoral or brachial approach.[15] In either case, right heart catheterization allows potentially valuable measurement of baseline and intraprocedure filling pressures and/or standby ventricular pacing. Based on our own experience, however, we seldom place *prophylactic* pacing catheters in patients undergoing coronary angioplasty.[16] Baseline angiograms are obtained of one or both coronary arteries, using either standard diagnostic catheters or the angioplasty guiding catheter. If the guiding catheter is used for angiography, it must be manipulated carefully, since the large diameter and nontapered tip of the guiding catheter increase the risk of ostial injury. Coronary injections should be repeated after the administration of 200 mcg of intracoronary nitroglycerin, to demonstrate that spasm is not a significant component of the target stenosis and to minimize the occurrence of coronary spasm during the subsequent angioplasty. Intravenous verapamil or sublingual nifedipine may be administered in addition to nitroglycerin. Baseline angiography also serves to evaluate any potential changes in angiographic appearance (interval development of total occlusion, thrombus formation) since the prior diagnostic catheterization, and to permit the selection of the angiographic views which allow optimal visualization of the stenoses and their surrounding branch vessels.

Following baseline angiography, the appropriate guiding catheter is introduced and positioned in the coronary ostium. The dilatation catheter and leading guide wire are then advanced into the guiding catheter through a sidearm device, which permits continued monitoring of pressure within and injection of contrast medium through the guiding catheter lumen. While the dilatation catheter remains within the tip of the guiding catheter, the steerable guide wire is advanced into the involved coronary artery, through the target stenosis, and into the distal vessel. Its position relative to vessel branches and lesions is evaluated by a series of contrast injections through either the guiding catheter or the dilatation catheter. Alternatively, the dilatation catheter need not be introduced into the guiding catheter until a bare exchange-length guide wire has been manipulated across the lesion. This approach allows more effective utilization of the guiding catheter lumen for contrast injection during wire advancement. In either case, the guide wire then serves as a track permitting safe advancement of the dilatation catheter through the lesion.

Once the dilatation catheter has been positioned within the target stenosis, the balloon is inflated progressively until it assumes its full cylindrical shape. In most cases this is associated with a transient "hourglass" appearance of the balloon due to its constriction by the coronary stenosis. This resolves abruptly once adequate distending pressure is developed. Current standard balloon catheters can tolerate inflation pressures of 10 to 12 atmospheres (150 to 180 psi),[17] at which full cylin-

drical inflation of the balloon is almost always possible. These polyethylene and polyester balloons tend to maintain their specified inflated diameters within ±10% at pressures between 6 and 10 atmospheres (90 to 150 psi), compared to older polyvinyl chloride balloons which tended to expand further (up to 20% over specified diameter) at high pressures. In *elastic* stenoses, however, the arterial wall tends to recoil partially once the balloon is deflated. Depending on the angiographic appearance of the dilated segment, the residual transstenotic pressure gradient measured between the guiding catheter and the tip of the dilatation catheter positioned beyond the stenosis, and the clinical condition of the patient, it may be necessary to repeat or prolong inflations (up to one minute in duration[18]) or to exchange the initial balloon for a larger-sized device to achieve the desired result. In contrast to the *elastic* (usually eccentric[19]) stenosis, the calcified or fibrotic *rigid* stenosis may resist expansion at conventional pressures, yielding only to application of pressures of 20 atm (300 psi), delivered with the use of special high-strength balloons (Fig. 26–3). In either event, it is almost always possible to reduce the severity of the stenosis by at least 20% to a residual stenosis <50%. While many operators still rely heavily on the transstenotic gradient as an index of dilatation adequacy, actual measurement of the gradient is complicated by the presence of the dilatation catheter within the stenosis and the small size of the dilatation catheter lumen.[9] Similarly, angiographic evaluation of the residual stenosis may be difficult, owing to eccentricity or poor definition of the lumen after angioplasty.[20] While complete normalization of the vessel lumen is the ideal end result of coronary angioplasty, the operator must bear in mind that the use of excessively large balloon sizes or inflation pressures in the pursuit of this goal may lead to extensive coronary dissection and vessel closure.[21,22] As our surgical colleagues often remark, "The enemy of good is better."

Once adequate dilatation is achieved, the balloon catheter is withdrawn into the guiding catheter. It is common practice in our labo-

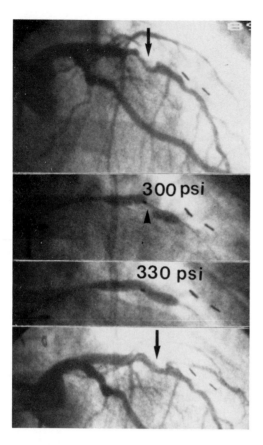

Fig. 26–3. Successful dilatation of a rigid calcific lesion. This rigid lesion (top) in the mid left anterior descending coronary artery of a post-bypass patient (note surgical clips) resisted dilatation at 300 psi (20 atmospheres), but yielded to an inflation pressure of 330 psi (22 atmospheres) with an excellent angiographic result (bottom panel). These pressures are obtainable only with special high-pressure balloon construction because standard angioplasty balloons have rated rupture pressures of only 150 to 180 psi (10 to 12 atmospheres).

ratory to leave an exchange-length guide wire across the dilated segment for several minutes while observing the vessel for angiographic deterioration. During this time, the dilatation catheter can be removed from the guiding catheter to allow high-quality angiographic visualization, in a situation where readvancement of the balloon over the guide wire would still provide easy access to the dilated segment. If the dilated segment remains stable, the guide wire is withdrawn and other significant lesions are dilated similarly, or the patient is transferred to a recovery area.

Although most laboratories once partially reversed the heparin administered during PTCA to allow removal of the femoral sheaths in the catheterization laboratory at the end of the procedure, it is now common practice to leave the sheaths in place until the heparin wears off spontaneously (usually 4 hours) or overnight during continuous heparin infusion, particularly if substantial intimal dissection is evident on the post-PTCA films.[23] In addition to the benefit of continued anticoagulation, this approach allows rapid reintroduction of catheters for the evaluation and management of the occasional patient who develops chest pain or electrocardiographic evidence of myocardial ischemia during the several hours following angioplasty.[23] If the sheath is left in place, it is important to perfuse its lumen adequately (20 ml/hr) and to monitor closely for limb ischemia.

The patient typically remains at bed rest for 18 to 24 hours after removal of the femoral sheath, then ambulates before discharge. The postangioplasty physiologic state should be evaluated by a maximal exercise test just before discharge, or within the week following discharge. The patient is discharged from hospital on aspirin, dipyridamole, a calcium channel blocker, and frequently a long-acting nitrate preparation. The latter two drugs are usually discontinued between 6 weeks and 3 months after the procedure, and dipyridamole is usually discontinued at 6 months after angioplasty. The patient is encouraged to return to full activity as soon as the femoral puncture site has healed and should expect to have no anginal symptoms. Return of anginal symptoms or deterioration in follow-up exercise test findings suggests restenosis of the dilated segment (see subsequent section entitled Immediate and Longterm Efficacy).

MECHANISM OF PTCA

According to the original explanation advanced by Dotter[1] and by Gruentzig,[3] the enlargement of the vessel lumen following angioplasty was ascribed to compression of the atheromatous plaque. In fact, compression accounts for only about 5% of the improvement.[24] Extrusion of liquid components from the plaque accounts for some improvement in soft plaques but contributes minimally to improvement in more fibrotic lesions, even when balloon inflation is prolonged to one minute.[18] The bulk of the improvement following PTCA seems to result from controlled overstretching of the vessel by the PTCA balloon, leading to fracture of the intimal plaque, partial disruption of the media and adventitia, and enlargement of the overall caliber of the vessel[24-26] (Fig. 26–4). This localized vessel trauma is apparent in the post-PTCA angiogram,[27] and histologic examination of post-mortem angioplasty specimens.[28] Fortunately, dislodgment and distal embolization of plaque fragments seems to be an infrequent event in both experimental studies[29] and clinical angioplasty procedures, although it has been described in

one patient undergoing dilatation of a saphenous vein bypass graft[30] and several patients with intracoronary thrombus adherent to the dilated lesion.[31] Vessel rupture is a theoretically possible but fortunately extremely rare consequence of vessel stretching during balloon angioplasty, unless significantly oversized balloons are used.[32,33]

IMMEDIATE AND LONG-TERM EFFICACY OF PTCA

Early published data on coronary angioplasty derive mostly from the NHLBI Angioplasty Registry, which collected all procedures performed between 1977 and September 1981.[5] These 3000 patients were the subject of reports on clinical success and complications.[34,35] Although case selection in the Registry focused on "ideal" PTCA candidates—

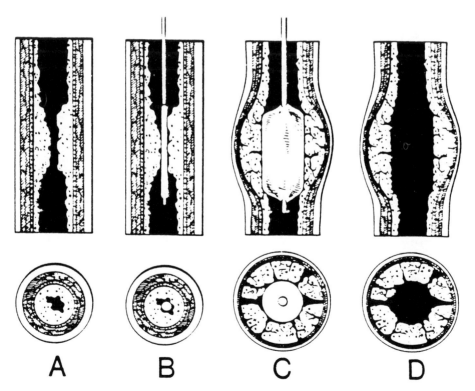

Fig. 26–4. Proposed mechanism of angioplasty. Inflation of the balloon catheter within the stenotic segment leads to cracking of the intimal plaque, stretching of the media and adventitia, and expansion of the outer diameter of the vessel. In contrast, compression of the plaque material and extrusion of liquid plaque components appear to contribute only slightly to the improvement in luminal diameter. (From Castaneda-Zuniga WR, et al: The mechanism of balloon angioplasty. Radiology 135:565, 1980.)

those with proximal, discrete, concentric, subtotal, noncalcified stenoses of a single vessel—the primary success rate of 63% would be considered disappointing by current standards. The main explanations for the low primary success rate in the registry were failure to cross the lesion with the dilatation system (29% of cases) and failure to dilate the lesion adequately once having crossed (12% of cases).[5] These failures were due to two factors: (1) the relative lack of experience of operators contributing cases to the Registry (the "learning curve") and (2) the use of original Gruentzig fixed-wire dilatation catheters with limited maneuverability, a comparatively high deflated balloon profile, and a low peak inflation pressure.

Despite the inclusion of patients with more difficult coronary anatomy, progressive improvement in equipment (with widespread availability of steerable guide wires since 1983 and ongoing reduction in balloon profile since 1985), as well as better operator experience and technique, have allowed progressive improvement in the primary success rate of coronary angioplasty to approximately 90%. This improvement in primary success has been evident both in single-center series,[36] and in a second PTCA Registry which enrolled patients at 14 centers between 1985 and 1986.[37] Moreover, analysis of complications in the 1985–1986 Registry[38] shows a concomitant reduction in the incidence of emergency bypass surgery (from 5.8 to 3.5%), and a reduction in the mortality for patients with single vessel disease (from 0.85 to 0.2%), although *overall* procedural mortality remained close to 1% because of the inclusion of more patients with multi-vessel disease in the 1985–1986 Registry. Follow-up of 838 patients with single-vessel disease in the 1985–1986 Registry[39] shows mortality in 1.6%, myocardial infarction in 1.9%, repeat angioplasty in 18.1%, and bypass surgery in 6.2%, within the first year after hospital discharge. Although patients with multivessel disease had a higher in-hospital mortality (1.7 vs. 0.2%), events within the first year after hospital discharge were only slightly more common (mortality in 2.8%, my-

ocardial infarction in 3.4%, repeat angioplasty in 18.8%, and late bypass surgery in 8.7%), partly because of the increased prevalence of unfavorable clinical covariates (age >65, prior MI, etc.) among the multivessel disease patients.

In patients undergoing angiographically successful PTCA, anatomic improvement correlates with elimination of anginal symptoms and improved function on atrial pacing or conventional exercise testing.[40,41] Studies using thermodilution, videodensitometric techniques,[42] and Doppler flow measurement[43] have shown restoration of nearly normal coronary flow reserve following successful coronary angioplasty.

These improvements are generally well maintained during follow-up ranging over several years,[44–46] but approximately 20% of patients redevelop anginal symptoms or exercise test evidence of ischemia as the result of restenosis of the dilated segment during the 1.5 to 6 months after successful PTCA.[42,48] An additional 10% of patients will have angiographic evidence of partial restenosis despite lack of symptoms and a negative exercise test.[49] Although several factors, including elastic recoil of the dilated segment,[19] focal vasoconstriction,[50] and local thrombus formation may contribute to early loss of lumen diameter, there is now little doubt that the main mechanism of restenosis after coronary angioplasty is *localized neointimal proliferation*[26,47–48,51] (Fig. 26–5). This probably results from early platelet adhesion to deep components of the fractured vessel wall, with release of potent smooth muscle mitogens such as platelet derived growth factor (PDGF),[47] and possible ongoing stimulation by locally produced mitogens.[52]

Clinical studies have identified several risk factors for the occurrence of restenosis after a successful dilatation procedure. These include *patient-related factors* (male sex, recent symptom onset, unstable or variant angina), *lesion-related factors* (severe stenosis, location [right coronary ostium or proximal left anterior descending, or vein graft], total occlusions, bifurcation lesions or lesions in bends), and *pro-*

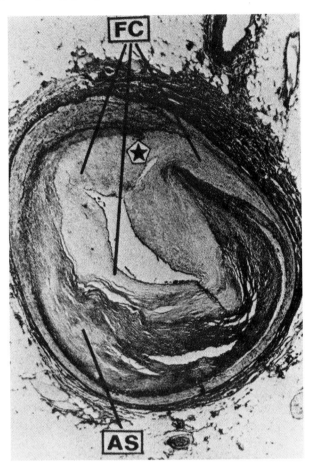

Fig. 26–5. Mechanism of restenosis: cross section of a restenotic lesion in the left anterior descending artery 5 months after initial coronary angioplasty shows the original atherosclerotic plaque (AS), the crack in the medial layer induced by the original procedure (star), and the proliferation of fibrocellular tissues (FC) which constitutes the restenotic lesion. (From Serruys PW, et al: Assessment of percutaneous transluminal coronary angioplasty by quantitative coronary angiography: diameter versus videodensitometric area measurements. Am J Cardiol 54:482, 1984.)

cedure-related factors (incomplete dilatation with residual stenosis/gradient, soft lesions that dilate without evident intimal tear).[53–55] In many cases, the restenosis process also appears to be detectable well before the recurrence of symptoms, through use of early thallium exercise tests.[56]

Efforts to reduce the restenosis rate by manipulating procedure-related variables (such as duration of balloon inflation[57]) have been largely unrewarding, although there is still a possibility that application of one of the new technologies for coronary intervention (stents, atherectomy, laser techniques—see Chapters 27 and 28) may be at least partly effective in this regard. Similarly, trials of numerous drug regimens (aspirin, nifedipine, ticlopidine, steroids, prolonged heparin administration) have shown no beneficial effect against restenosis.[14,26,48,58] Data regarding the use of n-3

fatty acids (fish oil) are still contradictory,[48,59–60] and a larger multicenter trial with fish-oil supplementation is now in progress.

Without an effective means of *preventing* restenosis, patients who develop recurrent symptoms after successful angioplasty should undergo repeat coronary angiography. If this discloses restenosis of the dilated segment, repeat dilatation (Fig. 26–6) can be performed during the same procedure with excellent acute results, although at least 30% of such patients go on to develop a *second* restenosis.[61] At particularly high risk are men with long lesions or associated disease progression at other sites, who present with recurrent stenosis within 5 months after the first dilatation. Subsequent restenoses can be treated by third, fourth, or even fifth dilatations,[62] although the restenosis rate appears to approach 50% as the number of repeat dilatations increases, leading many

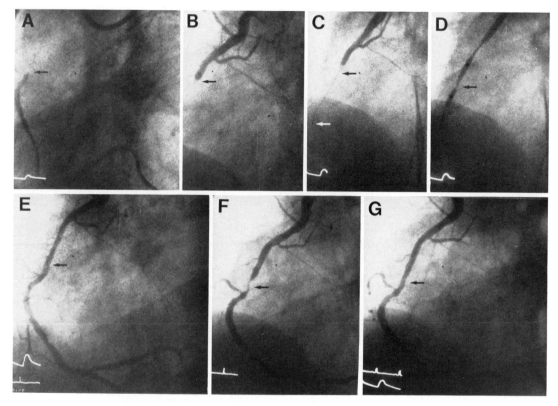

Fig. 26–6. Clinical restenosis. A to D, A totally occluded right coronary artery with filling of the distal vessel by way of left to right collaterals. E, The essentially normal appearance of the right coronary artery following successful angioplasty. F, The appearance 6 weeks later when angina had recurred. G, The appearance following successful re-PTCA. Restenosis developed again six weeks following the second PTCA, but the patient is now asymptomatic more than 6 years after a third PTCA procedure. (From Dervan JP, Baim DS, Cherniles J, Grossman W: Transluminal angioplasty of occluded coronary arteries: use of a moveable guide wire system. Circulation 68:776, 1983.)

patients with recurrent restenosis to ultimately choose the alternative of surgical revascularization.

Several other causes of recurrent symptoms after apparently successful coronary angioplasty should be considered. The first is coronary artery spasm, which may be exacerbated within the first six weeks after the procedure.[63] Most groups are now using calcium-channel blockers and nitrates during this period, particularly given the suggestion that uncontrolled spasm may increase the chance of organic restenosis.[54] A second cause of recurrent symptoms after several months is *persistence* of disease in undilated segments. Whereas cardiac surgeons routinely bypass all significant stenoses at the time of surgery, most angioplasty operators confine their efforts to the severe

(greater than 70%) stenoses,[64] leaving behind moderate lesions that are unlikely to cause persistent symptoms. The rationale for this approach is that dilatation of these milder lesions requires additional time and administration of contrast medium, exposes the patient to additional hazards of abrupt vessel closure, and may initiate progressive restenosis leading to a more severe lesion than was present initially.[65] On the other hand, failure to dilate significant and clinically relevant lesions in patients with multivessel disease may cause persistent symptoms, leading to subsequent need for revascularization[66–68] (Fig. 26–7). When symptoms recur more than 6 months after successful dilatation, *disease progression* is the most likely explanation,[69] although late-presenting restenosis is also possible. Late ste-

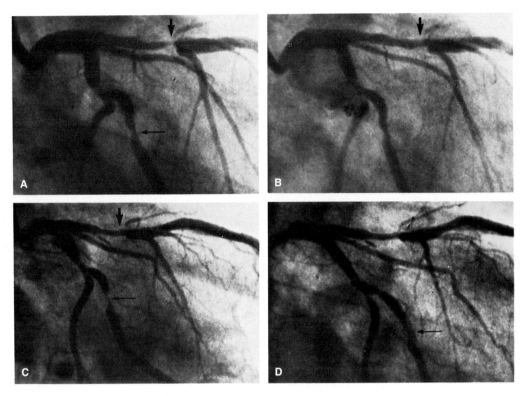

Fig. 26–7. Recurrent angina caused by progressive disease in a nondilated segment. Left coronary artery in RAO projection A, before and B, after successful dilatation of the middle left anterior descending artery. Despite the presence of a moderate lesion in the circumflex marginal branch, this patient had an entirely normal exercise tolerance test until the recurrence of symptoms one year later. C and D, Preserved patency of the LAD, but interval progression of the circumflex stenosis, which was then dilated successfully to restore an asymptomatic status. (From Baim, DS: Percutaneous transluminal coronary angioplasty—analysis of unsuccessful procedures as a guide toward improved results. Cardiovasc Intervent Radiol 5:186, 1982.)

nosis at the left or right coronary ostium (presumably the result of guiding catheter-induced injury) has also been reported as a rare cause of late symptom recurrence,[70] which is readily apparent on angiography restudy.

COMPLICATIONS

As a specialized form of cardiac catheterization, coronary angioplasty is attended by the usual risks related to invasive cardiac procedures.[13] The large-caliber angioplasty guiding catheter is more likely to result in damage to the proximal coronary artery than conventional coronary angiographic catheters, and subselective advancement of guide wires and dilatation catheters may lead to vessel injury if they are manipulated too aggressively. The

most common complications of coronary angioplasty, however, relate to local injury at the dilatation site.[71]

Coronary Artery Dissection. Although plaque dissection may be caused by overly vigorous attempts to pass the guide wire through a tortuous stenotic lumen, most dissections are the result of the "controlled injury" induced intentionally by inflation of the dilatation catheter.[24–26] In fact, localized dissections can be found routinely in animal or cadaveric models of angioplasty[25] and are evident angiographically in approximately one half of patients immediately after angioplasty.[27] When these dissections are small and nonprogressive and do not interfere with antegrade flow in the distal vessel, they have no clinical consequence other than transient mild pleuritic chest discomfort. Follow-up angiography as soon as 6 weeks after the angioplasty procedure usually demonstrates complete healing of the dissected segment (Fig. 26–8), although occasional localized formation of aneurysms has been described at the site of dissection[72,73] (Fig. 26–9).

In contrast, large progressive dissections may interfere with antegrade flow and lead to total occlusion of the dilated segment within 30 minutes of final balloon inflation (Fig. 26–10). This is usually the result of compression of the true lumen by the dissection flap,[74,75] although superimposed thrombus formation, platelet adhesion, or vessel spasm may contribute. This process can be reversed in up to one half of the patients with abrupt vessel reclosure by administration of intracoronary nitroglycerin or readvancement of the balloon dilatation catheter to "tack up" the dissection via repeated (Fig. 26–11)[23,76] or prolonged balloon inflations, up to 20 minutes in duration, using an auto-perfusion balloon[57] to limit ongoing ischemia. Failure to reopen the occluded vessel and the resultant severe myocardial ischemia mandate emergency coronary artery bypass surgery in approximately 3% of patients in whom angioplasty is attempted.[37–38,71,74–76] This makes it desirable to observe the patient both clinically and angio-graphically in the cardiac catheterization laboratory for several minutes after the dilatation and to perform elective coronary angioplasty only in a setting where the resources for prompt emergency bypass surgery are available. Most centers report an elapsed time of approximately two hours between the occurrence of an angioplasty-related vessel occlusion in the cardiac catheterization laboratory and the re-establishment of coronary perfusion (cross-clamp release) at the completion of an emergency bypass procedure.[76–78] Although the outcome of emergency surgery for abrupt closure is usually favorable, surgical mortality (6%) and perioperative infarction rates (50%) are significantly higher than those associated with *elective* coronary bypass procedures.[76] Complications of abrupt closure and emergency surgery are, in fact, the major contributors to the 0.3 to 0.6% mortality seen with elective coronary angioplasty.[38] In certain subgroups—those with extensive prior or ongoing myocardial damage, multivessel disease, a large myocardial territory perfused by the target stenosis, or prior coronary bypass surgery—procedure-related mortality may be several times higher,[38,79] requiring the most vigilant surgical standby and the immediate availability of intraaortic balloon counterpulsation. More recently, some laboratories have

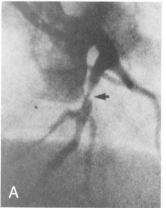 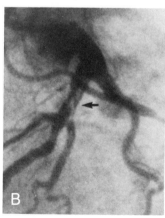 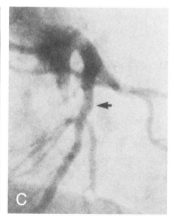

Fig. 26–8.   Normal healing of PTCA-related coronary dissection. Compared to the baseline angiogram (A), the immediate post-PTCA angiogram (B) shows enlargement of the LAD lumen with two small filling defects typical of an uncomplicated coronary dissection. C, Follow-up angiogram 3 months later shows preservation of luminal caliber with complete healing of the localized dissection. (From Baim DS: Percutaneous transluminal coronary angioplasty. *In* Braunwald E (ed): Harrison's Principles of Internal Medicine: Update VI, New York, McGraw-Hill, 1985.)

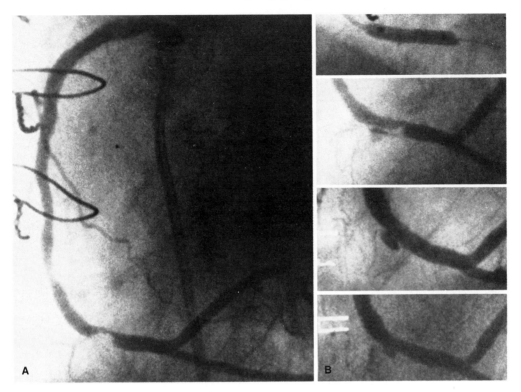

Fig. 26–9. Healing of coronary dissection resulting in formation of localized aneurysm. A, Baseline appearance of a distal right coronary stenosis in a patient with prior left coronary bypass. B (Top to bottom), the inflated 3.0 mm balloon within the stenosis, the appearance of a localized dissection immediately following PTCA, a localized coronary artery aneurysm 6 weeks after procedure, and partial normalization of this aneurysm 6 months after procedure.

begun using temporary percutaneous cardio-pulmonary support (CPS, C.R. Bard Inc.) by way of femoral arterial and venous introduction of 18 Fr cannulae (see Chapter 25) as a way to manage the hemodynamic embarrassment associated with abrupt vessel closure, either as a therapeutic measure during transport to the operating room or as a prophylactic measure during perceived "high-risk" dilatation procedures.[80] This means of support, however, carries its own potentially serious side effects, does not improve myocardial oxygen supply during vessel closure, and has not been shown to improve the outcome in patients who remain stable hemodynamically.

A promising innovation has been the perfusion or "bail-out" catheter, a 4.3 Fr catheter with multiple side-holes along its distal segment, similar to the design of an autoperfusion balloon.[57] When it is positioned over the guide wire so that it lies across an abruptly closed coronary segment, removal of the guide wire allows blood to enter the side holes proximal to the occlusion, flow through the catheter shaft, and exit the side holes distal to the occlusion. This maintains 60 to 80 ml/min of antegrade blood flow as the patient is being transported to the operating room, and this approach has been shown to reduce the incidence of transmural infarction during emergency surgery to approximately 10%.[81] Similar benefits might be expected with other systems that maintain antegrade flow (of blood or oxygenated perflurocarbon blood substitutes), or supply myocardial inflow by way of coronary sinus retroperfusion, but much less clinical experience is available with these alternative support techniques. Despite the apparent beneficial effect of the "bailout" catheter, it must be emphasized that it cannot be placed successfully in all cases of abrupt closure (because of loss of guide wire position in

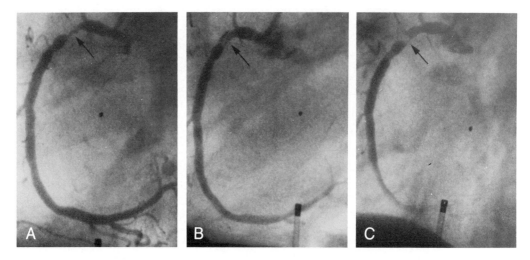

Fig. 26–10. Coronary dissection leading to abrupt reclosure. The appearance of a right coronary stenosis. A, prior to and B, immediately following coronary angioplasty, with an evident localized dissection. Within 15 minutes following removal of the dilatation catheter, the patient experienced chest pain associated with inferior ST segment elevation and angiographic evidence of progressive dissection with impeded antegrade flow (C). Although current practice would be to attempt to recross the lesion and ''tack down'' the dissection, standard management in 1980 consisted of emergency bypass surgery which was accomplished without complication. (From Baim DS: Percutaneous transluminal angioplasty—analysis of unsuccessful procedures as a guide toward improved results. Cardiovasc Intervent Radiol 5:186, 1982.)

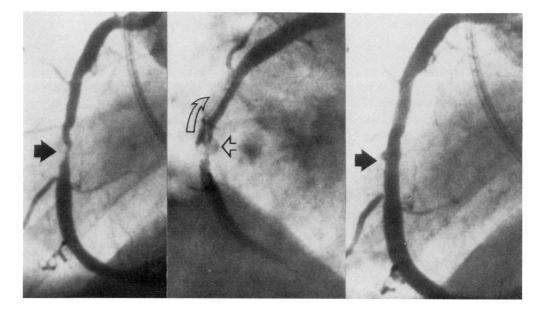

Fig. 26–11. Reversal of abrupt closure by repeat balloon inflation. Eccentric stenosis in the midright coronary artery (left panel, arrow) dilates with production of large dissection (middle panel, curved arrow), focal dye stain (open arrow), and retarded distal flow. Repeat inflations with a 0.5 mm larger balloon catheter, using inflation durations of up to 5 minutes, ''tacked up'' the dissection to provide a stable luminal appearance (right panel, dark arrow). Approximately 50% of abrupt closure events can be reversed in this manner.

the distal vessel, or proximal tortuosity precluding catheter passage), so that it *does not* provide a reliable alternative to ready availability of high-quality on-site surgical support during the performance of coronary angioplasty procedures.[81]

Independent of the above efforts to soften the deleterious effects of abrupt closure en route to the operating room, a series of new technologies (stents, laser balloon, etc.) seek to prevent or effectively reverse abrupt closure when it occurs (see Chapters 27 and 28). If this can be accomplished, the safety and acceptability of coronary angioplasty will be markedly enhanced.

Other Complications. A variety of other complications have been described as the result of coronary angioplasty. *Embolization of plaque constituents* is fortunately very rare,[30] but embolization of large thrombi that are adherent to the stenosis may occur[31] and should be taken into account during angioplasty of patients with unstable angina or acute myocardial infarction (see below).

Occlusion of branch vessels originating from within the stenosed segment occurs in 14% of vessels at risk during angioplasty of the main vessel, according to what has been termed the ''snowplow effect''[82] (Fig. 26–12). If the branch vessel is small, this event usually has no significant clinical sequelae and should not discourage attempted angioplasty. On the other hand, if a large branch vessel originates from within the stenosed segment, simultaneous dilatation of the main vessel and the involved branch with two separate dilatation systems (the ''kissing balloon'' technique) may be required for preservation of both vessels.[83] This originally required two separate guiding catheter/balloon dilatation catheter systems (Fig. 26–13), but can now be accomplished by insertion of two ultra-low profile fixed-wire dilatation systems through a single guiding catheter.[84] Alternatively, two *guide wires* can be inserted through a single guiding catheter (one guide wire placed into the main vessel and one into the involved side branch), allowing advancement of a balloon catheter into one and then the other vessel.[85] Although

the latter approach allows *sequential* rather than *simultaneous* balloon inflation, it is an effective means of protecting a large involved side branch from snowplow occlusion.

Perforation of the coronary artery with a stiff guide wire occurs rarely and does not necessarily have dire consequences. *Frank rupture of the coronary artery* due to use of too large a dilatation balloon leading to rapid tamponade and death has been described.[32,33] Tamponade may also result from perforation of the right atrium or right ventricle during placement of temporary pacemaker electrode catheters, particularly in angioplasty patients who are receiving antiplatelet therapy in addition to full heparinization. This potential complication and the infrequency (<1%) of severe bradycardic complications support our recommendation *against* prophylactic pacing during coronary angioplasty.[16]

Ventricular fibrillation occurs in approximately 1% of angioplasty procedures,[38] usually as the result of prolonged ischemia during balloon advancement or inflation. In addition to causing electrical instability, ischemia during balloon inflation may cause marked electrocardiographic changes,[86] abnormalities in regional left ventricular systolic and diastolic function,[86–88] and regional myocardial lactate production.[88]

Although angioplasty guide wires and catheters are extremely reliable devices, failures can occur when any device is subjected to severe operating stresses (i.e., when a guide wire is rotated repeatedly in a single direction while its tip is held fixed in a total occlusion, or when a balloon catheter is inflated past its operating pressure range in attempting to dilate a resistant stenosis). In a small percentage of cases, this may lead to detachment of a part of the wire or dilatation catheter, with a fragment remaining in the coronary artery.[89] To avoid the need for surgical removal, the angioplasty operator should be familiar with the techniques of catheter retrieval.[90] Finally, the operator must be careful to limit the amount of contrast material administered (usually to 3 or at most 4 ml/kg) to avoid renal toxicity, particularly during complex or multivessel procedures.

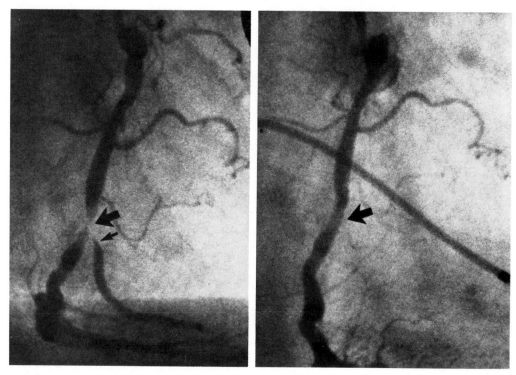

Fig. 26–12. The "snowplow" effect. Dilatation of mid-right coronary stenosis resulting in occlusion of a diseased right ventricular branch which originated from within the stenotic segment. There were no clinical sequelae. Approximately 14% of involved branches will suffer a similar fate. If the branch is large, use of a multiple guide wire technique (simultaneous advancement of one guide wire down the main artery and one guide wire down the diseased branch) should be considered as a means of preserving the patency of both vessels. (From Baim DS: Percutaneous transluminal angioplasty. In Braunwald E (ed): Harrison's Principles of Internal Medicine: Update VI. New York, McGraw-Hill, 1985.)

CURRENT INDICATIONS

With the improvements in equipment and technique described above, coronary angioplasty has grown progressively (Fig. 26–1), to the point where more than 200,000 procedures are performed annually. These procedures represent nearly half of the revascularizations (angioplasty plus bypass) performed in the United States each year.[4] Prospective studies at the Beth Israel Hospital in 1985 identified the facts that 60% of patients undergoing initial diagnostic catheterization for coronary artery disease were referred subsequently for revascularization, and that nearly half of those revascularizations were performed by angioplasty.[91] During this period of rapid growth, however, there has been no demonstrable fall in the use of bypass surgery. This suggests that the use of angioplasty is no longer restricted to patients who would otherwise be undergoing bypass surgery, as had been suggested in the original NHLBI Registry guidelines (Fig. 26–14).

Because the person who is responsible for case selection is often the person who will perform the angioplasty, operators need to be sure that only suitable patients are identified, based on: (1) a relatively compelling justification for revascularization, (2) anatomic lesions that can be approached with a reasonable level of safety and probability of successful dilatation, and (3) the fact that angioplasty compares favorably (or at least equally) with the other therapeutic options of bypass surgery or continued medical therapy. This evaluation process involves integration of complex clinical, patholophysiologic, and technical knowl-

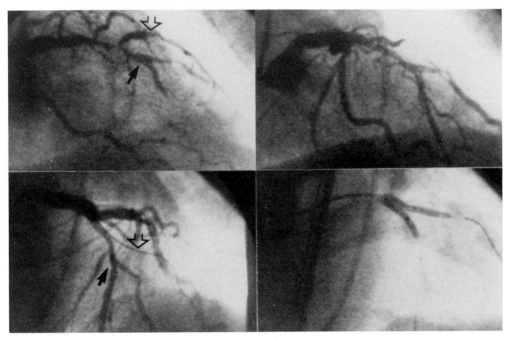

Fig. 26–13. Kissing balloon treatment of a bifurcation lesion. Upper left, a severe stenosis involves the bifurcation of the left anterior descending (dark arrow) and a large diagonal branch (open arrow). With conventional dilatation of the left anterior descending artery, the diagonal branch would have a 15% chance of "snowplow" occlusion, a complication that did occur (lower left). Note, however, a second guidewire (open arrow) that had been placed in the diagonal branch before LAD dilatation to allow "double wire" alternative dilatation of the LAD and diagonal branch. When this failed to provide adequate improvement in both vessels, a true "kissing balloon" procedure (simultaneous inflation of two balloon catheters) was performed (lower left), providing the result shown in the upper right (some luminal thrombus was present, but had resolved at follow-up angiography the next day).

edge to decide that a particular patient is or is not an "angioplasty candidate." Such decisions, therefore, are an important component of angioplasty operator training (see subsequent text). With the rapid growth of the technique, several cardiology organizations have recently prepared position statements that attempt to outline its "correct" utilization.[6,92] These statements are useful compilations that outline some well-accepted indications and contraindications for coronary angioplasty, but they each consign situations in which decisions are difficult and individualized to a "possibly indicated" category. In an effort to review some aspects of these evolving or controversial indications, we offer the following discussion of various anatomical clinical applications of coronary angioplasty.

Single-Vessel Coronary Disease. When the NHLBI Registry was formed in 1979, patients were considered to be candidates for coronary angioplasty if they had medically refractory angina, objective evidence of myocardial ischemia, and single-vessel coronary disease accessible to then-current angioplasty equipment.[5,34] Lesions considered appropriate for angioplasty were usually proximal, discrete, subtotal, concentric, and noncalcified.

Although these criteria continue to identify patients with a high likelihood of success, major improvement in equipment and technique have permitted the safe and effective application of coronary angioplasty in patients with less ideal anatomy. Steerable guide wires and dilatation catheters with smaller deflated profile have allowed most operators to attempt dilatation of more distal and diffusely diseased segments. The routine use of prolonged inflation at low pressure (50 to 60 psi) has allowed dilatation of eccentric stenoses,[93] and special devices[94] have been developed for dilatation of lesions located within curved vessel segments, which appear to be prone to dissection using standard balloons.

CLINICAL STATUS OF ELECTIVE PTCA

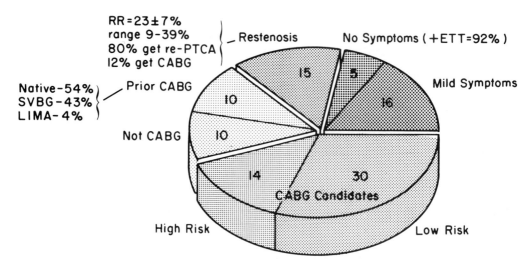

Fig. 26–14. Current utilization of coronary angioplasty. Pie chart shows the breakdown of PTCA indications according to a survey of experienced operators.[4] Although original angioplasty indications suggested that all patients be candidates for bypass surgery, only about half of the patients currently being referred for PTCA would meet this test. Of the remainder, some 20% would not be candidates due to age, poor left ventricular function, acute myocardial infarction (not CABG), or because of prior surgery (prior CABG) in which angioplasty is performed on a native vessel, saphenous vein graft (SVBG), or internal mammary artery graft (LIMA). An additional 21% would not have been candidates for surgery because of mild or absent symptoms on medical therapy, and a final 15% undergo angioplasty as a treatment for restenosis after prior angioplasty. These ''non-surgical'' indications account for the rapid growth in angioplasty without a corresponding decrease in the use of coronary bypass surgery (see Figure 26–1). (From Baim DS and Ignatius EJ: Use of percutaneous transluminal coronary angioplasty: Results of a current survey. Am J Cardiol 61:3G, 1988).

Total Coronary Occlusion. It is also now clear that many totally occluded vessels can be dilated successfully in patients with ongoing ischemic symptoms due to inadequate collateral flow (Fig. 26–15). To avoid vascular dissection or perforation, a series of guide wires (soft progressing to stiff-tipped) should be used to gently probe the stump of the occlusion until the latent vascular channel is entered. Once the guide wire has been passed into the distal vessel, the lesion can be crossed and dilated in the usual manner. The success rate of angioplasty in totally occluded vessels is clearly lower than in conventional stenotic vessels (60% versus 90% in our experience),[95] with most unsuccessful procedures resulting from inability to advance the guide wire transluminally into the distal vessel. Success is favored by the presence of a ''funnel'' entry to the total occlusion, a short totally occluded segment, and comparatively recent occlusion,[96] although chronic total occlusions of

several years' duration have been dilated successfully. Perhaps because of competitive flow by way of distal collaterals or other lesional characteristics, successfully dilated total occlusions appear to have a higher (40 to 50%) restenosis rate than do subtotal stenoses.[95–97]

Multivessel Coronary Disease. With the improved success rate in single-vessel coronary angioplasty, extension of the technique to patients with *multivessel* disease seems natural. In fact, many patients in the NHLBI Registry underwent single-vessel angioplasty in the setting of multivessel disease, with the hope that correction of the most severe lesions would control ischemic symptoms, even though milder lesions in other vessels remained untreated mechanically.[5,64] Although it is possible to attempt angioplasty on these *milder* residual lesions, experience has shown that these dilatations carry a significant risk of acute vessel occlusion and may initiate the restenosis process resulting in the formation of

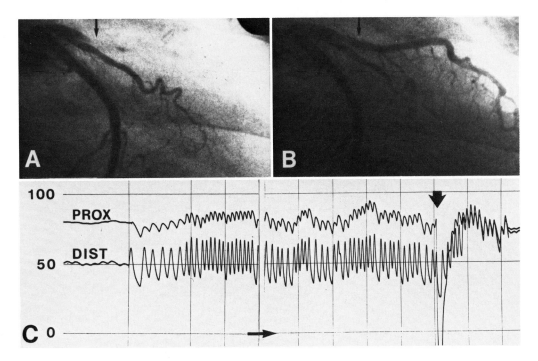

Fig. 26–15. Angioplasty of a totally occluded left anterior descending coronary artery. Panels A and B show the artery before and after angioplasty, and panel C shows the proximal (PROX) and distal (DIST) left anterior descending artery presence. This patient had normal anterior wall motion because of the presence of right to left collaterals capable of maintaining a distal occluded left anterior descending pressure of nearly 50 mmHg, but not capable of meeting flow requirements during exertion. (From Dervan JP, Baim DS, Cherniles J, Grossman W: Transluminal angioplasty of occluded coronary arteries: use of a movable guide wire system. Circulation 68:776, 1983.)

a severe stenosis within a matter of months.[65] In contrast, patients with *severe* stenosis of two or even all three coronary arteries are now increasingly being considered for true multivessel angioplasty.[37] Such procedures are technically more demanding than single vessel angioplasty and carry a higher risk of complication should vessel occlusion occur.[38] One possible exception is the "boot-strap" two-vessel procedure, in which a totally occluded artery is collateralized by a second vessel with a severe stenosis (Fig. 26–16). In this situation, the total occlusion can be dilated first without risk, thereby providing retrograde collateral flow to the stenotic vessel to improve the safety of the second dilatation. Because of concerns about incomplete revascularization, increased risk if abrupt closure develops, and increased restenosis, only about one third of the patients with multivessel disease at catheterization are found to be good candidates for coronary angioplasty (compared to nearly three quarters of those with single-vessel dis-

ease).[4] Patients with diffuse coronary disease, or those with significant (>50%) stenosis of the left main coronary artery[98] are still best treated by surgical bypass. Between these two extremes, several randomized trials are now in progress to establish the correct relative use of coronary angioplasty and bypass surgery in patients with symptomatic multivessel coronary artery disease.

Bypass Grafts. More than half of the patients who undergo bypass surgery using saphenous vein conduits will have occlusion or severe narrowing of those grafts within 10 years of surgery.[99] Internal mammary conduits have a better long-term track record, but many of these grafts also develop significant stenosis, particularly at the distal anastomosis. Finally, patients with previous bypass surgery may develop new or progressive disease beyond a graft insertion or in a nongrafted vessel. These problems may cause recurrent angina, which previously required repeat bypass surgery (a higher-risk procedure compared to ini-

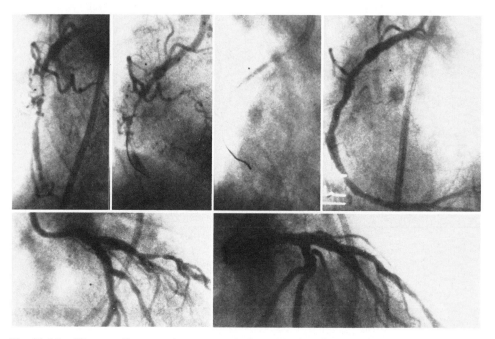

Fig. 26–16. "Boot-strap" two-vessel coronary angioplasty. Dilatation of a subtotally occluded right coronary (top) which received collaterals from a severely stenotic left anterior descending artery. Because the right coronary artery was protected by the left-to-right collaterals, it could be dilated at low risk. Once the right coronary was dilated, it served as a source of collateral flow to protect the left anterior descending artery during subsequent angioplasty of that vessel (bottom). Angioplasty of these two vessels in the opposite order (LAD first) would have carried significantly greater risk due to simultaneous jeopardy of both territories.

tial bypass). With the progressive growth of coronary angioplasty, however, many such patients can be managed by balloon dilatation of the diseased graft or a stenotic native vessel, so that angioplasty of postoperative patients accounts for approximately 10% of current volume.[4,100]

Vein graft stenoses that present within the first year after surgery are most commonly caused by intimal hyperplasia, and respond quite well to balloon dilatation.[28,100] In contrast, late vein graft stenoses are more commonly caused by diffuse atherosclerosis, which has a distinct tendency to fragment and/or embolize into the distal coronary bed during dilatation.[28,30] In either case, dilated graft lesions have a high (>40%) restenosis rate, particularly those in the mid-portion of the graft, or those that contain a large volume of thrombus. While the thrombus can be lysed with intracoronary thrombolytic infusion, allowing the underlying stenosis to be dilated,[101] poor

long-term patency gives such procedures only marginal utility.[102]

Internal mammary artery grafts are generally resistant to disease, with a 10-year patency rate >90%, but we have seen a number of patients with recurrent angina early (within 6 months) after bypass surgery, because of stenosis of the internal mammary-native artery anastomosis. These lesions can be dilated effectively using low-profile, trackable dilatation catheters,[103,104] with a moderate (35 to 40%) restenosis rate.

When attempting angioplasty in a patient with previous bypass surgery, the operator should keep in mind that the extensive mediastinal fibrosis and risk of injuring functional anterior grafts will prolong the time required for emergency surgery should a complication of angioplasty occur.[105] This fact and the common presence of multivessel disease and impaired left ventricular function increase the risk of angioplasty in this patient group.

Stable Angina. The initial group of patients who were candidates for coronary angioplasty were patients with stable but medically refractory angina pectoris and suitable coronary anatomy. Occasional patients with milder symptoms and ideal anatomy are candidates, if they willingly accept the 3 to 5% risk that angioplasty will lead to emergency bypass surgery.[106] In doing so, mildly symptomatic patients with single- or double-vessel disease should be aware that there are currently no controlled studies that demonstrate improved survival or freedom from infarction with angioplasty as opposed to medical therapy.[107]

Older patients (>70 years of age) with stable or unstable angina constitute an important category of angioplasty candidates. Unlike bypass surgery (which carries a higher risk and a longer recovery period in the elderly), angioplasty has almost as favorable an outlook in this group as it does in younger patients.[108]

Unstable Angina. Patients with unstable angina (including new onset angina) account for a large portion of current angioplasty practice.[109] Our own experience[110] suggests that more than 85% of patients admitted to the coronary care unit with this diagnosis are referred for revascularization, even if they respond to intensification of medical therapy. Revascularization is divided nearly equally between angioplasty (predominantly for patients with single- and double-vessel disease) and bypass surgery (predominantly for patients with triple-vessel and left main disease). To facilitate rapid treatment of unstable patients, many centers even perform the initial diagnostic catheterization with "angioplasty standby," so that suitable lesions can be treated by balloon dilatation during the same procedure.[111] We generally reserve this approach for patients whose anginal syndrome is sufficiently compelling to warrant treatment "on the spot" because the dilatation procedure may not go as smoothly without a chance to review the diagnostic cineangiograms and discuss the anatomy (and attendant risks) with the patient and family, particularly if the anatomy proves to be complex. Moreover, it is not clear if patients who respond to medical therapy (possibly including thrombolysis) still need to proceed with diagnostic catheterization and revascularization in the absence of recurrent angina or a positive predischarge exercise test—a question that is now the topic of the multicenter NIH-sponsored T3 Trial.

Acute Myocardial Infarction. The treatment of acute myocardial infarction has undergone a major revolution in the past decade, with the recognition that intracoronary thrombosis is the final mechanism of vessel occlusion, and the introduction of potent thrombolytic agents that are capable of opening more than 75% of these vessels within 90 minutes of intravenous administration.[112] A purely pharmacologic approach to the management of myocardial infarction has not proven satisfactory, however, because some vessels fail to open in response to thrombolytic therapy and up to 30% either reocclude during hospitalization or cause recurrent angina due to the persistence of an underlying high-grade atherosclerotic stenosis.

These shortcomings of thrombolysis have prompted several large clinical trials to explore the optimal strategy of combining thrombolysis with mechanical revascularization, using balloon angioplasty (if possible) or bypass surgery. A full discussion of this complex and still-evolving area would be beyond the scope of this chapter, but several trials[113] have demonstrated that *immediate* catheterization and angioplasty carries an increased risk and offers no additional benefit in terms of survival or recovery of left ventricular function. In fact, the TIMI IIB trial reported that even routine *delayed* catheterization (18 to 48 hours after thrombolysis) offered no additional benefit over a *conservative* strategy in which catheterization and angioplasty were reserved for patients with recurrent spontaneous or exercise-provoked ischemia.[114] On the other hand, some operators have reported excellent results using *primary angioplasty* rather than thrombolysis to open occluded vessels in the early hours of infarction.[115] In the absence of a randomized trial showing superiority of this approach to the conservative TIMI IIB strategy, we have reserved primary angioplasty for patients with infarctions that occur in hospital while awaiting catheterization or angioplasty, or in whom there is some contraindication to thrombolysis (elderly, uncontrolled hypertension, cerebrovascular disease, peptic ulcer disease, recent major surgical procedure, etc.).

FINANCIAL AND REGULATORY CONSIDERATIONS

Because coronary angioplasty is performed in a cardiac catheterization laboratory under local anesthesia, it is attended by substantially lower direct costs than coronary bypass surgery. Studies in our own institution[91] and at Emory University[116] confirm that the initial procedural cost for even multivessel coronary angioplasty is less than half that of bypass surgery—a cost difference that is maintained even when including the costs associated with repeat procedures for the treatment of restenosis within the first year. While this does not include all the hidden costs of maintaining surgical standby,[117] it seems clear that angioplasty affords the potential for a decrease in health care cost as well as patient morbidity when compared to bypass surgery.

Because of this net saving, and the perceived competitive benefits to the hospital and physician-operator offering angioplasty services,[118] there is continued pressure to involve more institutions and more operators in the performance of this procedure. From the institutional perspective, all current guidelines[6,92] make it clear that angioplasty should be limited to institutions that have on-site cardiac surgery capable of providing effective standby for emergency bypass operations resulting from angioplasty complications.

The issue of operator training and certification is still in evolution. Early angioplasty operators were exclusively physicians active in diagnostic catheterization who learned angioplasty techniques by attending live demonstration courses and watching or helping to perform a small number of procedures (i.e., 10 to 20) under the guidance of a knowledgeable operator. Given the ever-increasing complexity of the procedure, however, virtually all new angioplasty operators receive instead formal training, consisting of a third and/or fourth year of interventional fellowship following complete training in diagnostic coronary angiography. During the interventional fellowship, a trainee should perform a minimum of 125 procedures, including 75 as the primary operator.[6] Moreover, performance of complex procedures requires ongoing operator experience of 50 to 100 angioplasty procedures per year.[119] The results of operators with less experience suggest that, while they may have acceptable success rates with "simple" lesions, they have significantly poorer results on "complex" lesions than do operators with the suggested level of ongoing experience.[120] With the advent of a broad variety of new technologies for coronary intervention (see Chapters 27 and 28), and the introduction of new interventional techniques such as balloon valvuloplasty (Chapter 29), increasing functional specialization will be required of "interventional" cardiologists among the ranks of "invasive" cardiologists whose practices are limited to purely diagnostic cardiac catheterization.

REFERENCES

1. Dotter CT, Judkins MP: Transluminal treatment of arteriosclerotic obstruction: description of a new technique and a preliminary report of its application. Circulation 30:654, 1964.
2. Gruentzig A, Kumpe DA: Technique of percutaneous transluminal angioplasty with the Gruentzig balloon catheter. Am J Radiol 132:547, 1979.
3. Gruentzig AR, Senning A, Siegenthaler WE: Nonoperative dilatation of coronary artery stenosis—percutaneous transluminal coronary angioplasty. N Engl J Med 301:61, 1979.
4. Baim DS, Ignatius EJ: Use of percutaneous transluminal coronary angioplasty: Results of a current survey. Am J Cardiol 61:3G, 1988.
5. Kent KM, et al: Percutaneous transluminal coronary angioplasty: report from the registry of the National Heart, Lung, and Blood Institute. Am J Cardiol 49:2011, 1982.
6. Ryan TJ, et al: Guidelines for percutaneous transluminal coronary angioplasty—A report of the ACC/AHA Task Force on assessment of diagnostic and therapeutic cardiovascular procedures. J Am Coll Cardiol 12:529, 1988.
7. Avedissian MG, et al: Percutaneous transluminal coronary angioplasty: A review of current balloon

dilatation systems. Cathet Cardiovasc Diagn 18:263, 1989.

8. Simpson JB, Baim DS, Robert EW, Harrison DC: A new catheter system for coronary angioplasty. Am J Cardiol 49:1216, 1982.

9. Anderson HV, et al: Measurement of transstenotic pressure gradient during percutaneous transluminal coronary angioplasty. Circulation 73:1223, 1986.

10. Thomas ES, et al: Efficacy of a new angioplasty catheter for severely narrowed coronary lesions. J Am Coll Cardiol 12:694, 1988.

11. Lindsey RL, Kleist PC: Subselective intracoronary access guide catheters for use with the probe balloon on a wire coronary dilatation device. J Intervent Cardiol 2:9, 1989.

12. Dervan JP, McKay RG, Baim DS: The use of an exchange wire in coronary angioplasty. Cathet Cardiovasc Diagn 11:207, 1985.

13. Wyman RM, et al: Current complications of diagnostic and therapeutic cardiac catheterization. J Am Coll Cardiol 12:1400, 1988.

14. Schwartz L, et al: Aspirin and dipyridamole in the prevention of restenosis after percutaneous transluminal coronary angioplasty. N Engl J Med 318:1714, 1988.

15. Dorros G, et al: The brachial artery method to transluminal coronary angioplasty. Cathet Cardiovasc Diagn 8:233, 1982.

16. Harvey JR, Wyman RM, McKay RG, Baim DS: Use of balloon flotation pacing catheters for prophylactic temporary pacing during diagnostic and therapeutic cardiac catheterization. Am J Cardiol 62:941, 1988.

17. Abele J: Balloon catheters and transluminal dilatation: technical considerations. Am J Radiol 135:901, 1980.

18. Kaltenbach M, et al: Prolonged application of pressure in transluminal angioplasty. Cathet Cardiovasc Diagn 10:213, 1984.

19. Waller BF: The eccentric coronary atherosclerotic plaque: Morphologic observations and clinical relevance. Clin Cardiol 12:14, 1989.

20. Serruys PW, et al: Assessment of percutaneous transluminal coronary angioplasty by quantitative coronary angiography: diameter versus videodensitometric area measurements. Am J Cardiol 54:482, 1984.

21. Roubin GS, et al: Influence of balloon size on initial success, acute complications, and restenosis after percutaneous transluminal coronary angioplasty. Circulation 78:557, 1988.

22. Nichols AB, et al: Importance of balloon size in coronary angioplasty. J Am Coll Cardiol 13:1094, 1989.

23. Simpendorfer C, et al: Frequency, management and follow-up of patients with acute coronary occlusions after percutaneous transluminal coronary angioplasty. Am J Cardiol 59:267, 1987.

24. Castaneda-Zuniga WR, et al: The mechanism of balloon angioplasty. Radiology 135:565, 1980.

25. Sanborn TA, et al: The mechanism of transluminal angioplasty: evidence for formation of aneurysms in experimental atherosclerosis. Circulation 68:1136, 1983.

26. McBride W, Lange RA, Hillis LD: Restenosis after successful coronary angioplasty. N Engl J Med 318:1734, 1988.

27. Holmes DR, et al: Angiographic changes produced by percutaneous transluminal coronary angioplasty. Am J Cardiol 51:676, 1983.

28. Waller BF, et al: Morphologic observations after percutaneous transluminal balloon angioplasty of early and late aortocoronary saphenous vein bypass grafts. J Am Coll Cardiol 4:784, 1984.

29. Sanborn TA, et al: Transluminal angioplasty in experimental atherosclerosis: analysis for embolization using an in vitro perfusion system. Circulation 66:917, 1982.

30. Aueron F, Gruentzig A: Distal embolization of a coronary artery bypass graft atheroma during percutaneous transluminal coronary angioplasty. Am J Cardiol 53:953, 1984.

31. MacDonald RG, Feldman RL, Conti CR, Pepine CJ: Thromboembolic complications of coronary angioplasty. Am J Cardiol 54:916, 1984.

32. Saffitz JE, Rose TE, Oaks JB, Roberts WC: Coronary artery rupture during coronary angioplasty. Am J Cardiol 51:902, 1983.

33. Namay DL, et al: Saphenous vein rupture during percutaneous transluminal angioplasty. Cathet Cardiovasc Diagn 14:258, 1988.

34. Proceedings of the National Heart, Lung, and Blood Institute workshop on the outcome of percutaneous transluminal angioplasty (June 7–8, 1983), Kent KM, Mullin SM, Passamani ER (eds.). Am J Cardiol 53:1C, 1984.

35. Dorros G, et al: Percutaneous transluminal coronary angioplasty: report of complications from the National Heart, Lung, and Blood Institute PTCA Registry. Circulation 67:723, 1983.

36. Anderson HV, et al: Primary angiographic success rates of percutaneous transluminal coronary angioplasty. Am J Cardiol 56:712, 1985.

37. Detre K, et al: Percutaneous transluminal coronary angioplasty in 1985–1986 and 1977–1981: The NHLBI Registry. N Engl J Med 318:265, 1988.

38. Holmes DR, et al: Comparison of complications during percutaneous transluminal coronary angioplasty from 1977 to 1981 and from 1985 to 1986: the NHLBI PTCA Registry. J Am Coll Cardiol 12:1149, 1988.

39. Detre K, et al: One-year follow-up results of the 1985–1986 National Heart, Lung, and Blood Institute's percutaneous transluminal coronary angioplasty registry. Circulation 80:421, 1989.

40. Kent KM, et al: Improved myocardial function during exercise after successful percutaneous transluminal coronary angioplasty. N Engl J Med 306:441, 1982.

41. Hirzel HO, Neusch K, Gruentzig AR, Luetolf UM: Short- and long-term changes in myocardial perfusion after percutaneous transluminal coronary angioplasty assessed by thallium-201 exercise scintigraphy. Circulation 63:1001, 1981.

42. Zijlstra F, Reiber JC, Julliere Y, Serruys PW: Normalization of coronary flow reserve by percutaneous transluminal coronary angioplasty. Am J Cardiol 61:55, 1988.

43. Wilson RF, et al: The effect of coronary angioplasty on coronary flow reserve. Circulation 77:873, 1988.

44. Rosing DR, et al: Three year anatomic, functional, and clinical follow-up after successful percutaneous transluminal coronary angioplasty. J Am Coll Cardiol 9:1, 1989.

45. Talley JD, et al: Clinical outcome 5 years after attempted percutaneous coronary angioplasty in 427 patients. Circulation 77:820, 1988.

46. Gruentzig AR, et al: Long-term follow-up after percutaneous transluminal coronary angioplasty: The early Zurich experience. N Engl J Med 316:1127, 1987.

47. Liu MW, Rubin GS, King SB: Restenosis after coronary angioplasty: Potential biologic determinants and role of intimal hyperplasia. Circulation 79:1374, 1989.

48. O'Keefe JH, Hartzler GO: Restenosis after coronary angioplasty. J Inv Car 1:109, 1989.

49. Serruys PW, et al: Incidence of restenosis after successful coronary angioplasty: A time related phenomenon—a quantitative angiographic follow-up study of 342 patients. Circulation 77:361, 1988.

50. Fischell TA, Derby G, Tse TM, Stadius ML: Coronary artery vasoconstriction after percutaneous transluminal coronary angioplasty: A quantitative arteriographic analysis. Circulation 78:1323, 1988.

51. Essed CE, Van Den Brand M, Becker AE: Transluminal coronary angioplasty and early restenosis—fibrocellular occlusion after wall laceration. Br Heart J 49:393, 1983.

52. Libby P, Warner SJC, Salomon RN, Birinyi LK: Production of platelet-derived growth factor-like mitogen by smooth muscle cells from human atheroma. N Engl J Med 318:1493, 1988.

53. Leimgruber PP, et al: Restenosis after successful coronary angioplasty in patients with single vessel disease. Circulation 73:710, 1986.

54. Bertrand ME, et al: Relation of restenosis after percutaneous transluminal coronary angioplasty to vasomotion of the dilated arterial segment. Am J Cardiol 63:277, 1989.

55. Leimgruber PP, et al: Influence of intimal dissection on restenosis after successful coronary angioplasty. Circulation 72:530, 1985.

56. Breisblatt WM, Weiland FL, Spaccavento LJ: Stress thallium-201 imaging after coronary angioplasty predicts restenosis and recurrent symptoms. J Am Coll Cardiol 12:1199, 1988.

57. Quigley PJ, et al: Prolonged autoperfusion angioplasty: Immediate clinical outcome and angiographic follow-up (abstract). J Am Coll Cardiol 13:155A, 1989.

58. Whitworth HB, et al: Effect of nifedipine on recurrent stenosis after percutaneous transluminal coronary angioplasty. J Am Coll Cardiol 8:1271, 1986.

59. Dehmer GJ, et al: Reduction in the rate of early restenosis after coronary angioplasty by a diet supplemented in n-3 fatty acids. N Engl J Med 319:733, 1988.

60. Reiss GJ, et al: Randomized trial of fish oil for restenosis after coronary angioplasty. Lancet 2:177, 1989.

61. Black AJR, et al: Repeat coronary angioplasty: correlates of a second restenosis. J Am Coll Cardiol 11:714, 1988.

62. Tierstein PS, et al: Repeat coronary angioplasty: Efficacy of a third angioplasty for a second restenosis. J Am Coll Cardiol 13:291, 1989.

63. Holman J, et al: Coronary artery spasm at the site of angioplasty in the first two months after successful percutaenous transluminal coronary angioplasty. J Am Coll Cardiol 2:1039, 1983.

64. Wohlgelernter D, Cleman M, Highman HA, Zaret BL: Percutaneous transluminal coronary angioplasty of the "culprit lesion" for management of unstable angina in patients with multivessel coronary artery disease. Am J Cardiol 58:460, 1986.

65. Ischinger LT, et al: Should coronary arteries with less than 60% diameter stenosis be treated by angioplasty? Circulation 68:148, 1983.

66. Reeder GS, et al: Degree of revascularization in patients with multivessel coronary disease: A report from the NHLBI PTCA Registry. Circulation 77:638, 1988.

67. DiSciascio G, et al: Triple vessel coronary angioplasty: Acute outcome and long-term results. J Am Coll Cardiol 12:42, 1988.

68. Finci L, et al: Comparison of multivessel coronary angioplasty with surgical revascularization with both internal mammary arteries. Circulation 76:V–1, 1987.

69. Joelson JM, et al: Angiographic findings when chest pain recurs after successful percutaneous transluminal coronary angioplasty. Am J Cardiol 60:792, 1987.

70. Harper JM, Shah Y, Kern M, Vanadormael MG: Progression of left main coronary artery stenosis following left anterior descending coronary angioplasty. Cathet Cardiovasc Diagn 13:398, 1987.

71. Bredlau CE, et al: In-hospital morbidity and mortality in patients undergoing elective coronary angioplasty. Circulation 72:1044, 1985.

72. Hill JA, et al: Coronary arterial aneurysm formation after balloon angioplasty. Am J Cardiol 52:261, 1983.

73. Vassarelli C, et al: Coronary artery aneurysm formation after PTCA—A not uncommon finding at follow-up angiography. Int J Card 22:151, 1989.

74. Black AJR, et al: Tear or dissection after coronary angioplasty—morphologic correlates of an ischemic complication. Circulation 79:1035, 1989.

75. Ellis SG, et al: Angiographic and clinical predictors of acute closure after native vessel coronary angioplasty. Circulation 77:372, 1988.

76. Sinclair IN, McCabe CH, Sipperly ME, Baim DS: Predictors, therapeutic options and long-term outcome of abrupt reclosure. Am J Cardiol 61:61G, 1988.

77. Talley JD, et al: Coronary artery bypass surgery after failed elective percutaneous transluminal coronary angioplasty—A status report. Circulation 79:I126, 1989.

78. Kabbani SS, et al: Surgical experience following transluminal coronary angioplasty. Tex Heart Inst J 11:112, 1984.

79. Hartzler GO, et al: "High-risk" percutaneous transluminal coronary angioplasty. Am J Cardiol 61:33G, 1988.

80. Vogel RA, et al: Initial report of the National Registry of Elective Cardiopulmonary Bypass-Sup-

ported Coronary Angioplasty. J Am Coll Cardiol 15:23, 1990.

81. Sundrum P, et al: Benefit of the perfusion catheter for emergency coronary artery grafting after failed percutaneous transluminal coronary angioplasty. Am J Cardiol 63:282, 1989.

82. Meier B, et al: Risk of side branch occlusion during coronary angioplasty. Am J Cardiol 53:10, 1984.

83. Meier B: Kissing balloon coronary angioplasty. Am J Cardiol 54:918, 1984.

84. Myler RK, et al: Coronary bifurcation stenoses: The kissing balloon probe technique via a single guiding catheter. Cathet Cardiovasc Diagn 16:267, 1989.

85. Osterle SN, McAuley BJ, Buchbinder M, Simpson JB: Angioplasty at coronary bifurcations: single-guide, two-wire technique. Cathet Cardiovasc Diagn 12:57, 1986.

86. Wohlgelernter D, et al: Regional myocardial dysfunction during coronary angioplasty: evaluation by two-dimensional echocardiography and 12 lead electrocardiography. J Am Coll Cardiol 7:1245, 1986.

87. Bertrand ME, et al: Left ventricular systolic and diastolic dysfunction during acute coronary artery balloon occlusion in humans. J Am Coll Cardiol 12:341, 1988.

88. Serruys PW, et al: Left ventricular performance, regional blood flow, wall motion, and lactate metabolism during transluminal angioplasty. Circulation 70:25, 1984.

89. Hartzler GO, et al: Retained percutaneous transluminal coronary angioplasty equipment components and their management. Am J Cardiol 60:1260, 1987.

90. Serota H, et al: Improved method for transcatheter retrieval of intracoronary detached angioplasty guidewire segments. Cathet Cardiovasc Diagn 17:248, 1989.

91. Barbash GI, Rabkin MT, Kane NM, Baim DS: Coronary angioplasty under the prospective payment system—the need for a severity-adjusted payment system. J Am Coll Cardiol 8:784, 1986.

92. Bourassa MG, et al: Report of the Joint ISFC/WHO task force on coronary angioplasty. Circulation 78:780, 1988.

93. Meier B, et al: Does length or eccentricity of coronary stenoses influence the outcome of transluminal dilatation? Circulation 67:497, 1983.

94. Vivekaphirat V, Zapala C, Foschi AE: Clinical experience with the use of the angled-balloon dilatation catheter. Cathet Cardiovasc Diagn 17:121, 1989.

95. Safian RD, et al: Initial success and long-term follow-up of percutaneous transluminal coronary angioplasty in chronic total occlusions versus conventional stenoses. Am J Cardiol 61:23G, 1988.

96. Stone GW, et al: Procedural outcome of angioplasty for total coronary occlusion: An analysis of 971 lesions in 905 patients. J Am Coll Cardiol 15:849, 1990.

97. Ellis SG, et al: Risk factors, time course and treatment effect for restenosis after successful percutaneous transluminal coronary angioplasty of chronic total occlusion. Am J Cardiol 63:897, 1989.

98. O'Keefe JH, et al: Left main coronary angioplasty: Early and late results of 127 acute and elective procedures. Am J Cardiol 54:144, 1989.

99. Bourassa MG, et al: Long-term fate of bypass grafts—the coronary artery surgery study (CASS) and Montreal heart institute experiences. Circulation 72:V71, 1985.

100. Kussmaul WG: Percutaneous angioplasty of coronary bypass grafts—An emerging consensus. Cathet Cardiovasc Diagn 15:1, 1988.

101. McKeever L, et al: Prolonged selective urokinase infusion in totally occluded coronary arteries and bypass grafts. Cathet Cardiovasc Diagn 15:247, 1988.

102. de Feyter PJ, et al: Percutaneous transluminal angioplasty of a totally occluded venous bypass graft: a challenge that should be resisted. Am J Cardiol 64:88, 1989.

103. Pinkerton CA, et al: Percutaneous transluminal angioplasty in patients with prior revascularization surgery. Am J Cardiol 61:15G, 1988.

104. Shimshak TM, et al: Application of percutaneous transluminal coronary angioplasty to the internal mammary artery graft. J Am Coll Cardiol 12:1205, 1988.

105. Douglas JS, et al: Percutaneous transluminal coronary angioplasty in patients with prior coronary bypass surgery. J Am Coll Cardiol 2:745, 1983.

106. Bergin P, et al: Transluminal coronary angioplasty in the treatment of silent ischemia. Cathet Cardiovasc Diagn 15:223, 1988.

107. Ellis SG, et al: Comparison of coronary angioplasty with medical treatment for single- and double-vessel coronary disease with left anterior descending coronary involvement: Long term outcome based on an Emory-CASS registry study. Am Heart J 118:208, 1989.

108. Holt GW, et al: Results of percutaneous transluminal coronary angioplasty for unstable angina in patients 70 years of age and older. Am J Cardiol 61:994, 1988.

109. deFeyter PJ, et al: Emergency angioplasty in refractory unstable angina. N Engl J Med 313:342, 1985.

110. Leeman DE, et al: Use of percutaneous transluminal coronary angioplasty and bypass surgery despite improved medical therapy for unstable angina pectoris. Am J Cardiol 61:38G, 1988.

111. Feldman RL, et al: Coronary angioplasty at the time of initial catheterization. Cathet Cardiovasc Diagn 12:219, 1986.

112. The TIMI Study Group: The Thrombolysis in Myocardial Infarction (TIMI) trial—phase I findings. N Engl J Med 312:932, 1985.

113. Rogers WJ, Baim DS, Gore JM, et al: Comparison of immediate invasive, delayed invasive and conservative strategies after tissue-type plasminogen activator—results of the TIMI IIA trial. Circ 81:1457, 1990.

114. The TIMI Study Group: Comparison of invasive and conservative strategies after treatment with intravenous tissue plasminogen activator in acute myocardial infarction. N Engl J Med 320:618, 1989.

115. O'Keefe JH, et al: Early results and long-term outcome of direct coronary angioplasty for acute myocardial infarction in 500 consecutive patients. J Am Coll Cardiol 64:1221, 1989.

116. Black AJ, et al: Comparative costs of percutaneous coronary angioplasty and coronary artery bypass

grafting in multivessel coronary artery disease. Am J Cardiol 62:809, 1988.

117. Wilson JM, et al: The cost of simultaneous surgical standby for percutaneous transluminal coronary angioplasty. J Thorac Cardiovasc Surg 91:362, 1986.

118. Robinson JC, Garnick DW, McPhee SJ: Market and regulatory influences on the availability of coronary angioplasty and bypass surgery in U.S. hospitals. N Engl J Med 317:85, 1987.

119. Ryan TJ, et al: Clinical competence in percutaneous transluminal coronary angioplasty—ACP/ACC/AHA Task Force on clinical privileges in cardiology. Circ 81:2041, 1990.

120. Hamad N, et al: Results of percutaneous transluminal coronary angioplasty by multiple, relatively low frequency operators: 1986–1987 experience. Am J Cardiol 61:1229, 1988.

27

New Devices for Coronary Intervention: Intravascular Stents and Coronary Atherectomy Catheters

ROBERT D. SAFIAN and DONALD S. BAIM

Since the first successful coronary angioplasty in 1977,[1] the annual number of percutaneous transluminal coronary angioplasty (PTCA) procedures has increased steadily to more than 250,000.[2] Vast improvements in technology have permitted the application of PTCA to patients with increasingly complex coronary anatomy. Although reports from the original National Heart, Lung, and Blood Institute (NHLBI) Registry in 1979 suggested that PTCA should be reserved for patients with proximal, discrete, nontotal, and noncalcified lesions,[3] PTCA is now performed routinely in patients with total occlusions, calcified plaques, coronary artery bypass grafts, multivessel disease, and acute myocardial infarction[4-12] (see Chap. 26).

LIMITATIONS OF CONVENTIONAL BALLOON ANGIOPLASTY

Despite the broader application, improved success rate, and lower complication rate of current PTCA, several residual problems are associated with conventional balloon dilatation. These include: (1) failure to cross a stenosis or occlusion, (2) failure to dilate a lesion, (3) the development of abrupt closure, and (4) late restenosis. Considering the current array of guide wires, guiding catheters, and low-profile balloon catheters, *failure to cross* a lesion is mostly restricted to a chronic total coronary occlusion, where difficulty is encountered in crossing the lesion with a guide wire in up to 40 to 50% of total occlusions, particularly those more than 6 months in duration.[5,6]

Failure to dilate a lesion is usually a function of plaque eccentricity and/or rigidity. Dilatation of *rigid* calcified plaques may require special high-pressure balloon catheters. Dilatation of *eccentric* plaques may lead to suboptimal results because of the tendency to overstretch the normal-appearing wall rather than the plaque, leading to elastic recoil with significant residual stenosis or over-distension with dissection.[13] Poor immediate angiographic results in such lesions are also associated with a higher incidence of late restenosis.[14]

Abrupt closure and late restenosis remain the two most important limitations of balloon angioplasty in the coronary circulation. *Abrupt closure* occurs in 5 to 6% of patients, and necessitates emergency surgical revascularization in 2 to 3% of patients.[4,15] Despite the generally favorable results of emergency surgery, the perioperative mortality rate is higher (approximately 5 to 6%) than that of elective coronary bypass surgery.[16]

From a public health standpoint, the 17 to 40% incidence of late *restenosis* of the dilated segment is the most important limitation of PTCA.[14,17–22] Restenosis occurs even more commonly in certain situations such as PTCA of total coronary occlusions, proximal LAD disease, saphenous vein bypass grafts, and diffuse disease.[5,23–26]

POSSIBLE ROLES OF NEW TECHNOLOGIES

In an effort to solve these residual problems of conventional PTCA, several new interventional devices have been developed. These new devices fall into three broad categories: (1) intravascular stents, (2) atherectomy devices, and (3) lasers. By mid-1989, approximately 2000 coronary procedures had been performed using these new devices.[27]

Intravascular stents and atherectomy devices may have a role in solving some of the residual problems associated with conventional balloon dilatation, although their use in total occlusions is limited by the fact that most of these devices must still be passed coaxially over a guide wire. Certain atherectomy or ultrasound devices,[28,29] however, may prove useful in crossing total occlusions, as discussed below. Different *laser* technologies may also be able to address some of the limitations of PTCA, but are discussed separately (see Chap. 28).

INTRAVASCULAR STENTS

When Dotter and Judkins proposed the concept of transluminal angioplasty in 1964,[30] they simultaneously postulated that Silastic or plastic endovascular splints could help maintain vascular patency until reintimalization occurred. In 1969, Dotter and coworkers implanted stainless steel and Nitinol coils in the peripheral arteries of dogs and reported mixed results.[31,32]

Stent Designs

Since the studies of Dotter et al., three major stent designs have been introduced: (1) self-expanding (spring-loaded) stents, (2) balloon expandable stents, and (3) thermal memory stents. All current stent designs share the common goals of reducing the incidence of failure to dilate, abrupt closure, and restenosis by internally supporting the dilated segment, but there are major device-to-device differences with respect to stent flexibility, biocompatibility, radiographic visibility, and expandibility.

Early *self-expanding stents,* such as those described by Maass et al.[33] and Charnsangavej et al.,[34] were limited by geometric instability and stent migration. These early problems were virtually eliminated by the development of a wire mesh design consisting of several interwoven strands (Wallstent, Medinvent, Lausanne, Switzerland), as reported by Sigwart and coworkers.[35] This stent design is formed by braiding 16 stainless steel wire filaments, each 0.06 mm or 0.08 mm thick, into a flexible mesh tube 15 to 30 mm long with an expanded diameter of 3 to 6 mm (Fig. 27–1).

The Medinvent stent is delivered by compressing and constraining it on a specially designed delivery system, which consists of a small-diameter catheter surrounded by a retractable, doubled-over membrane. Once within the target lesion, the constraining membrane is pressurized with contrast and retracted, exposing the stent and allowing it to expand as it is released into the vascular lumen. Expansion continues until equilibrium is reached between the dilating force of the stent and the elastic constraint of the vessel wall, a point at which luminal cross-sectional area is increased significantly.[36] A stent-catheter system with an outer diameter of 1.57 mm can be used to deliver stents that expand up to a diameter of 6.5 mm, with the fully expanded stent selected to be 0.5 mm larger than the normal diameter of the stented vessel.

Balloon-expandable stents include the Schatz-Palmaz tubular mesh stent (Johnson

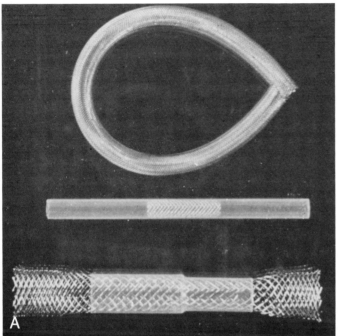

Fig. 27–1. Current stent designs. A, Spring-loaded stent (Medinvent). B, Balloon-expandable intravascular stent (Johnson & Johnson). C, Balloon-expandable flexible coil stent (Cook). (Reproduced, with permission, from Schatz RA: A view of vascular stents. Circulation 79:445, 1989, and from the American Heart Association, Inc.)

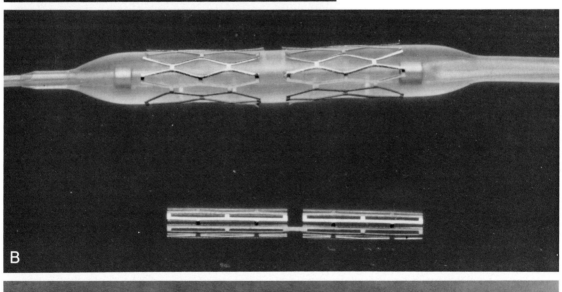

and Johnson, Inc., Somerville, NJ) and the Roubin-Gianturco flexible coil stent (Cook, Inc., Bloomington, IN). The Schatz-Palmaz stent consists of a rigid slotted stainless steel tube measuring 15 mm in length, 1.6 mm in diameter, and 0.08 mm in thickness.[37] This device has been further modified to create an "articulated" design, still formed from a single steel tube but consisting of two rigid steel segments (each 7 mm in length) joined by a flexible 1 mm bridge[38] (Fig. 27–1).

The Roubin-Gianturco flexible coil stent is a balloon-expandable stent that shares some features of the self-expanding stent. It is a serpentine coil made from a single strand of 0.006 inch (0.15 mm) surgical suture material, wrapped in a reversing pattern around a deflated standard balloon dilatation catheter. The stent thus assumes sequential U and inverted U configurations every 360 degrees of wrapping. Its ultimate diameter is determined by the diameter of the inflated delivery balloon[39] (Fig. 27–1).

Thermal memory stents expand from a small to a large diameter by virtue of the unique shape change that metals such as the nickel and titanium alloy known as Nitinol[32,40] undergo at a specific transition temperature. Use of such stents is particularly complex because they need to be refrigerated before implantation and chilled by cold saline infusion through the guiding catheter to prevent premature expansion in the guiding catheter before deployment. Although these stents have been used successfully in the peripheral circulation, there is little or no experience with them in the human coronary circulation.

Stent Characteristics

The ideal stent has yet to be designed, and data on the currently available designs fail to suggest clear superiority of any current device. Important to the immediate and long-term results of all stents, however, are certain characteristics, which include biocompatibility, flexibility, radiographic visibility, and expandability.[41]

In regard to intravascular stents, *biocom-*

patibility refers to the interaction of the metallic stent with blood. In a clinical context, biocompatibility consists of resistance both to thrombosis and corrosion. Most metals, including surgical-grade stainless steel, are positively charged and are therefore highly thrombogenic (i.e., they attract formed blood elements, which are negatively charged). The thrombogenicity of stainless steel stents can be reduced by *minimizing the metal surface area* and *using ultra-pure grades* of metal with a smooth polished surface. The biocompatibility of Nitinol stents is reported to be excellent, but overall clinical experience is limited because of problems discussed previously.[42,43]

The successful placement of intravascular stents is highly dependent upon *flexibility*. This feature is critically important in the coronary circulation, where the stent must overcome the shape and angulation of guiding catheters as well as the natural tortuosity of the coronary circulation itself. Experimental evidence, however, suggests that constant flexion *within* the stent may cause repeated injury to the neointima, possibly leading to late intimal proliferation and loss of luminal diameter.[44] Thus, the stent should be sufficiently flexible to pass through the guiding catheter and into the coronary circulation, but able to maintain a stable position without stimulating intimal proliferation.

Stent *visibility* during fluoroscopy is crucial to assure optimal placement, and is a function of the metal and metal thickness in the stent as well as the imaging system used in the catheterization laboratory. Metals such as gold and platinum are densely radiopaque but expensive and inelastic. Tantalum is more radiopaque than stainless steel and may be one alternative to steel as a material for constructing balloon expandable stents.[45–47]

Optimal stent delivery depends on reliable and predictable *expandibility*. Erratic expansion of self-expanding stents or thermal memory stents may cause either undersizing or oversizing of the vessel, as well as incomplete or premature stent deployment.[39,40,48,49] Balloon-expandable stents expand more precisely (to the inflated diameter of the delivery balloon), and their large expansion ratio (up to 6:1) permits them to be delivered through standard guiding catheters to treat target vessels up to 6 mm in diameter.

Stent Endothelialization and Thrombosis

Experimental studies in animals demonstrate that a thin layer composed of fibrin and platelets is deposited over the stent within the first few hours after implantation. Within 1 to 3 weeks, the stent is covered by a layer of immature neointima, which evolves within 8 weeks into a complete endothelial membrane comprised of collagen and normal, mature endothelial cells. Six months after implantation, the intimal layer thins slightly (to 150 to 500 μm) for vessels up to 5 mm in diameter (Fig. 27–2). Flow in branch vessels traversed by stent struts or wires is generally preserved.[37,39,48–53] After placement of self-expanding stents in dogs and sheep, slight thinning and fibrosis of the underlying media are usually seen histologically, as well as occasional rupture of the internal elastic lamina, cellular necrosis beneath the stent due to excessive mural pressure, or foreign body reaction, possibly indicating the potential for ongoing mural trauma.

Early experimental studies suggest that early thrombus formation precedes endothelialization and may influence subsequent neointimal growth. Maintenance of brisk antegrade flow by optimizing lumen geometry appears to be crucial for reducing the risk of thrombus formation and subsequent intimal hyperplasia. Palmaz et al.[54] have demonstrated that optimizing antithrombotic therapy is also crucial: the combination of dextran, heparin, aspirin, and dipyridamole results in less thrombus deposition after insertion of balloon-expandable stents in dogs, compared to other combinations of heparin, aspirin and dipyridamole without dextran (Fig. 27–3).

Techniques for Stent Placement

Self-Expanding Stent. To facilitate passage of the stent into the lesion, the vessel is first dilated using conventional balloon angioplasty. A stent diameter 15% larger than the diameter of the reference segment is chosen, and the length of the stent is selected to cover the entire dilated arterial segment, if possible. The initial PTCA balloon catheter is exchanged for the stent delivery system over a 0.014 inch guide wire through a standard 8 or 9 Fr guiding catheter, and the stent is deployed by pressurizing the constraining membrane to 3 atmospheres as it is retracted progressively to expose the stent. Once it is deployed, the inner surface of the stent may be smoothed further by brief inflations of a conventional PTCA balloon within the stented segment.

Balloon-Expandable Stents. The articulated Schatz-Palmaz stent is sufficiently flexible to traverse the bends in most conventional guiding catheters. After PTCA, the stent-balloon assembly is advanced en bloc over the guide wire and through the guiding catheter until it is positioned across the stenosis and delivered by inflating the balloon. The stented segment may then be expanded further using larger diameter balloons as necessary. If multiple stents are required, it is advisable to place the most distal stent first. In some cases, however, it may be necessary to place the proximal stent first to facilitate passage of additional stent(s) into the more distal segments. Before the development of a protective outer sheath, the exposed stent would occasionally snag on coronary intima or dissection flaps, impeding successful delivery. Following an unsuccessful placement attempt, withdrawal of the non-sheathed delivery system could lead to stripping of the stent from the delivery balloon with arterial embolization. Adoption of special 5 and 6 Fr stent delivery sheaths in 1990 allowed easier and more reliable stent implantation in a variety of native coronary vessels and bypass grafts.

The Gianturco-Roubin stent is also deployed by balloon inflation. After deflation of the delivery balloon, the catheter is advanced slightly to disengage the stent and removed.

Medications. To reduce the incidence of thromboembolic complications associated with intracoronary stents, a vigorous anti-

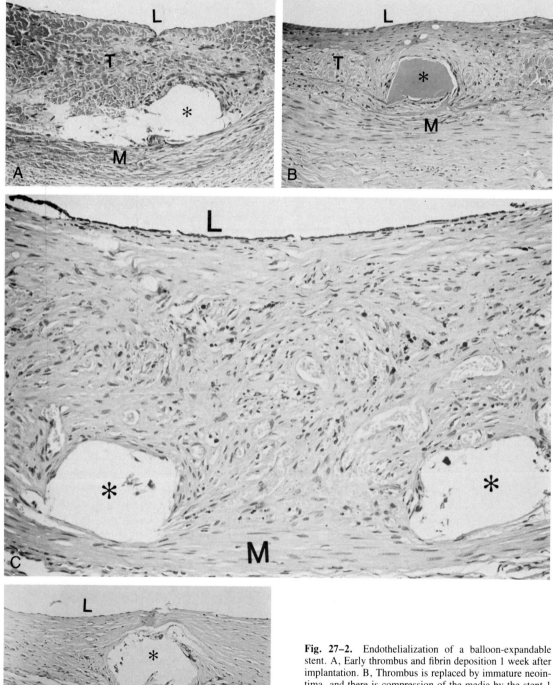

Fig. 27-2. Endothelialization of a balloon-expandable stent. A, Early thrombus and fibrin deposition 1 week after implantation. B, Thrombus is replaced by immature neointima, and there is compression of the media by the stent 1 to 3 weeks after implantation. C, By 8 weeks there is marked intimal proliferation and complete endothelialization with mature endothelial cells. D, By 6 months, there is thinning and fibrosis of the underlying media. L = lumen, M = media, T = thrombus, (*) = stent. (Reproduced, with permission, from Schatz RA, et al: Balloon-expandable intracoronary stents in the adult dog. Circulation 76:450, 1987, and from the American Heart Association, Inc.)

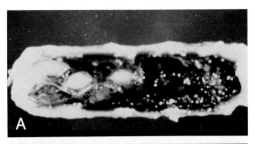

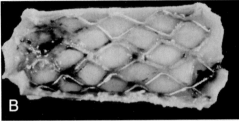

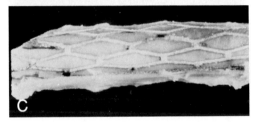

Fig. 27–3. Experimental stent thrombosis 3 hours after stent implantation. A, Severe thrombosis (no anticoagulation). B, Moderate thrombus formation (heparin, aspirin, and dipyridamole). C, Virtual absence of visible thrombus (heparin, aspirin, dipyridamole, and dextran). (Reproduced, with permission, from Schatz RA: A view of vascular stents. Circulation 79:445, 1989, and from the American Heart Association, Inc.)

thrombotic regimen is essential. The exact drug regimen is largely empiric, and requires a high degree of patient motivation and compliance. The importance of adherence to this drug regimen cannot be emphasized too strongly because early thrombosis is a clearly recognized hazard of stent placement.

For the Medinvent stent, patients are pretreated with aspirin, dipyridamole, sulfinpyrazone, and nifedipine beginning 24 hours before the procedure. During the catheterization procedure, intravenous heparin and intracoronary urokinase are administered. After completion of the procedure, intravenous heparin is continued until oral anticoagulation is achieved. Patients are discharged on aspirin (100 mg daily), dipyridamole (300 to 450 mg

daily), sulfinpyrazone (400 to 800 mg daily), nifedipine (30 to 60 mg daily), and acenocoumarin for 3 to 6 months.

For the Schatz-Palmaz stent, patients are premedicated with aspirin and dipyridamole for at least 24 hours before the procedure, with low molecular weight dextran (dextran-40, 100 cc/hr for 10 hours) begun 4 hours before the procedure. Prophylactic antibiotics (such as cefazolin, 1 gram every 8 hours) are administered just before stent placement and continued for 48 hours. After insertion of the arterial sheath, an intravenous heparin bolus (10,000 U) is administered and supplemented (usually 2500 U every 30 minutes) to maintain an activated clotting time (ACT) of 250 to 300 seconds. Heparin infusion is continued until a therapeutic prothrombin time (16 to 18 seconds) is achieved with oral Coumadin (warfarin). Patients are then discharged on aspirin (325 mg daily) and dipyridamole (200 mg daily) for 6 months, and oral Coumadin for 1 to 3 months.

Although endovascular infection has *not* been reported following stent placement, it is prudent to prescribe prophylactic antibiotics to guard against bacteremia associated with dental procedures and endoscopy that may be performed within 3 months of stent placement, before endothelialization is complete.

Possible Indications for Stent Use

Abrupt Closure. Abrupt closure occurs in approximately 5% of patients following PTCA, and is usually secondary to dissection, with or without associated thrombus and spasm.[4,15] Measures commonly used to reverse abrupt closure include long balloon inflations, low pressure inflations with a slightly oversized balloon, adjunctive therapy with thrombolytic or antiplatelet drugs (if thrombus is present), and administration of nitrates and calcium blockers to reverse coronary vasospasm.[15,55] These measures ultimately prove successful in establishing stable coronary patency in about half the patients with abrupt closure, so that the incidence of emergency bypass surgery has been reduced to 2 to 3%.[4,15]

New investigational approaches toward reversing abrupt closure include the use of mechanical stents to provide scaffold support for intimal flaps,[56,57] the use of laser balloon angioplasty for thermal welding of intimal tears,[58] and the use of atherectomy for excision of intimal flaps.[59] The use of lasers for abrupt closure is covered in Chapter 28, and the use of atherectomy devices subsequently in this chapter.

Several investigators have described their early experience with intracoronary stents for reversing abrupt closure. Sigwart et al.[56] successfully implanted 13 stents in 11 patients with abrupt closure: none required emergency bypass surgery or developed Q-wave myocardial infarction (Fig. 27–4), although 2 patients (18%) had evidence for non-Q-wave myocardial infarction based on minimal elevations of cardiac enzymes. The median time from initial vessel closure to stent implantation was 55 minutes. Short-term follow-up in these patients revealed late coronary bypass surgery in one patient because of acute occlusion of the stented segment.[56]

Roubin et al.[57] reported reversal of abrupt closure and reestablishment of normal antegrade flow in 6 patients after failed PTCA. In all patients, the Roubin-Gianturco stent was placed as a "bail-out" tactic immediately before emergency coronary bypass surgery, with no instances of Q-wave myocardial infarction or death.[57] There is still insufficient experience with the Schatz-Palmaz stent for treatment of abrupt closure to make any definitive comments at this time, but experience with other stents suggests that it will also prove useful for this indication.

Prevention of Restenosis. The most common limitation of conventional PTCA is the development of restenosis, which occurs in 17 to 40% of patients within 3 to 6 months of dilatation.[14,17–22] The histologic hallmark of restenosis is the presence of fibrointimal hyperplasia,[60,61] which appears to represent an excessive proliferative response of damaged endothelium and media to certain platelet-, fibroblast-, or endothelium-derived growth factors.[62,63] Intimal hyperplasia is not specific

for restenosis because it is also sometimes seen in de novo atherosclerotic lesions that have not been subjected to prior mechanical interventions,[64] or in the coronary arteries of patients during cardiac transplant rejection (Fig. 27–5).

Despite our understanding of the pathophysiology of the "restenosis lesion," no drug regimens yet developed prevent this process.[61] The persistent problem of restenosis has been the major impetus for the development of new interventional technologies for the treatment of coronary artery disease, in the hope that optimizing the initial result might substantially reduce late restenosis by either reducing the degree of intimal hyperplasia or providing a larger acute lumen that is better able to tolerate hyperplasia without the development of significant stenosis.

Preliminary Results of Stent Placement

Immediate Angiographic Results. The largest clinical experience with stent placement in human coronary arteries has been with the Medinvent stent in Europe[35,65,66] and the Schatz-Palmaz stent in the United States.[38,41,67,68] Sigwart and colleagues[66] have reported implantation of the Medivent stent in over 100 patients in Europe, including single stents in 85% of patients and 2 or more stents in 15% of patients. In the first 50 patients, the incidence of early in-hospital stent thrombosis was 16%. Other adverse effects were Q-wave myocardial infarction (4%), emergency coronary bypass surgery (4%), and death (2%). In their next 50 cases, however, improvements in selection criteria, operator experience, and antithrombotic regimen resulted in a much lower incidence of stent thrombosis (3%), and no instances of Q-wave myocardial infarction, emergency bypass surgery, or death.[66] Approximately 40 of these stents were placed in saphenous vein bypass grafts in several centers in Europe.[69,70]

In the United States, the Schatz-Palmaz stent has been implanted in 290 patients. After an initial series of 45 patients treated with only aspirin and dipyridamole at the time of hospital

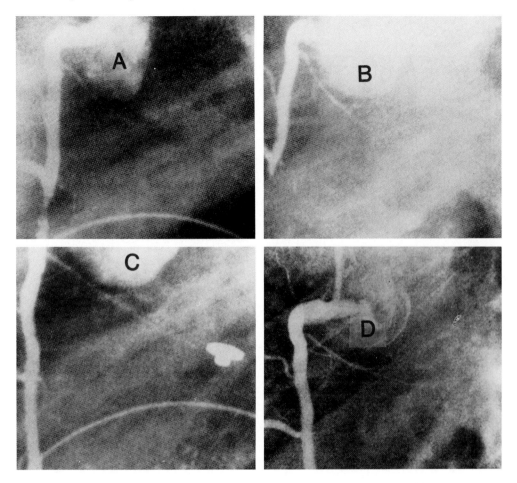

Fig. 27–4. Reversal of abrupt closure with a self-expanding stent. After conventional PTCA, there is a severe residual stenosis in the mid-RCA (A), which progresses to total occlusion (B). Successful implantation of tandem stents re-establishes normal antegrade flow (C), which still remains patent after 4 months (D). (Reproduced, with permission, from Sigwart U, et al: Emergency stenting for acute occlusion after coronary balloon angioplasty. Circulation 78:1121, 1988, and from the American Heart Association, Inc.)

discharge,[68] 245 patients were treated with chronic oral anticoagulants, aspirin, and dipyridamole at the time of hospital discharge. While there were *no* instances of acute stent thrombosis in the catheterization laboratory, subacute stent thrombosis (day 1 to 10) occurred in 16% of patients treated with aspirin and dipyridamole alone. In contrast, fewer than 0.6% of patients treated with the combination of aspirin, dipyridamole, and Coumadin developed subacute stent thrombosis. Patients on the less aggressive anticoagulant regimen had a higher incidence of myocardial infarction (13% versus 2.8%) and emergency bypass surgery (4.4% versus 0.8%), compared

to the 245 subsequent patients treated with the Coumadin regimen.

We have placed Schatz-Palmaz stents in more than 50 patients, all of whom were selected because of anatomic and/or clinical factors predictive of poor short-term or long-term outlook with conventional PTCA.[67] These factors included restenosis after PTCA in 57% of patients, marked lesion eccentricity in 46%, ulcerated lesions in 14%, and total occlusion in 5% (Fig. 27–6). Stent placement was successful in 96% of the vessels attempted, of which 7 received 2 stents, and 1 received 4 stents (Fig. 27–7). In about half of the patients, the initial stent delivery balloon was

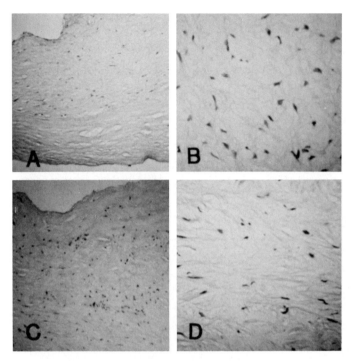

Fig. 27–5. Intimal proliferation in restenosis and de novo lesions as seen in specimens obtained during coronary atherectomy. A and B, Restenosis lesion following PTCA and laser balloon angioplasty shows marked intimal proliferation superimposed on atherosclerotic plaque (A, 6.3× and B, 16× magnification). C and D, Marked intimal proliferation from a de novo lesion, virtually indistinguishable from A and B (C, 6.3× and D, 16× magnification).

then exchanged for a larger balloon catheter, to achieve an optimal angiographic result.

Quantitative angiography revealed a baseline mean diameter stenosis of 83%, which decreased to 42% after PTCA and to −3% after stent placement. This corresponded to an increase in absolute lumen diameter from 0.59 mm at baseline to 1.91 mm after PTCA, and to 3.28 mm after stent placement (the corresponding reference segment measured 3.25 mm in diameter).

As expected, 54% of patients in this preselected high-risk subgroup had an inadequate result after conventional PTCA, including significant intraluminal haziness or irregularity in 14%, moderate localized dissection in 26%, and extensive dissection in 14%. Successful stent placement resulted in marked improvement in the angiographic result in two thirds of these patients, although one third of these patients still had a short segment of unstented disease or dissection distal to the stent.

These data suggest that stent placement significantly improves the absolute luminal dimensions and the appearance of the vessel wall compared to the typical results achieved after

conventional PTCA. These differences are even more striking in situations where PTCA is expected to offer less than optimal results.

Complications. The most important complication associated with stent implantation is *stent thrombosis,* discussed previously. Factors identified as possible predictors of subacute thrombosis after implantation of the Schatz-Palmaz stent include underdilatation of the stent, excessive overlap of multiple tandem stents, thrombocytosis, and omission of low molecular weight dextran or dipyridamole from the medical regimen.[68] Acute or subacute stent thrombosis can generally be managed by balloon angioplasty and thrombolytic therapy, without compromising the long-term clinical result. Late stent thrombosis (within 3 months of discharge) appears uncommon and is related to poor medical compliance or progressive intimal hyperplasia (restenosis) with secondary occlusion.

The incidence of *myocardial infarction* has been approximately 3%, and this generally occurs as a complication of stent thrombosis. *Emergency coronary bypass surgery* was required in 2 to 3% of patients undergoing place-

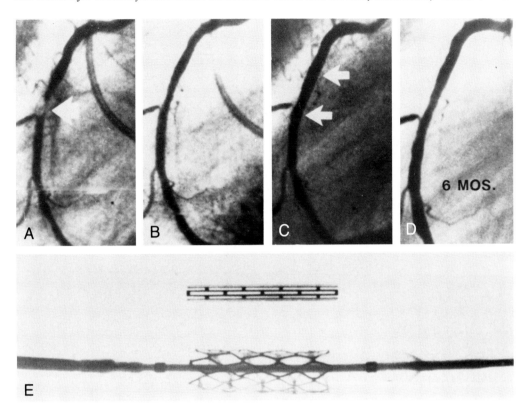

Fig. 27–6. Placement of a balloon-expandable Schatz-Palmaz intravascular stent in the mid-RCA. There is an eccentric restenosis lesion (A) which appears somewhat underdilated after conventional PTCA (B). Immediately after stent placement, the angiographic result is excellent (C), and the vessel remains patent at 6 months (D). The stent is shown in its collapsed and expanded states in E.

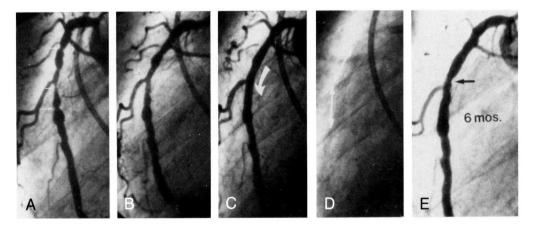

Fig. 27–7. Placement of tandem balloon-expandable Schatz-Palmaz stents in the mid-RCA. There is a diffusely diseased segment of restenosis (A) and the lumen still appears irregular after conventional PTCA (B). Immediately following implantation of 2 stents (C and D), the lumen is smooth, although there is mild focal intimal hyperplasia at 6 months (E), which may be secondary to stent overlap.

ment of the Medinvent stent, and was required in 0.8% of patients undergoing placement of the Schatz-Palmaz stent, usually because of problems with the guiding catheter or guide wire rather than the stent itself.[66,68]

Bleeding complications are more frequent after stent placement compared to conventional PTCA because of the aggressive anticoagulant regimen required. Bleeding complications are slightly more frequent after Medinvent stent implantation (9%) compared to Schatz-Palmaz stent implantation (5.7%), possibly because arterial sheaths are removed while patients were receiving full-dose heparin after placement of Medinvent stents. *Vascular injury* requiring surgical repair has occurred in approximately 5% of patients.[66,68]

Stent migration or embolization has not been reported with Medinvent stent implantation, but could be observed if the stent were significantly undersized. Stent embolization has been observed in three patients after unsuccessful attempts to deliver a rigid (nonarticulated) Schatz-Palmaz stent. After unsuccessful attempted placement, the stent was stripped from the delivery catheter during attempted withdrawal and embolized to the vasculature of the pelvis without clinical sequelae.

Fortunately, the incidence of procedure-related *death* is low (~1.0%), and seems to be similar to that of conventional PTCA. The incidence of *coronary vasospasm* after stent implantation is not known, but it is readily reversible and no sequelae have been reported.

Endovascular infection is a potential complication that has not yet been reported after stent implantation. Antibiotic prophylaxis is given routinely before implantation of Schatz-Palmaz stents, and we recommend appropriate antibiotics within the first 3 months of implantation for manipulations potentially associated with bacteremia.

Late Results. There is insufficient long-term clinical and angiographic follow-up to make definitive statements about the rate of restenosis following intracoronary stent placement. Preliminary findings suggest that stent placement may improve long-term patency in selected individuals, although the problem of restenosis has not been eliminated. Progressive stenosis may occur within the stent, or at the boundaries between the stent and the adjacent vessel wall. Experimental data[37,39,48–53] and tissue removed at the time of atherectomy (Simpson, personal communication) suggest that the cause of stent restenosis is fibrointimal hyperplasia, virtually indistinguishable from the intimal hyperplasia that occurs after conventional PTCA and other interventional procedures (Fig. 27–8).

Progressive stenosis at the boundaries of the stent has also been reported in a small number of patients. The cause of this type of lesion is not known, but it could be due to progression of unstented disease, restenosis of a dilated segment not covered by the stent, mechanical strain exerted by the stent on the vessel wall, or a combination of these factors.[71]

Preliminary follow-up angiographic data on the Medinvent stent suggests an 18% late angiographic restenosis rate for stents that are patent at discharge, similar to the 17% restenosis rate reported for single Schatz-Palmaz stents.[72,73] The restenosis rate, however, appears to be considerably greater (up to 50%) in patients with multiple tandem Schatz-Palmaz stents, possibly resulting from increased metal surface density within the overlap zone.[72]

After stent implantation, a thin layer of fibrin and thrombus forms on the metal and serves as a scaffold for subsequent endothelialization. Restenosis within the stent may then represent an exaggeration of the normal intimal response needed to completely cover the stent. Investigators have observed mild thickening of the neointima, accounting for a mild decrease in lumen diameter at late follow-up, even in the absence of anginal symptoms or provocable ischemia on exercise testing. The extent of intimal thickening at 6 months may vary from 300 to 500 μm, resulting in residual stenoses of about 30 to 40%[67] (see Figs. 27–6 and 27–7).

There are several potential approaches to the patient with stent restenosis. Conventional balloon angioplasty has been performed by Sigwart et al.[71] and Levine et al.[67] with excellent

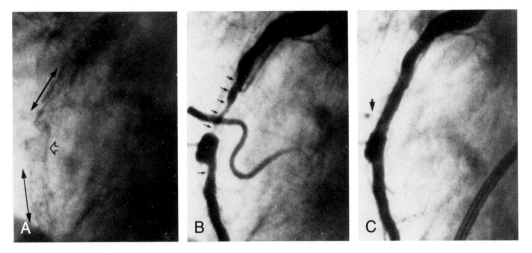

Fig. 27–8. Restenosis following intravascular stent placement. Tandem Schatz-Palmaz stents were placed in the mid-RCA (A). At 6 months after stent placement, there is marked intimal thickening (restenosis) within the proximal stent and an eccentric area of intimal thickening in the distal stent (B). The angiographic result following conventional PTCA is excellent (C).

immediate angiographic results and with a smooth appearance of the lumen (Fig. 27–8). Percutaneous coronary atherectomy has also been used in one patient with restenosis within a Medinvent stent (Simpson, personal communication). If appropriate, coronary bypass surgery should be considered.

CORONARY ATHERECTOMY

Several atherectomy devices have been introduced for application in the human coronary circulation. All of these devices share the goal of enlarging the coronary lumen by displacing or removing plaque, but differ in their fundamental designs. Ablative lasers might be considered as atherectomy devices (because plaque is removed by tissue vaporization), but these are discussed separately (see Chapter 28).

Atherectomy Catheter Designs

The different approaches to removing plaque all rely on high-speed rotation. Only four devices, however, actually remove atherosclerotic material from the body: (1) the directional coronary atherectomy catheter[74]; (2) the transluminal extraction catheter[75]; (3)

the flexible rotational atherectomy system[76,77]; and (4) the transluminal lysing system.[78] The other high-speed rotational devices rely on abrasion and pulverization techniques to debulk plaque, embolizing debris rather than removing plaque from the patient.[79,80]

The prototype of the *directional coronary atherectomy* catheter is the Simpson AtheroCath (Devices for Vascular Intervention, Inc., Redwood City, CA).[74] The catheter consists of several components: a double-lumen shaft with a guide wire lumen and a balloon inflation port, a windowed rigid stainless steel cylindric housing that contains a cup-shaped cutter, a 2.0 mm balloon affixed to the housing opposite the cutting window; and a nose-cone collection chamber for storage of excised tissue. The coronary device differs from the peripheral device in its smaller size and the hollow cutter torque-tubing that allows advancement over a movable 0.014-inch guide wire (Fig. 27–9).

Three different sizes are available for coronary use, with diameters of the stainless steel housing of 5.0, 6.0, and 7.0 Fr (1.7, 2.0, and 2.3 mm, respectively). The catheter shaft is braided, to provide torsional control for orienting the device within the stenosis. A separate battery-powered motor drive unit is avail-

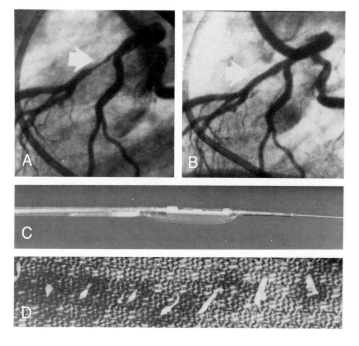

Fig. 27–9. Directional coronary atherectomy (Devices for Vascular Intervention). Left coronary angiography (lateral view) reveals a long eccentric stenosis in the mid-LAD (A). After atherectomy, the lumen is smooth, and there is no significant residual stenosis or dissection (B). A 7 Fr AtheroCath was used (C) and several pieces of atheroma were retrieved (D).

able that drives a cable to spin the cup-shaped cutter at approximately 2500 rpm. A small lever on the motor drive unit permits manual advancement to excise plaque, which is pushed down into the window during balloon inflation.

The *transluminal extraction catheter* (Interventional Technologies, Inc., San Diego, CA) consists of a motorized stainless steel element with a conical cutting head that rotates at 750 rpm. The cutting head is mounted on a flexible, hollow torque tube, which incorporates a vacuum system to aspirate atheroma fragments as the system is advanced down the diseased vessel over a 0.014-inch guide wire[75] (Fig. 27–10).

The *rotational atherectomy system (RAS)*

(C.R. Bard, Inc., Billerica, MA) consists of a flexible catheter (5 to 9 Fr), a special helical wire that serves as an auger device to capture atheromatous debris as the sharpened outer catheter is advanced across a lesion, and a motor drive unit, which rotates the outer catheter at 1200 rpm. The device is just entering clinical trials after preliminary animal and human postmortem studies.[76,77] Use of the *transluminal lysing system* seems feasible, but clinical experience is not available at this time.[78]

Other rotational devices rely on plaque abrasion and pulverization (rather than excision and removal), and include the high-speed rotary atherectomy device or *Rotablator* (Biophysics International, Bellevue, WA)[79–81] and

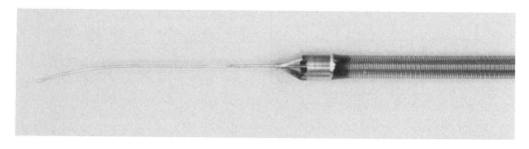

Fig. 27–10.   The transluminal extraction catheter (Interventional Vascular Technologies). See text for details.

the high-speed rotation dynamic angioplasty catheter or *Kensey catheter* (Theratek International, Miami, FL).[82,83] The Rotablator consists of an olive-shaped, stainless steel or brass burr, which is embedded with diamond chips measuring 30 to 120 μm in diameter. The burr is attached to a hollow flexible drive shaft which permits passage of a steerable, movable 0.009-inch guide wire. The drive shaft is encased within a Teflon sheath and a compressed air turbine rotates the drive shaft at 100,000 to 120,000 rpm. During rotation, sterile saline is pumped into the sheath to lubricate and cool the drive shaft and burr. Use of the device results in pulverization of the plaque into particles varying from approximately 2 to 10 μm with the 3.0 mm burr, and up to 15 to 20 μm with the 4.5 mm burr (Fig. 27–11), but larger particles may be produced. Larger particles can interfere with flow through the distal coronary microcirculation, leading to possible transient myocardial dysfunction or even infarction. Other complications and long-term patency have not yet been reported.

The *Kensey catheter* consists of a flexible polyurethane catheter ranging in size from 5 to 9 Fr, with an attached rotating cam. A metal cam at the catheter tip is driven at speeds up to 100,000 rpm by an internal torsion drive wire, which is powered by a direct current electric motor. Irrigation fluid, pressurized by air cylinders, flows through a channel in the catheter and exits at the base of the cam as a fine jet spray, creating a vortex. This spray is directed laterally against the vessel wall and serves to cool and lubricate the rotating cam, dilate the vessel, and maintain coaxial alignment. The combination of the high-speed rotation and the vortex serve to pulverize atheromatous material into particles ranging from 5 to 10 μm in diameter. The jet spray and the speed of rotation are controlled from a separate console (Fig. 27–12).

Other potentially useful recanalization de-

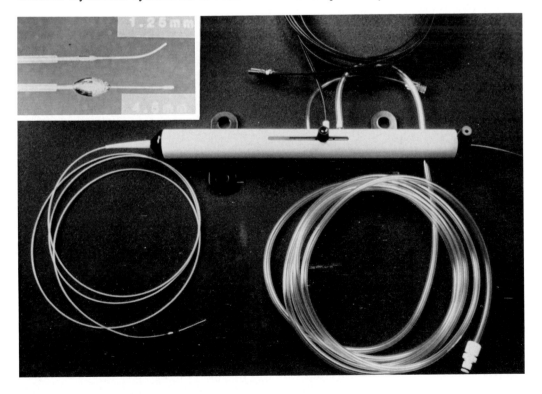

Fig. 27–11. The high-speed rotational atherectomy system (Rotablator, Biophysics International). (Reproduced, with permission, from Zacca NM, et al: Treatment of symptomatic peripheral atherosclerotic disease with a rotational atherectomy device. Am J Cardiol 63:77, 1989.)

Kensey Catheter

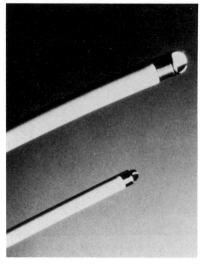

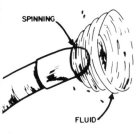

Fig. 27–12. The high-speed rotational dynamic angioplasty catheter (Kensey device, Theratek International), in 5 and 8 Fr sizes. Diagram at right illustrates the functional vortex created by the high speed rotational cam. (Reproduced, with permission, from Wholey MH: Advances in balloon technology and reperfusion devices for peripheral circulation. Am J Cardiol 61:87G, 1988.)

vices, particularly for chronic total peripheral occlusions, are the *atherolytic reperfusion guide wire* (Medrad)[84] and the *low-speed rotational angioplasty catheter.*[85] The atherolytic guide wire is a 0.035-inch wire with an olive-shaped tip. The proximal end of the wire may be attached to a hand-held, battery-operated power pack, which rotates the wire at 200 to 2000 rpm (Fig. 27–13). The low-speed rotational angioplasty catheter measures 2.2 mm in diameter and consists of 4 coiled steel wires with a rounded tip covered by a polyolefin or Teflon shrinking tube. The rotating catheter is

attached to a motor that spins at 200 rpm, and an inner lumen allows passage of a 0.35-inch exchange wire for further definitive therapy (Fig. 27–13).

Atherectomy Procedure

Considerable experience has been achieved with many of the currently available atherectomy catheters in the treatment of *peripheral* vascular disease.[76,81,83] The largest experience with atherectomy in the *coronary* circulation, however, has been obtained with the Simpson

Atherolytic Wire

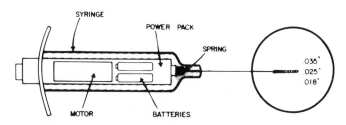

Fig. 27–13. The atherolytic reperfusion guide wire (Medrad) and the low-speed rotational angioplasty catheter. (Reproduced, with permission, from Wholey MH: Advances in balloon technology and reperfusion devices for peripheral circulation. Am J Cardiol 61:87G, 1988.)

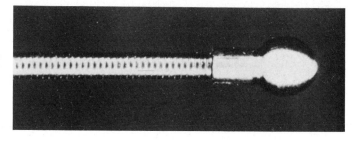

AtheroCath (over 1000 cases were performed in the United States alone by the end of 1989).

In using this device, we generally perform baseline right and left heart catheterization and coronary angiography using standard catheters for conventional PTCA. Standard PTCA guiding catheters, however, are *not* suitable for coronary atherectomy due to their acute angulations and comparatively small lumen. Thus, special 11 Fr guiding catheters (Devices for Vascular Intervention, Redwood City, California) have been constructed with gentle curves rather than sharp angles to facilitate passage of the rigid housing (Fig. 27–14).

Medications. Patients are treated with standard medications appropriate for PTCA, including aspirin 325 mg daily and dipyridamole 50 mg 4 times daily, starting at least 24 hours before the procedure and continuing indefinitely after discharge. After insertion of the arterial sheath, 10,000 units of heparin are administered, and additional heparin is given throughout the procedure (2500 units every 30 minutes) to maintain the activated clotting time between 250 and 300 seconds.

Device Selection and Use. The size of the normal vessel adjacent to the stenosis (the reference segment) is the major factor that determines the size of the atherectomy device. Generally, we use a 6 Fr device when the reference diameter is less than 3.0 mm, and a 7 Fr device is recommended when the reference diameter is larger than 3.0 mm or when there is a residual stenosis after use of the 6 Fr device with balloon inflation pressures up to 40 psi. Only rarely (e.g., subtotal lesions in calcified or moderately tortuous vessels) is the smaller 5 Fr device used to partially debulk the plaque, and facilitate passages of a larger device. It is not advisable to predilate the lesion before atherectomy because balloon dilation may make recovery of tissue during subsequent atherectomy more difficult.

After the central lumen is flushed and the balloon lumen filled with dilute contrast, the device is passed into the guiding catheter through a large-bore rotating hemostatic valve. The maneuvers necessary to advance the device across the target lesion are *different* from those used to advance a balloon catheter during conventional PTCA. Once the guiding catheter has been positioned and the lesion has been crossed with the 0.014-inch guide wire, the device is gently advanced until its nose cone passes into the proximal portion of the vessel. Gentle lifting on the guiding catheter helps align the device with the long axis of the vessel, and eases insertion. The device can then usually be advanced across the lesion by combining gentle forward pressure with continuous rotation. If these maneuvers are unsuccessful, predilatation or use of a smaller device may be necessary.

If the device does not pass easily, attempts to force it into the lesion or around curves in the vessel should be avoided because forceful advancement of the rigid device through a stiff, tortuous vessel could traumatize the vessel wall. Likewise, seating the guiding catheter deeply, a common maneuver in PTCA, should be avoided during atherectomy because the 11 Fr guiding catheter itself may cause injury to the coronary ostium.

Once the device is in position, it should be oriented under fluoroscopy so that the cutting window is seen in profile and is directed toward eccentric plaque deposits. Initial balloon

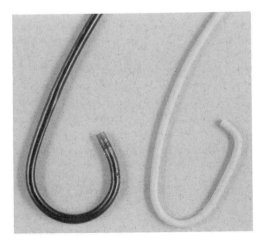

Fig. 27–14. Guiding catheters for directional coronary atherectomy (Devices for Vascular Intervention) are constructed with gentle curves rather than sharp angles. Left, the 11 Fr JCL 3.5 guiding catheter for coronary atherectomy; Right, the 9 Fr JL 4 guiding catheter for conventional PTCA.

inflation pressures of 10 to 20 psi are used to press the cutting window against the plaque as the motor-driven cutter is advanced slowly across the window. After each cut, the balloon is deflated and the device rotated 90 degrees to reorient the window within the lesion. The balloon is then inflated to 10 psi to prevent embolization of plaque as the cutter is retracted back to its starting position. Once the cutter is in its original position, the balloon is again inflated fully, allowing another cut to be made.

The device and guide wire should be removed from the patient every 4 to 6 cuts so that the collection chamber can be emptied completely. The number of passes and the final size of the device are determined based on the size of the reference segment and the presence of angiographic residual stenosis. Atherectomy is considered successful if there is tissue removal, the residual stenosis is less than 50% without resorting to PTCA after atherectomy, and there are no major complications (death, Q-wave myocardial infarction, or emergency coronary bypass surgery).

Preliminary Results of Atherectomy

Acute Angiographic Results. Over 1000 coronary atherectomy procedures have been performed with the Simpson AtheroCath with success in 85 to 90% of lesions. Coronary atherectomy may be particularly useful in situations in which clinical and anatomic features suggest an unfavorable short- or long-term outcome with conventional PTCA. Such features include a history of previous restenosis (which accounts for nearly half the patients referred for atherectomy at our institution), vein graft disease, ulcerated and eccentric plaques, long (>20 mm) or angulated lesions, and ostial location or total occlusion. Despite these unfavorable baseline characteristics, successful atherectomy typically results in a smooth-appearing lumen, without angiographic evidence for dissection[64,86,87] (Fig. 27–15).

At Beth Israel Hospital, we have performed coronary atherectomy in more than 100 patients. In our first year of experience, we had a success rate of 88%; a smooth lumen was present in 78% of cases after atherectomy, with mild focal dissection in only 3.9%. Successful atherectomy resulted in a decrease in diameter stenosis from 80% to 5% and an increase in absolute lumen diameter from 0.6 to 2.9 mm, compared to the reference segment of 3.1 mm. The absolute lumen diameters for the 6 Fr and 7 Fr devices were 2.6 mm and 3.7 mm respectively.[64]

The most common reason for unsuccessful atherectomy has been failure to cross the lesion with the atherectomy device because of tortuosity or calcification of the vessel proximal to the stenosis (10 to 15%). In one case of aorto-ostial graft stenosis, the initial atherectomy result was unsatisfactory, necessitating subsequent balloon dilatation.[64,86]

Complications. Based on data on more than 750 patients from a multicenter registry group, the incidence of complications following coronary atherectomy seems to be similar to that of conventional PTCA.[86] *Abrupt closure* requiring emergency bypass surgery occurred in approximately 3.1% of patients (usually secondary to dissection), but fell to less than 2% after an initial "learning curve." The incidence of *myocardial infarction* was approximately 5.1%, although Q-wave myocardial infarction occurred in 1.2% of patients. *Death* related to the procedure is rare and has been reported in one patient.

Despite the fact that deep arterial wall components are commonly seen on histological examination of atherectomy specimens, *coronary arterial perforation* is rare (< 0.5%), although it may occur and lead to coronary arteriovenous fistulae or pericardial tamponade requiring pericardiocentesis.

Distal embolization of plaque has occurred in 2 to 3% of patients, particularly in the setting of disease involving old saphenous vein bypass grafts. *Air embolization* occurred in 3% of patients in one study, and seems to have been related to leaks in the balloon, a problem with the early prototypes that appears to have been resolved.[64] Both of these problems may be managed acutely with intracoronary nitroglycerin and narcotic analgesics, and generally resolve within 10 to 15 minutes without sub-

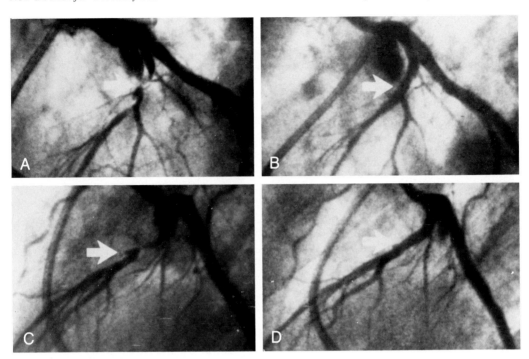

Fig. 27–15. Successful directional coronary atherectomy of a lesion unsuitable for conventional PTCA. A severe, eccentric, ulcerated lesion in the mid-LAD is shown in the LAO-cranial (A) and lateral projections (C). Following atherectomy (B and D), the lumen is smooth and there is no residual stenosis.

sequent sequelae. Prolonged ischemia may occur, however, and sometimes leads to non-Q-wave infarction.

Transient side branch occlusion has occurred in about 3 to 4% of patients after atherectomy, compared to 2% of patients after conventional PTCA.[3] It is generally recognized before the patient leaves the catheterization laboratory, and can be managed by conventional PTCA. *Thrombus formation* without impairment in flow occurred in 1.3% of patients, and coronary vasospasm (possibly caused by the vibration of the housing or rotation of the guide wire) occurred in 2.7% of patients and was readily relieved by intracoronary nitroglycerin.

Femoral vascular injury requiring blood transfusion or surgical repair under local anesthesia is a clear risk because of the large size of the arterial sheath, and has been seen in up to 4% of patients. Other complications, such as dysrhythmias, vagal reactions, and contrast reactions, occur with a frequency similar to that of conventional PTCA.

There have been a few cases of late *coronary aneurysm* formation following successful coronary atherectomy.[64] Similar angiographic findings have been reported after conventional balloon angioplasty, and may be secondary to thinning and stretching of the media, leading to weakening of the arterial wall.[88]

Late Follow-up. The initial hope was that coronary atherectomy would leave a large, smooth arterial lumen, resulting in a lower incidence of restenosis compared to conventional PTCA. Although long-term follow-up is limited for all of the new interventional devices, actuarial 6-month follow-up suggests that the overall restenosis rate following atherectomy is still 30%.[64] This restenosis rate may be somewhat lower than might be expected in similar patients who undergo conventional PTCA (~35 to 40%),[64] but controlled clinical trials are needed to evaluate this further. The restenosis rate following atherectomy of saphenous vein bypass grafts is high, and may approach 50% (Fig. 27–16).

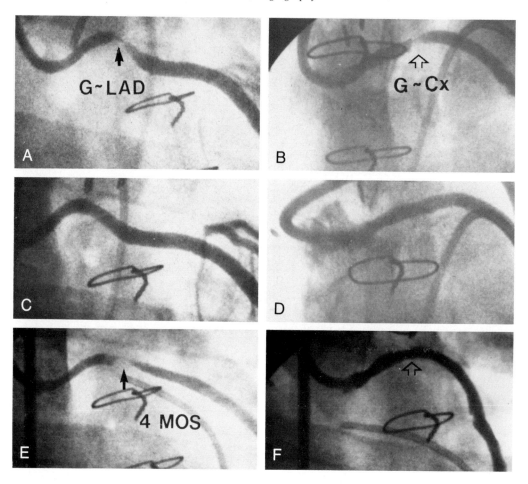

Fig. 27–16. Directional coronary atherectomy of saphenous vein graft lesions. Baseline angiography (A and B) reveals severe stenoses in the saphenous vein grafts to the LAD (A) and to the LCX (B). Successful atherectomy was performed on both grafts (C and D); 4 months later, restenosis occurred in the LAD graft, but the LCX graft remained patent (E and F). Atherectomy was repeated and follow-up angiography at 6 months (not shown) revealed continued patency of both grafts.

Clinical and angiographic factors that may be associated with a higher incidence of restenosis following atherectomy include the number of prior interventions on the treated vessel, the presence of diffuse disease, ostial location of the lesion, and stenosis involving a saphenous vein bypass graft. The depth of the atherectomy cut, manifested by the retrieval of deep wall components such as media and adventitia, may influence the subsequent development of restenosis.[64,89] Procedures characterized by more tissue removal rather than balloon dilatation seem to have a better long-term prognosis (see subsequent text).

Angiographic follow-up in patients without recurrent symptoms suggests that there may be mild proliferative intimal hyperplasia evident as slight loss in absolute lumen diameter by 6 months, corresponding to intimal thickening of approximately 500 to 600 μm.[64] It is not clear whether intimal hyperplasia will progress further over time.

Tissue Analysis. Atherectomy provides a unique opportunity for studying atherosclerosis in human coronary arteries. Standard light microscopy suggests that atherosclerotic plaque (94%), media (67%), and adventitia (27%) are commonly recovered, with an incidence that appears to be similar for primary and secondary lesions. It is remarkable, however, that retrieval of deep wall components including media and adventitia seems to be well tolerated,[64,90] with only rare occurrence of acute coronary artery perforation or late aneurysm formation.[64]

Study of tissue recovered during atherectomy has also provided some insight into the histology of restenosis. Our data suggest that intimal hyperplasia is present in 97% of restenosis-type lesions, but is also observed in 33% of primary lesions (see Fig. 27–5). These data suggest that intimal hyperplasia is highly correlated with restenosis, regardless of the type of procedure initially performed (PTCA, previous atherectomy, laser balloon angioplasty).[64]

In patients without prior intervention, the development of similar-appearing intimal hyperplasia may occur as a consequence of platelet or smooth muscle cell secretion of mitogenic factors similar to platelet-derived growth factors (PDGF) in response to a variety of arterial injuries, which might include such diverse insults as mechanical catheter interventions, immune response to transplanted tissue, or spontaneous plaque rupture or ulceration.

Insights into Mechanism

Conventional balloon dilatation results in cracking and disruption of atherosclerotic plaque, which separates plaque from the media and permits stretching of the vessel wall. These changes have been described as the "controlled injury" of successful balloon angioplasty.[61]

In contrast, atherectomy was designed to excise atherosclerotic plaque rather than to simply stretch the vessel wall. Preliminary observations using Doppler coronary stenosis velocity ratio measurements suggest that the cross-sectional area after atherectomy is larger than that following conventional PTCA.[91]

It is important, however, to point out that not all of the improvement in vessel lumen may be because of plaque removal alone. To study the relative contributions of tissue removal and balloon dilatation, we weighed tissue removed during our atherectomy procedures, which averaged approximately 20 mg. As a point of reference, complete atherectomy of an occluded vessel segment measuring 1 cm in length and 3.0 mm in diameter should require removal of tissue with a weight of approximately 70 mg, given a plaque specific gravity of 1 mg/ml.

These data suggest that part of the luminal enlargement following successful atherectomy is caused by "facilitated angioplasty" rather than pure atherectomy.[64] Excision of plaque and media during atherectomy may cause disruption of the internal elastic lamina and thinning of the vessel wall, increasing the radial compliance of the vessel. Subsequent balloon inflations may then cause focal stretching of the vessel wall in regions of increased radial compliance, further enlarging the lumen. Although the angiogram may demonstrate a large and smooth lumen, it fails to detect the presence of small amounts of residual plaque, and will not distinguish between complete plaque removal and partial balloon dilatation (Fig. 27–17). An "atherectomy index," the ratio of the removed tissue weight to the measured improvement in lumen volume, might provide data on the relative contributions of tissue removal and balloon dilatation in any given patient. This "atherectomy index" may be important in evaluating the subsequent course of the patient, particularly with regard to the potential for restenosis, but further study is needed. New intraluminal imaging techniques, such as angioscopy and ultrasound, may also prove to be useful adjuncts in the performance and evaluation of acute coronary atherectomy results.

Other Approaches to Atherectomy

Compared to that with the Simpson AtheroCath, experience with other atherectomy devices outside the peripheral circulation has remained quite limited. Fourrier and coworkers have reported their initial experience with the high-speed rotatory atherectomy device (Rotablator) in the coronary circulation.[80]

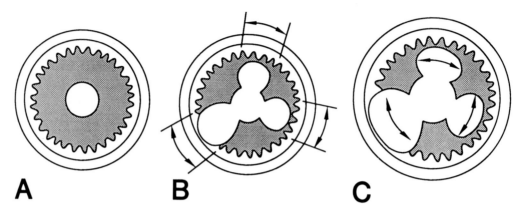

Fig. 27–17. Schematic representation of mechanism of directional coronary atherectomy and the concept of "facilitated angioplasty." A, Concentric stenosis in a coronary artery. The shaded area represents intimal plaque contained within the internal elastic lamina (wavy line). B, Excision of plaque and media at 8 o'clock results in thinning of the vessel wall; subsequent cuts at 1 and 4 o'clock do not penetrate the media. C, With disruption of the internal elastic lamina, radial compliance increases so that subsequent balloon inflations cause focal stretching of the vessel wall within the channels produced by previous atherectomy cuts ("facilitated angioplasty"). The resulting lumen appears smooth and free of residual stenosis in any angiographic projection, despite only partial atherectomy with the continued presence of residual intimal plaque.

Of the 12 patients treated, there were 2 failures and 5 additional patients had significant residual stenoses requiring conventional PTCA. The procedures were well tolerated, and no patients developed chest pain, ECG changes, or elevations in cardiac enzymes.

The *transluminal extraction catheter* has been used as both a primary revascularization technique and an adjunct to conventional balloon angioplasty in the peripheral circulation, with a success rate exceeding 90%. Improvement in luminal dimensions has been associated with objective improvement in ankle-brachial indices, with a low incidence of thrombosis, distal embolization, and perforation. In small groups of patients, the incidence of restenosis in peripheral vessels appears to be 20 to 30% at 6 months.[75] Preliminary results in the coronary circulation of the first 100 patients suggest the need for adjunctive PTCA in 50%, with a success rate of 93% and an angiographic restenosis rate of 43%.[92] Preliminary results are also encouraging with the BARD rotary atherectomy system in peripheral vessels, although it has not yet reached clinical trials in the coronary circulation.

Other rotational devices relying on plaque abrasion and pulverization have been used in patients with peripheral vascular disease. Initial postmortem studies of the Rotablator demonstrated luminal enlargement and recanalization of obstructed superficial femoral, popliteal, and tibial arteries.[79] Initial in vivo human studies were reported in a group of 7 patients with subtotal occlusion of one or more peripheral vessels, immediately before operative bypass. Nine vascular segments were treated successfully, leaving residual stenoses of less than 50%, without complications.[81]

The initial studies of the Kensey catheter reported use in 23 patients with symptomatic disease of the superficial femoral artery, including total occlusion in 10 patients. Successful revascularization was accomplished in 10 of 13 patients with subtotal occlusion and in 4 of 10 patients with total occlusion, but 11 of the 14 patients with successful results required concomitant conventional balloon angioplasty. No serious complications were reported after use of the Kensey catheter, although thrombosis and distal embolization occurred after subsequent balloon angioplasty,[83] and perforation is recognized as a potential complication.

Despite the encouraging immediate results with the Rotablator and the Kensey catheter in patients with peripheral vascular disease, a major concern with the use of these devices in the coronary circulation is the potential for distal embolization of pulverized plaque. Experimental studies have demonstrated that the particles are generally less than 10 μm in diameter, but the impact of showers of such particles to the distal coronary tree is not known.[79,80,82] Distal embolization, however, will certainly be better tolerated in the peripheral circulation, in which these devices may be more widely used.

CONCLUSION

Although intravascular stents and atherectomy devices appear to be promising new treatments for coronary artery disease, their ultimate role is still unknown. Early results indicate that these new technologies can be used safely, with complication rates similar to those associated with conventional PTCA. Immediate angiographic results are encouraging and show immediate luminal improvement and qualitative appearance often superior to those with conventional PTCA. Because of the predictability of these excellent angiographic results, these devices may come to be used selectively in lesions that appear to be unfavorable for conventional balloon dilatation, such as eccentric, ulcerated, or rigid plaques. Intravascular stents will almost certainly find an important application in the reversal of abrupt closure after PTCA.

The broader role of these new devices in the prevention and treatment of restenosis remains unknown. Despite early enthusiasm for the idea that devices that create a large, smooth lumen would lower the incidence of restenosis, the problem of restenosis remains. The relative merits of these devices in preventing this complication still needs to be established by randomized trials in large numbers of patients with adequate angiographic follow-up. In the meantime, the overall utility of these new investigational devices may be viewed with cautious optimism.

REFERENCES

1. Gruentzig AR, Senning A, Siegenthaler WE: Nonoperative dilatation of coronary artery stenosis—percutaneous transluminal coronary angioplasty. N Engl J Med 301:61, 1979.
2. Baim DS, Ignatius EJ: Use of percutaneous transluminal coronary angioplasty: results of a current survey. Am J Cardiol 61:3G, 1988.
3. Kent KM, et al: Percutaneous transluminal coronary angioplasty: Report from the registry of the National Heart, Lung, and Blood Institute. Am J Cardiol 41:2001, 1982.
4. Detre K, et al: Percutaneous transluminal coronary angioplasty in 1985–1986 and 1977–1981. N Engl J Med 318:265, 1988.
5. Safian RD, McCabe CH, Sipperly ME, McKay RG, Baim DS: Initial success and long-term follow-up of percutaneous transluminal coronary angioplasty in chronic total occlusions versus conventional stenoses. Am J Cardiol 61:23G, 1988.
6. Kereiakes DJ, et al: Angioplasty in total coronary artery occlusion: experience in 76 consecutive patients. J Am Coll Cardiol 6:526, 1985.
7. Reeder GS, et al: Angioplasty for aortocoronary bypass graft stenosis. Mayo Clinic Proc 61:14, 1986.
8. Douglas JS, et al: Percutaneous transluminal coronary angioplasty in patients with prior coronary bypass surgery. J Am Coll Cardiol 2:745, 1983.
9. Vlietstra RE, et al: Balloon angioplasty in multivessel coronary artery disease. Mayo Clin Proc 58:563, 1983.
10. Vandormael MG, et al: Immediate and short-term benefit of multi-lesion coronary angioplasty: Influence of degree of revascularization. J Am Coll Cardiol 6:983, 1985.
11. Topol EJ, et al: A randomized trial of immediate versus delayed elective angioplasty after intravenous tissue plasminogen activator in acute myocardial infarction. N Engl J Med 327:581, 1987.
12. The TIMI Study Group: Comparison of invasive and conservative strategies after treatment with intravenous tissue plasminogen activator in acute myocardial infarction. N Engl J Med 320:618, 1989.
13. Meier B, Gruentzig AR, Hollman J, Ischinger T, Bradford JM: Does length or eccentricity of coronary stenoses influence the outcome of transluminal dilatation? Circulation 67:497, 1983.
14. Leimgruber PP, et al: Restenosis after successful coronary angioplasty in patients with single vessel disease. Circulation 73:710, 1986.
15. Sinclair IN, McCabe CH, Sipperly ME, Baim DS: Predictors, therapeutic options, and long-term outcome of abrupt closure. Am J Cardiol 61:61G, 1988.
16. Bredlau CE, et al: In-hospital morbidity and mortality in patients undergoing elective coronary angioplasty. Circulation 72:1044, 1985.
17. Kaltenbach M, Kober G, Scherer D, Vallbracht C: Recurrence rate after successful coronary angioplasty. Eur Heart J 6:276, 1985.
18. Levine S, Ewels CJ, Rosing DR, Kent KM: Coronary angioplasty: clinical and angiographic follow-up. Am J Cardiol 55:673, 1985.
19. Holmes DR, et al: Restenosis after percutaneous transluminal coronary angioplasty (PTCA): A report from the PTCA registry of the National Heart, Lung, and Blood Institute. Am J Cardiol 53:77C, 1984.
20. Mabin TA, et al: Follow-up clinical results in patients

undergoing percutaneous transluminal coronary angioplasty. Circulation 71:754, 1985.

21. Ernst SMPG, et al: Long-term angiographic follow-up, cardiac events, and survival in patients undergoing percutaneous transluminal coronary angioplasty. Br Heart J 57:220, 1987.

22. Guiteras VP, et al: Restenosis after successful percutaneous transluminal coronary angioplasty: the Montreal Heart Institute experience. Am J Cardiol 60:50B, 1987.

23. Pinkerton CA, Slack JD, Orr CM, VanTassel JW, Smith ML: Percutaneous transluminal angioplasty in patients with prior myocardial revascularization surgery. Am J Cardiol 61:15G, 1988.

24. Ernst SMPG, et al: Percutaneous transluminal coronary angioplasty in patients with prior coronary artery bypass grafting. J Thorac Cardiovasc Surg 93:268, 1987.

25. Myler RK, et al: Multiple vessel coronary angioplasty: classification, results, and patterns of restenosis in 494 consecutive patients. Cathet Cardiovasc Diagn 13:1, 1987.

26. Cowley MJ, et al: Coronary angioplasty of multiple vessels: short-term outcome results. Circulation 72:1314, 1985.

27. Baim DS, Detre K, Kent K: Problems in the development of new devices for coronary intervention—Possible role for a multicenter registry. J Am Coll Cardiol 14:1389, 1989.

28. Siegel RJ, et al: Ultrasonic plaque ablation—A new method for recanalization of partially or totally occluded arteries. Circulation 78:1443, 1988

29. Rosenschein U, et al: Experimental ultrasonic angioplasty: Disruption of atherosclerotic plaques and thrombi in vitro and arterial recanalization in vivo. J Am Coll Cardiol 15:711, 1990.

30. Dotter CT, Judkins MP: Transluminal treatment of arteriosclerotic obstructions. Circulation 30:654, 1964.

31. Dotter CT: Transluminally placed coil-sprint endarterial tube grafts: long-term patency in canine popliteal artery. Invest Radiol 4:329, 1969.

32. Dotter CT, Buschmann RW, McKinney MK, Rosch J: Transluminal expandable nitinol coil stent grafting: Preliminary report. Radiology 147:259, 1983.

33. Maass D, et al: Transluminal implantation of self-adjusting expandable prostheses: Principles, techniques, and results. Prog Artif Org 2:979, 1983.

34. Charnsangavej C, et al: Stenosis of the vena cava: preliminary assessment of treatment with expandable metallic stents. Radiology 161:295, 1986.

35. Sigwart U, et al: Intravascular stents to prevent occlusion and restenosis after transluminal angioplasty. N Engl J Med 316:701, 1987.

36. Serruys PW, et al: Additional improvement of stenosis geometry in human coronary arteries by stenting after balloon dilatation. Am J Cardiol 61:71G, 1988.

37. Schatz RA, et al: Balloon-expandable intracoronary stents in the adult dog. Circulation 76:450, 1987.

38. Schatz RA, Palmaz JC, Tio F, Garcia O: Report of a new articulated balloon expandable intravascular stent (ABEIS). Circulation 78(Suppl II):II-449, 1988 (abstr).

39. Roubin GS, et al: Early and late results of intraco-

ronary arterial stenting after coronary angioplasty in dogs. Circulation 76:891, 1987.

40. Cragg A, et al: Nonsurgical placement of arterial endoprostheses: A new technique using nitinol wire. Radiology 147:261, 1983.

41. Schartz, RA: A view of vascular stents. Circulation 79:445, 1989.

42. DePalma VA, et al: Investigation of three surface properties of several metals and their relation to blood compatibility. J Biomed Mater Res Symp 3:37, 1972.

43. Baier RE, Dutton RC: Initial events in interaction of blood with a foreign surface. J Biomed Mater Res Symp 3:191, 1969.

44. Leung DY, Glagov S, Matthews MB: Cyclic stretching stimulates synthesis of matrix components by arterial smooth muscle cells in vitro. Science 191:475, 1976.

45. Schatz RA, Palmaz JC, Tio F, Garcia O: Report of a new radiopaque balloon expandable intravascular stent (RBEIS) in canine coronary arteries. Circulation 78(Suppl II):II-448, 1988 (abstr).

46. White CJ, et al: A new percutaneous balloon expandable stent. Circulation 78(Suppl II):II-409, 1988 (abstr).

47. White C, Chokshi SK, Isner JM: Pathologic findings after in-vivo placement of percutaneous balloon expandable tantalum stents. J Am Coll Cardiol 13:224A, 1989 (abstr).

48. Wright KC, et al: Percutaneous endovascular stents: An experimental evaluation. Radiology 156:69, 1985.

49. Rousseau H, et al: Self-expanding endovascular prosthesis: An experimental study. Radiology 164:709, 1987.

50. Palmaz JC, et al: Atherosclerotic rabbit aortas: Expandable intraluminal grafting. Radiology 160:723, 1986.

51. Palmaz JC, et al: Normal and stenotic renal arteries: Experimental balloon-expandable intraluminal stenting. Radiology 164:705, 1987.

52. Duprat G, et al: Flexible balloon-expanded stent for small vessels. Radiology 162:276, 1987.

53. Duprat G, et al: Self-expanding metallic stents for small vessels: an experimental evaluation. Radiology 162:469, 1987.

54. Palmaz JC, et al: Balloon expandable intra-arterial stents: effect of anticoagulation on thrombus formation. Circulation 76(Suppl IV):IV-45, 1987 (abstr).

55. Quigley PJ, et al: Myocardial protection during coronary angioplasty with an autoperfusion balloon catheter in humans. Circulation 78:1128, 1988.

56. Sigwart U, et al: Emergency stenting for acute occlusion after coronary balloon angioplasty. Circulation 78:1121, 1988.

57. Roubin GS, et al: Intracoronary stenting for acute closure following percutaneous transluminal coronary angioplasty (PTCA). Circulation 78(Suppl II):II-407, 1988 (abstr).

58. Sinclair IN, et al: Acute closure post PTCA successfully treated with laser balloon angioplasty. Circulation 80(Suppl II): II-476, 1989 (abstr).

59. Maynar M, et al: Percutaneous atherectomy as an alternative treatment for postangioplasty obstructive intimal flaps. Radiology 170:1029, 1989.

60. Austin GE, et al: Intimal proliferation of smooth mus-

cle cells as an explanation for recurrent coronary artery stenosis after percutaneous transluminal coronary angioplasty. J Am Coll Cardiol 6:36, 1985.

61. McBride W, Lange RA, Hillis LD: Restenosis after successful coronary angioplasty. N Engl J Med 318:1734, 1988.
62. Fuster V, Adams PC, Badimon JJ, Chesebro JH: Platelet-inhibitor drugs: role in coronary artery disease. Prog Cardiovasc Dis 29:325, 1987.
63. Libby P, Warner SJC, Salomon RN, Birinyi LK: Production of platelet-derived growth factor-like mitogen by smooth muscle cells from human atheroma. N Engl J Med 318:1493, 1988.
64. Safian RD, et al: Coronary atherectomy: Clinical, angiographic, and histologic findings and some observations regarding mechanism. Circulation 82:69, 1990.
65. Serruys PW, et al: Stenting of coronary arteries—Are we the sorcerer's apprentice? European Heart J 10:774, 1989.
66. Sigwart U, Urban P, Sadeghi H, Kappenberger, L: Implantation of 100 coronary artery stents: Learning curve for the incidence of acute early complications. J Am Coll Cardiol 13:107A, 1989.
67. Levine MJ, et al: Clinical and angiographic results of quantitative balloon-expandable intra-coronary stents in right coronary artery stenoses. J Am Coll Cardiol 16:332, 1990.
68. Schatz RA, et al: Short-term clinical results and complications with the Palmaz-Schatz coronary stent. J Am Coll Cardiol, July–August 1990 (Abstr).
69. Urban P, et al: Intravascular stenting for stenosis of aortocoronary venous bypass grafts. J Am Coll Cardiol 13:1085, 1989.
70. Serruys PW, et al: Stent implantation for the treatment of coronary artery bypass graft stenosis. J Am Coll Cardiol 13:107A, 1989.
71. Sigwart U, Urban P: Use of coronary stents following balloon angioplasty. *In* Braunwald E, ed. Heart Disease—Update. Philadelphia, WB Saunders, 1988, p 111.
72. Ellis SG, et al: Intracoronary stenting to prevent restenosis: Preliminary results of a multicenter study using the Palmaz-Schatz stent suggest benefit in selected high risk patients. J Am Coll Cardiol 15:118A, 1990 (abstr).
73. Urban P, Sigwart U, Kaufmann U, Kappenberger L: Restenosis within coronary stents: Possible effect of previous angioplasty. J Am Coll Cardiol 13:107A, 1989 (abstr).
74. Simpson JB, et al: Transluminal atherectomy for occlusive peripheral vascular disease. Am J Cardiol 61:96G, 1988.
75. Greenfield JC, Jr: An explosion of technology. Am J Cardiol 62(Part II):3F, 1988.
76. Smalling RW, et al: Initial experience with a flexible rotational atherectomy system designed for removal of coronary and small peripheral artery atheromas. J Am Coll Cardiol 13:223A, 1989 (abstr).
77. Battler A, et al: Bard rotary atherectomy system (BRAS) in normal canine coronary arteries. J Am Coll Cardiol 13:223A, 1989 (abstr).
78. Leyser LJ, et al: Evaluation of a coronary lysing system: Results of a preclinical safety and efficacy study. Cath Cardiol Diag 12:246, 1986.
79. Ahn SS, Auth D, Marcus DR, Moore WS: Removal of focal atheromatous lesions by angioscopically guided high-speed rotary atherectomy. J Vasc Surg 7:292, 1988.
80. Fourrier JL, et al: Percutaneous coronary rotational atherectomy in humans. Preliminary report. J Am Coll Cardiol 14:1278, 1989.
81. Zacca NM, et al: Treatment of symptomatic peripheral atherosclerotic disease with a rotational atherectomy device. Am J Cardiol 63:77, 1989.
82. Kensey KR, Nash JE, Abrahams C, Zarins CK: Recanalization of obstructed arteries with a flexible, rotating tip catheter. Radiology 165:387, 1987.
83. Snyder SO, et al: The Kensey catheter: Preliminary results with a transluminal atherectomy tool. J Vasc Surg 8:541, 1988.
84. Wholey MH: Advances in balloon technology and reperfusion devices for peripheral circulation. Am J Cardiol 61:87G, 1988.
85. Valbracht C, et al: Results of low speed rotational angioplasty for chronic peripheral occlusion. Am J Cardiol 62:935, 1988.
86. Vlietstra RE, et al: Complications with directional coronary atherectomy. Experience at eight centers. Circulation 80(Suppl II):II-582, 1989 (abstr).
87. Kaufmann UP, et al: Coronary atherectomy: First 50 patients at the Mayo Clinic. Mayo Clin Proc 64:747, 1989.
88. Hill JA, et al: Coronary arterial aneurysm formation after balloon angioplasty. Am J Cardiol 52:261, 1983.
89. Simpson JB, et al: Restenosis following successful directional coronary atherectomy. Circulation 80(Suppl II):II-582, 1989 (abstr).
90. Garratt KN, et al: Safety of percutaneous coronary atherectomy with deep arterial resection. Am J Cardiol 64:538, 1989.
91. White N, Jr: Greater improvement in coronary flow velocity with atherectomy compared to angioplasty. J Am Coll Cardiol 13:108A, 1989 (abstr).
92. Stack RS, et al: Multicenter registry of coronary atherectomy using the transluminal extraction-endarterectomy catheter. J Am Coll Cardiol 15:196A, 1990 (abstr).

28

Laser Angioplasty

ARLENE B. LEVINE and J. RICHARD SPEARS

L aser is an acronym for light amplification by stimulated emission of radiation. The conceptual framework was initially described by Albert Einstein in his thesis on the theory of light in 1917[1] and refined by the Nobel laureates Charles Hard Townes and Arthur L. Shawlow in 1958. In 1960, Theodore H. Maiman was the first to actually construct a laser using a synthetic ruby crystal.[2] Applications of lasers in medicine followed quickly, with laser technology finding uses in ophthalmology, dermatology, gastroenterology, gynecology, otolaryngology, neurology, urology, pulmonology, and general surgery. The laser's potential for relieving obstructive atherosclerotic vascular disease was seen almost immediately, but testing and application were delayed until advances in fiber optic technology allowed the transluminal delivery of laser irradiation to the target site.

LASER ENERGY

A laser is basically an optical resonator cavity containing a lasing medium. An energy source pumps energy into the lasing medium. The atomic or molecular species in this medium absorb the incident energy and are raised to an excited state. Once excited, they may return to a lower energy state by either of two distinctive mechanisms: (1) The excited species may emit light energy spontaneously; (2) They may emit energy when triggered by elec-

tromagnetic radiation of the proper frequency. The second process is described as "stimulated emission," and requires that the triggering radiation be of the same wavelength as the light that the lasing medium would emit spontaneously. Interestingly, photons produced by stimulated emission propagate in the same direction as the stimulating wave and are identical in polarization and phase *(coherent)*.

Most atoms or molecular species in any substance reside in a low energy ground state, and turn absorbed light into heat. What distinguishes a lasing medium from other substances is that the pumping energy forces a substantial number of atoms or molecules into an excited (high energy) state, leaving lower energy states relatively depopulated. This is termed "population inversion," a situation that makes it possible for an incident photon of proper frequency to trigger the emission of stimulated photons. If the lasing medium is placed within an optical resonator cavity (bounded by parallel mirrors at either end), the emitted electromagnetic radiation will reflect and oscillate between the mirrors as additional stimulated emission occurs, and the light builds in intensity. If one of the mirrors is partially transmissive, some of the light will escape as a beam that is *monochromatic* (one wavelength) and both temporally and spatially coherent. Such a light energy source can be focused to small spots that have extremely high power density, making laser irradiation a suitable in-

492

strument for ablating plaque and recanalizing obstructive vascular disease.[3]

Laser Tissue Interactions

A vast array of continuous wave and pulsed, ultraviolet, visible, near and mid infrared lasers have been investigated for applications in ablative angioplasty. To assess the effect of various wavelengths and different dosimetries of laser irradiation on the target tissue, the following processes need to be examined: (1) the distribution of laser light in tissue, (2) the rate of heat generation in tissue due to light absorption, (3) the dissipation of heat to cooler regions, (4) thermal tissue injury, and (5) tissue ablation.[4]

Light distribution in tissue caused by laser irradiation is expressed as fluence rate $I = (W/cm^2)$, a function of both the laser beam (the spot size, divergence, and wavelength) and the optical properties of the tissue (absorption and scattering).[5]

Absorbed light is converted to heat in tissue with the rate of heat generation (W/cm^3) equal to the tissue absorption coefficient A (1/cm) times the fluence rate I. Deposited heat causes increased tissue temperature, which leads to conductive heat transfer to cooler tissue regions, and to dehydration and cellular water vaporization as tissue temperatures reach 100°C. More rapid temperature increases may result in a nonequilibrium reaction with superheating to temperatures in excess of 100°C before actual ablation.[4,6]

About 4% of the incident beam is reflected, with the remainder of the beam transmitted into tissue and variably absorbed or scattered. The degree of absorption and scattering is a function of the laser beam wavelength relative to the tissue optical properties. *Ultraviolet* irradiation is highly absorbed by tissue, leading to direct excitation of electronic transitions in proteins with molecular disruption. At *visible* wavelengths, tissue absorption is low and is determined by the absorption spectra of specific chromophores. In the *infrared,* tissue absorption is primarily determined by tissue water content. Thus, wavelengths in both the ultraviolet (193 nm, 248 nm, and 308 nm excimer lasers) and mid and far infrared (2.94 μm erbium:YAG and 10.6 μm CO_2 lasers) are highly absorbed with penetration depths ranging between 1 to 20 μm, and insignificant scattering.[5]

For lasers in the visible range (between 450 nm and 590 nm) including the flashlamp-pumped dye laser (480 nm) and argon ion laser (488 to 514 nm), absorption and scattering coefficients are of equal magnitude so that laser light penetrates to approximately 0.5 to 2.5 mm as it is multiply scattered. Backscattering accounts for up to 40% of the incident beam.

In the near infrared (from 590 nm to 1.5 μm, including the 1.06 μm and 1.32 μm Nd:YAG laser), scattering predominates and tissue penetration depth ranges from 2 to 15 mm. Backscattering may account for up to 80% of the incident beam.[5]

Continuous wave (CW) ablation refers to continuous irradiation at any wavelength, as well as to exposure durations or pulse frequencies at which thermal diffusion determines tissue temperature. Depending on irradiation conditions, preablation plaque surface temperatures as high as 300°C have been recorded. At visible and near infrared continuous wave irradiation, maximal tissue temperatures develop just beneath the surface because of conductive cooling of the tissue surface itself. The critically heated subsurface tissue may evaporate explosively, and be blown out of the tissue, creating mechanical tissue tears.[7] The histology of CW ablation is also characterized by variable degrees of crater carbonization, subjacent vacuolization, and tissue coagulation (Fig. 28–1).[7,8] The size of the surrounding zone of thermal injury is inversely related to tissue light absorption.

Efforts to lower the risk of vessel perforation by excessive local thermal injuries have focused on using the highly absorbed CO_2 laser. Conventional silica fiber optics do not transmit CO_2 laser irradiation, but recently developed nontoxic, flexible, and insoluble silver halide fibers (AgCl:AgBr) have been used successfully to transmit CO_2 laser light transluminally

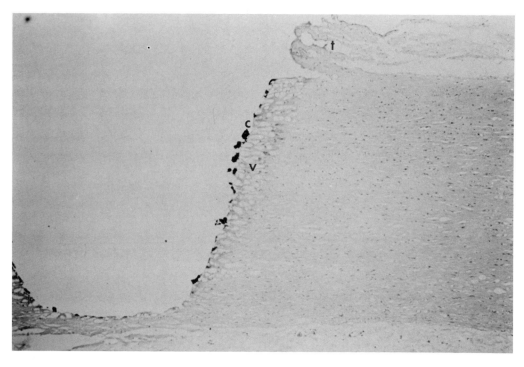

Fig. 28–1. Normal human aorta irradiated by 488 to 514.5 nm argon ion laser irradiation delivered by 400 μm fiber optic in air. The ablation crater is surrounded by discrete carbonization (c), vacuolization (v) with subjacent coagulation, and extensive subsurface tissue tears (t).

and ablate plaque in human atherosclerotic xenografted arteries implanted in dogs.[9–11]

Alternatively, *pulsed laser* ablation has been shown by Deckelbaum, Isner, and Clarke[12,13] to minimize or eliminate thermal boundary injury, irrespective of laser wavelength as long as optimal dosimetry is used. Specifically, peak power density must be sufficiently high to achieve ablation and pulse repetition rate must be sufficiently low to prevent tissue heating.[12,13] Such optimized dosimetry results in pulse-per-pulse complete ablation of the irradiated tissue volume with sufficient heat dissipation between pulses to minimize surrounding thermal injury.[14–16]

Additional nonthermal mechanisms that may play a role in pulsed laser tissue ablation are photoablation and photodisruption. Photoablation may contribute to tissue removal with pulsed ultraviolet irradiation, where sufficient photon energy is deposited in tissue to disrupt peptide bonds and cause ejection of molecular fragments. Photodisruption may

cause tissue fragmentation by plasma-generated shock waves created by high peak power pulses.[5,17,18] This phenomenon has been observed with the microsecond pulsed flashlamp-pumped dye laser. The resulting histology, although free of characteristic thermal injury, may reveal significant tissue tearing. Proper dosimetry of a pulsed laser is thus essential to effect a clean tissue cut. Inappropriate dosimetry has been shown to result in excessive thermal or mechanical tear injuries (Fig. 28–2).

The four most important excited dimer (i.e., excimer) gases are ArF, KrF, XeCl, and XeF, which have wavelengths of 193, 248, 308, and 355 nm respectively. Although 193 nm irradiation produces the cleanest, most knife-like tissue ablation, existing fiber technology cannot transmit sufficient pulse energies at that wavelength for ablation. Furthermore, concern about the mutagenic and carcinogenic potential at 193 nm has steered investigators toward longer ultraviolet wavelengths. The XeCl excimer laser at 308 nm (Advanced Interven-

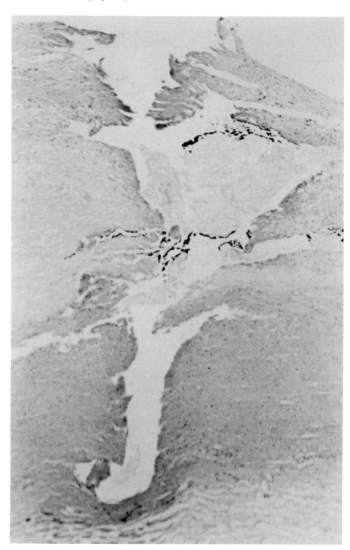

Fig. 28–2. Diseased human aorta irradiated under normal saline with 2.1 μm holmium:YAG laser irradiation. In addition to a 200 to 300 μm zone of surrounding coagulative thermal injury, the ablation crater is marked by extensive tissue tears.

tional Systems, Inc., Irvine, CA) has been studied extensively for laser angioplasty. Although the threshold for ablation of calcific plaque is higher than for normal tissue, 308 nm excimer laser light can effectively cut through even calcified tissue.[19,20] Stretching the pulse duration (from 15 nsec to 100 to 250 nsec) has allowed higher energy densities to be transmitted fiberoptically.[21] The initial clinical results with this laser in peripheral and coronary arteries have been promising.[22,23]

The microsecond pulsed flashlamp pumped dye laser (MCM, Mountain View, CA) effectively ablates atheromatous and calcific target tissue as well as venous thrombi.[24–26] The as-

sociated plasma formation and secondary photodisruption may cause significant mechanical trauma to tissue even in the absence of thermal injury.

Efforts to reproduce the clean tissue ablation of excimer lasers by infrared pulsed lasers (and avoid potential ultraviolet-associated carcinogenicity) remain in the investigational phase. The near infrared-pulsed laser systems have the additional advantages of being less expensive, more compact, rugged, and easier to handle than excimer laser systems. At 2.94 μm, the erbium:YAG laser is highly absorbed by tissue water. Surprisingly, erbium:YAG laser cuts are surrounded by a 10 to 50 μm thermal injury zone. Narrower, 5 to 10 μm injury zones were encountered with the Q-switched erbium:YAG.[16,27,28] Unfortunately, currently available silica fiber optics do not transmit 2.94 μm irradiation. Investigations with the 2.1 μm holmium:YAG laser are currently being pursued, and other pulsed infrared lasers, particularly around the 1.9 μm water absorption peak, may prove promising in the future.

In summary, efforts at optimizing laser-tissue interactions to control intravascular radiative injuries suggest the use of a highly absorbed laser wavelength, delivered in pulsed fashion at sufficiently high power density and slow repetition rate to maximize ablation and minimize heating. Pulsed delivery has the additional advantage of delivering high peak powers, which are more effective at ablating heavily calcified lesions. At present, a near ultraviolet or infrared pulsed laser appears to be the most attractive laser source for effective ablation.

ABLATIVE LASER ANGIOPLASTY

The last decade has seen the overwhelming growth and success of percutaneous transluminal coronary angioplasty (PTCA). Growing clinical experience and technological refinements have rendered even complex multivessel coronary artery disease amenable to PTCA. Expensive laser technology will play a role only in instances when conventional PTCA techniques may fail, namely, in the recanalization of chronic total occlusions, the treatment of diffuse atherosclerotic disease, the recanalization of severely stenosed or occluded coronary artery bypass grafts, and possibly the prevention of the 25% to 35% angioplasty restenosis rate.[29,30]

Early work by Macruz,[31] Choy,[32] and Lee et al.[33] demonstrated successful plaque ablation using fiberoptically transmitted Argon laser light. Despite the extravagant initial expectations for laser angioplasty, early in vivo experience in both the animal lab and the clinical setting resulted in sobering complications. A high incidence of perforation (Fig. 28–3), both mechanical and radiative in origin, has

been observed during experimental canine coronary angioplasty procedures[34,35] as well as during early clinical coronary laser angioplasty procedures.[36,37] Restenosis occurred in all patients studied by Choy et al. 25 days postprocedure.[36] Aneurysm formation was reported by Lee.[38] Mechanical and laser-induced perforations, vessel spasm, procedural pain, and vessel reocclusion were also observed in the initial clinical trials for peripheral arterial disease[39–41] using continuous wave irradiation by means of bare fiber optics.

Several approaches have sought to improve the safety and efficacy of ablative laser angioplasty. These approaches have focused on the following areas: Fiber optic catheter modifications; targeting approaches and imaging techniques; and attempts to optimize laser tissue interactions.

Fiber Optic Catheter Modifications

Sanborn and Cumberland pioneered an alternative approach to the use of bare fiber optics for laser recanalization.[42] The distal tip of a 300 micron core silica fiber optic was encased in a bullet-shaped metal alloy (Laserprobe, Trimedyne, Santa Ana, CA) to render the fiber optic catheter tip radiopaque and mechanically atraumatic (Fig. 28–4).[42,43] Activation of a continuous wave argon or Nd:YAG laser source results in heating of the metal tip to approximately 400°C.[7] It was hoped that probe heating would be less damaging than uncontrolled radiative deposition of laser energy in vascular tissue.

In practical applications, a ''cold'' Laserprobe catheter is often capable of recanalizing total occlusions by simple mechanical stiffness. When the probe is heated, careful application of pressure enhances its ablative potential by compressing the vacuolated, coagulated tissue and decreasing the probe-tissue thermal resistance.[7] The Laserprobe, however, is likely to stick to the vessel wall during its heating and cooling phases (between 100 and 200°C), and must therefore be moved to and fro continually. If probe sticking occurs, it can be reversed by briefly reheating the

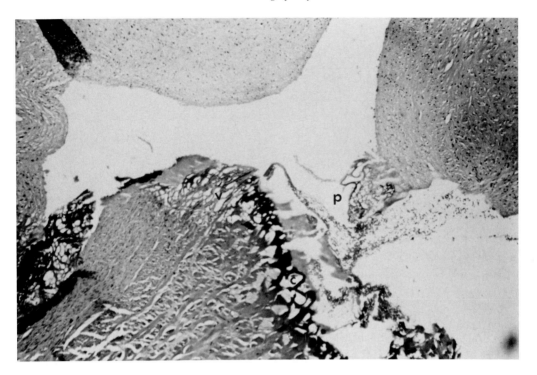

Fig. 28–3. Perforation in a subtotally occluded miniswine iliac artery following 60 J of argon ion laser irradiation delivered by 1.5 mm silica ball-tip fiber optic. The site of perforation (p) is marked by the extravasation of red blood cell debris. It is surrounded by an extensive zone of carbonization (c) and extensive vacuolization (v) and coagulation.

probe.[7,44,45] Importantly, the operator must limit the amount of thermal energy transmitted conductively into tissue; otherwise, nonablative heating will result in extensive radial vascular thermal injury.[44]

In the largest published series using percutaneous peripheral laser thermal angioplasty followed by balloon dilation, Sanborn et al. achieved a 77% success rate in recanalizing subtotal and total femoral-popliteal occlusions. Uniform success was seen for short (1 to 3 cm) total occlusions, 70% success for medium-length (4 to 7 cm), and 66% success for long (over 7 cm) occlusions. Although a 4% vessel perforation rate was encountered, no patient required emergency surgery. The 1-year cumulative clinical patency rate was 77%, broken down as 95% and 93% for stenoses and short occlusions respectively, 76% for medium-length occlusions, and 58% for long total occlusions.[46] These 1-year patency rates compared favorably to historical balloon PTA controls and appeared to confirm earlier impressions derived from animal studies which suggest less restenosis with thermal as compared to balloon angioplasty.[43]

Laser thermal coronary angioplasty, using a wire-guided approach, has had a lower success rate and a higher incidence of complications.[47–49] Spasm, myocardial infarction, side branch occlusion, procedural vessel wall adhesion of the fiber optic probe, and perforation have been observed. These clinical observations are not surprising in view of numerous in vitro studies documenting tissue adhesion of the heated tip, endothelial charring with extensive subjacent coagulation, and increased vasoreactivity following the thermal insult.[7,50] Furthermore, the thermal probe is incapable of ablating calcific plaque which mechanically deflects the probe and contributes to coronary perforation.[51,52]

Alternative radiofrequency, catalytic and electrical energy sources for thermal angioplasty have been developed.[53] A hybrid probe (Spectraprobe, Trimedyne, Santa Ana, CA)

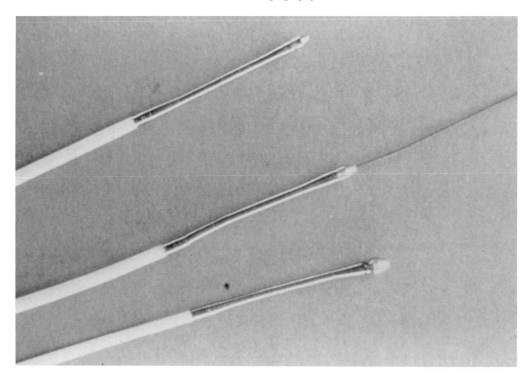

Fig. 28–4. Newer generation metal-tipped fiber optic Laserprobes, 1.3, 1.6, and 1.9 mm in size.

features a sapphire lens near the tip of the probe to combine both optical and thermal means of revascularization, and has been introduced into clinical use.[54]

More recently, sapphire tips have been affixed to the distal end of a fiber optic. The artificial sapphire crystal (Al_2O_3) has been used in surgical practice for delivery of Nd:YAG laser light for incision and hemostasis. The sapphire contact probe (Surgical Laser Technologies, Malvern, PA) has good mechanical strength, a high melting point (2,040°C), and low thermal conductivity.[55,56] Sapphire tips, typically of rounded configuration, are connected to the fiber optic catheter. Distal saline perfusate serves to protect the fiber optics. Depending on tip geometry, sapphire probes have been reported to absorb up to 10% to 50% of incident Nd:YAG laser energy. As they age, they become even less transmissive to laser light.[55] Thus, sapphire tips may reach temperatures as high as 250°C in vitro, suggesting that the mechanism of sapphire probe tissue ablation may be similar to the Laserprobe's thermal effect.[57]

Clinically, sapphire tip adhesion to tissue has been a less prominent problem, although procedural discomfort has been noted by patients. The sapphire tip has been used primarily in conjunction with the continuous wave Nd:YAG laser as energy source, although the pulsed Nd:YAG laser has been used successfully as well. The most extensive clinical experience with peripheral sapphire tip angioplasty has been in Europe, where comparable success rates (78% and 82%) have been obtained in the recanalization of total occlusions of femoral or popliteal arteries using either the Laserprobe or sapphire tip devices respectively. The patency rate at 6 months was 84%, and perforations occurred in 14% and 8% for the two tips.[58,59]

A bilaterally convex sapphire lens, emitting a 40° divergent beam, has been used by the Lastac System (GV-Medical, Inc., Minneapolis, MN), with an argon laser source. The fiber optic is centered by a coaxial balloon catheter. Blood is replaced by saline irrigation at 10 to 50 cc/min, while noncontact irradiations are performed at 10 W for 1 to 2 seconds with the lens tip positioned 2 mm from the target tissue. The system has been used clinically in the recanalization of both peripheral and coronary vessels as well as saphenous vein bypass grafts.[60–62] To date, approximately 1000 peripheral and 110 coronary laser procedures have been performed on subtotal and total occlusions, with 84% success in peripheral and 77% in coronary recanalizations. Perforations occurred in 2.1% in the periphery.

Although the Lastac System has been successful clinically, the laser wavelength, dosimetry, and noncontact approach are suboptimal for the ablation of complex calcific disease. The system does not incorporate wire guidance; substantial amounts of flush fluid may be required during prolonged procedures, and only total occlusions can be accessed that allow vessel occlusion by the centering balloon catheter in the proximal vessel portion for substantial amounts of time.

Fused silica ball-tipped optical fibers (Fig. 28–5) in coaxial array with a balloon catheter have been used in experimental animal and limited clinical studies of laser-assisted balloon angioplasty (Fig. 28–6). In 10 patients, a flashlamp-pumped pulsed dye laser at 480 nm was used with a 3 mm ball-tipped quartz fiber, achieving successful recanalization in 7 of 10 patients.[63] Using a pulsed Nd:YAG laser and a 1.5 mm ball-tipped 320 μm silica fiber optic catheter, we successfully recanalized 6 of 9 ileofemoral total occlusions in 8 patients at our institution with continued patency at 3 months' follow-up in all successful patients (Fig. 28–7). The ball-tipped fiber is advanced with mild to moderate pressure into the total

occlusion, with a balloon catheter as a centering device. In the limited number of cases studied, there was no device adhesion to the vessel wall, no associated vessel spasm, thrombosis, or patient discomfort. No perforations were observed.

This lens-tipped fiber optic catheter concept, although of value in straight-segment ileofemoral disease, has limited applicability in tortuous below-the-knee trifurcation vessel disease or in the coronary circulation because of lack of steerability or guide wire availability. Additionally, a significant drawback of lens-tip fibers appears to be tip damage incurred by back-reflected and backscattered light at poorly absorbed laser wavelengths. Because such tip damage alters the optical and thermal properties of the lens device, a feedback feature warning the operator of lens damage may have to be incorporated in these devices. The atraumatic rounded design of catheter tips has dramatically reduced the incidence of vessel perforation, and appears to improve intraluminal tracking of the device. Additionally, the fiber optic tip allows the size of the ablation neolumen to exceed the fiber optic diameter by means of thermal or optical effects.

Wire guidance is an important safety feature, but (except for recent modifications in the Laserprobe) none of the lens-tipped catheters described incorporate this feature. In animal studies, an early prototype wire-guided fiber optic appeared to increase fiber optic catheter steerability and decrease the perforation risk by enhancing coaxial alignment with the vessel lumen.[64]

More sophisticated, multifiber laser cathe-

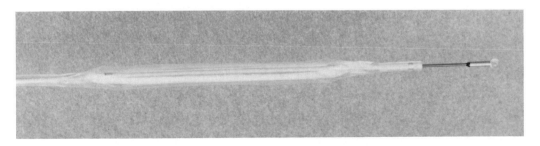

Fig. 28–5. 1.5 mm fused silica ball-tipped 300 μm fiber optic in coaxial array with a 5 mm Schwarten balloon catheter.

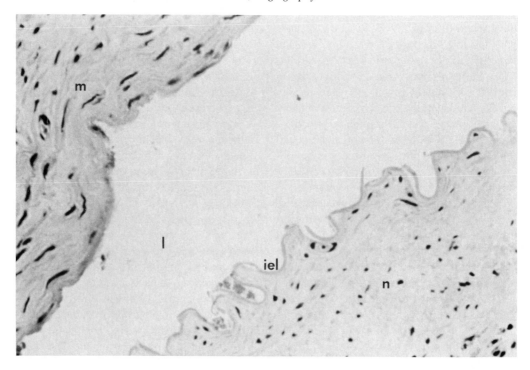

Fig. 28–6. Vessel lumen (l) created by serial 50 J pulse trains of 1.09 μm Nd:YAG laser irradiation delivered by means of 1.5 mm silica ball-tipped fiber optic catheter in a total iliac artery occlusion of a hypercholesterolemic miniswine. There is minimal thermal injury along the vessel neolumen. Interestingly, the fiber optic passed along the internal elastic lamina (iel) separating the normal media (m) from the occlusive neo-intima (n), following a path of least mechanical resistance.

ters with central guide wire lumina have been developed with the aim of increasing laser neoluminal diameter. Argon, and more recently holmium:YAG laser irradiation, delivered by means of four fiber optics, has been used in peripheral and coronary recanalization work (U.S.C.I., Inc., Billerica, MA).[65] Twelve 200 μm optical fibers surrounding a central guide wire channel in a 5 Fr catheter (Fig. 28–8) have been used to deliver 308 nm XeCl excimer laser irradiation for peripheral and coronary revascularization with 118 of 143 successful coronary and 54 of 72 successful peripheral procedures (Advanced Interventional Systems, Irvine, CA) at the time of this writing. Two and 2.4 mm diameter multifiber catheters are similarly in investigational use, increasing the percentage of "stand-alone" procedures not requiring follow-up balloon dilatations. Similar multifiber catheter systems have been developed by Spectranetics (Colo-

rado Springs, CO) for use with an XeCl laser. A 14 fiber, flexible 4.8 Fr catheter, over a regular or fiber optic guide wire, has been used to deliver the 480 nm flashlamp-pumped dye laser in initial coronary revascularization procedures (MCM Laboratories, Inc., Mountain View, CA).

The multifiber array catheters allow excellent catheter flexibility and steerability. Mechanisms to increase effective spot size, however, must be developed to avoid the necessity of follow-up balloon or mechanical endarterectomy angioplasty.

Imaging and Targeting Approaches

Single and biplane fluoroscopic imaging clearly do not adequately delineate the course of a totally occluded vessel, although they have been useful in guiding percutaneous revascularization attempts in straight, totally oc-

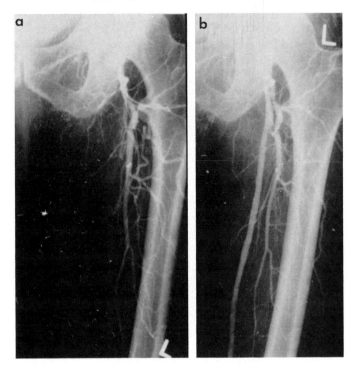

Fig. 28–7. a, Angiogram demonstrating total occlusion of the superficial femoral artery in a patient before laser-assisted angioplasty. b, Angiogram at 3 months following pulsed Nd:YAG laser-assisted angioplasty performed by retrograde popliteal approach demonstrating continued patency of the successfully recanalized superficial femoral artery.

cluded peripheral and coronary vascular segments. Additional targeting and imaging techniques must be developed to assist the operator in recanalizing curvilinear or tortuous total occlusions, particularly in the coronary circulation, where perforation may be fatal.

Targeting approaches appear to be attractive. If a laser wavelength were found to ablate selectively only atheroma, with no effect on normal vessel wall, arterial perforation could be avoided without the requirement for sophisticated, expensive imaging techniques.

Studies comparing the optical properties of plaque and normal vessel wall have disappointingly failed to reveal any significant differences in their absorption spectra.[6] Prince et al. identified a window of increased light absorption by yellow plaque between 420 to 530 nm,[26] because of the chromophore carotene. Using a 482 nm flashlamp-pumped dye laser, they found a lower ablation threshold for plaque versus normal vessel. Unfortunately, this selectivity applies only to fibrofatty yellow plaque, and is of limited value in the clinical setting.

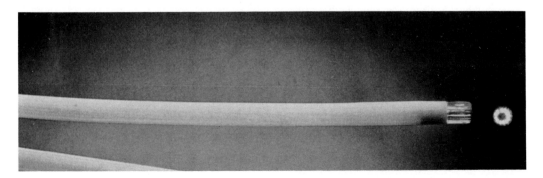

Fig. 28–8. Multifiber laser catheter with central guide wire lumen. Twelve 200 μm optical fibers in circular array within a 5 Fr catheter surround a central channel to accommodate a 0.018″ guide wire.

Different investigators have sought to alter exogenously the optical properties of plaque. Hematoporphyrin derivative (HPD), a photosensitive material producing cytotoxic singlet oxygen upon light exposure,[66] has been found to be taken up selectively by plaque.[67] Despite initially promising results in animal models,[68,69] photodynamic therapy via diffuse 631 nm intravascular irradiation has not found clinical application. Interestingly, Pollock and Berns found a significantly lower ablation threshold for HPD-labled plaque versus normal vessel tissue at the argon wavelength.[70] The requirement for prolonged systemic loading with HPD and the resultant systemic photosensitization detract from the appeal of this targeting approach. Other compounds selectively taken up by plaque have been tetracycline, beta carotene, and psoralenes.[71,72]

Because of failure of effective tissue targeting, alternative approaches to guide laser ablation are currently under investigation. These include angioscopic imaging, fluorescence spectroscopy, and endovascular ultrasonography. Angioscopy, pioneered by Spears,[73] has been used in conjunction with laser angioplasty to visualize atheromatous target tissue pre- and postablation.[74–76] Currently available angioscopes are sufficiently miniaturized (4.3 Fr), and incorporate lumina for guide wires, occlusive balloon, flushing, and illumination and imaging fiber bundles (ACS, Santa Clara, CA). Angioscopy can detect the presence of intraluminal thrombus, ulcerated plaque, dissection planes,[77] and tissue charring following thermal angioplasty.[75,76] Nonlinear magnification and geometric image distortion, however, preclude the use of angioscopy for quantitative applications.[73] Most importantly, angioscopy visualizes only the inner vessel lumen, and is incapable of estimating plaque or vessel wall thickness, or of delineating the course of a totally occluded vessel segment. These considerations limit the clinical applicability of angioscopically assisted laser angioplasty.

Interrogation of the autofluoresence spectrum of normal and diseased vessel wall as elicited by a variety of low-power laser sources (nitrogen, He-Cd and argon laser) has been shown to discriminate between normal wall, thrombus, and atheroma both in vitro and in vivo.[78,79] Importantly, during ablation with a cleanly cutting laser source, repeated spectroscopic feedback of target autofluorescence allows continued ablation in the presence of atheroma, with cessation on detection of normal media.[80–83] This ''test and ablate'' sequence is currently in clinical use combining a ''diagnostic'' low-power He-Cd laser with a ''therapeutic'' high-power flashlamp-pumped dye laser (MCM, Mountain View, CA). Importantly, the same fiber optics perform both the interrogation and the ablation sequence.

Currently, operation of such sophisticated on-line spectroscopic imaging is laborious and time-consuming. Furthermore, this technology does not guide the ablating catheter in coaxial alignment with the vessel lumen. Its aim is rather to prevent imminent perforation. Disappointingly, initial clinical experience with the system suggests that it has not reduced the incidence of perforations.[84]

Recently, miniaturized 20 MHz catheter tip echocardiographic transducers have been used for endovascular ultrasonographic imaging (Fig. 28–9). Computer reconstructions provide cross-sectional images of the arterial wall, providing information on plaque and wall thickness as well as on lesion composition.[85–88] To date, this approach appears to hold the greatest promise for use as a guidance system. Further device miniaturization, enhanced imaging, and incorporation into a laser catheter may permit vessel recanalization with continuous visualization of vessel wall boundaries.

Targeting approaches to selective ablation of atheromata have so far remained elusive. Of the various imaging techniques under current investigation, both fluorescence spectroscopy and, more especially, endovascular ultrasonographic imaging hold the greatest promise for the development of a practical guidance system.

Overview of Laser Ablation

Over the past decade, a bewildering array of laser sources, delivered through a similarly

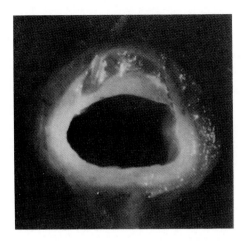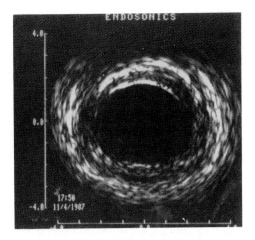

Fig. 28–9. Computed intraluminal sonogram derived by a 20 MHz phased array ultrasonic tip transducer. Shown on the left is the pathologic appearance of the diseased vessel segment. The ultrasonic image on the right shows bright reflections from the eccentric plaque with characteristic shadowing.

bewildering array of fiber optic catheter configurations at varying dosimetries, has been used to cause variable degrees of thermal and mechanical injury to irradiated tissue. The clinical experience gained with currently available laser angioplasty systems suggests that laser technology may play a role in the recanalization of total occlusions in peripheral and coronary arteries. Clean ablation of atheroma with pulsed near ultraviolet laser sources holds the greatest promise for benign vessel healing. Current multifiber over-the-wire fiberoptic catheters have the greatest appeal. Refinements of techniques to identify target tissue composition and wall thickness will be essential to enable any irradiative or mechanical revascularizing system to successfully negotiate total occlusions in the coronary vasculature. Ablative laser technology may be used initially as a recanalizing mechanism with subsequent balloon dilation. Only the demonstration of a significantly improved long-term patency rate would warrant the expense of pursuing complete laser endarterectomy.

LASER BALLOON ANGIOPLASTY (LBA)

During LBA, heat and pressure are applied simultaneously to the arterial wall in an attempt to improve luminal diameter and mor-

phology beyond those achievable with pressure alone.[89] Heat is generated by a Nd:YAG laser (wavelength 1.06 micron), whose output is diffused within a modified angioplasty balloon and then absorbed by adjacent normal and atheromatous tissues to a depth of 2–3 mm (Fig. 28–10). Laser dosimetry is adjusted to produce a tissue temperature approaching 100°C, well below the threshold for vaporization of solid components of tissue. The combination of heat and pressure generated by balloon inflation results in fusion of separated tissue layers, reduction of arterial recoil, and rapid desiccation of thrombus.

Arterial Dissection

Photothermal energy has been used clinically for decades to repair retinal tears, coagulate retinal tissue, and assist in the control of bleeding during resection of vascular tissues. Potentially relevant to LBA, successful creation of "sutureless" anastomoses for a variety of soft tissues with laser/thermal energy has been described.[90] At an appropriate level of coagulation, structural detail is preserved (as assessed by light microscopy) and continuity of stromal layers across juxtaposed tissues is seen acutely after successful fusion of tissues. Local inflammatory responses compare favorably with those associated with con-

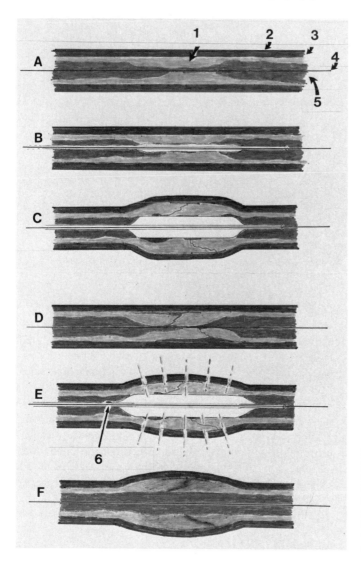

Fig. 28–10. Laser balloon angioplasty. Nd:YAG laser energy may be useful for fusing disrupted elements of the arterial wall following conventional PTCA. An acoustic sensor could be used to detect high frequency sounds generated by tissue vaporization to automatically terminate the laser exposure.

ventional suture technique, providing impetus to the development of laser-based methods for small vessel and nerve anastomoses.

Spears and colleagues adapted this concept to the laser/thermal fusion of separated layers of human postmortem atheromatous aortic sections, using a threshold temperature of 80 to 90°C for a least 10 seconds during the application of some tissue pressure (0.5 atm).[91] The use of a penetrating radiation, such as the 1.06 μm wavelength Nd:YAG laser, was also necessary to fuse tissues to a depth of 1 mm. Although layers of complex atheromatous plaques, including heavily calcified ones, could also be effectively fused to adjacent arterial tissues, the most problematic aspect of the procedure was the great variability of the weld strength achieved, related in part to variation in the adequacy of the topographic match between juxtaposed tissues at both the gross and ultrastructural level.

Arterial Recoil

After conventional angioplasty, luminal diameter is nearly always less than that of the fully inflated balloon, suggesting an element of arterial recoil. Within 30 minutes of PTCA, evidence of increased vasomotor tone has also been observed.[92] During LBA in various animal models, thermal remodeling of elastic tissue and loss of smooth muscle cell viability have been found to result in an increased luminal diameter by 0.3 mm to 0.5 mm compared to that of a 3.0 mm conventional angioplasty balloon. This increased diameter is sustained in normal arteries unless an excessively high laser dose results in a peak tissue temperature above 120°C. Such inappropriately high laser doses appear to produce late perivascular fibrosis and increased neointimal thickening.

Desiccation of Thrombus

Conventional angioplasty of thrombotic lesions frequently produces a suboptimal acute result. The relatively strong absorption of laser radiation over a wide range of wavelengths by thrombus, compared to other soft tissues, results in the rapid desiccation of thrombus by an LBA laser dose sufficient to fuse separated layers of tissue. Because water comprises most of the mass of thrombus, the latter can be effectively debulked by desiccation, and simultaneous application of heat and pressure remodels the desiccated thrombus into a smooth, nonobstructing film adherent to the luminal surface. The optimal laser dose for LBA treatment of thrombus has yet to be defined, however.

Adverse Biologic Reactivity

After mechanical injury to the arterial wall, exposed subendothelial tissues may render the luminal surface thrombogenic. Loss of the endothelial lining layer causes deposition of platelets, but deeper mural tears expose a variety of proteins such as collagen (types I and III), thromboplastin, fibronectin, and necrotic plaque material, promoting local thrombus formation in conjunction with the irregular luminal geometry associated with mural disruption. The recent angioscopic observation of the frequent presence of thrombus shortly after PTCA[93] supports the notion that thrombogenicity of the luminal surface may play an important role in both short-term and long-term success of PTCA.

Thermal fixation of tissue with microwave energy has been shown by Login et al.[94] to simulate the protein cross-linking effects of glutaraldehyde, which reduces the thrombogenicity of heterograft valves. It is attractive to hypothesize that the appropriate thermal fixation of tissue might confer a similar benefit to the mechanically injured arterial wall, or that thermal denaturation of thrombin might reduce its inherent thrombogenicity. Experimental evidence for such potentially favorable effects is currently limited, and the optimal laser dose required may differ from that currently used to improve luminal geometry.

Some workers feel that vasoconstriction is a potential contributor to restenosis.[95] Thermal destruction of smooth muscle cell viability by LBA results in a loss of vasoconstrictor potential. Repopulation of the arterial wall with smooth muscle cells may occur, in addition to probable fibroblast infiltration noted experimentally one month after LBA, but a spatially synchronized contraction is not likely to be possible, given the random alignment of cells at this time.

Smooth muscle cell proliferation appears to be the fundamental cause of PTCA restenosis. Interestingly, neointimal thickening still occurs after LBA doses that would ensure loss of smooth muscle cell viability.[96] Thus, the possibility exists that initial thermal destruction of this cell type may not produce any long-term benefit.

Clinical Studies

An LBA catheter was developed for a percutaneous coronary application (USCI Div. of C.R. Bard, Inc.) along with a continuous wave Nd:YAG laser (1.06 μm) delivery system (Quantronix, Inc.). This over-the-wire catheter is similar to that of a conventional angioplasty balloon catheter in terms of flexibility, profile, trackability, and balloon material (polyethylene terephthalate). A third channel within the body of the catheter permits passage of a 100 μm core silica fiber optic, which terminates in a helical diffusing tip surrounding the central shaft. The diffusing tip used in the first 200 patients provided an uneven distribution of laser energy axially, with a 30 to 50% variation circumferentially. Recent refinements have resulted in a more uniform cylindrical pattern of radiation from the diffusing tip. The materials of the balloon components are relatively transparent to the radiation, so that tissue heating results solely from direct absorption of laser energy.

Currently, PTCA is performed initially with a balloon of the same dimensions (2.5 mm, 3.0 mm, or 3.5 mm; 20 mm length) to facilitate a comparison of LBA and PTCA in the same patient in terms of improvement in minimum luminal diameter achieved. LBA is then performed in the same manner as PTCA, except

that a maximum balloon pressure of 4 atm is used and normal saline at 37°C is infused through the #8 Fr guiding catheter and the central channel of the LBA balloon immediately before and during a 20-second laser exposure. A relatively high laser power is used during the first 5 seconds of exposure, with a step-wise reduction over the remaining 15 seconds to quickly achieve and maintain a target tissue temperature of 80 to 105°C, at a depth of 0.5 to 1.0 mm into the arterial wall.

Preliminary results suggest that technical success in the performance of LBA can be achieved in 95% of patients and that the complication rate is lower than that associated historically with PTCA.[97] Computerized image analysis of cineangiograms shows that the minimum luminal diameter is increased by a mean value of 0.5 mm ± 0.3 mm over the initial conventional PTCA results (Fig. 28–11). More importantly, the improvement

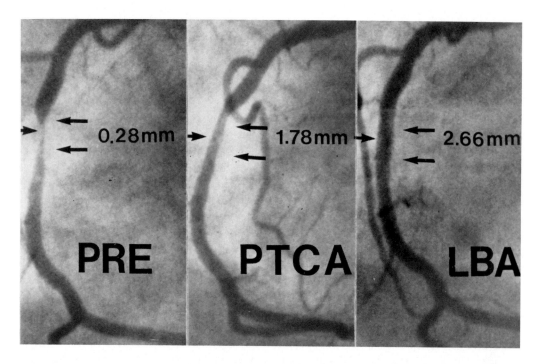

Fig. 28–11. Lumen diameters (in mm) shown before (PRE) and after conventional PTCA with a 3.0 mm diameter balloon, demonstrating substantial elastic recoil. After treatment with the same size laser balloon catheter (peak laser dose 25 W), recoil is diminished and nearly the entire balloon diameter is recovered. (Photo courtesy of Robert D. Safian, M.D.)

afforded by LBA over PTCA has been found to be inversely proportional to the post-PTCA stenotic diameter, so that the largest improvement in dimension is provided by LBA when the conventional PTCA result is poorest (such as in the setting of PTCA-induced acute closure).[98] The mechanisms responsible for the improvement appear to be a reduction of arterial recoil, desiccation and remodeling of thrombus, and fusion of separated tissue layers. While the first two tissue effects appear to be predictable, the ability to completely seal PTCA-induced dissections has been less reliable, with an approximate 50% success rate. Because LBA has appeared to be effective in the prevention of propagation of dissections, a potentially more effective means of performing the procedure may consist of a laser exposure during the initial balloon inflation, which reduces the chance of initiation of dissection.

To date, the only clinical problem associated with LBA has been a relatively high incidence of restenosis in the first series of 30 patients treated with a high laser dose. Lower laser doses used in all subsequent patients appear to be equally effective in improving minimum luminal diameter with an incidence of clinical restenosis similar to that reported for conventional PTCA.

With the recent availability of an LBA catheter that emits a more uniform cylindric pattern of radiation, the effect of laser dosimetry on each of the multiple proposed beneficial tissue reactions can be studied more appropriately, both experimentally and clinically. The proper application of thermal energy relies on the results of such studies, which include observational trials of LBA and randomized trials of LBA versus PTCA, the primary endpoint of which is the acute and chronic angiographic minimum luminal diameter.

REFERENCES

1. Einstein A: Zur Quantentheorie der Strahlung. Phys SZ 18:121, 1917.
2. Maiman TH: Stimulated optical irradiation in ruby. Nature 187:493, 1960.
3. Bass M: Lasers for use in medicine. Endoscopy 18:2, 1986.
4. Welch AJ, Valvano JW, Pearce JA, et al: Effect of laser radiation on tissue during laser angioplasty. Lasers Surg Med 5:251, 1985.
5. Welch AJ, van Gemert MJC, Bradley AB: Optical and thermal events in laser angioplasty. In: Primer on Laser Angioplasty; Ginsburg R, White JC (eds). Mt Kisco, NY, Futura Publications, 1989.
6. van Gemert MJC, Welch AJ, Bonnier JJM, et al: Some physical concepts in laser angioplasty. Semin Intervent Radiol 3:27, 1986.
7. Welch AJ, Bradley AB, Torres JH, et al: Laser probe ablation of normal and atherosclerotic human aorta in vitro: A first thermographic and histologic analysis. Circulation 76:1353, 1987.
8. Abela GS, Normann S, Cohen D, et al: Effects of carbon dioxide, Nd-YAG, and argon laser irradiation on coronary atheromatous plaque. Am J Cardiol 50:1199, 1982.
9. Eldar M, Battler A, Neufeld HN, et al: Transluminal carbon dioxide-laser catheter angioplasty for dissolution of atherosclerotic plaques. J Am Coll Cardiol 3:135, 1984.
10. Zeevi B, Gal D, Abramovici A, et al: Carbon dioxide fiber optic laser for treatment of coarctation of the aorta. Am Heart J 113:1518, 1987.
11. Battler A, Gal D, Eldar M, et al: CO_2 laser catheter angioplasty in human atherosclerotic xenograft arteries. J Intervent Cardiol 2:29, 1989.
12. Deckelbaum LI, Isner JM, Donaldson RF, et al: Reduction of laser-induced pathologic tissue injury using pulsed energy delivery. Am J Cardiol 56:662, 1985.
13. Deckelbaum LI, Isner JM, Donaldson RF, et al: Use of pulsed energy delivery to minimize tissue injury resulting from carbon dioxide laser irradiation of cardiovascular tissues. J Am Coll Cardiol 7:898, 1987.
14. Kramer JR, Bott-Silverman C, Ratliff NB, et al: Removal of atherosclerotic plaque using multiple short exposures of argon ion laser light. Am Heart J 113:1038, 1987.
15. Strikwerda S, Bott-Silverman C, Ratliff NB, et al: Effects of varying argon ion laser intensity and exposure time on the ablation of atherosclerotic plaque. Lasers Surg Med 8:66, 1988.
16. Walsh JT, Flotte JT, Deutsch TF: Er:YAG laser ablation of tissue: effect of pulse duration and tissue type on thermal damage. Lasers Surg Med 9:314, 1989.
17. Cross FW, Bowker TJ: The physical properties of tissue ablation with excimer lasers. Med Instrumentation 21:226, 1987.
18. Bowker TJ, Cross FW, Fox KM, et al: Laser assisted coronary angioplasty. Eur Heart J 9(suppl C):25, 1988.
19. Grundfest WS, Litvack F, Forrester JS, et al: Laser ablation of human atherosclerotic plaque without adjacent tissue injury. J Am Coll Cardiol 5:929, 1985.
20. Murphy-Chutorian D, Selzer PM, Kosek J, et al: The interaction between excimer laser energy and vascular tissue. Am Heart J 112:739, 1986.
21. Litvack F, Grundfest WS, Goldenberg T, et al: Pulsed laser angioplasty; wavelength power and energy dependencies relevant to clinical application. Lasers Surg Med 8:60, 1988.

22. Litvack F, Grundfest W, Hickey A: Percutaneous coronary excimer laser angioplasty in animals and humans. J Am Coll Cardiol 13:61A, 1989.
23. Wollenek G, Laufer G, Grabenwoeger F: Percutaneous transluminal excimer laser angioplasty in total peripheral artery occlusion in man. Lasers Surg Med 8:464, 1988.
24. Prince MR, LaMuraglia GM, Teng P, et al: Preferential ablation of calcified arterial plaque with laser-induced plasmas. J Quant Electron QE-23:1783, 1987.
25. LaMuraglia GM, Anderson RR, Parrish JA, et al: Selective laser ablation of venous thrombus: Implications for a new approach in the treatment of pulmonary embolus. Lasers Surg Med 8:486, 1988.
26. Prince MR, Deutsch TF, Shapiro AH, et al: Selective ablation of atheromas using a flashlamp-excited dye laser at 465 nm. Proc Nat Acad Sci USA 83:7064, 1986.
27. Esterowitz L, Hoffman CA, Tran DC, et al: Advantages of the 2.94 μm wavelength for medical laser applications. In: Technical Digest: Conference on Lasers and Electro-optics. Washington, DC: Optical Society of America, 1986, p 122.
28. Walsh JT, Deutsch TF: Er:YAG laser ablation of tissue: Measurement of the ablation rate. Lasers Surg Med 9:327, 1988.
29. Kent KM, Bentivoglio LG, Block PC, et al: Percutaneous transluminal coronary angioplasty: report from the registry of the National Heart, Lung, and Blood Institute. Am J Cardiol 49:201, 1982.
30. Holmes DR, Vlietstra RE, Smith HC, et al: Restenosis following percutaneous transluminal coronary angioplasty: Report from the NHLBI registry. Am J Cardiol 53:77C, 1984.
31. Macruz R, Martins JRM, Tupinamba A, et al: Possibilidades terapeuticas do raio laser em arteromas. Arq Bras Cardiol 34:9, 1980.
32. Choy DSJ, Stertzer S, Rotterdam HZ, Bruno MS: Laser coronary angioplasty: Experience with 9 cadaver hearts. Am J Cardiol 50:1209, 1982.
33. Lee G, Ikeda RM, Kozina J, Mason DT: Laser dissolution of coronary atherosclerotic obstruction. Am Heart J 102:1074, 1981.
34. Crea F, Fenech A, Smith W, et al: Laser recanalization of acutely thrombosed coronary arteries in live dogs: Early results. J Am Coll Cardiol 6:1052, 1985.
35. Crea F, Abela GS, Fenech A, et al: Transluminal laser irradiation of coronary arteries in live dogs: An angiographic and morphologic study of acute effects. Am J Cardiol 57:17, 1986.
36. Choy DSJ, Stertzer SH, Myler RK, et al: Human coronary laser recanalization. Clin Cardiol 7:377, 1984.
37. Crea F, Davies G, McKenna W, et al: Percutaneous laser recanalization of coronary arteries. Lancet 11:215, 1986.
38. Lee G, Ikeda RM, Theis J, et al: Acute and chronic complications of laser angioplasty: vascular wall damage and formation of aneurysms in the atherosclerotic rabbit. Am J Cardiol 53:290, 1984.
39. Ginsberg R, Wexler L, Mitchell RS, Profitt D: Percutaneous transluminal angioplasty for treatment of peripheral vascular disease. Radiology 156:619, 1985.
40. Geschwind H, Boussignac G, Teisseire B, et al: Percutaneous transluminal laser angioplasty in man. Lancet 1:844, 1984.
41. Fourrier JL, Brunetaud JM, Prat A, et al: Percutaneous laser angioplasty with sapphire tip. Lancet 1:105, 1987.
42. Cumberland DC, Sanborn TA, Tayler DL, et al: Percutaneous laser thermal angioplasty: Initial clinical results with a laser probe in total peripheral artery occlusions. Lancet 1:1457, 1986.
43. Sanborn TA, Haudenschild CC, Garber GR, et al: Angiographic and histologic consequences of laser thermal angioplasty: Comparison with balloon angioplasty. Circulation 75:1281, 1987.
44. Rosenthal E, Montarello JK, Palmer T, Curry PVL: Thermal effects of stationary "hot tip" laser coronary probes: An in vitro assessment. Lasers Surg Med 9:229, 1989.
45. Crea F, Davies G, McKenna WJ, et al: Laser recanalization of coronary arteries by metal capped optical fibers: Early clinical experience in patients with stable angina pectoris. Br Heart J 59:168, 1988.
46. Sanborn TA, Cumberland DC, Greenfield AJ, et al: Percutaneous laser thermal angioplasty: Initial results and 1-year follow-up in 129 femoropopliteal lesions. Radiology 168:121, 1988.
47. Keogh B, Crea F, Davies G, Taylor K, et al: Angioscopy and intra-operative coronary laser angioplasty. Lancet 2:969, 1987.
48. Linnemeier TJ, Cumberland DC: Percutaneous laser coronary angioplasty without balloon angioplasty. Lancet 1:154, 1989.
49. Rosenthal E, Montarello JK, Palmer T, Curry PVL: Coronary artery thermal damage during percutaneous "hot tip" laser-assisted angioplasty. Am J Cardiol 64:116, 1989.
50. Morcos NC, Berns M, Henry WL: Effect of laser-heated tip angioplasty on human atherosclerotic coronary arteries. Lasers Surg Med 8:22, 1988.
51. White RA, White GH, Vlasak J, et al: Histopathology of human laser thermal angioplasty recanalization. Lasers Surg Med 8:469, 1988.
52. Tobis J, Smolin M, Mallery J, et al: Laser-assisted thermal angioplasty in human peripheral artery occlusions: Mechanism of recanalization. J Am Coll Cardiol 13:1547, 1989.
53. Grundfest W, Litvack F, Hickey A, et al: Radiofrequency thermal angioplasty for the treatment of peripheral vascular occlusive disease: Preliminary results of a clinical trial. J Am Coll Cardiol 13:14A, 1989.
54. Cumberland DC, Belli AM, Myler RK, et al: Combined laser/thermal recanalization of peripheral artery occlusions. J Am Coll Cardiol 13:13A, 1989.
55. Verdaasdonk RM, Cross FW, Borst C: Physical properties of sapphire fibretips for laser angioplasty. Lasers Med Sci 2:183, 1987.
56. Geschwind HJ, Blair JD, Mongkolsmai D, et al: Development and experimental application of contact probe catheter for laser angioplasty. J Am Coll Cardiol 9:101, 1987.
57. Isner JM, Steg PG, Clark RH: Current status of cardiovascular laser therapy, 1987. IEEE J Quant Electron 23:1756, 1987.
58. Pilger E, Lammer J, Kleinert R, et al: Laser angio-

plasty with a contact probe for the treatment of peripheral vascular disease. Cardiovasc Res 22:149, 1988.

59. Lammer J, Karnel F: Percutaneous transluminal laser angioplasty with contact probes. Radiology 168:733, 1988.

60. Nordstrom LA, Castaneda-Zuniga WR, Lindeke CC, et al: Laser angioplasty: Controlled delivery of argon laser energy. Radiology 167:463, 1988.

61. Nordstrom LA, Castaneda-Zuniga WR, Young EG, et al: Direct argon laser exposure for recanalization of peripheral arteries: early results. Radiology 168:359, 1988.

62. Foschi A, Myers G, Crick WF, et al: Laser angioplasty of totally occluded coronary arteries and vein grafts: Preliminary report on a current trial. Am J Cardiol 63:9F, 1989.

63. Murray A, Wood RF: Peripheral laser angioplasty with the pulsed dye laser and ball-tipped optical fibres. Lancet 1:324, 1989.

64. Anderson HV, Zaatari GS, Roubin GS, et al: Steerable fiber optic catheter delivery of laser energy in atherosclerotic rabbits. Am Heart J 111:1065, 1986.

65. Cote G, Stertzer SH, Myler RK, et al: Early clinical experience with percutaneous transluminal argon laser coronary angioplasty. J Am Coll Cardiol 13:61A, 1989.

66. Weishaupt KR, Gomber CJ, Dougherty TJ: Identification of singlet oxygen as the cytotoxic agent in photoinactivation of a murine tumor. Cancer Res 36:2326, 1976.

67. Spears JR, Serur J, Shropshire D, Paulin S: Fluorescence of experimental atheromatous plaques with hematoporphyrin derivative. J Clin Invest 71:395, 1983.

68. Spears JR, et al: Effect of hematoporphyrin derivative photodynamic therapy on the normal and atheromatous rabbit aorta. J Clin Invest 71:395, 1983.

69. Litvack F, Grundfest WS, Forrester JS, et al: Effects of hematoporphyrin derivative and photodynamic therapy on atherosclerotic rabbits. Am J Cardiol 56:667, 1985.

70. Pollock ME, Eugene J, Hammer-Wilson M, Berns MW: Photosensitization of experimental atheromas by porphyrins. J Am Coll Cardiol 9:639, 1987.

71. Murphy-Chutorian D, Kosek J, Mok W, et al: Selective absorption of ultraviolet laser energy by human atherosclerotic plaque treated with tetracycline. Am J Cardiol 55:1293, 1985.

72. Prince MR, LaMuraglia GM, McNichol EF: Increased preferential absorption in human atherosclerotic plaque with oral beta carotene: implications for laser endarterectomy. Circulation 78:338, 1988.

73. Spears JR, Spokoyne A, Marais HJ: Coronary angioscopy during cardiac catheterization. J Am Coll Cardiol 6:93, 1985.

74. Lee G, Ikeda RM, Stobbe D, et al: Laser irradiation of human atherosclerotic obstructive disease: Simultaneous visualization and vaporization achieved by a dual fiber optic catheter. Am Heart J 105:163, 1983.

75. Abela GS, Seeger JM, Barbieri E, et al: Laser angioplasty with angioscopic guidance in humans. J Am Coll Cardiol 8:184, 1986.

76. Richens D, Rees M, Watson DA: Laser coronary angioplasty under direct vision. Lancet 2:683, 1987.

77. Sherman CT, Litvack G, Grundfest W, et al: Coronary angioscopy in patients with unstable angina pectoris. N Engl J Med 315:15, 1986.

78. Sartori M, Sauerbrey R, Kubodera S, et al: Autofluorescence maps of atherosclerotic human arteries—A new technique in medical imaging. IEEE J Quant Electron QE-23:1794, 1987.

79. Deckelbaum LI, Lam JK, Cabin HS, et al: Discrimination of normal and atherosclerotic aorta by laser-induced fluorescence. Lasers Surg Med 7:330, 1987.

80. Leon MB, Lu DY, Prevosti LG, et al: Human arterial surface fluorescence: Atherosclerotic plaque identification and effects of laser atheroma ablation. J Am Coll Cardiol 12:94, 1988.

81. Deckelbaum LI, Stetz ML, O'Brien KM, et al: Fluorescence spectroscopy guidance of laser ablation of atherosclerotic plaque. Lasers Surg Med 9:205, 1989.

82. Cutruzzola FW, Stetz ML, O'Brien KM, et al: Change in laser-induced arterial fluorescence during ablation of atherosclerotic plaque. Lasers Surg Med 9:109, 1989.

83. Bartorelli AL, Bonner R, Almagor V, et al: Enhanced recognition of plaque composition in vivo using laser-excited fluorescence spectroscopy. J Am Coll Cardiol 13:54A, 1989.

84. Geschwind HJ, Dubois-Rabde JL, Poirot G, et al: Guided percutaneous pulsed laser angioplasty. Results and follow-up. J Am Coll Cardiol 13:13A, 1989.

85. Tobis JN, Mallery JA, Mahon D, et al: Intravascular ultrasound visualization of atheroma plaque removal by atherectomy. J Am Coll Cardiol 13:222A, 1989.

86. Graham SP, Brands D, Savakus A, et al: Utility of an intravascular ultrasound imaging device for arterial wall definition and atherectomy guidance. J Am Coll Cardiol 13:222A, 1989.

87. Hodgson JM, Graham SP, Savakus AD, et al: Clinical percutaneous imaging of coronary anatomy using an over-the-wire ultrasound catheter system. Int J Card Imaging 4:187, 1989.

88. Gussenhoven EJ, Essed CE, Lancee CT, et al: Arterial wall characteristics determined by intravascular ultrasound imaging: An in vitro study. J Am Coll Cardiol 14:947, 1989.

89. Spears JR: Method and apparatus for angioplasty. U.S. Patent 4,799,479.

90. Jain KK, Gorisch W: Repair of small blood vessels with the Neodymium-YAG laser: A preliminary report. Surgery 85:684, 1979.

91. Hiehle JF, et al: Nd:YAG laser fusion of human atheromatous plaque-arterial wall separations in vitro. Am J Cardiol 56:953, 1985.

92. Fischell TA, Derby G, Tse TM, Stadius ML: Coronary artery vasoconstriction routinely occurs after percutaneous transluminal coronary angioplasty. Circulation 78:1323, 1988.

93. Kyoichi M, et al (National Defense Medical College, Saitama, Japan): Evaluation of coronary thrombi after PTCA by angioscopy. Circulation 80(suppl II): II-523, 1989.

94. Login GR, Dvorak AM: Microwave energy fixation for electron microscopy. Am J Pathol 120:230–243, 1985.

95. Bertrand ME, Lablanche JM, Fourrier JL, Gommeaux A, Ruel M: Relation to restenosis after percutaneous transluminal coronary angioplasty to va-

somotion of the dilated coronary arterial segment. Am J Cardiol 63:277, 1989.

96. Jenkins RD, et al: Laser balloon angioplasty vs balloon angioplasty in normal rabbit iliac arteries. Lasers Surg Med, in press.

97. Spears JR, et al and the LBA Study Group, Harper Hospital/Wayne State University, Detroit MI: Laser balloon angioplasty: Angiographic results in a multicenter trial. Circulation 80(suppl II):II-476, 1989.

98. Sinclair IN, et al, and the LBA Study Group: Acute closure post PTCA successfully treated with laser balloon angioplasty. Circulation 80(suppl II):II-476, 1989.

29

Balloon Valvuloplasty

RAYMOND G. MCKAY and WILLIAM GROSSMAN

Percutaneous balloon valvuloplasty is a relatively new catheter technique that involves the dilatation of stenotic cardiac valves with large-diameter balloon catheters introduced percutaneously in the cardiac catheterization laboratory. The procedure has been used to treat pulmonic stenosis since 1982, mitral stenosis since 1984, congenital aortic stenosis since 1984, acquired aortic stenosis since 1985, and tricuspid stenosis since 1987. While the United States Food and Drug Administration has recently approved pulmonic valvuloplasty for clinical use, balloon valvuloplasty for other valves is still an experimental technique whose overall clinical utility remains under active investigation.

The efficacy and safety of the balloon valvuloplasty procedure varies according to which cardiac valve is being dilated, the underlying etiology of the stenotic lesion (i.e., congenital, rheumatic, senile degenerative), the pathologic characteristics of the specific valve, prior experience of the operator, and the specific valvuloplasty technique used. Multiple mechanisms of successful balloon valvuloplasty have been identified, including separation of commissural fusion, fracture of calcific nodules, annular and leaflet stretching, tearing of leaflets, and annular fracture. These same mechanisms, however, may contribute to the complications associated with the procedure. As a result, enthusiasm generated from early reports describing significant short-term hemodynamic and symptomatic improvement following balloon valvuloplasty has been offset by more recent studies citing dramatic valvuloplasty complications and poor short- and long-term hemodynamic results, particularly with aortic stenosis.

Over the last several years, there has been a rapid ongoing evolution of valvuloplasty equipment, techniques, complications, and indications for the procedure. At least four different types of balloon catheters have been developed, including single, modified single, double, and trefoil balloon catheters. In addition, recent improvements in balloon technology have resulted in major changes in second- and third-generation valvuloplasty catheters, including reduction in the profiles of deflated balloons, increases in balloon burst strength, and lowered inflation-deflation times. The effects of these changes on the efficacy and safety of the procedure are currently under investigation.

With respect to valvuloplasty technique, numerous balloon dilatation techniques have been described for all four cardiac valves. These have included both single and double balloon techniques, the use of "undersized" and "oversized" balloon diameters with respect to the diameter of the valvular annulus, and the use of both antegrade and retrograde approaches to valves. The relative merits of each approach and modifications of each approach are still unknown. A major technical question that remains unanswered is the maximum balloon size that can be used safely in any given patient to provide optimal enlargement of either the aortic or mitral valve orifice.

With respect to complications, both major and minor complications have been reported by virtually all groups doing valvuloplasty. Although some of these complications may be inherent to the technique, it is likely that many of them will decrease following operators' initial learning curves. In addition, potential future improvements in valvuloplasty catheters may reduce several common valvuloplasty complications, including local vascular trauma, creation of atrial septal defects, and perforation of the left ventricle.

Finally, indications for the use of balloon valvuloplasty are not settled. Stenotic valvular disease represents a significant proportion of heart disease in both industrialized and non-industrialized countries. Although surgical intervention with either commissurotomy or prosthetic valve replacement has proven effective, the higher risk of open heart surgery in certain populations has been an ongoing impetus for the development of a catheterization-based method of relieving valvular stenosis. In addition, other patients who would normally be considered good surgical candidates would prefer to avoid surgery if a safe and efficacious catheterization-based method existed to palliate or cure their valvular disease. Whether balloon valvuloplasty may actually compete with surgical therapy for the general population of patients with valvular stenosis or whether this technique should be reserved for limited subgroups of patients will be ascertained only with large multi-center clinical trials, some of which are currently in operation.

This chapter will attempt to summarize the advances in this rapidly evolving field over the last several years.

PULMONIC VALVULOPLASTY

Historical Developments

Recognition of the potential use of balloon dilatation to treat congenital pulmonic stenosis was a natural consequence of the early surgical experience with mechanical dilatation of stenotic pulmonary valves. In particular, the earliest reports on the surgical treatment of congenital pulmonic stenosis involved the use of the Brock procedure.[1] In this operation, a valvulotome was introduced through a small cut in the right ventricle and advanced to the pulmonic valve, where incisions were made through the congenitally fused valvular commissures. The commissural incisions were enlarged subsequently using a graded series of bougies, and the valvotomy was then completed with a hinged dilator. Although the subsequent development of cardiopulmonary bypass allowed the direct surgical treatment of pulmonary valve stenosis, with incision of the commissures under direct vision, the early success of the Brock procedure and its long-term effectiveness suggested that stenotic pulmonic valves might be opened adequately using simple mechanical dilatation. Accordingly, in 1979 Semb and co-workers[2] reported the first successful use of a balloon catheter in a critically ill patient with pulmonary valve stenosis and tricuspid regurgitation. Using a Berman angiographic catheter positioned in the pulmonary artery, the balloon catheter was inflated with carbon dioxide and then pulled back across the pulmonic valve, reducing the systolic pressure gradient from 29 mmHg to 6 mmHg.

Following Semb's initial success, large fixed-diameter polyethylene balloon-tipped catheters became available for the first time (Medi-Tech, Watertown, MA). The balloon catheters ranged in size from 10 to 20 mm in diameter when inflated fully, and could be inserted percutaneously over a guide wire. Using this equipment, Kan et al.[3] in 1982 described the first use of percutaneous balloon dilatation to treat pulmonic stenosis in an 8-year-old child. Using a 14 mm balloon catheter advanced antegrade over an exchange guide wire from the right femoral vein to the level of the pulmonary valve, balloon dilatation to a pressure of 3 atmospheres and for 20 seconds resulted in an immediate decrease in the pulmonic gradient from 48 to 14 mmHg. The procedure was complicated only by a transient period of sinus bradycardia immediately following balloon inflation. Following dilatation, the patient's systolic ejection murmur was less harsh and was decreased in intensity, and serial electrocardiograms obtained at 1 and 4 months postprocedure showed a decrease in right ventricular hypertrophy. In addition, repeat catheterization at 4 months after the procedure demonstrated a 20 mmHg residual gradient, with no change in cardiac output. Kan performed balloon valvuloplasty subsequently for pulmonic stenosis in four additional children 3 months, 18 months, 3 years, and 14 years old. In all four cases, the procedure was performed without complications and resulted in an immediate reduction in the pulmonic gradient and the ratio of right ventricular pressure to systemic arterial pressure.

The first balloon valvuloplasty for pulmonic valve stenosis in an adult was performed by Pepine in 1982.[4] Using a 20 mm balloon inflated to 5 atmospheres, balloon valvuloplasty resulted in improvement in pulmonary valve area from 0.3 to 1.0 cm[2] in a 59-year-old woman with congenital pulmonic stenosis who was severely limited by dyspnea and fatigue. The procedure resulted in a marked reduction in the intensity of the murmur of pulmonic stenosis and significant improvement in the patient's exercise tolerance. Of note, however, a residual infundibular pressure gradient developed in the patient following relief of valvular obstruction. This infundibular gradient was noted subsequently to regress 10 days after valve dilation.

A substantial series of pulmonic valvuloplasty patients was reported by Lababidi in 1983.[5] Using 12 to 15 mm valvuloplasty balloons, he performed pulmonic valvuloplasty in 18 patients ranging in age from 11 months to 19 years. Valve dilatation resulted in a decrease in mean pulmonary valve gradient from 81 ± 31 to 23 ± 11 mmHg, a fall in right ventricular pressure from 106/5 $\pm$ 31/2 to 50/6 $\pm$ 12/2 mmHg, and no change in cardiac output. The procedure was associated with no significant complication in any of the 18 patients.

Lababidi's series was complemented by a report from Walls and Curtis in 1984.[6] They described 39 patients with congenital pulmonic stenosis who underwent balloon dilatation with valvuloplasty balloons ranging between 12 and 20 mm and for whom transvalvular pressure gradient decreased from 85 ± 35 to 30 ± 15 mmHg. Repeat catheterization in 11 patients 5 to 16 months after the dilatation procedure demonstrated that transvalvular gradients remained significantly lower than prevalvuloplasty values (pre: 69 ± 31 mmHg, post: 21 ± 10 mmHg, follow-up: 23 ± 12 mmHg). Once again, no significant complications were associated with the procedure.

Following initial reports on the success of balloon pulmonic valvuloplasty, an important observation that influenced the technique of pulmonic valvuloplasty was made, namely, that oversized balloon catheters equal in size to, or even larger than, the pulmonic annulus could be used to enhance gradient reduction. In particular, in 1984 Lock's group reported animal experiments in newborn lambs indicating that balloon sizes up to 30% larger than the pulmonary valve annulus results in only minor trauma to the right ventricular outflow tract.[7] This observation led subsequent investigators to use "oversized" balloons in clinical trials.

In this regard, the first attempted use of a double-balloon technique to achieve successful pulmonic valvuloplasty was published by Ali Kahn in 1986.[8] Balloon sizes that were 2 mm larger in diameter than the pulmonic annulus were used in 32 patients, ranging in age from 6 months to 12 years. Two balloons were used simultaneously in patients with a pulmonary artery annulus larger than 25 mm. Using this technique, Ali Kahn reported reduction of the pulmonic gradient from 99 ± 23 mmHg to 23 ± 11 mmHg, with no significant complications. Subsequent follow-up at a mean of 10 months demonstrated marked clinical improvement in two thirds of the patients. In addition, repeat catheterization in 14 patients at 6 months demonstrated no significant valvular restenosis.

A final variation in the technique for percutaneous pulmonary balloon valvuloplasty was published by Meier in 1986, who described the use of a trefoil balloon catheter for dilatation of stenotic pulmonic valves.[9] The trefoil balloon consists of three identical 15 mm balloons mounted on a single catheter shaft. Using this catheter, Meier was able to achieve successful gradient reduction in four adolescents with congenital pulmonic stenosis.

Pathophysiologic Mechanisms

Based on early surgical experience with the Brock procedure, the mechanism of successful gradient reduction with pulmonic valvuloplasty was assumed to be mechanical separation of congenitally fused commissures. Subsequent investigation, however, has revealed that balloon dilatation commonly results in tearing or avulsion of valve leaflets. At the time of surgery, for example, Lababidi noted balloon-induced tears in pulmonic leaflets in a patient with tetralogy of Fallot who underwent an initial pulmonic valvuloplasty followed by total surgical repair.[5] Similarly, Walls noted commissural splitting, mid-leaflet tears, and occasionally avulsion of cusps from the pulmonic annulus in seven patients who had undergone pulmonary valvuloplasty and required surgery because of additional cardiac anomalies.[6] The use of oversized balloons to effect pulmonic gradient reduction is presumably associated with a higher incidence of tearing of valve tissue. In addition, loss of valve infrastructure presumably results in significant pulmonary insufficiency.

Regardless of the effect of balloon inflation on the structure of the pulmonic valve, it is notable that this procedure, like surgical valvotomy, may be associated with the development of an infundibular gradient. This gradient may resolve with time secondary to regression of right ventricular hypertrophy. In some cases, however, this gradient may represent the development of critical infundibular obstruction. In 1985, Ben-Shackar described a 14-month-old boy with suprasystemic right ventricular pressure secondary to pulmonary valvular stenosis who underwent successful

valvuloplasty with a 12 mm balloon.[10] Immediately after valvuloplasty, right ventricular pressure nearly doubled. A post-valvuloplasty right ventriculogram demonstrated severe systolic infundibular obstruction not present before valve dilatation, and the patient subsequently required surgical relief of the obstruction.

Technical Aspects

Pulmonic balloon valvuloplasty is currently performed in adults in our laboratories using either a single- or double-balloon technique, depending on the pulmonic annulus size. Balloon catheters are specifically chosen to dilate with a balloon size 20 to 40% larger than the annular diameter. In patients with an annular diameter less than 25 mm, a single balloon is used, and two balloons are used for patients with larger diameters.

After administration of a local anesthetic, the patient is instrumented with a 5 Fr arterial monitor line in the radial or femoral artery, and two 8 Fr vascular sheaths in the left and right femoral veins. A 7 Fr balloon-tipped end-hole catheter which can accommodate an 0.038 inch guide wire (Critikon) is passed from the left femoral vein to the pulmonary artery, and a 7 Fr pigtail catheter is passed from the right femoral vein to the right ventricle. Following measurement of baseline hemodynamics including right atrial, right ventricular, pulmonary artery, pulmonary capillary wedge and systemic arterial pressures, and cardiac output, a biplane right ventricular cineangiogram is recorded in the anteroposterior and lateral projections. The annular diameter is subsequently measured at the valve hinge points from the lateral view. Next, the pigtail catheter is removed and replaced with a second 7 Fr balloon-tipped catheter, which is advanced from the femoral vein to the pulmonary artery. In patents in whom a single valvuloplasty balloon is used for pulmonary valve dilatation, one of the 7 Fr balloon-tipped catheters is exchanged for a valvuloplasty catheter while the second is used for monitoring pulmonary artery pressure during inflation;

in patients in whom a double balloon technique is used, both 7 Fr balloon-tipped catheters are exchanged for valvuloplasty catheters.

Balloon dilatation is accomplished by exchanging either one or both of the 7 Fr balloon-tipped catheters for an 0.038 inch guide wire, the tip of which is placed in the pulmonary artery, and advancing the valvuloplasty catheter(s) over the guide wire(s) to the level of the pulmonic valve. A 10 to 15 second inflation is then performed with a hand injection of a saline-contrast mixture to a maximum pressure of 5 to 6 atmospheres until a "waist" caused by the stenotic valve disappears. During inflation, it is very common for the dilating balloon(s) to move forward into the pulmonary artery with the force of right ventricular contraction; as a result, care must be taken to maintain the balloon position within the valve orifice to achieve effective dilatation.

Following balloon dilatation, the valvuloplasty catheter(s) is (are) removed and repeat measurements of the transvalvular and subvalvular gradients and cardiac output are made. A second right ventricular cineangiogram is also performed to look for changes in the severity of the subvalvular stenosis.

Clinical Results, Complications, and Long Term Follow-Up

Statistics gathered by a 15-center valvuloplasty registry at the Mansfield Scientific Corporation (Mansfield, MA) have shown that over 800 pulmonic balloon valvuloplasties have been performed in children and adults.[11] Successful reduction of the transpulmonic gradient has been achieved in nearly 90% of patients. The only reported complications associated with the procedure have been arrhythmias and hypotension during balloon inflation and catheter exchanges in preparation for dilatation, the development of an infundibular gradient, and transient right bundle branch block. To date, no deaths have been associated with use of the procedure after the first month of life.

More reports on pulmonic valvuloplasty have identified other isolated complications as-

sociated with the procedure. In 1987, Attia reported rupture of tricuspid valve papillary muscle during pulmonic valvuloplasty.[12] In 1988, Lo described a case of persistent complete heart block in a patient with congenital pulmonic stenosis who underwent balloon valvuloplasty.[13] In addition, femoral vein thrombosis and an ischemic cerebrovascular accident were both noted in a series by Rey in 1988.[14]

Long-term clinical follow-up of pulmonic valvuloplasty patients has been described in several reports. Mullins reported on 30 pulmonic valvuloplasty patients studied at a mean of 13 months after dilatation, and found no significant differences in pulmonic gradients measured by Doppler examination immediately after valvuloplasty and at follow-up.[15] Of note, no significant pulmonary regurgitation was detected. Rocchini[16] reported similar results in patients studied by Doppler echocardiography up to 4 years after balloon dilatation for pulmonic stenosis. Repeat cardiac catheterization studies have been performed by Rey in 19 patients[14] and by Shrivasta in 21 patients[17] up to 17 months after pulmonic valve dilatation with no evidence of valvular restenosis.

As a result of the immediate and late follow-up studies performed to date, the Food and Drug Administration (FDA) has approved pulmonic balloon valvuloplasty for use in both children and adults. Based on the available results, pulmonic balloon valvuloplasty is now considered the treatment of choice for children and adults with congenital pulmonic stenosis. Additional follow-up, however, will be needed to assess the long-term effect of the procedure on right ventricular function, patients' clinical status, and life expectancy.

MITRAL VALVULOPLASTY

Historical Development

As with pulmonic valvuloplasty, early surgical experience with the treatment of mitral stenosis provided the conceptual framework for the use of a percutaneously introduced balloon catheter to effect mechanical dilatation of the stenotic valve.[18–22] In particular, reports dating from as early as 1920 by Cutler,[18] Souter, Bailey,[21,22] Harken[19] and their associates on the various techniques of closed and open mitral commissurotomy using valvulotomes and simple finger fracture suggested that fused mitral commissures could be separated with simple mechanical dilatation. On the basis of this experience, successful use of a balloon technique for opening stenotic mitral valves might have been predicted. Similarly, early surgical experience with mitral commissurotomy had predicted the potential complications of balloon mitral valvuloplasty in regard to embolic phenomena, valvular regurgitation, and valvular restenosis.

Equally important in the development of the technology for balloon mitral valvuloplasty was the development of two techniques, transseptal heart catheterization[23] and balloon atrial septotomy.[24] Both of these procedures are an integral part of the technique that currently is used most commonly to dilate stenotic valves with balloon catheters.

In 1984, Inoue provided the first report of successful mitral valvuloplasty using a balloon catheter.[25] With use of a single balloon with an outer diameter ranging between 23 to 26 mm, six patents with critical mitral stenosis underwent mitral valvuloplasty by way of a transseptal approach. Balloon dilatation caused a reduction of the mean mitral valve gradient from 18 mmHg to 7 mmHg. The procedure was associated with a significant decrease in left atrial pressure and no major complications.

In 1985, Lock extended Inoue's findings, and described results in eight children and young adults with rheumatic mitral stenosis who underwent percutaneous balloon mitral valvuloplasty.[26] In Lock's series, the atrial septum was traversed by needle puncture by way of a standard transseptal approach and subsequently dilated with an 8 mm angioplasty balloon advanced over a guide wire. Following atrial septal dilatation, valvuloplasty balloon catheters ranging from 18 to 25 mm in diameter were used to dilate the mitral valve. Valve dilatation resulted in a decrease of the mean mitral gradient from 21 ± 4 mmHg to 10 ± 5 mmHg, an increase in cardiac output from 3.8 ± 1.0 to 4.9 ± 1.3 liters/minute, and an increase in calculated mitral valve area index from 0.73 ± 0.29 to 1.34 ± 0.32 cm²/ M². The intensity of the murmur diminished immediately after balloon commissurotomy in all patients. Of note, the greatest reduction in pressure gradient was achieved with the largest balloon diameter, i.e. 25 mm. Mitral valvuloplasty resulted in minimum mitral regurgitation in only one patient. Follow-up catheterization at 2 to 8 weeks demonstrated persistence of hemodynamic improvement, with evidence of partial restenosis in only one patient.

Following Lock's report, Al Zaibag reported the successful use of a double-balloon technique for treating rheumatic mitral valve stenosis in adolescents.[27] Successful valvuloplasty was achieved in seven of nine patients with severe mitral stenosis, with improvement in the mitral valve area from 0.7 ± 0.2 to 1.5 ± 0.2 cm², cardiac index from 2.6 ± 0.5 to 3.0 ± 0.9 L/min/M², and mean transmitral gradient from 15 ± 3 to 5 ± 3 mmHg. The technique described by these investigators involved two transseptal punctures, followed by dilatation of the interatrial septum with an 8 mm balloon, followed subsequently by placement of two 15 mm balloons across the mitral valve. The effect of balloon valvuloplasty on mitral valve competency was minimal, with no change in mitral regurgitation in four patients and an increase in mitral regurgitation from trace to 1+ in the remaining five.

Reports of Inoue, Lock, and Al Zaibag[25–27] were essentially limited to young patients with no evidence of calcific mitral valve disease or mitral regurgitation at baseline. The first reports of successful balloon mitral valvuloplasty in adult patients with calcific mitral stenosis were made simultaneously by our laboratory[28] and by Palacios et al.[29] In our study, a 75-year-old man with long-standing rheumatic mitral stenosis and marked valve calcification, mild mitral regurgitation, and severe pulmonary hypertension underwent valvuloplasty with a single 25 mm balloon. This brought about reduction of the mean mitral valve gradient from 18 to 12 mmHg, an increase in cardiac index from 1.7 to 2.5 liters/minute/M^2 and an increase in mitral valve area from 0.6 to 1.4 cm^2. Mitral regurgitation increased from mild (1+) to moderate (2+). Repeat catheterizations 6 and 12 months after valvuloplasty showed essentially complete resolution of pulmonary hypertension and no evidence of valvular restenosis or worsening mitral regurgitation. It is notable, however, that the procedure did result in an atrial septal defect with a pulmonary-to-systemic blood flow ratio of 1.8/1.0.

Palacios et al.[29] similarly described successful mitral valvuloplasty in a 57-year-old man, also with calcific mitral stenosis. Dilatation with a single 25 mm balloon resulted in a decrease in mitral gradient from 20 to 4 mmHg, an increase in cardiac output from 3.4 to 5.7 liters/minute and an increase in mitral valve area from 0.7 to 2.5 cm^2. The procedure was not associated with significant increase in mitral regurgitation or creation of an atrial septal defect.

Since these initial reports of the use of balloon mitral valvuloplasty in adult patients, several larger series have appeared in the literature. Palacios et al. reported results in 35 patients with severe mitral stenosis, including 16 with mitral valve calcification.[30] In this series, balloon dilatation resulted in a reduction of the mean mitral gradient from 18 ± 1 to 7 ± 1 mmHg, an increase in cardiac output from 3.9 ± 0.2 to 4.6 ± 0.2 L/min/minute, and an increase in mitral valve area from 0.8 ± 0.1 to 1.7 ± 0.2 cm^2. Complications included death of one patient, an embolic episode in one patient, the development of moderate to severe mitral regurgitation in one patient, and complete heart block requiring temporary ventricular pacing in two patients.

Charles McKay and coworkers reported similar results using a double-balloon technique in 12 patients with rheumatic mitral stenosis.[31] In this series, the mean mitral gradient decreased from 16 ± 6 to 5 ± 2 mmHg, cardiac output increased from 4.4 ± 1.2 to 5.5 ± 1.4 L/min, and mitral valve area increased from 1.0 ± 3.3 to 2.4 ± 0.8 cm^2. Mitral regurgitation did not increase in any patient and no embolic episodes occurred. Oximetry demonstrated small left-to-right shunts in 2 of the 12 patients.

Numerous modifications in mitral valvuloplasty technique have been introduced over the last several years. The first use of a retrograde approach to valve dilatation was reported by Babic in 1986.[32] In three patients with moderate mitral stenosis, a balloon catheter was inserted percutaneously from the left femoral artery over a long guide wire and advanced retrograde to the level of the mitral valve and inflated; the guide wire which was used had been previously introduced into the right femoral vein and advanced transseptally through a Brockenbrough catheter to the left ventricle, where it was subsequetly drawn out of the body through the left femoral artery using an intravascular retriever set. Successful balloon dilatation was achieved in all three patients without increases in mitral regurgitation or emboli.

Another modification of the retrograde approach to mitral valvuloplasty involving retrograde left atrial catheterization and not requiring transseptal catheterization was reported in 1989 by Orme.[33] Using this technique in three patients, the authors were able to perform double-balloon valvuloplasty in all three patients without significant complications.

Use of a trefoil balloon for mitral dilatation in a large cohort of patients was described by Vahanian in 1988.[34] Balloon valvuloplasty was attempted in 130 patients and was successful in 121, using either a single trefoil balloon or a double trefoil balloon. Valvuloplasty resulted in an increase in mitral valve area from 1.1 ± 0.2 to 2.2 ± 0.5 cm^2. Complications described in the study group included air embolism in one patient and left ventricular perforation in two.

Still another modification of the mitral valvuloplasty technique that has been reported is use of the Inoue "self-positioning" balloon.[35] This was developed by Inoue and involved a single balloon that inflated distally first, followed by inflation of the proximal portion of the balloon. Its use allows more stable placement of the balloon catheter within the mitral orifice, and prevents slippage during inflation. In a preliminary report on 515 patients, use of this balloon resulted in an increase in valve area from 1.2 ± 0.4 to 1.9 ± 0.5 cm^2, with an incidence of complications of cerebral embolism in 0.5%, severe mitral regurgitation in 2%, and atrial septal defect in 15%.

Various factors have been identified that influence the ability to perform a successful mitral valvuloplasty. Herrmann et al.[36] analyzed 60 consecutive mitral dilatation procedures and found an increase in mitral valve area from 0.8 ± 0.04 to 1.6 ± 0.11 cm^2 with a decrease in valve gradient from 18 ± 1 to 7 ± 0.4 mmHg. Of note, 21 of the 60 patients (35%) had a suboptimal result, defined as a postprocedure valve area less than 1 cm^2, an increase in valve area less than 25%, or a final gradient of 10 mmHg or more. Patients in whom such a result was obtained were those with severe valve leaflet thickening or immobility and an extreme amount of subvalvular thickening and calcification by echocardiogram. A too-small balloon dilating area and atrial fibrillation also predicted a poorer result.

Palacios, Block, and coworkers subsequently developed a score, based on the echocardiogram, that seems to help predict outcome.[37,46] Leaflet mobility, leaflet thickening, subvalvular thickening, and calcification are each rated on a scale of 1 to 4 with the last two factors being the most important. Based on echo score and clinical parameters, a good candidate is defined as having a total echo score less than 8, young age, and normal sinus rhythm. Likewise, a poor candidate is one who is older than 70 years, with long-standing atrial fibrillation, and an echo score greater than 11. Data from Reid et al.[38] have confirmed these results, noting that patients having rigid leaflets, subvalvular disease, and calcification tend to have poorer results with balloon dilatation of the mitral valve.

Pathophysiologic Mechanisms

The mechanism of successful balloon valvuloplasty was first described by Inoue, who noted separation of fused commissures on direct vision in patients who had undergone percutaneous mitral valvuloplasty and subsequently underwent mitral valve replacement.[25] This finding was corroborated in our laboratory, which described the results of balloon valvuloplasty in postmortem specimens of the mitral valve.[39] Postmortem balloon dilatation caused an increased valve orifice area in all valves that were dilated. The mechanism of successful valve dilatation involved separation of fused commissures, as well as increased leaflet mobility secondary to balloon-induced fractures through calcific nodules in the leaflets. Of note, in no case did balloon dilatation result in tearing of valve leaflets, disruption of the mitral ring, or liberation of potentially embolic debris. Similar results have been noted by Block et al.[40] and Kaplan and co-workers.[41]

Technical Aspects

Currently, both single- and double-balloon techniques are used in our laboratories to dilate stenotic mitral valves. After administration of a local anesthetic, the left femoral artery and left and right femoral veins are instrumented with 8 Fr vascular sheaths. Routine left and right heart catheterization using a 7 Fr pigtail catheter and a 7 Fr balloon-flotation pacing catheter, respectively, is performed from the left groin. During the right heart catheterization, a diagnostic oxygen saturation series is obtained. After placement of the left and right heart catheters, systemic arterial, left ventricular, pulmonary capillary wedge, and pulmonary artery pressure, and Fick cardiac output are measured. Pulmonary capillary wedge pressure is confirmed by aspirating blood from the wedge position and subsequently documenting an arterial oxygen saturation. Oxygen consumption is measured using a metabolic rate meter (Waters). Left ventriculography is then performed in the routine manner.

After prevalvuloplasty measurements, transseptal catheterization is accomplished by standard technique using an 8F Mullins transseptal sheath and dilator and Brockenbrough needle. After entry into the left atrium, the needle and dilator are removed and a 7 Fr balloon-tipped end-hole catheter that can accommodate an 0.038 inch guide wire (Critikon) is advanced from the sheath into the left atrium. Left heart pressures and the transvalvular pressure gradient are then measured. The 7 Fr balloon catheter is then advanced through the mitral valve into the left ventricle, followed by insertion of an 0.038 inch, 300 cm long Teflon-coated exchange wire into the flow-directed catheter. Alternatively, the 7 Fr balloon catheter (with balloon inflated) may be advanced to the LV apex, curved to reverse direction, advanced across the aortic valve and placed in the descending thoracic aorta. The sheath and balloon catheter are then removed, leaving only the guide wire in place (Fig. 29–1).

Next, an 8F angioplasty catheter with an 8 mm balloon (Medi-Tech) is advanced over the guide wire to the level of the interatrial septum and inflated to dilate the septal opening (Fig. 29–1A). After removal of this catheter, a 9 Fr balloon dilatation catheter with a 25 mm balloon (Medi-Tech) is advanced across the septum to the left atrium and then to the position of the mitral annulus. Under fluoroscopic control, the balloon is subsequently inflated for 10 to 15 seconds with a mixture of saline and radiographic contrast medium (Fig. 29–1). Repeat inflations are made until the waist in the balloon at the level of the mitral valve disappears. Immediately after balloon valvuloplasty, all hemodynamic measurements are repeated, including determination of the transvalvular pressure gradient and the cardiac output (Fig. 29–2). Left ventriculography and right heart oximetry are also repeated to document changes in the degree of mitral regurgitation and to search for evidence of a new left-to-right shunt, respectively. Mitral valve areas before and after valvuloplasty are calculated by the Gorlin formula, using systemic blood flow in the presence of a left-to-right shunt.

In patients who do not have sufficient gradient reduction with a single-balloon technique, a double-balloon technique is used. In these patients, after placement of the first guide wire through the mitral orifice as described previously, a second guide wire is similarly placed using a double lumen 7F exchange catheter (Medi-Tech) designed by Drs. Block and Palacios to accommodate two guide wires. The exchange catheter is removed subsequently and 18 and 20 mm or two 20 mm dilatation balloons are then positioned over the two guide wires in the mitral apparatus before simultaneous inflation to effect valve dilatation.

All patients are treated with a total of 10,000 units of IV heparin immediately after transseptal catheterization.

Clinical Results

Between October 1, 1985 and January 1, 1989, percutaneous mitral valvuloplasty was attempted in 120 patients with mitral stenosis at the Beth Israel Hospital, Boston, Mass. The study group has consisted of 89 women and 31 men with a mean age of 59 years (range 27 to 83). All patients were symptomatic with congestive heart failure and were classified as NYHA Class II, III, or IV. Sixteen percent of patients had coronary artery disease, 53% had significant valvular calcification, and 38% were in atrial fibrillation. Mitral regurgitation was absent in 35% of patients, mild in 40% of patients, moderate in the remaining 25% of patients. Fourteen patients in this group had previously undergone mitral commissurotomy.

Of the patients in whom balloon mitral valvuloplasty was attempted, 54% were considered poor surgical candidates and the remaining 46% refused surgery as their initial therapy. Patients were classified as poor surgical candidates for the following reasons: age over 70 (32%), severe pulmonary hypertension (34%), need for extensive additional surgery including aortic valve replacement and/or coronary bypass surgery (12%), moribund clinical state (7%), severe chronic obstructive lung disease (2%), severe left ventricular dysfunction (2%), morbid obesity (1%), pregnancy (2%), and religious objection (Jehovah's witness) (1%).

Balloon mitral valvuloplasty was successful in 110 patients (92%) and unsuccessful in the remaining 10 (8%). The 10 unsuccessful pro-

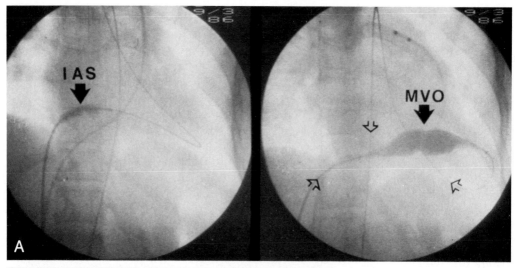

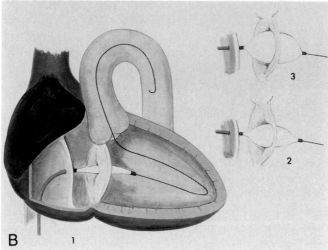

Fig. 29–1. Mitral balloon valvuloplasty (A) in a woman with severe mitral stenosis. The procedure involved dilatation of the interatrial septum (IAS) followed by placement of a 25 mm dilatation balloon across the mitral orifice (dark arrow, MVO). A guide wire (white arrows) is looped in the left ventricular apex and its tip is positioned in the descending thoracic aorta. B shows a schematic representation of the procedure. Reproduced with permission from McKay RG, Grossman W: Balloon valvuloplasty for treating pulmonic, mitral, aortic, and prosthetic valve stenoses. *In* Braunwald E, Heart Disease Update, Suppl 1. Philadelphia: WB Saunders, 1988, pp 1–13, and McKay RG, et al: Balloon dilatation of mitral stenosis in adult patients: Postmortem and percutaneous mitral valvuloplasty studies. J Am Coll Cardiol 9:723, 1987.

cedures included death in one patient secondary to guide wire perforation of the left ventricle, mitral valve disruption with severe valvular regurgitation in two patients, left atrial perforation in three, inability to dilate the interatrial septum in three, and a severe vagal reaction in one.

In the 110 patients in whom the procedure was successfully completed, there was improvement in mitral valve area (1.0 ± 2.0 to 1.9 ± 0.8 cm^2), mean mitral gradient (14 ± 7 to 6 ± 3 mmHg), and cardiac output (4.3 ± 1.3 to 5.1 ± 1.8 L/min). There were also significant decreases in left atrial pressure (24 ± 3 to 16 ± 2 mmHg), mean pulmonary

artery pressure (39 ± 5 to 31 ± 3 mmHg), and pulmonary vascular resistance (335 ± 120 to 277 ± 120 dynes-sec-cm-5). There were no significant changes in left ventricular systolic or diastolic pressure, mean right atrial pressure, or heart rate.

Complications that occurred in the 120 procedures included the mentioned procedural death secondary to guide wire perforation, 1 patient; in-hospital death secondary to a pulmonary embolus, 1 patient; mitral valve disruption requiring urgent mitral valve replacement, 2; cardiac tamponade secondary to left atrial perforation, 3; cerebrovascular events including one stroke and one transient ischemic

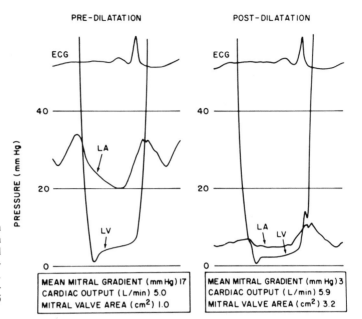

PRE-DILATATION · POST-DILATATION

ECG

PRESSURE (mm Hg)

40 · 20 · 0

LA · LV

MEAN MITRAL GRADIENT (mmHg) 17
CARDIAC OUTPUT (L/min) 5.0
MITRAL VALVE AREA (cm^2) 1.0

MEAN MITRAL GRADIENT (mmHg) 3
CARDIAC OUTPUT (L/min) 5.9
MITRAL VALVE AREA (cm^2) 3.2

Fig. 29–2. Hemodynamic result in a young woman undergoing balloon valvuloplasty for treatment of mitral stenosis. Left atrial (LA) and left ventricular (LV) pressures are shown. The gradient was practically eliminated in this patient with a single 25 mm balloon.

attack, 2; atrial septal defect postprocedure, 19; transient dysrhythmias, 13; and need for transfusion, 3.

Clinical outcome in the patients who underwent 110 successful procedures is as follows. At a mean follow-up of 16 months, 87 patients remained symptomatically improved. Fourteen patients had developed recurrent symptoms. Seven of these underwent early or late mitral valve replacement, four were treated medically, and three underwent repeat balloon mitral valvuloplasty at a mean of 17 months after initial dilatation. Of these three patients, two have subsequently died, one of complications related to peripheral vascular surgery and one of lung cancer. The third patient remains symptomatically improved 13 months following repeat dilatation. There have been 10 other deaths, at a mean of 10 months following valvuloplasty, for a total of 12 deaths in patients who underwent a successful procedure. Causes of late death include progressive heart failure because of uncorrected tricuspid regurgitation, 1 patient; progressive heart failure from multivalvular and coronary artery disease, 1; stroke in the setting of inadequate anticoagulation, 1; tamponade from pacemaker insertion, 1; urosepsis, 1; COPD, 2; cancer, 2; noncardiac surgery, 2.

Doppler echocardiographic follow-up data showed immediate improvement in mitral valve area (0.9 to 1.7 cm^2) and mitral valve gradient (12 to 6 mmHg). Follow-up echoes ranging to 12 months postprocedure demonstrated a mild decrease in mitral valve area to 1.5 cm^2.

Repeat cardiac catheterization at a mean of 12 months following valve dilatation has been performed in 24 patients, including 7 who had recurrent symptoms. For the entire group as a whole, the mitral valve areas increased from 0.9 to 1.8 cm^2 immediately after valvuloplasty, and remained significantly elevated at 1 year following valvuloplasty at 1.4 cm^2. Actuarial survival by standard life-table analysis demonstrates a 91% probability of survival at 1 year postprocedure and 86% at 2 years. In terms of recurrence of symptoms, mitral valve replacement, or death, the probability of event-free survival was 85% at 1 year.

Complications

It is notable that all early series of balloon mitral valvuloplasty have demonstrated both major and minor complications. Perhaps the most serious complication is cerebrovascular accident secondary to an embolic event. Emboli complicating closed surgical mitral commissurotomy have been estimated to range from 4 to 8%,[42] and will probably remain a definite complication of both surgical and balloon mitral valvuloplasty. In our laboratories, patients with evidence of left atrial thrombus on echocardiographic examination or those who have had a history of prior embolic events are excluded from mitral valvuloplasty. In addition, all patients are anticoagulated with coumadin for a period of 4 to 6 weeks before intervention. Nevertheless, dislodgement of left atrial thrombus not detected by prevalvuloplasty echocardiographic examination, or release of calcific debris following balloon dilatation, could potentially lead to embolism. Recent studies have suggested that transesophageal echocardiography may be more sensitive than standard 2D echocardiography in detecting left atrial thrombi, and may help to decrease the incidence of embolic valvuloplasty complications by eliminating patients at risk.[43] A second potentially life-threatening complication of mitral valvuloplasty is acute, severe mitral regurgitation. This complication presumably results either from tearing of valve leaflets that may occur with an over-sized balloon(s), or secondary to improper positioning of the dilatation balloon through mitral chordae tendinae. In our laboratories, mitral valvuloplasty is performed with a nitroprusside mixture, an intra-aortic balloon console, and cardiac surgery all on stand-by in the event of balloon-induced massive mitral regurgitation.

Still another potential complication is cardiac perforation, leading to cardiac tamponade. The transseptal approach is, by itself, associated with a small but finite risk of cardiac perforation. In addition, improper positioning of the mitral valvuloplasty guide wire could lead to left ventricular perforation.

Creation of a significant atrial septal defect secondary to septal dilatation is perhaps the most common complication of mitral valvuloplasty. Thus far, no acute hemodynamic deterioration has been described in patients with a balloon-induced atrial septal defect, and preliminary work has failed to identify any long-term deleterious effects of these interatrial

shunts.[44] In our series, the incidence of defect creation is higher with a single (25 mm)-balloon technique rather than the double-balloon technique, suggesting that the profile of the deflated balloon is an important factor in this complication. Potential improvements in balloon technology to produce lower profile balloons will probably decrease the incidence of this complication.

All of these complications could potentially result in death of the patient during the procedure, and any true assessment of the safety of balloon mitral valvuloplasty will obviously have to measure an actual procedural mortality rate. It will be important, however, to assess this mortality rate in terms of the patient population in which the procedure is performed. Mitral valvuloplasty may, for example, become the procedure of choice in treating very elderly patients with long-standing mitral stenosis complicated by severe pulmonary hypertension—a subgroup of patients who may previously have been considered inoperable or at high risk for operation.[45] The risk of balloon mitral valvuloplasty in these patients would presumably be significantly higher than in other candidates, and cannot be compared simply to the extremely low mortality rates currently cited for mitral valve surgery.

Long-Term Follow-up

To date, only limited information has been reported on the long-term results of balloon mitral valvuloplasty. Because the incidence of restenosis after surgical valvuloplasty has been estimated to range from 2 to 60%, with approximately 10% of patients requiring reoperation within 5 years and 60% within 10 years,[45] it seems likely that significant rates of restenosis will also occur after balloon mitral valvuloplasty.

In 1989, Palacios published data on 100 consecutive mitral valvuloplasty patients who were followed a mean of 13 months after dilatation, and demonstrated that valvular restenosis and postprocedure mortality were directly related to the prevalvuloplasty echo score.[46] Patients with low echo scores tended to have better results with lower NYHA class on follow-up, less restenosis detected by catheterization and Doppler studies, and a lower mortality rate.

Al Zaibag[47] published echocardiographic results on 41 patients who had undergone double-balloon valvuloplasty, and found no significant change in mitral valve area between 6 weeks and 1 year following the procedure (pre: 0.8 ± 0.2 cm^2; 6 weeks: 1.6 ± 0.3 cm^2; 1 year: 1.7 ± 0.3 cm^2). Predilation, 29% of patients were NYHA Class II and 71% of patients were either NYHA Class III or IV. One year postdilatation, all patients were alive, 88% were NYHA Class I, and 12% were NYHA Class II.

Conclusions

Early studies indicate that balloon mitral valvuloplasty can be accomplished successfully in both children and adults with rheumatic mitral stenosis, including patients with moderate to severe calcification, mild to moderate mitral regurgitation, and severe pulmonary hypertension. Significant lessening of symptoms may result from improvement in valvular function. The mechanism of successful valve dilatation involves separation of fused commissures and fracture of nodular calcium. Major complications associated with the procedure include embolic phenomena, acute mitral regurgitation, left ventricular perforation, creation of an atrial septal defect, and death. Based on these early results, our current indications for mitral valvuloplasty include two groups of patients: those who are considered high-risk candidates for surgical intervention because of severe pulmonary hypertension, biventricular heart failure, advanced age, and/or associated medical conditions such as chronic pulmonary or renal failure; and those who would not be optimum candidates for either chronic anticoagulation or placement of a porcine bioprosthesis (e.g., young women who wish to become pregnant). As more information becomes available on the long-term follow-up of mitral valvuloplasty in this latter group, the procedure may be extended to larger

groups with mitral stenosis as an alternative to surgical intervention.

AORTIC VALVULOPLASTY

Historical Development

Unlike reports on the treatment of pulmonic and mitral stenosis, early reports on the surgical therapy of aortic stenosis did not predict a favorable response to mechanical valvular dilatation. And although early reports on balloon aortic valvuloplasty have often demonstrated dramatic hemodynamic and clinical improvement, the disappointing early surgical experience has been predictive of the late hemodynamic results, with mortality and restenosis rates associated with percutaneous balloon dilatation.

The earliest reports on the mechanical dilatation of aortic stenosis included studies on closed aortic commissurotomy.[48-54] In the 1950s, both Bailey and Harken experimented with the transventricular and retrograde insertion of various valvulotomes designed to incise the stenotic aortic valve somewhat indiscriminately. They found, however, that the procedure usually resulted in acute aortic regurgitation. In Bailey's first clinical case, he inserted a Brock valvulotome through the left ventricular apex and antegrade through the valve of a severely symptomatic 26-year-old woman with rheumatic aortic stenosis. When he drew the blade back through the valve, the heart slowed immediately and the patient died soon afterward. At autopsy, it was found that the noncoronary leaflet had been divided and was flail, resulting in severe incompetence. Realizing that the cusps must be preserved and only commissures divided, Bailey and others worked on several aortic dilators that were inserted either through the left ventricular apex or retrograde through the innominate artery. Operative mortality, however, remained high. As a result, closed aortic valvotomy for calcific aortic stenosis was largely abandoned soon after the development of open aortic valve surgery.

Valvulotomy under direct vision for congenital aortic stenosis was first described in 1956 and subsequently performed using both an inflow occlusion technique and cardiopulmonary bypass.[55] Late follow-up of patients undergoing open valvulotomy has revealed a high rate of restenosis requiring aortic valve replacement, as well as a significant incidence of major complications including aortic regurgitation, infective endocarditis, and embolization.[56] Similar results have been noted with mechanical decalcification/debridement procedures performed in adult patients with calcific aortic stenosis.[57] Nonetheless, open valvulotomy has remained the operation of choice for infants and children with critical aortic stenosis.

Percutaneous balloon aortic valvuloplasty was first performed in 23 children and young adults by Lababidi and Walls in 1984.[58] Patients ranged in age from 2 to 17 years and all were thought to have congenital aortic stenosis. Balloons 10 to 20 mm in diameter were advanced retrograde from the femoral artery and positioned in the aortic valve. Subsequent balloon dilatation resulted in a decrease in the peak aortic gradient from 113 ± 48 mmHg to 32 ± 15 mmHg with no change in the cardiac output. Labadidi's results were soon confirmed by Ruprath, who demonstrated the efficacy of this technique in infants and adolescents.[59]

Successful balloon valvuloplasty in adult patients with calcific aortic disease was first reported in 1986 by Cribier[60] and our laboratory.[61] In Cribier's report, three elderly patients (aged 68, 77, and 79) with calcific aortic stenosis were treated with percutaneous balloon dilatation. Valvuloplasty resulted in a reduction in peak aortic gradient from approximately 75 mmHg to 33 mmHg and an increase in calculated aortic valve area from 0.5 to 0.8 cm². Balloon dilatation produced no significant increase in aortic regurgitation or emboli, and brought about striking clinical improvement. Our initial report described two elderly patients (aged 93 and 85 years) with longstanding calcific aortic stenosis who underwent balloon dilatation with 12 to 18 mm balloons. Again, balloon valvuloplasty resulted in a substantial reduction in the peak aortic pressure

gradient and a significant increase in aortic valve area. In our first patient (Fig. 29–3), a 93-year-old woman with recurrent pulmonary edema, balloon dilatation resulted in elimination of symptoms of heart failure and angina and a subsequent increase in left ventricular ejecton fraction from 28 to 58% over 2 months. In the second patient, balloon dilatation brought about a significant improvement in congestive heart failure, but the patient continued to experience unstable angina. Coronary angiography revealed the presence of severe obstruction of the left main coronary artery and three-vessel coronary artery disease, and the patient subsequently underwent successful aortic valve replacement and coronary artery bypass grafting.

Following the initial reports of successful balloon aortic valvuloplasty in elderly patients, several larger series have appeared. In 1987, Cribier reported their experience with 92 adult patients with severe calcific aortic stenosis.[62] The mean age of Cribier's study group was 75 years. Valvuloplasty was performed using catheter balloon sizes of 15, 18, and 20 mm (Fig. 29–4), and resulted in a reduction of the mean systolic pressure gradient from 75 ± 26 to 30 ± 13 mmHg and an increase in the mean calculated aortic valve area from 0.49 ± 0.17 to 0.93 ± 0.36 cm². Immediately after the procedure, the ejection fraction increased from 48 ± 16 to $51 \pm 16\%$. In general, there were only minor increases in the severity of aortic regurgitation, except in two patients in whom it increased from 1 to 3 +. Subsequent follow-up showed marked improvement in symptoms of heart failure, angina, and syncope in most patients, although there were three in-hospital deaths and eight late deaths. Catheterization performed in 12 patients 4 to 24 weeks following the procedure showed that the hemodynamic improvement persisted.

Similar results were noted by Schneider and coworkers in a series of six patients in whom aortic valve area increased from 0.6 ± 0.1 cm² to 0.8 ± 0.1 cm² using 15 to 18 mm balloons.[63]

Several modifications of the percutaneous retrograde balloon aortic valvuloplasty tech-

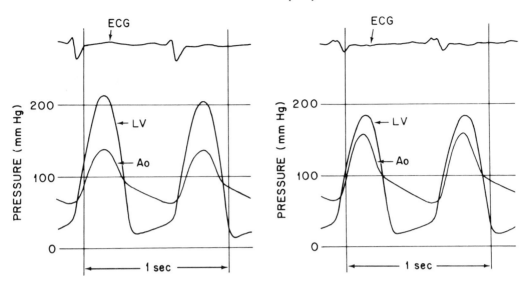

Fig. 29–3. Balloon valvuloplasty in a 93-year-old woman with severe aortic stenosis and congestive heart failure. Left ventricular (LV) and aortic (Ao) pressures are shown. Even though aortic valve area only increased from 0.4 cm^2 to 0.6 cm^2, LV ejection fraction by radionuclide technique rose from 28% prevalvuloplasty to 40% at 48 hours and 58% at 6 weeks after valvuloplasty.

nique have been described. The performance of balloon aortic valvuloplasty by way of a transseptal approach involving antegrade positioning of aortic valvuloplasty balloons advanced over a guide wire from the femoral vein has been described by Block and Palacios.[64] Use of a surgical cutdown to achieve femoral arterial access for valvuloplasty balloons has been described in patients by Isner and colleagues.[65] Both of these reports have provided possible alternative techniques to avoid the vascular trauma associated with percutaneous insertion of valvuloplasty catheters. Finally, use of a double-balloon technique for performing aortic valvuloplasty has been described by Dorros et al.[66] Using a combined

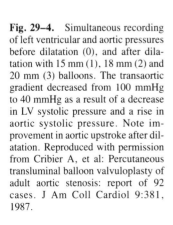

Fig. 29–4. Simultaneous recording of left ventricular and aortic pressures before dilatation (0), and after dilatation with 15 mm (1), 18 mm (2) and 20 mm (3) balloons. The transaortic gradient decreased from 100 mmHg to 40 mmHg as a result of a decrease in LV systolic pressure and a rise in aortic systolic pressure. Note improvement in aortic upstroke after dilatation. Reproduced with permission from Cribier A, et al: Percutaneous transluminal balloon valvuloplasty of adult aortic stenosis: report of 92 cases. J Am Coll Cardiol 9:381, 1987.

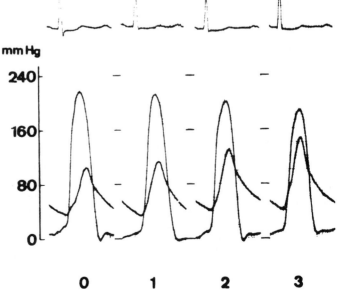

brachial and femoral artery approach to insert two valvuloplasty catheters simultaneously, successful valvuloplasty was achieved in 10 patients with a decrease in peak systolic gradient from 77 ± 28 to 27 ± 15 mmHg and an increase in aortic valve area from 0.6 to 1.0 cm^2.

Pathophysiologic Mechanisms

The mechanism of balloon aortic valvuloplasty has been studied from post-mortem and intraoperative dilatations performed in our laboratory (Fig. 29–5). In a study of 39 specimens,[67] the cause of aortic stenosis included degenerative nodular calcification in 28 cases, calcific bicuspid stenosis in 8, and rheumatic heart disease in 3. Balloon dilatation was performed with 15 to 25 mm balloons under direct vision. Following balloon dilatation, the dimensions of the valve orifice and mobility of the leaflets increased in all specimens. The mechanism of successful dilatation included fracture of calcified nodules in 16 aortic valves (Fig. 29–5), separation of fused commissures in 5 valves, both in 6 valves, and grossly inapparent microfractures in 12 valves. Liberation of calcific debris, valve disruption or mid-leaflet tears did not occur in any valve, although leaflet avulsion occurred in one after inflation with a clearly oversized balloon.

Given the range of possible mechanisms of aortic valvuloplasty (i.e., fracture of calcific nodules, commissural splitting, leaflet stretching) and the range of possible etiologies of aortic stenosis (i.e., senile degenerative, congenital bicuspid, and rheumatic), it is understandable that heterogenous results have been

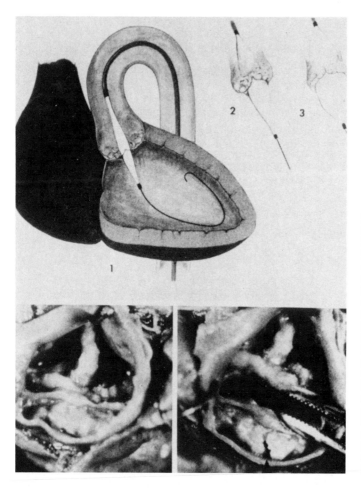

Fig. 29–5. Schematic representation of technique of retrograde balloon aortic valvuloplasty is illustrated in the upper panel. One mechanism of action of aortic valvuloplasty (fracture of calcific nodules) is seen in the lower panel of a postmortem specimen before (lower left) and after (lower right) in vitro balloon dilatation. Reproduced with permission from McKay RG, Grossman W: Balloon valvuloplasty for treating pulmonic, mitral, aortic, and prosthetic valve stenoses. *In* Braunwald E, Heart Disease Update, Suppl 1. Philadelphia, WB Saunders, 1988: 1–13; and Safian RD, et al: Postmortem and intraoperative balloon valvuloplasty of calcific aortic stenosis in elderly patients: Mechanisms of successful dilatation. J Am Coll Cardiol 1987 9:655, 1987.

associated with percutaneous valve dilatation, with some patients demonstrating little or no change in aortic valve area and others exhibiting marked increases. The variation in mechanism of dilatation and etiology of valvular stenosis may also be an important factor in the time course of valvular restenosis in any given patient.

Technical Aspects

In our laboratories, balloon aortic valvuloplasty is currently performed using a single-balloon advanced retrograde from the femoral artery. Patients initially undergo placement of a percutaneous radial cannula for blood pressure monitoring, right heart catheterization from the left femoral vein using a 7 Fr balloon-tipped flotation catheter, and left heart catheterization from the right femoral artery using a 7 Fr pigtail catheter. An 0.038 inch, straight-tipped guide wire is used initially to cross the aortic valve. After placement of left and right heart catheters, measurements are made of systemic arterial, left ventricular, pulmonary arterial, and pulmonary capillary wedge pressures, as well as Fick cardiac output. Aortic valve area is determined using the Gorlin formula.

Following prevalvuloplasty measurements, a 300 cm 0.038 inch exchange guide wire is advanced through the left heart catheter into the left ventricle, and the left heart catheter is removed. An additional curve is placed in the distal tip of the exchange wire to minimize trauma to the endocardium with subsequent balloon inflations and exchanges. A 12 Fr dilator (UMI) is inserted over this guide wire to dilate the femoral artery. Balloon dilatation is performed subsequently with valvuloplasty catheters inserted percutaneously and advanced retrograde over the exchange wire (Fig. 29–5). The initial valvuloplasty balloon used in most patients is a 20 mm balloon. In patients in whom the aortic valve area is less than 0.5 cm^2, the initial balloon used is a 15 mm, followed by an 18 or 20 mm balloon depending on the results of the initial dilatation. The largest balloon size used in our laboratory is 23 mm. This balloon is used only if inflations with a 20 mm balloon are tolerated without evidence of hypotension. The duration of inflation of each balloon is variable (range 20 to 60 seconds), depending on the degree of hypotension induced by left ventricular outflow tract obstruction from the fully inflated balloon. After the balloon dilatation, the valvuloplasty catheter is removed and replaced by the 12 Fr sheath to control bleeding from the femoral artery, and the pigtail catheter is exchanged over the guide wire into the left ventricle. Repeat measurements of pressures and cardiac output are made. All patients receive 5000 units of heparin.

Following the procedure, patients are monitored in the coronary care unit for at least 24 hours. The femoral artery sheath is removed approximately 4 hours after the procedure.

Clinical Results

Preliminary reports from two multicenter national studies currently under way have described hemodynamic results in large groups of aortic valvuloplasty subjects. The Mansfield Balloon Aortic Valvuloplasty Registry (Mansfield Scientific, Mansfield, MA) was established in 1986 and consists of 27 clinical centers across the United States that studied 492 patients who underwent balloon aortic valvuloplasty between 12/1/86 and 10/30/87.[68] The study group consisted of 273 females and 219 males with a mean age of 79 ± 8 years (range 22 to 95). All patients were symptomatic with congestive heart failure (92%), angina (54%), and/or syncope (22%), with 82% of patients classified as either New York Heart Class III or IV. All patients were considered to have an increased surgical risk for aortic valve replacement by virtue of advanced age (87%), severe coexisting medical condition (69%), severe left ventricular dysfunction (30%), and/or severe coronary artery disease requiring coronary artery bypass surgery (22%).

Balloon aortic valvuloplasty was performed from a femoral approach (92%), brachial approach (6%), or transseptal approach (2%). A single-balloon technique was used in 72% of patients, and a double-balloon technique in the remaining 28%. The largest balloon size was 20 mm in 54% of patients, with only 8% of patients having smaller balloon sizes (15 mm, 18 mm) and the remaining 38% having larger balloon sizes (23 mm, 25 mm, or double balloon combination).

Balloon aortic valvuloplasty resulted in an increase in aortic valve area from 0.50 ± 0.18 to 0.81 ± 0.18 cm^2, a decrease in mean aortic valve gradient from 60 ± 24 to 30 ± 14 mmHg, and an increase in cardiac output from 3.86 ± 0.55 to 4.01 ± 0.51 L/min. The overall complication rate for the procedure was 22.6%, including procedural death (4.9%), death within 7 days of the procedure (2.6%), embolic phenomenon (2.2%), ventricular perforation resulting in tamponade (1.4%), massive aortic insufficiency (1%), significant arrhythmia (0.8%), and myocardial infarction (0.2%). Emergency aortic valve replacement was done in 1.2% of the study group, and there was an 11% incidence of local vascular injury, with surgical repair required in 5.7% of the patients.

A second multicenter that has published preliminary aortic valvuloplasty results is the National Heart Lung and Blood Institute Balloon Valvuloplasty Registry.[69] This registry consists of 24 clinical centers enrolling aortic valvuloplasty patients as part of a planned 2-year study between November 1, 1987 and November 1, 1989. Preliminary results in 501 patients enrolled between November 1, 1987 and December 15, 1988 have been presented. The mean age of the study group was 79 years, including 43% women and 57% men. Congestive heart failure was present in 92% of patients, angina in 45% of patients, and prior syncope in 35%. The valvuloplasty technique was retrograde in 94% and transseptal in 3%; in the remaining 3%, the procedure was uncompleted. A single-balloon technique was used in 94% of the study group, including 3.2% of patients with balloon sizes less than 20 mm, 59% with a 20 mm balloon, and 34% with a 23 or 25 mm balloon. A double-balloon technique was used in 15% of patients, in-

cluding 7% in whom a single-balloon technique was also used.

Balloon aortic valvuloplasty resulted in an increase in aortic valve area from 0.5 ± 0.2 to 0.8 ± 0.5 cm^2, a decrease in aortic valve gradient from 57 ± 30 to 29 ± 13 mmHg, and an increase in cardiac output from 3.9 ± 1.2 to 4.1 ± 1.2 L/min. Major complications associated with the procedure including procedural death (2%), cardiac arrest (5%), emergency aortic valve replacement (1%), left ventricular perforation with tamponade (2%), cerebrovascular accident (1%), systemic embolus (1%), emergency temporary pacing (5%), persistent conduction defect (5%), and ventricular arrhythmia requiring countershock (3%).

Complications

As with balloon mitral valvuloplasty, major life-threatening complications can occur with aortic valvuloplasty. Major embolic events have been reported in isolated patients, and presumably represent dislodgement of calcific or thrombotic debris during the valvuloplasty procedure. A major increase in aortic regurgitation has likewise been reported on rare occasion, and may result from leaflet tearing or leaflet avulsion. The incidence of this complication as well as aortic rupture is presumably greater with the use of oversized balloons.[70] Ventricular perforation leading to tamponade has been reported in small numbers in several series. Vascular trauma requiring surgical repair has occurred as the most common complication in all series. Technical improvements in catheter design and construction to decrease the profiles of the deflated balloon may reduce the incidence of this complication. Conduction defects, primarily left bundle branch block, may occur but are usually transient.

Follow-up

There are sufficient follow-up data to confirm that restenosis and/or death are common in the first year after balloon aortic valvuloplasty. This is not surprising in view of surgical reports on open and closed aortic commissurotomy. As a result, use of the procedure in our hospitals is completely limited to patients with severe aortic stenosis in whom the risk of open heart surgery is high because of advanced age or concurrent illness.

Between October 1, 1985 and October 1, 1988, 193 patients (mean age 77 years) with critical aortic stenosis underwent balloon aortic valvuloplasty at the Beth Israel Hospital in Boston.[71] All were symptomatic with congestive heart failure, approximately one half had angina, and approximately one third experience syncope. Balloon aortic valvuloplasty was performed with 12 to 23 mm balloons from either the femoral (n = 182), brachial (n = 10), or transseptal approach (n = 1). Balloon dilatation resulted in an increase in cardiac output from 4.4 ± 1.4 to 4.8 ± 1.6 L/min, an increase in aortic valve area from 0.6 ± 0.2 to 0.9 ± 0.3 cm², and a decrease in peak aortic valve gradient from 71 ± 28 to 36 ± 15 mmHg. Major complications associated with the procedure included procedural death (n = 1), in-hospital death (n = 6), major increase in aortic regurgitation (n = 2), left ventricular perforation and tamponade (n = 3), vascular injury requiring surgical repair (n = 17), myocardial infarction (n = 1), and transient conduction abnormalities (n = 20).

Of the 193 consecutive procedures, 191 were completed successfully, with two procedures aborted due to intercurrent complications including ventricular perforation in one patient and iliac artery perforation in the second. Of the remaining patients, seven died before hospital discharge and seven underwent aortic valve replacement, including four because of a poor hemodynamic result and three because of concomitant coronary artery disease and persistent angina. The causes of in-hospital death included bradyarrhythmia, progressive heart failure, renal failure, ventricular perforation, ventricular tachycardia, and increased aortic regurgitation. A total of 178 patients were subsequently discharged from the hospital, with improvement in symptoms of heart failure, angina, and syncope in virtually all patients.

These 178 patients were followed clinically for a mean of 14 months after valvuloplasty.[71] Of these patients, 48 (28%) have died at a mean of 9.6 months post valvuloplasty, 35 (18%) have required aortic valve replacement a mean of 8 months postdilatation, and 27 (14%) have required repeat valvuloplasty at a mean of 10 months after initial valvuloplasty. The remaining 77 patients (40%) have had persistent symptomatic improvement. The predominant cause of late death was progressive congestive heart failure, with a small number of deaths from noncardiac causes. A Kaplan-Meir plot of survival and event-free survival has demonstrated a 1-year mortality of 28% and a 51% chance of having persistent clinical improvement without aortic valve replacement or repeat valvuloplasty.[71]

The clinical improvement associated with balloon aortic valvuloplasty may be accompanied by major improvement in systolic and diastolic left ventricular function. Safian et al.[72] published results on 25 patients with aortic stenosis and a depressed left ventricular ejection fraction in whom serial changes in left ventricular performance were assessed by radionuclide ventriculography before, immediately after, and 6 weeks after balloon aortic valvuloplasty.[72] Fourteen patients demonstrated progressive increases in left ventricular ejection fraction (36 to 49 to 59%) and in left ventricular peak filling rate (1.8 to 1.9 to 2.2 EDV/sec), while progressive decreases occurred in left ventricular end-diastolic volume index (138 to 119 to 99 ml/M²). The remaining 11 patients showed no change in left ventricular ejection fraction, peak filling rate, or left ventricular end-diastolic volume, but experienced significant clinical improvement. Of note, serial echocardiographic-Doppler assessment in this last group of patients showed significant decreases in mitral regurgitation, possibly offsetting a potential increase in left ventricular ejection fraction.

Conclusions

Balloon aortic valvuloplasty in children appears to be an effective and safe technique for treating congenital aortic stenosis, although additional follow-up is needed. Balloon aortic valvuloplasty in adults with calcific disease is a purely palliative procedure that often leads to marked symptomatic improvement but only a relatively small increase in aortic valve area and a high rate of restenosis. Potential mechanisms of balloon aortic valvuloplasty include fracture of calcific nodules, separation of fused commissures, and stretching of valve leaflets. Major complications of death, embolism, acute aortic regurgitation, and ventricular perforation are uncommon, although the risk of local vascular trauma requiring surgical repair is substantial. In adults, the procedure should be limited to high-risk patients who are deferred from surgical intervention.

There are several specific uses of balloon aortic valvuloplasty which are currently under investigation in our laboratories. First, in selected patients in whom surgery is considered a high risk because of poor left ventricular function, balloon valvuloplasty may be used as a preparative technique to improve cardiac output, left ventricular filling pressures, and left ventricular ejection fraction before aortic valve replacement. This may reduce surgical mortality and morbidity. Second, in patients who have both critical aortic stenosis and a second medical condition requiring surgical intervention (e.g., resection of a malignancy, fixation of a hip fracture, surgery for gastrointestinal bleeding, etc.), balloon aortic valvuloplasty may be performed first to increase the safety of general anesthesia and surgery for the second medical problem, followed by aortic valve replacement as definitive therapy for the aortic stenosis. Third, in patients with critical aortic stenosis characterized by a low aortic valve gradient with a low cardiac output, balloon aortic valvuloplasty may be used to assess the patient's left ventricular response to decreased afterload following valve dilatation, and thus to aid in deciding whether to proceed to aortic valve replacement.

TRICUSPID VALVULOPLASTY

To date, there have been only a few isolated reports on the successful use of balloon val-

vuloplasty to treat tricuspid stenosis. Al Zaibag first documented the technique in 1987 in a 27-year-old woman with rheumatic tricuspid stenosis.[73] The procedure was performed using a double-balloon technique (20 mm and 20 mm) and resulted in an increase in tricuspid valve area and in cardiac output, and marked symptomatic relief.

Khalilullah documented a second case of successful tricuspid valvuloplasty in a 36-year-old woman whose valve was dilated with two 20 mm balloons.[74] The procedure resulted in an increase in tricuspid valve area from 1.2 to 2.6 cm^2, and was associated with transient complete heart block which disappeared approximately twelve hours after the procedure.

In spite of the limited data on tricuspid valvuloplasty, it is expected that balloon dilatation will offer a feasible and effective percutaneous method for treating this condition. Given the most common rheumatic etiology of the disease, separation of fused commissures appears to be the underlying mechanism of success. A double-balloon technique will presumably be needed to achieve effective dilatation, given the size of the tricuspid annulus in most adults. In addition, given the proximity of the atrioventricular conduction system to the tricuspid valve, complete heart block is also expected to be a complication of the procedure.

VALVULOPLASTY FOR PROSTHETIC VALVE STENOSIS

Percutaneous dilatation of prosthetic valve stenosis is perhaps the most recent and most experimental of valvuloplasty techniques. Waldman published results of balloon dilatation of bioprosthetic valves in four children with a stenotic bioprosthetic porcine valve in right ventricle-to-pulmonary artery conduits.[75] The average gradient was reduced from 47 to 27 mmHg. Obstruction at the connection between the conduit and the pulmonary artery became apparent after dilatation of the valve. These distal stenoses were also dilated. Balloon dilatation was also tested in vitro with the use of nonstenotic valves and fresh conduits.

No damage to the valve or conduit was found when oversized balloons were used in a standard fashion or intentionally inflated until rupture.

The use of balloon valvuloplasty for stenosis of a Hancock porcine bioprosthesis in the tricuspid position was reported by Feit.[76] The tricuspid valve area increased from 0.69 to 1.22 cm². Balloon dilatation was associated with significant clinical improvement, markedly increased exercise tolerance, and decreased peripheral edema.

REFERENCES

1. Brock R: The surgical treatment of pulmonic stenosis. Br Heart J 23:337, 1961.
2. Semb BKH, Tjonneland S, Stake G, Aabyholm G: Balloon valvotomy of congenital pulmonary valve stenosis with tricuspid insufficiency. Cardiovasc Radiol 2:239, 1979.
3. Kan J, White RI, Mitchell SE, Gardner TJ: Percutaneous balloon valvuloplasty: A new method for treating congenital pulmonary valve stenosis. N Engl J Med 307:540, 1982.
4. Pepine CJ, Gessner JH, Feldman RL: Percutaneous balloon valvuloplasty for pulmonic valve stenosis in the adult. Am J Cardiol 50:1442, 1982.
5. Lababidi Z, Wu JR: Percutaneous balloon valvuloplasty. Am J Cardiol 52:560, 1983.
6. Walls JT, Curtis JJ: Assessment of percutaneous balloon pulmonary and aortic valvuloplasty. J Thorac Cardiovasc Surg 88:352, 1984.
7. Ring JC, Kulik TJ, Burke BA, Lock JE: Morphologic changes induced by dilation of the pulmonary valve annulus with over-large balloons in normal newborn lambs. Am J Cardiol 55:210, 1984.
8. Ali Khan MA, Yousef SA, Mullins CE: Percutaneous transluminal balloon pulmonary valvuloplasty for the relief of pulmonary valve stenosis with special reference to double-balloon technique. Am Heart J 112:158, 1986.
9. Meier B, Friedli B, Oberhaeush I, Belenger J, Fuici L: Trefoil balloon for percutaneous valvuloplasty. Cathet Cardiovasc Diagn 12:277, 1986.
10. Ben-Shachar G, Mark MH, Sivakoff MC, Portman MA, Riemenschneider TA, Van Heeckeren DW: Development of infundibular obstruction after percutaneous pulmonary balloon valvuloplasty. J Am Coll Cardiol 5:754, 1985.
11. Lock JE: Personal communication.
12. Attia I, Weinhaus L, Walls JT, Lababidi Z: Rupture of tricuspid valve papillary muscle during balloon pulmonary valvuloplasty. Am Heart J 114:1233, 1987.
13. Lo RNS, Clau K, Leung MP: Complete heart block after balloon dilatation for congenital pulmonary stenosis. Br Heart J 59:384, 1988.
14. Rey C, Marache P, Francart C, Dupuis C: Percutaneous transluminal balloon valvuloplasty of congenital pulmonary valve stenosis, with a special report on infants and neonates. J Am Coll Cardiol 11:815, 1988.
15. Mullins CE, et al: Balloon valvuloplasty for pulmonic valve stenosis—two year follow-up: Hemodynamic and doppler evaluation. Cathet Cardiovasc Diagn 14:76, 1988.
16. Rocchini AP, Beekman RH: Balloon angioplasty in the treatment of pulmonary valve stenosis and coarctation of the aorta. Texas Heart Inst J 13:377, 1986.
17. Shrivastava S, Sundar AS, Mukhopadhyaya S, Rajani M: Percutaneous transluminal balloon pulmonary valvuloplasty—long term results. Int J Cardiol 17:303, 1987.
18. Cutler EC, Beck CS: The present status of the surgical procedures in chronic valvular disease of the heart. Arch Surg 18:403, 1929.
19. Harken DE, Ellis LB, Ware PF, Norman LR: The surgical treatment of mitral stenosis. I. Valvuloplasty. N Engl J Med 239:801, 1948.
20. Glover RP, Bailey CP, O'Neill TJE: Surgery of stenotic valvular disease of the heart. JAMA 144:1049, 1950.
21. Bailey CP: The surgical treatment of mitral stenosis (mitral commissurotomy). Dis Chest 15:377, 1949.
22. Bailey CP, Glover RP, O'Neill TJE: The surgery of mitral stenosis. J Thorac Surg 19:16, 1950.
23. Brockenbrough EC, Braunwald E: A new technique for left ventricular angiocardiography and transseptal left heart catheterization. Am J Cardiol 6:1062, 1960.
24. Rashkind WJ, Miller WW: Creation of an artrial septal defect without thoracotomy: A palliative approach to complete transposition of the great vessels. JAMA 196:991, 1966.
25. Inoue K, Owaki T, Nakamura T, Kitamura F, Miyamoto N: Clinical application of transvenous mitral commissurotomy by a new balloon catheter. J Thorac Cardiovasc Surg 87:394, 1984.
26. Lock JE, Khalilullah M, Shrivasta S, Bahl V, Keane JF: Percutaneous catheter commissurotomy in rheumatic mitral stenosis. N Engl J Med 313:1515, 1985.
27. Al Zaibag M, Kasab SA, Ribeiro PA, Fagih MR: Percutaneous double balloon mitral valvotomy for the rheumatic mitral valve stenosis. Lancet 1:757, 1986.
28. McKay RG, Lock JE, Keane JF, Safian RD, Aroesty JM, Grossman W: Percutaneous mitral valvuloplasty in an adult patient with calcific rheumatic stenosis. J Am Coll Cardiol 7:1410, 1986.
29. Palacios IF, Lock JE, Keane JF, Block PC: Percutaneous transvenous balloon valvotomy in a patient with severe calcific mitral stenosis. J Am Coll Cardiol 7:1416, 1986.
30. Palacios I, et al: Percutaneous balloon valvotomy for patients with severe mitral stenosis. Circulation 75:778, 1987.
31. McKay CR, Kawanishi DT, Rahimtoola SH: Catheter balloon valvuloplasty of the mitral valve in adults using a double balloon technique. JAMA 257:1753, 1987.
32. Babic UU, Pejic P, Djurisic Z, Vucinic M, Grujicic SM: Percutaneous transarterial balloon valvuloplasty for mitral stenosis. Am J Cardiol 57:1101, 1986.
33. Orme EC, Wray RB, Mason JW: Balloon mitral valvuloplasty via retrograde left atrial catheterization. Am Heart J 117:680, 1989.

34. Vahanian A, et al: Percutaneous mitral commissurotomy. A propros of 130 cases. Arch Mal Coeur 81:755, 1988.
35. Inoue K, Nobuyoshi M, Chen C, Hung JS: Advantage of Inoue-balloon (self-positioning) in percutaneous mitral commissurotomy. Circulation 78:II-490, 1988.
36. Hermann HC, Wilkins GT, Abascal VM, Weyman AE, Block PC, Palacios IF: Percutaneous balloon mitral valvotomy for patients with mitral stenosis. J Thorac Cardiovasc Surg 96:33, 1988.
37. Block PC: Who is suitable for percutaneous balloon mitral valvuloplasty? Int J Cardiol 20:9, 1988.
38. Reid CL, McKay CR, Chandraratna PAN, Kawanishi DT, Rahimtoola SH: Mechanisms of increase in mitral valve area and influence of anatomic features in double-balloon, catheter balloon valvuloplasty in adults with rheumatic mitral stenosis. Circulation 76:628, 1987.
39. McKay RG, et al: Balloon dilation of mitral stenosis in adults: Post-mortem and percutaneous mitral valvuloplasty studies. J Am Coll Cardiol 9:723, 1987.
40. Block PC, Palacios IF, Jacobs ML, Fallon JT: Mechanism of percutaneous mitral valvuloplasty. Am J Cardiol 59:178, 1987.
41. Kplan JD, et al: In-vitro analysis of mechanisms of balloon valvuloplasty of stenotic mitral valves. Am J Cardiol 59:318, 1987.
42. Mullins EM, Glancy EL, Higgs LM, Epstein SE, Morrow AG: Current results of operation for mitral stenosis. Clinical and hemodynamic assessments in 124 consecutive patients treated by closed commissurotomy, open commissurotomy or valve replacement. Circulation 46:298, 1972.
43. Seward JB, et al: Transesophageal echocardiography: technique, anatomic correlations, implementation, and clinical applications. Mayo Clin Proc 63:649, 1988.
44. Erny RE, Diver DJ, Safian RD, Come PC, Grossman W, McKay RG: Hemodynamic results and follow-up of patients with iatrogenic atrial septal defects following balloon mitral valvuloplasty. J Am Coll Cardiol 13:70A, 1989.
45. Ellis LB, Singh JB, Morales DD, Harken DE: Fifteen to twenty-year study of one thousand patients undergoing closed mitral valvuloplasty. Circulation 48:357, 1973.
46. Palacios IF, Block PC, Wilkins GT, Weyman AE: Follow-up of patients undergoing percutaneous mitral valvotomy. Analysis of factors determining restenosis. Circulation 79:573, 1989.
47. Al Zaibag M, et al: One year follow-up after percutaneous double balloon mitral valvotomy. Am J Cardiol 63:126, 1989.
48. Bailey CP, Glover RP, O'Neill TJE, Ramirez HPR: Experiences with the experimental surgical relief of aortic stenosis. J Thorac Surg 20:516, 1950.
49. Smithey HG, Parker EF: Experimental aortic valvulotomy. A preliminary report. Surg Gynecol and Obstet 84:625, 1947.
50. Brock RC: The arterial route to the aortic and pulmonary valves. The mitral route to the aortic valve. Guy's Hosp Report 99:236, 1950.
51. Bailey CP, Redondo-Ramirez HP, Larzelere HB: Surgical treatment of aortic stenosis. JAMA 150:1647, 1952.
52. Larzelere HB, Bailey CP: Aortic commissurotomy. J Thorac Surg 26:31, 1953.
53. Larzelere HB, Bailey CP: New instrument for cardiac valvular commissurotomy. J Thorac Surg 25:78, 1953.
54. Bailey CP, Bolton HE, Jamison WL, Nichols HT: Commissurotomy for rheumatic aortic stenosis. 1. Surgery. Circulation 9:23, 1954.
55. Abelmann WH, Ellis LB: Severe aortic stenosis in adults: Evaluation by clinical and physiologic criteria and results of surgical treatment. Ann Intern Med 51:449, 1959.
56. Hsieh Kai-sheng, Keane JF, Nadas AS, Bernhard WF, Castaneda AR: Long-term follow-up of valvotomy before 1968 for congenital aortic stenosis. Am J Cardiol 58:338, 1986.
57. King RM, Pluth JR, Giuliani ER, Piehler JM: Mechanical decalcification of the aortic valve. Ann Thorac Surg 42:269, 1986.
58. Lababidi Z, Wu JR, Walls JT: Percutaneous balloon aortic valvuloplasty: Results in 23 patients. Am J Cardiol 53:194, 1984.
59. Rupprath G, Neuhaus KL: Percutaneous balloon valvuloplasty for aortic valve stenosis in infancy. Am J Cardiol 55:1655, 1985.
60. Cribier A, Savin T, Saondi N, Rocha P, Berland J, Letac B: Percutaneous transluminal valvuloplasty of acquired aortic stenosis in elderly patients. An alternative to valve replacement? Lancet 1:63, 1986.
61. McKay RG, Safian RD, Lock JE, Mandell VS, Thurer RL, Schmitt SJ, Grossman W: Post-mortem, intraoperative, and percutaneous valvuloplasty studies. Circulation 74:119, 1986.
62. Cribier A, Savin T, Berland J, Rocha P, Mechmeche R, Saoudi N, Behar P, Letac B: Percutaneous transluminal balloon valvuloplasty of adult aortic stenosis: Report of 92 cases. J Am Coll Cardiol 9:381, 1987.
63. Schneider JF, Wilson M, Gallant TE: Percutaneous balloon aortic valvuloplasty for aortic stenosis in elderly patients at high risk for surgery. Ann Intern Med 106:696, 1987.
64. Block PC, Palacios IF: Comparison of hemodynamic results of antegrade versus retrograde percutaneous balloon aortic valvuloplasty. Am J Cardiol 60:259, 1987.
65. Isner JM, et al: Treatment of calcific aortic stenosis by balloon valvuloplasty. Am J Cardiol 59:313, 1987.
66. Dorros G, Lewin RF, King JF, Janke LM: Percutaneous transluminal valvuloplasty in calcific aortic stenosis: The double balloon technique. Cathet Cardiovasc Diagn 13:151, 1987.
67. Safian RD, et al: Postmortem and intraoperative balloon valvuloplasty of calcific aortic stenosis in elderly patients: Mechanisms of successful dilation. J Am Coll Cardiol 9:655, 1987.
68. McKay RG, for the Mansfield Scientific Aortic Valvuloplasty Registry: Balloon aortic valvuloplasty in 285 patients: Initial results and complications. Circulation 78:II-594, 1988.
69. McKay RG, for the NHLBI Aortic Valvuloplasty Registry: Clinical outcome following balloon aortic valvuloplasty for severe aortic stenosis. J Am Coll Cardiol 13:1218, 1989.
70. Lewin RF, Dorros G, King JF, Seifert PE, Schmahl TM, Auer JE: Aortic annular tear after valvuloplasty:

The role of the aortic annulus echocardiographic measurement. Cathet Cardiovasc Diagn 16:123, 1989.

71. Safian RD, et al: Balloon aortic valvuloplasty in 170 consecutive patients. N Engl J Med 319:125, 1988.

72. McKay RG, et al: Assessment of left ventricular and aortic valve function after aortic balloon valvuloplasty in adult patients with critical aortic stenosis. Circulation 75:192, 1987.

73. Al Zaibag M, Ribeiro P, Al Kasab S: Percutaneous balloon valvotomy in tricuspid stenosis. Br Heart J 57:51, 1987.

74. Khalilullah M, Yadav BS, Lochan R: Double balloon valvuloplasty of tricuspid stenosis. Am Heart J 114:1232, 1987.

75. Waldman JD, et al: Balloon dilatation of porcine bioprosthetic valves in the pulmonary position. Circulation 76:109, 1987.

76. Feit F, Stecy PJ, Nachame MS: Percutaneous balloon valvuloplasty for stenosis of a porcine bioprosthesis in the tricuspid valve position. Am J Cardiol 58:363, 1983, 1986.

30

Pediatric Interventions

STANTON B. PERRY, JOHN F. KEANE, and JAMES E. LOCK

The list of transcatheter interventions available for treating patients with congenital and acquired heart disease continues to grow. Among these procedures are creation of interatrial defects by balloon and blade septostomy,[1,2] balloon dilation of stenotic vessels and valves, and closure of unwanted intra- and extracardiac defects and vessels. This chapter focuses on the technical aspects of eight interventions: percutaneous balloon pulmonary valvotomy; aortic valvotomy; angioplasty of aortic coarctation and of pulmonary artery stenosis; coil embolization of unwanted vessels, and double umbrella closure of patent ductus arteriosus (PDA), atrial septal defects (ASD), and ventricular septal defects (VSD).

BALLOON DILATION VALVULOPLASTY AND ANGIOPLASTY

When choosing a balloon dilation catheter for a particular procedure, one must consider both the lesion to be dilated and the various characteristics of the catheter. Choosing the most appropriate catheter is important not only to maximize the likelihood of successful dilation but also to avoid or minimize complications. The most common type of balloon dilation catheter has a single, cylindric balloon mounted on a shaft, and is delivered to the stenotic lesion over a guide wire. This type of

catheter has the advantages of distributing wall stress equally around the circumference and folding to a relatively small profile in its collapsed state. They do, however, tend to obstruct blood flow completely during inflation. Catheters with two or three balloons mounted on the same shaft help overcome this problem, but their failure to distribute wall stress evenly may engender clinical consequences. Other specialized balloons include Inoue's unique balloon for dilating mitral stenosis, and a variety of balloons designed for coronary angioplasty such as those mounted directly on a guide wire (see Chap. 26).

It is important to know the maximal pressure to which balloons can be inflated before rupture. This pressure varies with the material in the balloon and inversely with the balloon diameter. High pressures are rarely needed when dilating valves, for example, but are essential for dilating most pulmonary artery stenoses. Balloons are designed to rupture longitudinally. If the rupture is transverse, as occurs occasionally, part of the balloon may be sheared off the shaft and lost in the body during removal. For this reason and to minimize the risk of vessel rupture,[3] intentional balloon rupture should be avoided. A pressure gauge should be used to monitor inflation pressure when dilating lesions that require a high pressure.

Balloons are manufactured to achieve certain maximal diameters. The actual inflated diameter varies slightly for each balloon and with inflation pressure. It is therefore important to record the inflation on videotape and measure the balloon to be sure the desired diameter has been achieved. The balloon length, by convention, refers to the flat part of the balloon excluding the taper at either end. Most balloons (other than those used for coronary angioplasty) are 2, 3, 4, or 5.5 cm long. Long balloons are more stable during inflation and easier to keep positioned as the heart contracts and ejects. As the balloon straightens during inflation in a curved structure, however, the distal ends of a long balloon may damage adjacent structures. Examples include damage to the right ventricular outflow tract when dilating valvar pulmonary stenosis.[4] Therefore, 2 or 3 cm balloons are used for most lesions. An exception is aortic valvuloplasty in older patients, in whom use of a long balloon is necessary to avoid its ejection from the valve orifice during inflation. The balloon profile, defined as the diameter of the deflated balloon, can be several Fr sizes larger than the shaft, depending on balloon size and material. High profile balloons are more likely to damage vessels at the entry site, and may have difficulty in crossing tight stenoses. Balloons also vary in terms of the length of the shoulders at each end of the balloon. While a longer taper may make entry at the groin easier, the taper, when combined with the distal tip, may prevent centering the balloon in the lesion. For example, the stenotic orifice in mitral stenosis is near the left ventricular apex and a long taper and tip may prevent the balloon from being advanced far enough to allow dilation of the stenosis.

Most angioplasty balloons are mounted on shafts ranging from 4 to 9 Fr. A large shaft offers the potential advantages of increased stiffness and larger guide wire and inflation lumens. The large shaft, however, is more likely to damage the femoral vessels, the most common complication in pediatric patients undergoing balloon dilation. Therefore, we generally choose the smallest shaft size available. Stiffer shafts make groin entry easier and help to stabilize the balloon position during infla-

tion, but may make following the guide wire around sharp turns more difficult. The tip of the catheter, the part of the shaft that extends beyond the balloon, varies in length and degree of tapering. While longer tips with more gradual taper are easier to pass through the groin, the long tip may prevent proper positioning of the balloon. It is important to have a close match between guide wire and catheter lumen to prevent entrapping tissue at the tip of the catheter. Because the most difficult part of most procedures is obtaining stable wire position across the stenosis using specialized catheters and guide wires, one must sometimes choose the balloon catheter based on the wire one has been able to position.

Two balloons may be positioned and inflated simultaneously to achieve a larger effective diameter than is possible with a single balloon. We use Yeager's formula[5] for calculating the effective combined diameter of 2 balloons.

PERCUTANEOUS BALLOON PULMONARY VALVOTOMY

Reports of using blade or balloon catheters to perform pulmonary valvotomies appeared as early as 1953.[6,7] The static balloon technique, reported by Kan et al. in 1982,[8] was the first to be applied widely. Results[9–12] have demonstrated the safety and effectiveness of this technique and established it as the treatment of choice for children and adults with isolated pulmonary stenosis (see Chap. 29).

Technique

A complete precatheterization Doppler echocardiogram defines valve morphology, measures the pulmonary annulus, and rules out associated defects. Using routine sedation, a 7 Fr sheath is placed percutaneously in the femoral vein and a balloon-tipped end-hole catheter is used to measure right heart oxygen saturations and pressures. After placement of a small pigtail in the femoral artery for monitoring arterial pressure, the patient is heparinized. The gradient across the pulmonary outflow is measured, and the location of the valve is defined using fluoroscopy and a right ventriculogram in the anteroposterior and lateral projections. The pulmonary annulus is measured at the hinge points of the valve and the balloon diameter is chosen to be 1.2 to 1.4 times that of the annulus (Fig. 30–1). Animal studies[4] and results in patients[9] have demonstrated that use of such oversize balloons is safe and yields improved results. When the annulus is >20 mm, overdilation requires use of two balloons.

An end-hole catheter is advanced to the distal right or left pulmonary artery and the venous catheter and sheath removed over an exchange wire. The balloon dilation catheter is purged first with carbon dioxide and then with dilute contrast in the inferior vena cava. Once the balloon has been centered across the pulmonary valve, it is inflated rapidly until the waist disappears, and then deflated and withdrawn to the inferior vena cava. At least two inflations are performed and videotapes are reviewed to ensure proper balloon position and size.

The balloon dilation catheter is exchanged for a sheath and end-hole catheter. A pressure pullback is performed to measure the transvalvar gradient and to look for a subvalvar gradient, which may develop following dilation. A residual transvalvar gradient >20 to 30 mm Hg is unusual, and suggests improper position of the balloon during dilation, improper balloon size, or a dysplastic valve. If the subvalvar gradient is >30 mm Hg, a right ventriculogram is performed. The cardiac output is measured to calculate valve area.

Patients with critical pulmonary stenosis may not tolerate having a catheter across the valve because of further reduction in valve area. In patients with systemic right ventricular pressure, we perform the initial right ventriculogram before crossing the valve. If the patient deteriorates when the valve has been crossed, the catheter is removed without measuring a gradient and only the exchange wire is left in place. In these patients, a relatively small balloon is frequently used for the initial dilation, followed by an oversized balloon for subsequent dilations.

Neonates presenting with critical pulmonary stenosis are commonly cyanotic because of right-to-left atrial level shunts, and ductus-dependent for pulmonary blood flow. Because of the atrial and ductal shunts, both systemic and pulmonary blood flow tend to be maintained during balloon inflation. Crossing the valve can be difficult because of both the small, hy-

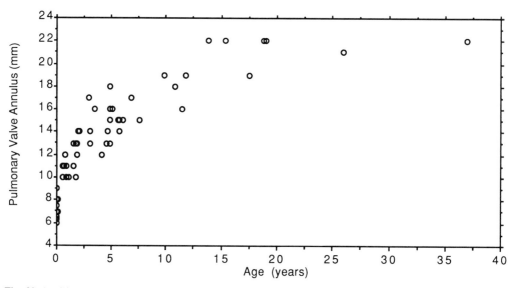

Fig. 30–1.   The pulmonary valve annulus diameter measured from angiograms versus patient age.

pertrophied right ventricle and the pinhole opening in the valve. We attempt to cross the valve with a balloon-tipped end-hole catheter, but if unsuccessful use a 3 or 4 Fr multipurpose catheter (60 to 90 degrees preformed, short bend at the distal end). This catheter is manipulated to the right ventricular outflow tract. If it does not cross the valve directly, a soft guide wire is used to probe the outflow tract until the valve is crossed. Using these techniques, failure to cross the valve occurs in less than 10% of cases. Once across the valve, we dilate initially with a small balloon and then with a balloon 20 to 40% larger than the annulus.

Results

Except for neonates, the first 66 patients undergoing balloon pulmonary valvotomy at our institution included 9 who had undergone previous surgical valvotomy—most for critical pulmonary stenosis as neonates. In these 9 patients, the transvalvar gradient was decreased from 60 ± 18 to 9 ± 10 mm Hg using a balloon-to-annulus ratio of 1.24 ± 0.19, with no significant complications. In the remaining 57 patients, 54 were successfully dilated with a balloon-to-annulus ratio of 1.27 ± 0.16. The transvalvar gradient decreased from 74 ± 26 to 15 ± 8 mm Hg and the right ventricular pressure from 101 ± 31 to 50 ± 22 mm Hg, with no significant change in cardiac output. The postdilation, transvalvar gradient in the 54 successes was <30 mm Hg regardless of the predilation gradient or age. Small subvalvar gradients are common, but 4 of 54 patients had subvalvar gradients >30 mm Hg (45, 60, 75, and 80 mm Hg). The subvalvar gradient resolved in each case within 1 year. There were four failures in three patients with severely dysplastic valves. No cases of significant restenosis have been identified. The only significant complication occurred early in the series in a patient who developed transient complete heart block.

In 15 consecutive neonates with critical pulmonary stenosis, the valve was crossed and dilated in 14. After dilation with a low-profile 5 or 6 mm balloon, a larger balloon was used in 13 of the 14 cases. Because of the presence of a patent ductus arteriosus in 10, transvalvar gradients were unreliable indicators of obstruction, but right ventricular pressures decreased from 118 ± 17 mm Hg to 61 ± 22 mm Hg. The right ventricular-to-systemic pressure ratio (systolic) decreased from 1.6 ± 0.3 to 0.8 ± 0.3. The balloon-to-annulus ratio for the largest balloon used was 1.25 ± 0.15. On follow-up, the only patient with a gradient >35 mm Hg was dilated with a balloon-to-annulus ratio of <1. Complications included persistent right bundle branch block in one patient and obstruction of the iliac vein in another.

Our results, combined with those from other centers, demonstrate that balloon pulmonary valvotomy, using oversized balloons, is safe and effective in relieving pulmonary valve stenosis in all age groups and in patients who have undergone surgical valvotomies. We currently attempt balloon pulmonary valvotomy in any patient with a transvalvar gradient >40 mm Hg and in neonates with critical pulmonary stenosis.

PERCUTANEOUS BALLOON AORTIC VALVOTOMY

Balloon aortic valvotomy was first reported in 1983 in a child with congenital aortic stenosis,[13] and has subsequently been performed in large numbers of patients with both congenital and acquired stenosis.[14-16] Although initial results in adults with calcific stenosis were encouraging, the modest relief of stenosis combined with high rates of early restenosis has limited its use in this group of patients. Most adult centers now reserve balloon valvotomy for patients who are high-risk candidates for valve replacement. For most younger patients with congenital aortic stenosis, the alternative to balloon dilation is surgical valvotomy. Because results of balloon valvotomy appear comparable to surgical valvotomy in terms of relief of obstruction and restenosis rate, we continue to use this procedure in younger patients.

Technique

Using routine sedation, a femoral vein and artery are entered percutaneously and the patient heparinized. The venous catheter measures right heart pressures and cardiac output pre- and postdilation. Although aortic valves can be dilated using a transspetal approach, the retrograde femoral arterial approach is preferred. We start with an appropriately sized sheath in the artery and a pigtail catheter 1 Fr smaller than the sheath. This allows simultaneous pressure measurements through the sheath and pigtail. The intrinsic gradient of the system is determined with the pigtail first in the iliac artery and then in the ascending aorta.

The easiest technique for crossing the aortic valve retrograde is to advance the soft end of a straight wire out of a thin-walled pigtail catheter and use it to probe for the valve orifice (see Chap. 5). This probing need not be entirely random in that precatheterization echocardiograms should define the valve morphology and position of the orifice. In addition, in congenitally stenotic valves, even unicommissural valves, the commissure between the left and noncoronary cusp is almost always open. Thus, at the same time as one is probing with the wire, the pigtail catheter is manipulated to direct the wire posteriorly and to the left. The probing must be done gently to avoid perforating a cusp or damaging the coronary arteries. When the left ventricle is entered, a transvalvar gradient is measured using the pigtail and femoral sheath. If the valve was easy to cross, a pressure pullback is performed, followed by an aortogram for aortic regurgitation. A left ventriculogram is performed and the aortic annulus measured at the hinge points of the valve.

The balloon diameter is chosen to be 75 to 90% of the annulus diameter (Fig. 30–2). Animal and clinical studies[17,18] demonstrate balloon/annulus ratios >1.0 are more likely to be associated with damage to the outflow tract and increased aortic regurgitation. A double balloon technique is used when the annulus is larger than 22 mm. The pigtail catheter and femoral sheath are exchanged for the dilation catheter over an exchange wire and the balloon is flushed with carbon dioxide and dilute contrast in the thoracic aorta. The balloon is centered across the valve, inflated and deflated rapidly, and pulled back to the descending aorta. Videotapes are reviewed to check balloon size and position.

In older patients, a second pigtail catheter is placed in the other femoral artery prior to dilation. With two arterial catheters, the gradient can be measured without a pullback. Alternatively, a pullback following dilation can be performed using a pigtail catheter equipped over the wire with a side-arm adaptor to avoid losing wire position. If the residual gradient is high and an aortogram performed with the second pigtail shows no significant increase in regurgitation, a larger balloon is used to redilate. Finally, a pressure pullback and aortogram are performed.

It can be difficult to keep the inflated balloon positioned in the valve during left ventricular ejection. A stiff catheter shaft, long balloon, and stiff or extra-stiff exchange wire will help to stabilize the position. In addition, balloon ejection is hindered by advancing the catheter so that it lies along the top of the arch rather than around the underside of the arch. Finally, the double-balloon technique, which does not totally obstruct flow, makes it easier to maintain balloon position.

Although the overall approach is similar to that used in older patients (see Chap. 29), several special techniques are useful in neonates. The umbilical artery can usually be used in the first week of life. Catheter manipulation is more difficult from the umbilical artery, but its use avoids the risk of damage to the femoral artery. We therefore try the umbilical artery approach before using the femoral artery. The venous catheter is advanced across the foramen ovale to the left ventricle and used for measuring pressure and performing ventriculograms. To cross the aortic valve retrograde, a 3 or 4 Fr pigtail catheter with the tail partially cut off is used to direct the guide wire posteriorly and to the left to the open commissure. Because neonatal valves are easy to perforate

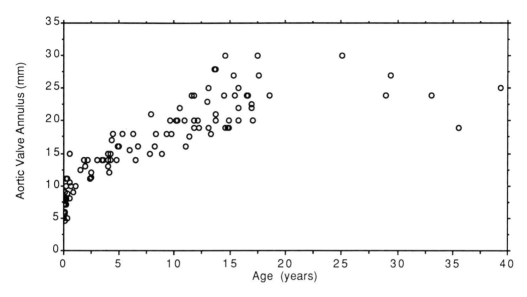

Fig. 30–2. The aortic valve annulus diameter measured from angiograms versus patient age.

with the guide wire, any difficulty in getting the pigtail or balloon catheter to follow the wire across the valve should suggest cusp perforation.

Results

We have performed 154 balloon aortic valvotomies in 149 patients. The results and complications are considered in 2 groups: neonates (<1 month) and older patients. In the 122 older patients, the transvalvar gradient was reduced from 76 ± 22 to 33 ± 16 mm Hg or $56 \pm 21\%$. The valve area index increased $51 \pm 47\%$ from 0.53 ± 0.20 to 0.80 ± 0.27 cm^2/m^2. The percent gradient reduction was unrelated to age (1 month to 39 years), history of prior surgical valvotomy (n = 18), predilation gradient, or final balloon/annulus ratio (mean 0.98 ± 0.11, range 0.71 to 1.33). Aortic regurgitation, on a scale of 0 to 5, increased from grade 0.57 ± 0.64 to grade 1.18 ± 0.80. We have previously shown an inverse relationship between gradient reduction and increased regurgitation.[14] The risk of a greater than 1 grade increase in regurgitation was 11% (6/55) when the balloon/annulus ratio was ≤1.0, versus 30% (6/20) when the ratio was >1.0. No deaths occurred in these older patients. Com-

plications included pulse loss in 30% of patients (60% in patients <2 years of age (including neonates), and 15% in patients >2 years), which was permanent in 10%. The femoral artery was torn in one patient and a pseudoaneurysm developed in a second. Transient left bundle branch block occurred in 15% and ventricular arrhythmias requiring cardioversion in 3%. During average follow-up of 6 ± 6 months, there have been no significant changes in transvalvar gradients or regurgitation.[14]

Neonates are different in terms of results and complications. We have dilated 27 consecutive neonates with critical valvar aortic stenosis regardless of clinical condition, valve morphology, left ventricular size or function or degree of mitral regurgitation. They ranged from 1 to 30 days of age and from 2.2 to 5 kg. Unicommissural valves were present in 17 and bicommissural in 10. The left ventricular volume was >80% of predicted normal in 16, 60 to 80% of normal in 7 and <60% of normal in 4. Using a balloon-to-annulus ratio of 0.90 ± 0.14, the peak systolic ejection gradient was reduced from 58 ± 27 to 27 ± 19 and the left ventricular end-diastolic pressure was also reduced significantly. New aortic regurgitation developed in 11 and was mild in 8 and severe in 3 who died. Because of poor ventricular function and the common presence of a PDA with right-to-left flow, however, gradients are an unreliable indicator of the degree of obstruction and outcome. If failure is defined as death (n = 9) or need for stage I palliation for hypoplastic left heart syndrome (n = 2), there were 11 failures with 9 occurring in the 11 patients with left ventricular volumes <80% of normal.

We currently dilate congenitally stenotic aortic valves in patients with transvalvar gradients >55 mm Hg and no more than mild aortic regurgitation and in neonates with critical aortic stenosis.

PERCUTANEOUS BALLOON ANGIOPLASTY OF COARCTATION AND POSTOPERATIVE AORTIC OBSTRUCTIONS

Percutaneous balloon angioplasty of coarctation was first described in 1982[19] and has since been used in large numbers of patients with native coarctation (unoperated) and postoperative recoarctation.[20–23] A study of experimental coarctation in lambs[25] demonstrated that relief of obstruction occurs by tearing the intima and media. Short- and longterm complications seen in that study, including perforation resulting in death and late aneurysm formation, have now been described in patients.

Technique

Using routine sedation, the femoral vein and artery are entered percutaneously and the patient is heparinized. Coarctations have been dilated using an antegrade approach, but the retrograde femoral arterial approach is preferred. Right and left heart hemodynamics are measured, including cardiac output and a careful pullback performed to localize gradients. Biplane aortograms are performed in either anteroposterior and lateral or right anterior oblique and long axial oblique projections. More than one aortogram may be required to profile the lesion. The diameters of the nar-

rowest area of coarctation and of the normal proximal and distal aorta are measured.

The balloon is chosen to be approximately 2.5 to 3 times the narrowest area, but not greater than 1.5 times the normal proximal or distal aorta. Double balloons are used when balloon diameters >20 mm are required. Relatively long balloons can be used in distal coarctations, but short balloons should be used in the transverse arch. High inflation pressures are often required in recoarctations. The balloon dilation catheter is advanced over an exchange wire and purged with carbon dioxide and dilute contrast in the descending aorta. It is centered across the coarctation, inflated until the waist disappears or to maximal inflation pressure, and deflated. Videotapes are reviewed to ensure proper position and balloon size. The balloon catheter is exchanged for a pigtail and a pullback gradient can be measured using the single pigtail over the wire with a side-arm adaptor or by placing a second arterial line. The dilated area should be crossed only over a guide wire because of the danger of perforation. An aortogram is performed after dilation to determine diameter of the narrowing and to look for tears, aneurysms or dissections. If significant obstruction remains despite disappearance of the balloon waist during inflation, a larger balloon can be used. Chest pain is common during balloon inflation, but persistent pain suggests aortic rupture or dissection.

Results

Of 64 angioplasties in 62 patients ranging in age from 3 days to 67 years, 5 had native and 59 postoperative coarctations.[26] The gradient was reduced from 39 ± 17 to 13 ± 11 mm Hg, and the diameter of the lesion increased from 4.9 ± 3.0 to 8.2 ± 4.3 mm. Procedures are considered successful if the gradient is reduced ≥50% and the diameter is increased ≥30%. Based on these criteria, 54 (83%) were successful. The balloon-to-lesion ratio was 3.0 ± 1.0 for the successful group and 1.6 ± 0.7 for the failures. The failures had significantly lower predilation gradients and significantly larger predilation lesion diameters, and were significantly older. Because of the relatively large predilation diameters in the failed group, use of larger balloons, which might improve gradient reduction, would risk injuring the normal aorta. Results in recoarctations are unrelated to the type of previous surgery. An additional 18 balloon angioplasties have been performed in patients with aortic obstructions following surgical repair of interrupted aortic arch (12 in 10 patients) and hypoplastic left heart syndrome (6 in 6 patients). Using the same criteria as with coarctation, 15 of the 18 procedures were successful.

The most common complication is transient loss of the arterial pulse, and one baby died following iliac artery rupture and a retroperitoneal hemorrhage. The only other significant short-term complication in our series was an aortic dissection immediately following dilation in a 67-year-old woman with a native coarctation. During follow-up, three patients were found to have small asymptomatic aneurysms (two postoperative interrupted aortic arches and one following dilation of a native coarctation).

Aneurysm formation following dilation of recoarctation or, more commonly, native coarctation, has been reported by several groups. At present, we dilate recoarctations or other postoperative aortic obstructions and native coarctations only in patients who are high surgical risks. Other investigators dilate selected native coarctations which are discrete or membranous and report minimal residual gradients and a low incidence of complications and aneurysms.[21–23] Defining the indications in terms of gradient and coarctation diameter is difficult, but our results suggest that dilation is unlikely to be successful in patients with low gradients and relatively large coarctation diameters.

PERCUTANEOUS BALLOON ANGIOPLASTY OF BRANCH PULMONARY ARTERY STENOSIS

Branch pulmonary artery stenosis or hypoplasia may be acquired (e.g., at sites of shunts,

bands, or conduits) or congenital. Anatomy ranges from single stenotic areas to multiple stenoses to diffuse hypoplasia. Successful dilation generally results in tearing of the intima and media.[3] Indications for angioplasty include near-systemic or higher right ventricular pressure, hypertension in unaffected portions of the vascular bed, marked decrease in flow to an affected portion, and/or symptoms.

Technique

Pulmonary arteries are most commonly dilated from the femoral veins, but can be dilated from the subclavian or internal jugular veins or from the femoral arteries in patients with systemic to pulmonary artery shunts. A small pigtail is placed in the femoral artery to monitor pressure and the patient is heparinized. Right heart hemodynamics are measured and the magnitude and location of gradients in the pulmonary arteries are determined. Pulmonary angiograms should include selective injections (AP and lateral) in each lung and in affected lobes or segments. This is most efficiently accomplished using a cut-off pigtail over a guide wire with a side-arm adaptor. This arrangement allows pressure measurements and angiograms to be performed without losing wire position. Angiograms that opacify both lungs are generally not useful. Lower lobe stenoses, in particular, are often better seen on the lateral projection, and with the lungs superimposed it may not be possible to visualize stenoses or differentiate the right from the left lung.

An exchange wire should be positioned in the largest vessel distal to the stenosis to minimize the risk of aneurysm formation, which most commonly follows overdilation of small distal vessels. In vessels that are difficult to enter, a stiff exchange wire or the stiff end of a wire may be needed to get the balloon catheter to follow the wire. The ideal balloon has a low profile, a short distal tip, and a high maximal inflation pressure. The balloon diameter is chosen to be 3 to 4 times the diameter of the lesion but not more than 2 times the diameter of the normal vessel on either side.[27,28] The balloon is inflated until the waist disappears or until maximum inflation pressure is reached. If the waist does not disappear at low inflation pressures, a pressure gauge is used. Inflation time ranges from 10 to 60 seconds depending on the response of the waist and how well the cardiac output is maintained. Following dilation, the balloon catheter is exchanged over the guide wire for a pigtail catheter with part of the tail cut off and pressure measurements are repeated. Successful dilation may result in a decrease in proximal pressures, a decrease in the gradient or an increase in the pressure distal to the stenosis. Angiograms are repeated to measure the diameter of the stenosis and to look for tears and aneurysms. If the waist in the balloon caused by the lesion disappeared during inflation but significant obstruction persists, a larger balloon may be used.

Multiple lesions can be dilated at the same procedure, but care is taken not to cross previously dilated areas because of the risk of dissection or perforation at the site of an intimal tear. In general, when multiple lesions are present, distal lesions are dilated before proximal lesions and severe stenoses before milder stenoses. It is safest to use balloon-tipped catheters and soft torque-controlled wires.

Results

We have dilated 218 branch pulmonary artery stenoses in 135 patients.[27] Success was defined as an increase in diameter of >50%, an increase in flow in the affected segment of >20%, and/or a decrease of >20% in the systolic right ventricular to aortic pressure ratio. Based on these criteria, the overall success rate was 58%. With dilation, the diameter of the lesions increased from 3.8 ± 1.7 to 5.5 ± 2.1 mm (Fig. 30–3). The balloon-to-lesion ratio was significantly higher in successful (4.2) than in failed (3.0) dilations. Outcome did not correlate with patient age, but was better in surgically induced than in native stenoses. The incidence of restenosis was 16%. Complications included four deaths, two caused by vessel rupture in the early postoperative period. Consequently, dilation within 4 to 6 weeks of surgery should be avoided. Transient pulmonary edema in the dilated segment occurred in four patients. Aneurysms occurred in 11, most commonly in small vessels distal to the stenosis. With positioning of the wire in the largest vessel distal to the stenosis and avoiding distal migration of the balloon, the incidence of aneurysms has been decreased.

We compared results and complications before and after 1986. Before 1986, the success rate was 49% and the mortality 5%, and aneurysms occurred in 13%. After 1986, the success rate was 60% and the mortality 1%, and aneurysms occurred in 3% This appears to be caused primarily by technical modifications, including use of larger balloon-to-lesion ratios,

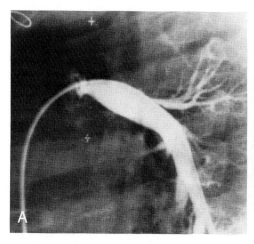
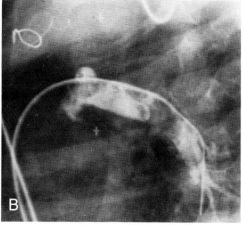

Fig. 30–3.   A selective left pulmonary artery injection A, before and B, after balloon dilation of the stenotic origin.

balloons with higher inflation pressure, and avoiding dilations in the early postoperative period and in small distal vessels. It should be kept in mind that most of these lesions are too distal to be dealt with surgically.

COIL EMBOLIZATION OF CONGENITAL AND ACQUIRED THORACIC VESSELS

Therapeutic embolization of unwanted thoracic vessels was first reported in 1974.[29] Various materials and devices have been used to successfully occlude aortopulmonary collaterals, arteriovenous malformations, Blalock-Taussig shunts, venous collaterals, and venae cavae, and coronary artery fistulae.[30,31] This section will discuss the use of Gianturco coils,[32,33] the device that has been used most frequently.

Coils (occluding spring emboli, Cook, Bloomington, Indiana) are stainless steel wires, either 0.025 or 0.038 inch, embedded with Dacron strands to promote thrombosis. The coil is delivered by positioning a catheter in the vessel to be embolized and extruding the coil from the catheter using a guide wire. As the wire coil is extruded from the catheter, it coils to a predetermined diameter, most commonly 2, 3, 5, 8, 10, or 12 mm. The length of the wire coil is 1.2, 2, 2.5, 3, 4, or 5 cm before coiling.

Technique

Routine sedation is used and intravenous heparin (100 units/kg body weight) is given when vascular access has been obtained. Patients are given an antibiotic (usually cefazolin) before coil embolization and for 24 hours after embolization.

Vascular access for coil embolization depends on which vessels are to be embolized. Most aortopulmonary collaterals and shunts are closed using the femoral or, rarely, the axillary artery. Various catheters are used to perform angiograms, test-occlude vessels, and deliver the coils, and therefore a sheath in the artery is helpful. On the other hand, a major advantage of coils in pediatric patients is that they can be delivered through catheters as small as 3 Fr. Thus, in small patients we sacrifice the convenience of a sheath for the safety of small catheters. Venous collaterals, venae cavae, and pulmonary arteriovenous malformations are closed from the venous side using the femoral, subclavian or internal jugular veins.

To decide whether to close a particular vessel, one needs to know the hemodynamic consequences of closure and the technical feasibility of embolization. The hemodynamic consequences of closure depend on the vessel to be closed, the presence of other defects and what surgery the patient has undergone.

Closure of aortopulmonary collaterals, a source of pulmonary blood flow, in patients with cyanotic congenital heart disease causes increased cyanosis if the intracardiac defects are unrepaired. If there are multiple collaterals or other sources of pulmonary blood flow, such as shunts, however, closure of some collaterals before complete repair may be possible. This is tested by balloon-occluding each collateral and measuring the systemic oxygen saturation. If a collateral is the only source of pulmonary blood flow to a segment of lung (no supply by the native pulmonary arteries), embolization may lead to pulmonary infarction. Absence of dual supply, however, is rare in our experience. As with collaterals, test balloon occlusion of surgically created systemic-to-pulmonary artery shunts is required before embolization unless intracardiac defects have been corrected.

Most veins considered for embolization are in patients with Glenn- or Fontan-like procedures. These veins are associated with right-to-left shunts, diminished pulmonary blood flow, and systemic desaturation. Closure will eliminate the systemic desaturation, but can raise pulmonary artery or right heart pressures, and this can be tested with balloon occlusion. Similarly, occlusion of a left superior vena cava in the absence of an innominate or adequate connecting veins can critically raise pressure above the occlusion, and this should be assessed by test occlusion. Finally, the presence and anatomy of branches must be defined. For example, when embolizing a left superior vena cava, one must be careful to position the coils so that the hemiazygous vein does not drain to the left heart.

The difficult part of most procedures is entering the vessel to be embolized. The availability of a variety of preformed catheters and specialty wires including tip deflectors and soft torque control wires has made this task easier. Once in the vessel, selective angiograms define the length, the proximal and distal anatomy, the presence of stenoses, and the diameter of the vessel. It is important to realize that the diameter may increase once the vessel is occluded. This is rarely a problem in arteries, but veins are more distensible, and it is therefore best to perform angiograms with the vessels balloon occluded. Failure to do so can lead to migration of the coils as the vessel enlarges after embolization. Criteria for proceeding with embolization include availability of an appropriately sized coil and a vessel long enough to accept the coil. The presence of distal stenoses decreases the risk of distal migration. The length and shape of the coil when embolized depend on a number of factors including the ratio of coil-to-vessel diameter, the distensibility of the vessel, and the diameter of the wire in the coil. Thus, if the coil diameter is too large for a vessel, it straightens rather than coils and pushes the catheter out of the vessel. We choose the first coil to be about 10 to 40% larger than the vessel diameter and can theoretically embolize vessels between approximately 1.8 and 10 mm in diameter.

The type of catheter used to deliver the coil depends on the anatomy of the vessel to be embolized, but attempts are made to avoid acute angles in the catheter course (which make passage of the coil through the catheter difficult) and to fix the position of the catheter tip during delivery of the coil by either inflating the balloon on a balloon-tipped catheter or using preformed curves in the catheter. Coils are soaked in topical thrombin (Thrombin, Topical (Bovine), USP. Armour Pharmaceutical Co. Kankakee, IL) before embolization of high-flow vessels. Coils are extruded from the catheter using the soft end of appropriately sized

guide wires. Occasionally, particularly with tortuous catheter courses, the coil cannot be extruded. If it is still entirely within the catheter, the catheter and coil are removed. If the coil is partially out of the end of the catheter but appropriately positioned, the coil is delivered by rapidly flushing the catheter with saline using a 1 cc tuberculin syringe.

If the vessel remains patent 5 to 10 minutes after coil placement, additional coils, often smaller than the first, are placed or blood flow in the vessel is interrupted using balloon occlusion to promote thrombosis. The procedure is terminated when the vessel is completely occluded or when no space remains for additional coils.

Modified Blalock-Taussig shunts (Gore-tex tubes), as a group, are technically difficult to coil-embolize for several reasons. Most vessels expand or bulge in response to the coil, a property that tends to fix the coil. Rigid Gore-tex tubes do not, and this, combined with the high flow and common lack of distal stenoses, increases the risk of distal migration. Also, coils that are even slightly too large straighten and may push the catheter out of the shunt. If this happens, the coil may be pulled out of the shunt and embolize to a systemic artery. For these reasons, we choose coils 10% larger than the shunt and, in some cases, occlude the distal end of the shunt with a balloon dilation catheter in the pulmonary artery during coil delivery.

Coronary artery fistulae can be closed either retrograde from the aorta or from the venous side by entering the distal opening, which is commonly into the right atrium. Although standard coronary catheters can be used, the fistulae can be entered easily with balloon-tipped, flow-directed catheters because of their size and high flow. Angiograms should demonstrate multiple distal openings, the presence of stenoses, and the location of normal coronary branches so that one can decide where to position the coils. Test-occluding at that site with a balloon before coil embolization is prudent.

Results

We have coil-embolized 191 vessels in 112 patients. Of 141 aortopulmonary collaterals embolized in 66 patients, 115 were completely occluded, 21 had minimal residual flow, and 5 were partly occluded (Fig. 30–4). An average of 2.6 coils was used in each collateral. Complications included migration of two coils to the pulmonary arteries and one to the aorta, and asymptomatic rupture of one vessel. Of 24 Blalock-Taussig shunts embolized, 18 were occluded completely, 5 subtotally, and 2 partially. One failed. Complications included migration of three coils to the pulmonary artery and one malposition requiring retrieval. With increased experience and pulmonary artery balloon occlusion at the distal end of the shunt, no migrations have occurred in the last 14 shunts embolized. Of the 15 veins embolized in 10 patients, 5 were SVCs, 1 was an IVC, and 9 were systemic venous-to-atrial collaterals causing right-to-left shunts and cyanosis. All were completely occluded. The only complication was extravasation of contrast while attempting to enter an LSVC, which was eventually closed. Coronary artery fistulae in seven of eight patients have been successfully occluded, five with coils. The retrograde approach was used to embolize three. Of the three fistulae not coil-embolized, one was found to be occluded after prolonged catheter manipulation, presumably by an intimal flap. In another, multiple distal openings into the

right atrium precluded embolization. Finally, one was too large for coils and was occluded with a double umbrella at its entrance to the right atrium. With the exception of the asymptomatic intimal flap, there have been no complications in this group.

DOUBLE UMBRELLA CLOSURE OF PDA, ASD, AND VSD

Transcatheter closure of the patent ductus arteriosus was first reported by Porstmann et al. using a plug, and this technique is still used successfully in some centers.[34,35] King reported the successful closure of atrial septal defects using a double-disk device.[36] The single umbrella of Rashkind was developed to close atrial septal defects but its use was associated with multiple problems and few successes.[37] The double umbrella, in various sizes and modifications, has proven to be the most versatile device for closing intra- and extracardiac defects. The double umbrella was initially developed by Rashkind to close PDAs and has been used successfully in numerous patients.[38] Most recently, Lock modified the PDA double umbrella to close atrial and ventricular septal defects.[34–36] In addition to closing PDAs, ASDs, and VSDs, double umbrel-

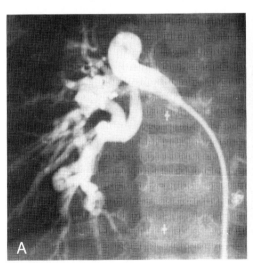 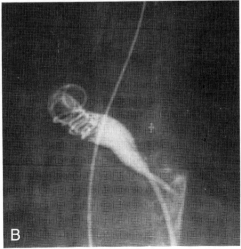

Fig. 30–4. An aortopulmonary collateral from the descending aorta to the right lung A, before and B, after coil embolization.

las have been used to close a coronary artery fistula, left ventricular apex to descending aorta conduits, SVC to right atrial communications following Glenn shunts, SVC and azygous veins, Potts anastomoses, large aortopulmonary collaterals, and large arteriovenous malformations.[39]

Double-umbrella systems include the double umbrella, a cylinder for straightening the umbrellas and loading them into the delivery catheter, and the delivery catheter. To load the umbrella for delivery, it is first connected to the release wire in the delivery catheter. The umbrellas, which have foam or Dacron on spring-loaded arms, are collapsed using the loading cylinder and then pulled into the pod at the end of the delivery catheter using the release wire. Before loading the umbrella, a long sheath is positioned across the defect to be closed. Originally, the system was designed so that the umbrella would be positioned and opened using the pod at the end of the delivery system. In practice, it is easier to advance the delivery system into the sheath and then advance the umbrella out of the pod into the sheath using the release wire. The umbrella is advanced to the distal end of the long sheath which is across the defect. The sheath is then retracted until the distal arms and umbrella spring open. The entire system, delivery catheter, umbrella, and sheath are then pulled back until the distal arms begin to evert as they are pulled against the distal side of the defect to be closed. Without moving the umbrella, the sheath is retracted farther until the proximal umbrella springs open on the proximal side of the defect. At this point, the umbrella is still connected to a release wire in the delivery system and can be retrieved. Before releasing the device, the position can be checked with angiograms, echocardiograms, or by manipulating the device. That is, with gentle pulling of the umbrella the distal arms evert as they are pulled against the defect and with pushing, the proximal arms evert against the proximal side of the defect. Failure of the arms to move appropriately could indicate that both umbrellas are on the same side of the defect or that part of an umbrella is on the wrong side. If the position is satisfactory, the umbrella is released using the release mechanism at the proximal end of the delivery system.

PDA Occlusion

The double umbrella used for PDA closure (Bard PDA Umbrella, USCI Division, C. R. Bard, Billerica, MA) has two circular, foam umbrellas and comes in two sizes (Fig. 30–5). The smaller device is 12 mm in diameter and has six arms, three distal and three proximal. This device requires an 8 Fr long sheath for delivery. The 17 mm device has four arms supporting each umbrella and requires an 11 Fr sheath for delivery. In general, the 12 mm device is used for ducts <4 mm in diameter and the 17 mm device for ducts between 4 and 8 mm in diameter.

Technique. Most PDA closures are performed as outpatient procedures. Precatheterization evaluation includes a complete physical examination and Doppler echocardiogram to ensure the presence of the PDA, evaluate its anatomy, and to rule out other defects. The sedation/anesthetic regimen includes morphine as a premedication and ketamine at the time the device is delivered to prevent any movement by the patient. The patient is given three doses (one before and two after closure) of antibiotics, usually cefazolin.

At catheterization, a femoral vein and femoral artery are entered percutaneously. The patient is not heparinized. A 7 Fr sheath and balloon-tipped end-hole catheter are placed in the femoral vein and used to measure right heart oxygen saturations and pressures. A pigtail catheter is placed in the femoral artery and used to monitor pressure and perform descending aortograms. Because the patient is not heparinized, a relatively small pigtail is used and not advanced to the ascending aorta or left ventricle, and every effort is made to keep the procedure as short as possible.

The PDA is not crossed until a descending aortogram has been performed to determine the PDA size, morphology, and location. This is done to avoid catheter-induced spasm in the PDA and consequent underestimation of PDA size. In most patients, the straight lateral pro-

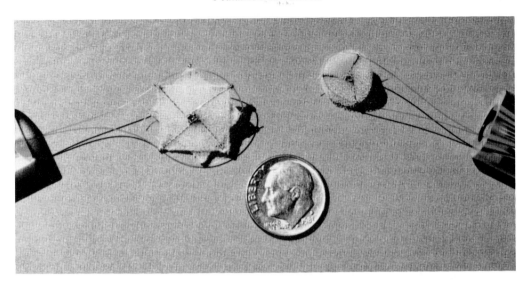

Fig. 30–5. The 12 mm and 17 mm Bard PDA Umbrella. (Courtesy of USCI Division, C. R. Bard, Billerica, MA.)

jection demonstrates the anatomy best. The narrowest area of restrictive ducts, usually at the pulmonary end, is commonly superimposed on the tracheal shadow in the lateral projection. On the basis of these angiograms, the appropriate umbrella size is chosen.

The PDA is crossed from the venous side using the catheter or a guide wire, and the catheter is advanced to the descending aorta. The catheter and venous sheath are removed over an 0.038 exchange guide wire. Before placing the long sheath, the groin is predilated with a dilator 1 Fr larger than the sheath to be used. This helps prevent damage to the tip of the sheath, which may make advancing it through the duct difficult. The umbrella is not loaded into the pod at the end of the delivery system until the sheath is through the duct and in the descending aorta. For most ducts, we soak the umbrella in topical thrombin before loading to promote closure, but not all centers do this.

The wire is withdrawn from the dilator and the dilator pulled inside the sheath. The sheath is pulled until it points straight posteriorly toward the posterior wall of the aorta. An angiogram is performed with a hand injection through the sheath and dilator to determine the anatomy, which may be distorted by the large sheath. The dilator is removed and replaced

with the delivery system, which is advanced to the IVC-RA junction. The umbrella is advanced out of the loading pod and across the PDA to the end of the sheath. The center of the umbrella is positioned at the aortic end of the duct (using previous angiograms and landmarks such as the trachea) and the distal arms opened by retracting the sheath over the umbrella. The entire system is pulled back until the distal (aortic) arms begin to evert and the center of the umbrella is at the narrowest area of the duct. The proximal arms are opened by retracting the sheath without moving the umbrella. If properly positioned, the proximal arms open on the pulmonary side of the duct.

Position is checked before release by gently moving the umbrella back and forth. It should be emphasized that the tension one feels when advancing and retracting the system is mostly because of sheath entrapment at the groin and not the umbrella in the duct, making it possible for the umbrella to be pulled through the duct into the main pulmonary artery. This is especially true of the 12 mm umbrella because of its smaller size and weaker arms. Position can also be checked with an angiogram (using the pigtail), but again the risks of undue delays leading to umbrella dislodgement must be weighed against the benefits of knowing exactly where the umbrella is. The release wire may occasionally become entrapped in the foam when the umbrella is released. If this occurs, the sheath is readvanced, pinning the umbrella against the pulmonary artery and allowing retraction of the release wire without pulling on the umbrella.

Following release, an aortogram is performed to check position and closure. Trivial leaks are common because of the porous nature of the foam and almost always close (based on color flow Doppler studies) within hours to days. If more than a trivial leak is present, a balloon on an end-hole catheter is used to tamponade the pulmonary side of the umbrella for 10 to 15 minutes.

If a PDA is too small to cross with the sheath and it is felt important to close it, the PDA can be dilated with a 3 or 4 mm balloon dilation catheter. Rarely, a PDA cannot be crossed from the pulmonary side, but most PDAs are easily crossed from the aortic side. Although the PDA can be closed from the aortic side, the disadvantage of this approach is putting the large sheath in the femoral artery. Alternatively, one can snare the aortic wire, pull it out through the venous side, and close the PDA from the venous side. In patients with pulmonary artery hypertension or complex congenital heart disease, it may be useful to test occlude the PDA with a balloon before closure.

Results. In a multicenter trial, several hundred patients have had their PDA closed with the double umbrella (Fig. 30–6). The patients have ranged from 4 kg infants to 70-year-old adults. The overwhelming majority of these patients had restrictive ducts and continuous murmurs and were asymptomatic. The primary indication for closure was prevention of bacterial endarteritis. In this group, closure, defined as disappearance of the continuous murmur, can be expected in over 95% of patients. Although trivial leaks are common immediately following placement, follow-up color flow Doppler studies have demonstrated complete closure in over 95%. A smaller group of patients was symptomatic. They either had large ducts or were elderly patients who developed ischemic heart disease and no longer

tolerated the volume load. Significant residual leaks are most common in ducts >6 mm in diameter. Several PDAs with persistent leaks have been successfully closed with a second umbrella at a second procedure. Leaks are also occasionally seen in small ducts with unusual courses or shapes in which the umbrella does not fit well. In addition, the temptation to use the 17 mm device in small ducts should be avoided. Although the 12 mm device is harder to deliver, the 17 mm device tends to distort small ducts, which can lead to a poor fit and residual leaks.

The most common complication has been migration of the device to the pulmonary arteries or, less commonly, to the aorta. Most migrations occurred early in the experience, when techniques were being refined. Some investigators have left the device in the pulmonary artery, and follow-up angiograms have demonstrated patency of the pulmonary artery. Some devices were removed surgically and some using transcatheter techniques. We have now retrieved four devices using grabbers or baskets and have placed a second device successfully at the same procedure. Migrations due to malposition of the device at the time of release should be avoidable. The system is designed so that even when both umbrellas are open, the device can be pulled back into the sheath, and we have done this on several occasions. We did, however, lose one device while attempting this maneuver when the release mechanism broke. Migration may also occur if the duct is too large for the device. Overall, the incidence of migration is about 2%, and no long-term sequelae have resulted from migration. No device has migrated after the patient left the catheterization laboratory.

Closure of Atrial and Ventricular Septal Defects

The Bard PDA Umbrella was used to close a few small atrial and ventricular defects, but clearly a different and larger device was needed if these defects were to be closed routinely. Lock, in conjunction with USCI, has now modified the PDA umbrella, yielding the

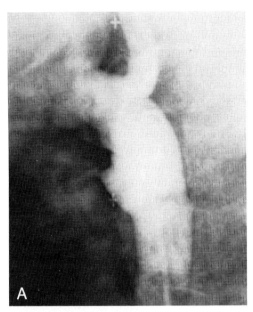

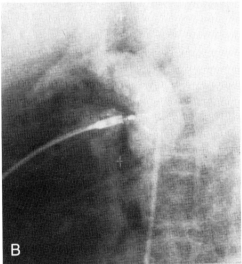

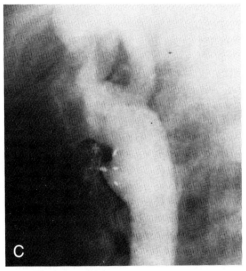

Fig. 30–6. A, An aortogram demonstrating a small PDA. B, An aortogram demonstrating a 12 mm PDA umbrella with both sets of arms open, connected to the delivery system. C, Complete occlusion of the PDA after release of the umbrella.

Bard Clamshell Septal Umbrella (Bard PDA Umbrella, USCI Division, C. R. Bard, Billerica, MA) (Fig. 30–7). This device has longer arms with springs in the middle of each arm, which cause the distal and proximal arms and umbrellas to overlap partially.[40] This design helps center the device in defects and promotes opposition of the umbrellas to the septal surfaces and complete closure. The device has square Dacron umbrellas and is currently available in 17, 23, 28, 33, and 40 mm sizes. Each requires an 11 Fr long sheath for delivery.

Technique. A precatheterization echocardiogram should define the number, type, location, and size (in more than one plane) of atrial defects. Distances between the edge of the defect and the vena cava, the pulmonary veins and atrioventricular valves should be measured. Early experience demonstrates that centrally located secundum-type defects with circumferential septal rims and patent foramens are the best candidates for closure. Primum defects are not candidates because they abut the atrioventricular valves. Defects with

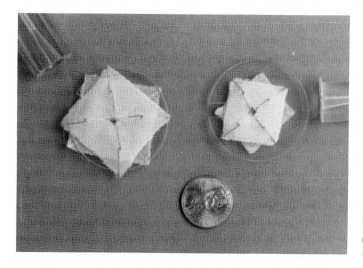

Fig. 30–7. A 27 mm and 40 mm Bard Clamshell Septal Umbrella. (Courtesy of USCI Division, C. R. Bard, Billerica, MA.)

multiple fenestrations can occasionally be closed with a single device, but multiple, widely spaced defects are more difficult.

Initially, the catheterization was performed with sedation followed by ketamine at the time of umbrella delivery. Intubation and general anesthesia are more commonly used now that transesophageal echo is being used in most cases. A 7 Fr sheath and balloon-tipped end-hole catheter are placed percutaneously in the femoral vein and a small pigtail for pressure monitoring in the femoral artery. The patient is heparinized and right heart hemodynamics are measured. The ASD is crossed and a left atrial angiogram performed in the hepatoclavicular view. In patients with right-to-left shunts, the defect is test-occluded with a balloon and the systemic oxygen saturation measured.

The defect is balloon-sized, yielding the "stretched" diameter. For small defects, standard balloon-tipped catheters can be used. For larger defects, special sizing balloons are required. Balloon sizing is performed by passing the balloon both right to left and left to right across the defect over a guide wire in the left atrium or pulmonary vein. For example, the balloon is overinflated in the left atrium, gently pulled back against the septum, and then gradually deflated until it pops through the defect. A circumferential indentation can be seen in the balloon as it comes through the defect. Because a balloon much smaller than

the defect can get caught on the septal rim, seeing the indentation is important. A clamshell is placed on the patient's chest before balloon-sizing so that the balloon indentation and device can be compared on the same image (it is necessary to allow for different magnifications).

The stretched diameter, which is commonly 30 to 40% larger than the diameter measured by echo, is used to choose umbrella size. Ideally, the clamshell diameter should be two times the stretched diameter of the defect, although ratios as low as 1.5 have been used. Although this is not absolute, the largest defects closed routinely are 20 mm in diameter. It may not be possible to close smaller defects if the appropriate clamshell is likely to impinge on vital structures such as the atrioventricular valves.

When the decision to proceed with closure has been made, a 0.035 exchange wire is placed in the left atrium or pulmonary vein. The groin and femoral vein are dilated with a 12 Fr dilator. An 11 Fr sheath and dilator with side arm adaptor are placed on the wire and flushed outside the body to remove air. The sheath and dilator are advanced over the wire to the left atrium. The clamshell is loaded into the delivery system. As the wire and dilator are removed slowly from the sheath, saline or dilute contrast is infused through the sidearm to fill the sheath and prevent air from being sucked into the sheath. The attention to detail required to prevent air embolism in the left atrium cannot be overemphasized. The delivery system is loaded into the sheath and the umbrella is pushed out of the loading pod to the distal end of the sheath in the left atrium. The distal umbrella is opened in the left atrium and the entire system withdrawn until the arms start to evert as they contact the atrial septum. It is important not to be fooled by extension of the arms as they get hung up on the right pulmonary veins or other structures. It is also important to realize that the heart and atrial septum can move several centimeters during the respiratory cycle. For these reasons, transesophageal echo during delivery is helpful. The proximal umbrella is then opened on the right atrial side.

Position, before release, can be checked with echo and angiograms, or by moving the device and watching arm motion. After release, camera angles are adjusted so that one is parallel to the plane of the umbrellas and the other is perpendicular. The former helps one determine if all eight arms are positioned on the correct sides of the septum. The latter view demonstrates the relationship of the device to systemic and pulmonary veins and AV valves on subsequent angiograms. A right atrial angiogram is performed and the contrast

followed through to the levophase. Residual, mild shunts are common because it takes hours to days for the pores in the Dacron to close.

Results. We have now closed 69 atrial septal defects in 73 patients ranging from 6 months to 73 years of age (Fig. 30–8). ASD closure in nine additional patients was not performed because they were too large, had partial anomalous pulmonary venous connections, or had an interrupted IVC. The defects ranged from 3 to 26 mm. Complications included two strokes, one probably caused by air embolism. The other occurred immediately after placement of the sheath in an elderly, high-risk patient who was cyanotic and had had multiple previous strokes. The ASD was closed, but the patient died 1 week later. In four patients, the umbrella embolized several hours to 3 days following placement; three went to the aorta and one was ensnared in the tricuspid valve. One patient had a brief run of ventricular tachycardia, presumably as the device went through the systemic ventricle, but the rest were asymptomatic. The devices migrating to the aorta were retrieved in the catheterization laboratory. In each of these cases, the ASD was either large or eccentrically positioned. Follow-up shows complete closure in 78%,

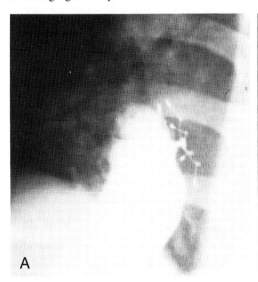 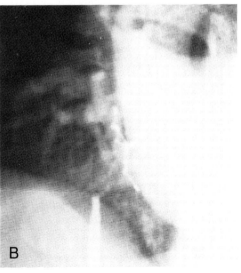

Fig. 30–8. A, A right atrial injection with B, levophase demonstrating complete closure of a secundum atrial septal defect with a 27 mm clamshell umbrella.

trace residual leaks in 15%, and small residual leaks in 7%.

The initial experience suggests that most small to moderately sized,. centrally located defects (ASD secundum and patent foramen ovale) can be closed using the clamshell device with few complications. Large defects have been closed successfully but with a higher rate of residual leaks and complications. The availability of larger devices may improve results in this latter group.

Technique. Precatheterization Doppler echocardiograms should define the number, location, and size of the VSDs and the relationship of these defects to the atrioventricular and semilunar valves.

A VSD is usually easier to cross from the left to the right ventricle than from the right ventricle. This is because of the smooth left ventricular surface and the left-to-right shunt in most defects. The left ventricle can be entered retrograde from the aorta or antegrade from the venous side transseptally and across the mitral valve. The choice depends on patient size and VSD location. If the retrograde approach is used, a 7 Fr sheath is placed in the artery. A 7 Fr sheath and balloon-tipped end-hole catheter are placed in the femoral vein. Right and left hemodynamics are measured and a left ventriculogram is performed in a projection most likely to profile the VSD. The decision must then be made as to what venous access to use for device delivery. A muscular VSD is easier to close using the internal jugular vein, because the approach is straighter and the sheath is less likely to kink. The VSD is crossed and an exchange wire advanced out through that catheter, snared, and drawn out through the skin at the venous site to be used for closure. It is important to avoid getting the wire entangled in the tricuspid valve apparatus. This wire now runs from either the femoral vein or artery through the heart across the VSD and out, for example, the internal jugular vein. Traction on this wire can damage the heart or induce aortic or mitral regurgitation, depending on its course. This wire is used to take selective pictures in the VSD using a pigtail

catheter and Y-arm adaptor and for balloon sizing of the defect.

As with atrial defects, the umbrella should be at least twice the diameter of the defect. In choosing the umbrella size, one must also consider the distances between the defect and valves and from the septum to the free wall of the left ventricle. The venous site is predilated with a 12 Fr dilator and the long 11 Fr sheath and dilator are advanced through the right ventricle and across the VSD to the left ventricle. The umbrella is loaded into the delivery system and the wire and dilator removed from the sheath. The umbrella is advanced to the end of the sheath and delivered as for PDA and ASD closure. Because of the thickness of the septum and the presence of trabeculae, the right ventricular arms do not always open completely. If the left ventricular arms fail to open, entrapment in the free wall or other vital structures should be ruled out before release.

Results. Lock et al. reported the first transcatheter closure of ventricular septal defects and demonstrated the feasibility of the technique.[41] We have now closed an additional 15 ventricular septal defects in 14 patients[42] (Fig. 30–9). Patients ranged in weight from 2 to 89 kg and the defects from 4 to 14 mm in diameter. The defects were muscular in 11, perimembranous in 1, and at the margin of a surgical patch in 3. Flow was abolished (13 of 15) or significantly reduced in all. All devices remained in stable position. Complications included femoral vein thrombosis (n = 1), asymptomatic hemothorax (n = 1), and umbrella impingement on the septal leaflet of tricuspid valve (n = 1). In the latter patient, the arm was repositioned at surgery the next day at the time of transposition repair.

The results demonstrate the feasibility of transcatheter closure of ventricular septal defects. Although the experience is limited, the clearest indication at present is for closure of muscular defects. These defects are difficult to close surgically and often require a left ventriculotomy. At the same time, these defects and some defects at the margins of surgical patches are particularly suitable for device closure because they are usually not close to the

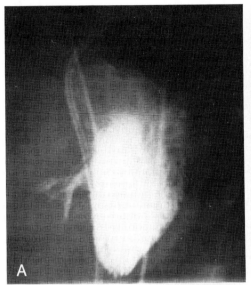

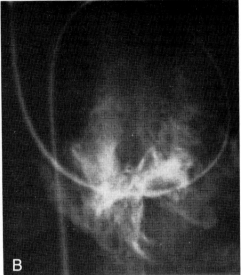

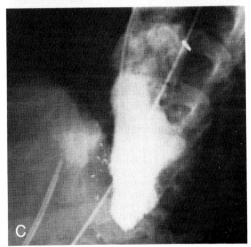

Fig. 30–9. A, A left ventriculogram demonstrating a midmuscular VSD. B, A selective injection in the VSD with a pigtail over a wire from the femoral vein through the atrial septum and VSD and out the SVC and internal jugular vein. C, A left ventriculogram after umbrella placement demonstrates complete closure. The contrast in the right ventricle is from a malalignment VSD, which was closed surgically.

atrioventricular or semilunar valves. Conoventricular, perimembranous, and AV-canal (or inlet) type defects are, on the other hand, usually too close to the valves to be closed with currently available devices. Several patients with multiple ventricular septal defects have now had muscular defects closed with 1 or more umbrellas and then gone to the operating room to have perimembranous or other defects repaired.

REFERENCES

1. Rashkind WJ, Miller WW: Creation of an atrial septal defect without thoracotomy: Palliative approach to complete transposition of the great arteries. JAMA 196:991–992, 1966.
2. Park SC, Zuberbuhler JR, Neches WH, Lenoa CC, Zoltun RA: A new atrial septostomy technique. Cathet Cardiovasc Diagn 1:195–201, 1975.
3. Edwards BS, Lucas RV, Lock JE, Edwards JE: Morphologic changes in the pulmonary arteries after percutaneous balloon angioplasty for pulmonary arterial stenosis. Circulation 71:195–201, 1985.
4. Ring JC, Kulik TJ, Burke BA, Lock JE: Morphologic changes induced by dilation of the pulmonary valve annulus with overlarge balloons in normal newborn lambs. Am J Cardiol 55:210–214, 1984.
5. Yeager S: Letter. J Am Coll Cardiol 9:467–468, 1987.
6. Rubio-Alvarez V, Limon RL, Soni J: Valvulotomias intracardiacas por medio de un cateter. Arch Inst Cardiol Mex 23:183–192, 1953.
7. Semb BKH, Tjonneland S, Stake G, Aabyholm G: Balloon valvulotomy of congenital pulmonary valve

stenosis with tricuspid valve insufficiency. Cardio-vasc Radiol 2:239–241, 1979.

8. Kan JS, White RI Jr, Jitchell SE, Gardner TJ: Percutaneous balloon valvuloplasty: A new method for treating congenital pulmonary valve stenosis. N Engl J Med 307:540–542, 1982.

9. Radkte W, Keane JF, Fellows KE, Lang P, Lock JE: Percutaneous balloon valvotomy of congenital pulmonary stenosis using oversized balloons. J Am Coll Cardiol 8:909–915, 1986.

10. Ali Khan MA, Yousef SA, Mullins CE: Percutaneous transluminal balloon pulmonary valvuloplasty for the relief of pulmonary valve stenosis with special reference to double-balloon technique. Am Heart J 112:158–166, 1986.

11. Stanger P, Cassidy SC, Girod DA, et al: Balloon pulmonary valvuloplasty: Results of the valvuloplasty and angioplasty of congenital anomalies registry. Am J Cardiol 65:775–783, 1990.

12. Perry SB, Keane JF, Lock JE: Interventional catheterization in pediatric congenital and acquired heart disease. Am J Cardiol 61:109G–117G, 1986.

13. Lababidi Z: Aortic balloon valvuloplasty. Am Heart J 106:751, 1983.

14. Sholler GF, Keane JF, Perry SB, et al: Balloon dilation of aortic stenosis: Results and influence of technical and morphological features on outcome. Circulation 78:351–360, 1988.

15. Rocchini P, Beekman RH, Schachar GB, et al: Balloon aortic valvuloplasty: Results of the valvuloplasty and angioplasty of congenital anomalies registry. Am J Cardiol 65:784–789, 1990.

16. Cribier A, Savin T, Berland J, et al: Percutaneous transluminal balloon valvuloplasty of adult aortic stenosis: Report of 92 cases. J Am Coll Cardiol 9:381–386, 1987.

17. Helgason H, Keane JF, Fellows KE, et al: Balloon dilation of the aortic valve: Studies in normal lambs and in children with aortic stenosis. J Am Coll Cardiol 9:816–822, 1987.

18. Waller BF, Girod DA, Dillon JC: Transverse aortic wall tears in infants after balloon angioplasty for aortic valve stenosis: Relation of aortic wall damage to diameter of inflated angioplasty balloon and aortic lumen in 7 necropsy cases. J Am Coll Cardiol 4:1235–1241, 1984.

19. Singer MI, Rowen M, Dorsey TJ: Transluminal aortic balloon angioplasty for coarctation of the aorta in the newborn. Am Heart J 103:131–132, 1982.

20. Saul JP, Keane JF, Fellows KE, Lock JE: Balloon dilation angioplasty of postoperative aortic obstructions. Am J Cardiol 59:943–948, 1987.

21. Morrow WR, Vick GW, Nihil MR, et al: Balloon dilation of unoperated coarctation of the aorta: Short- and intermediate-term results. J Am Coll Cardiol 11:133, 1988.

22. Beekman RH, Rocchini AP, Dick M: Percutaneous balloon angioplasty for native coarctation of the aorta. J Am Coll Cardiol 10:1078, 1987.

23. Tynan M, Finley JP, Fontes V, et al: Balloon angioplasty for the treatment of native coarctation: Results of the valvuloplasty and angioplasty of congenital anomalies registry. Am J Cardiol 65:790–792, 1990.

24. Hellenbrand WE, Allen HD, Golinko RJ, et al: Bal-loon angioplasty for aortic recoarctation: Results of the valvuloplasty and angioplasty of congenital anomalies registry. Am J Cardiol 65:793–797, 1990.

25. Lock JE, Niemi T, Burke B, Einzig S, Castaneda-Zuniga W: Transcutaneous angioplasty of experimental aortic coarctation. Circulation 66:1280–1286, 1982.

26. Perry SB, Zeevi B, Keane JF, Lock JE: Interventional catheterization of left heart lesions, including aoretic and mitral valve stenosis and coarctation of the aorta. Cardiol Clin 7:341–349, 1989.

27. Rothman A, Perry SB, Keane JF, Lock JE: Early results and follow-up of balloon angioplasty for branch pulmonary artery stenosis. J Am Coll Cardiol 15:1109–1117, 1990.

28. Kan JS, Marvin WJ, Bass JL, et al: Balloon angioplasty-branch pulmonary artery stenosis: Results from the valvuloplasty and angioplasty of congenital anomalies registry. Am J Cardiol 65:798–801, 1990.

29. Zuberbuhler JR, Anker E, Zoltun R, et al: Tissue adhesive closure of aortic-pulmonary communications. Am Heart J 88:41, 1974.

30. Barth KH, White RI, Kaufman SL, et al: Embolotherapy of pulmonary arteriovenous malformations with detachable balloons. Radiology 142:599, 1982.

31. Perry SB, Radtke W, Fellows KE, et al: Coil embolization to occlude aortopulmonary collateral vessels and shunts in patients with congenital heart disease. J Am Coll Cardiol 13:100–108, 1989.

32. Gianturco C, Anderson JH, Wallace S: Mechanical devices for arterial occlusion. Am J Roentgenol 124:428–435, 1975.

33. Anderson JH, Wallace S, Gianturco C, Gerson LP: ''Mini'' Gianturco stainless steel coils for transcatheter vascular occlusion. Radiology 132:301–303, 1979.

34. Portsmann W, Wierny L, Warnke H, et al: Catheter closure of patent ductus arteriosus, 62 cases treated without thoracotomy. Radiol Clin North Am 9:203–218, 1971.

35. Sato K, Fujino M, Kozuka T, et al: Transfemoral plug closure of patent ductus arteriosus. Circulation 51:337–341, 1975.

36. King TD, Mills NL: Secundum atrial septal defects: Nonoperative closure during cardiac catheterization. JAMA 235:2506–2509, 1976.

37. Rashkind WJ: Transcatheter treatment of congenital heart disease. Circulation 67:711–716, 1983.

38. Rashkind WJ, Mullins CE, Hellenbrand WE, Tait MA: Nonsurgical closure of patent ductus arteriosus: Clinical application of the Rashkind PDA occluder system. Circulation 5:583–592, 1987.

39. Lock JE, Cockerham JT, Keane JF, et al: Transcatheter umbrella closure of congenital heart defects. Circulation 75:593–599, 1987.

40. Lock JE, Rome JJ, Davis R, et al: Transcatheter closure of atrial septal defects: Experimental studies. Circulation 79:1091–1099, 1989.

41. Lock JE, Block PC, McKay RG, et al: Transcatheter closure of ventricular septal defects. Circulation 78:361–368, 1988.

42. Goldstein SAN, Perry SB, Keane JF, et al: Transcatheter closure of congenital ventricular septal defects. J Am Coll Cardiol 15:240A (Abstr), 1990.

Part VIII

Profiles of Hemodynamic and Angiographic Abnormalities in Specific Disorders

31

Profiles in Valvular Heart Disease

WILLIAM GROSSMAN

The cardiac valves have as their function the maintenance of unidirectional flow, thus ensuring that the energy released during myocardial contraction is transformed efficiently into the circulation of blood around the body. When the valves become diseased, compensatory mechanisms are brought into play to maintain the circulation commensurate with the metabolic needs of the body. These mechanisms, chief among which are dilatation and hypertrophy, are not without clinical costs, and it is these costs that are responsible for the major manifestations of valvular heart disease.

Valvular disease results in either incompetence of the valve with regard to its function of maintaining unidirectional flow (i.e., valvular insufficiency and regurgitation), or obstruction to the forward and natural course of the circulation (i.e., stenosis). Although mixed stenosis and insufficiency, both of moderate degree, frequently coexist in a particular valve, severe stenosis and severe insufficiency are almost never present in the same valve. Thus, the 0.5 cm^2 valvular orifice of a patient with severe calcific aortic stenosis may barely allow 50 to 60 ml to be ejected from the left ventricle during systole, and this only at a left ventricular systolic pressure of 200 to 300 mmHg. The tiny fixed orifice cannot be ex-

Note: some material in this chapter has been retained from the first and second editions, to which Dr. Lewis Dexter had contributed.

pected to permit more than mild regurgitation in the subsequent diastole, where the driving force is an aortic diastolic pressure of 80 mmHg.

I have seen an exception to this general rule in a middle-aged woman with rheumatic aortic stenosis and insufficiency. Aortography demonstrated severe aortic regurgitation; nevertheless, there was a resting transaortic systolic gradient of approximately 60 mmHg. The explanation was apparent on close examination of the aortic valve during cineaortography. Although two leaflets were heavily calcified and immobile, the third was thickened but mobile. During diastole this leaflet prolapsed freely into the left ventricular cavity, whereas during systole its opening motion was limited or checked by apparent abutment against the free edges of the calcific, immobile leaflets. Another example of mixed, severe stenosis and aortic insufficiency is described later in this chapter and illustrated in Figure 31–9.

Valvular heart disease may be considered to impose two different types of stress on the cardiac chamber proximal to the lesion. These are either pressure overload (increased afterload) or volume overload (increased preload). The former is generally the result of a valvular stenosis, and the latter of valvular insufficiency. Both pressure and volume overload serve as stimuli for the heart to call upon compensatory mechanisms. As mentioned, chief among these mechanisms are hypertrophy (which allows the generation of greater systolic force and at the same time tends to normalize wall stress by increasing wall thickness), and dilatation (which enables increased strength and extent of shortening by the Frank-Starling mechanism). These mechanisms preserve the circulation at the cost of increased myocardial oxygen needs and elevated ventricular filling pressures, leading to clinical evidence of ischemia and congestive heart failure.

In this chapter, I shall discuss the hemodynamic and angiographic findings in patients with valvular heart disease. I have found it useful to apply the general physiologic principles discussed above in the interpretation of catheterization data obtained in patients with disordered valve function. This approach will generally enable the physician to unravel even the most complicated of problems.

MITRAL STENOSIS

The orifice area of the normal mitral valve is about 4.5 cm². As a result of chronic rheumatic heart disease, the orifice becomes progressively smaller. This leads to two circulatory changes.[1] The first is the development of a pressure gradient across the valve, the left ventricular mean diastolic pressure remaining at its normal level of about 5 mmHg and the left atrial mean pressure rising progressively, reaching about 25 mmHg when the orifice of the mitral valve is reduced to approximately 1.0 cm² (Fig. 31–1). The second circulatory change is a reduction of blood flow across the valve—i.e., cardiac output. The normal resting output of 3.0 L/min/m² usually falls to about 2.5 L/min/m² when the valve size is 1.0 cm². A rise of left atrial pressure necessitates a similar rise of pressure in pulmonary veins and pulmonary capillaries, and pulmonary edema occurs when the pulmonary capillary pressure exceeds the oncotic pressure of normal plasma, which is about 25 mmHg.

Pulmonary vascular complications practically never occur in mitral stenosis until the mitral valve area approaches 1.0 cm², i.e., when the resting left atrial pressure approaches

25 mmHg. After this point, reactive changes in the pulmonary arteriolar bed frequently develop and pose a progressive obstruction to blood flow through the lungs.

As pulmonary vascular obstruction becomes increasingly severe, the pulmonary arterial pressure rises and occasionally may exceed the systemic pressure. In the extreme, the pulmonary vascular resistance can rise to 25 or 30 times normal. Despite substantial hypertrophy, the right ventricle cannot cope with the enormous pressure load imposed upon it, and dilates and fails.

The "Second Stenosis." Thus, in mitral stenosis, two "stenoses" eventuate—first at the mitral valve and second in the arterioles of the lung. The hemodynamic findings in patients with tight mitral stenoses with and without major pulmonary vascular disease are illustrated in Figure 31–2. As can be seen, the *second stenosis* (Fig. 31–2, bottom panel) has resulted in a 70-mmHg mean pressure gradient across the lungs, giving a pulmonary vascular resistance of 1866 dynes-sec-cm⁻⁵. Workup of the patient with mitral stenosis should include an assessment of both of these obstructions.

Catheterization Protocol

The usual indication for cardiac catheterization in patients with mitral stenosis is that the patient is being considered a candidate for corrective surgery by the clinician. Catheterization should be a combined right and left heart procedure, in which the following measurements and calculations are made:

1. Simultaneous left ventricular diastolic pressure, left atrial (or pulmonary capillary wedge) diastolic pressure, heart rate, diastolic filling period and cardiac output. From these, the size of the orifice of the mitral valve may be calculated (see Chapter 11 for details of the orifice area calculation).

2. If the transmitral pressure difference is less than 5 mmHg, the error of calculation of the mitral valve orifice area is appreciable. The circulatory measurements should be repeated under circumstances of stress (ex-

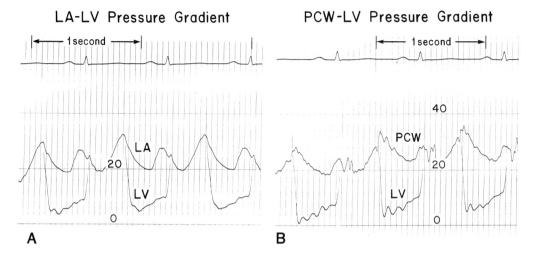

Fig. 31–1. Simultaneous left atrial (LA) and left ventricular (LV) pressures (A) and pulmonary capillary wedge (PCW) and LV pressures (B) in a patient with tight mitral stenosis and a mean PCW pressure of approximately 25 mmHg. LV end diastolic pressure is normal at 10 mmHg. Note the presence of *"a"* waves in the LA and PCW trace which are not transmitted to the LV because of the damping effect of the stenotic mitral valve. Reproduced from Lange RA et al, J Am Coll Cardiol 13:825, 1989, with permission.

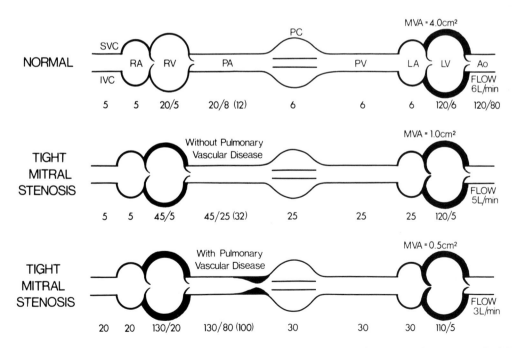

Fig. 31–2. Diagrammatic representation of the circulation in patients with normal hemodynamics (upper panel), tight mitral stenosis (middle panel), and tight mitral stenosis with pulmonary vascular disease and the development of a *second stenosis* at the pulmonary arteriolar level (bottom panel). See text for discussion.

ercise, tachycardia induced by isoproterenol or pacing) to increase the pressure difference across the mitral valve.

3. Simultaneously, or in close order, pulmonary arterial mean pressure, left atrial (or pulmonary capillary wedge) mean pressure, and cardiac output for the calculation of pulmonary vascular resistance.

4. Right ventricular systolic and diastolic pressures for assessment of right ventricular function.

5. If *other lesions* are suspected (e.g., mitral regurgitation, aortic valve disease, left atrial myxoma), they too must be evaluated. In this regard, it should be pointed out that certain lesions tend to occur in combination with mitral stenosis. In my experience, many (if not most) patients with severe mitral stenosis have had some degree of **aortic regurgitation.** Also, although it is rare, **tricuspid stenosis** should always be looked for in the patient with severe mitral stenosis, because it is seen only in association with this condition. Another condition that may be associated with mitral stenosis is **atrial septal defect** with left-to-right shunt. The combination of mitral stenosis and atrial septal defect is known as Lutembacher's syndrome. Thus, as with standard right heart catheterization, described in Chapters 4 through 6, the operator should obtain screening blood samples from superior vena cava and pulmonary artery for oximetry determination. This has taken on added importance in the present era when balloon mitral valvuloplasty (see Chapter 29) has become a standard treatment for mitral stenosis. Balloon mitral valvuloplasty generally requires transseptal catheterization and involves limited dilatation of the interatrial septum; thus the procedure may create an atrial septal defect,[2] thereby producing Lutembacher's syndrome.

The following case studies illustrate the different clinical and hemodynamic syndromes seen in patients with mitral stenosis. The first is a typical example of a symptomatic patient

with "tight" mitral stenosis, normal pulmonary vascular resistance, and a normal-sized heart (stage II, Fig. 31–3). The second is an example of a relatively asymptomatic patient with more severe mitral stenosis, a five- to tenfold increase of pulmonary vascular resistance, and an enlarged heart caused principally by enlargement of the right ventricle (stage III, Fig. 31–3). The third represents terminal mitral stenosis with an extreme degree of pulmonary vascular resistance, pulmonary hypertension and right ventricular failure (stage IV, Fig. 31–3).

Case 1

Tight Mitral Stenosis with Normal Pulmonary Vascular Resistance. A.R., a 35-year-old woman, had chorea as a child and was thereafter asymptomatic until two years prior to admission, when she noted the onset of exertional dyspnea. This progressed to the point of her having to stop after climbing one flight of stairs slowly. She had had one recent episode of hemoptysis. Her most troublesome symptom had been paroxysmal atrial fibrillation over a period of several months. She had had orthopnea and one episode of paroxysmal nocturnal dyspnea.

On physical examination, she was in no ap-

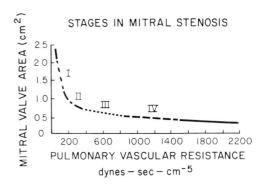

Fig. 31–3. Stages in the natural history of mitral stenosis. As the mitral orifice progressively narrows, pulmonary vascular resistance increases. This increase is slow at first, but when the mitral valve area becomes "critical" (less than 1 cm²), the increase is rapid, reflecting the development of a second stenosis at the level of the precapillary pulmonary arterioles. Clinical correlations are discussed in the text.

parent distress. Blood pressure was 130/70 mmHg and pulse rate was 80 beats/min and regular. There was no jugular venous distension, lungs were normal, and the PMI was in the fifth interspace in the midclavicular line. S_1 was accentuated. At the apex, there was a grade 1 pansystolic murmur, an opening snap, and a grade 2 diastolic rumble with presystolic accentuation. The liver edge was at the costal margin, and there was no edema.

The ECG was within normal limits.

The chest roentgenogram showed a normal-sized heart, an enlarged left atrium, a mild degree of pulmonary vascular redistribution, and no calcification in the region of the mitral valve, and was otherwise normal.

Cardiac catheterization revealed the following:

Body surface area, m^2	1.78
O$_2$ consumption, ml/min	180
A-V O$_2$ difference, ml/L	40
Cardiac output, L/min	4.5
Heart rate/min	76, NSR
Pressures, mmHg:	
Brachial artery	130/70, $\overline{90}$
Left ventricle	130/8
Diastolic mean	6
Diastolic filling period, sec/beat	0.42
Pulmonary capillary wedge, mean	24
Diastolic mean	20
Pulmonary artery	40/22, $\overline{28}$
Right ventricle	40/6
Right atrium, mean	4
Pulmonary vascular resistance, dynes-sec-cm^{-5}	71
Calculated mitral valve area, cm^2	1.0

Cineangiography of the left ventricle revealed no mitral regurgitation.

Interpretation. This patient was symptomatic because of her increased left atrial pressure and atrial arrhythmia. She had not yet developed the ''second stenosis'' at the precapillary pulmonary arteriolar level, discussed previously. Thus, her pulmonary artery pressure elevation was purely a consequence of the increased left atrial and pulmonary venous pressures, and the pulmonary vascular resistance was normal (<120 dynes-sec-cm^{-5}). In the spectrum of patients with mitral stenosis, she would fall into stage II of Figure 31–3.

Case 2

Severe Mitral Stenosis, Moderately Elevated Pulmonary Vascular Resistance, Few Symptoms, Fatigue Syndrome. E.C., a 42-year-old woman, had no history of acute rheumatic fever. She was asymptomatic until she was 19 years old, when during the last month of her first pregnancy, she developed pulmonary congestion. She responded well to therapy and remained asymptomatic thereafter, even during three subsequent pregnancies. However, during her fifth pregnancy at age 37, dyspnea, orthopnea, paroxysmal nocturnal dyspnea, and one episode of hemoptysis of pure red blood occurred at the seventh month, necessitating hospitalization through term. Thereafter she improved but became progressively tired with loss of energy and drive. She became less thorough in her housework and in her attention to the children's clothes and lost her previous meticulousness. If she pushed herself, she would become somewhat short of breath on a flight of stairs, but it was fatigue more than breathlessness that bothered her.

On examination, she was well-nourished and had a malar flush. Her blood pressure was 115/70 mmHg; her pulse, 90 beats/min and irregularly irregular. Respirations were 15. There was no pulmonary or peripheral congestion. The neck veins were just visible at the clavicles with the patient sitting upright. The PMI was in the fifth interspace just outside the midclavicular line. The impulse was normal. A prominent parasternal heave was present. S_1 was accentuated. No apical systolic murmur was present. There was an opening snap and a grade 2 apical diastolic rumble.

The ECG showed right ventricular hypertrophy and atrial fibrillation.

Chest radiographs showed the heart to be moderately enlarged because of enlargement of the left atrium and right ventricle. The pulmonary arteries were prominent, and there was a moderate degree of pulmonary vascular redistribution.

The findings at cardiac catheterization were as follows:

Body surface area, m^2	1.41
O$_2$ consumption, ml/min	188
A-V O$_2$ difference, ml/L	51
Cardiac output, L/min	3.7
Heart rate/min	85, AF
Pressures, mmHg:	
Brachial artery	120/62, $\overline{84}$
Left ventricle	120/7
Diastolic mean	5
Diastolic filling period, sec/beat	0.38
Pulmonary capillary wedge, mean	27
Diastolic mean	23
Pulmonary artery	82/32, $\overline{51}$
Right ventricle	82/10
Right atrium, mean	8
Pulmonary vascular resistance, dynes-sec-cm^{-5}	520
Calculated mitral valve area, cm^2	0.7

Interpretation. This patient's symptoms were initially caused by elevated left atrial pressure when, during her fifth pregnancy, she developed hemoptysis, orthopnea, and paroxysmal nocturnal dyspnea. Subsequently, however, her major symptom was fatigue, associated with a reduced cardiac output and an increased arteriovenous O$_2$ difference. The orthopnea and paroxysmal dyspnea had receded somewhat despite the fact that her pulmonary capillary pressure was at the pulmonary edema level. This is a common, although poorly understood, phenomenon in patients with mitral stenosis when pulmonary vascular disease begins to occur. Thus, this patient was beginning to develop the "second stenosis" discussed previously, and this is apparent from the elevated pulmonary vascular resistance (520 dynes-sec-cm^{-5}). In the spectrum of patients with mitral stenosis, she would be representative of stage III of Figure 31–3.

Case 3

Terminal Mitral Stenosis With Severe Pulmonary Hypertension. C.A., a 47-year-old woman, had had acute rheumatic fever at 8 years of age and a murmur ever since. She did well thereafter until 5 years ago, when she noticed exertional dyspnea and paroxysmal nocturnal dyspnea. Four years ago, these symptoms worsened. Orthopnea and ankle edema appeared. Her symptoms then improved for nearly two years, only to return about two months prior to admission. Since then, despite a good cardiac regimen, she had had to lead a bed-chair-bathroom existence.

On examination, she was cachectic, dyspneic, and orthopneic. Acrocyanosis was evident. Blood pressure was 96/72 mmHg; pulse rate, 90 beats/min and irregularly irregular; respirations, 32. Neck veins were distended to the angle of the jaw, "V" waves were prominent, and there were bibasilar rales over the lung fields. The PMI was in the anterior axillary line. The apex impulse was normal, but a parasternal heave was present. S$_1$ was loud. Systole was silent. An opening snap was present, and there was a barely audible mitral diastolic murmur with appreciable presystolic accentuation. The pulmonary component of S$_2$ was loud and palpable. The liver was two fingerbreadths below the right costal margin and was tender. There was considerable pitting edema to the knees.

The ECG showed atrial fibrillation, right axis deviation, and right ventricular hypertrophy.

Chest roentgenogram showed a large heart with prominent left atrium, right ventricle, pulmonary arteries, pulmonary vasculature, and Kerley B lines.

Cardiac catheterization revealed the following:

Body surface area, m^2	1.4
O$_2$ consumption, ml/min	201
A-V O$_2$ difference, ml/L	110
Cardiac output, L/min	1.8
Pulse rate/min	92, AF
Pressures, mmHg:	
Brachial artery	108/70

Left ventricle	108/12
Diastolic mean	10
Diastolic filling period, sec/beat	0.36
Pulmonary capillary wedge, mean	33
Diastolic mean	31
Pulmonary artery	125/65; $\overline{75}$
Right ventricle	125/20
Right atrium, mean	19
Pulmonary vascular resistance, dynes-sec-cm^{-5}	1838
Calculated mitral valve area, cm^2	0.3

Interpretation. This patient had symptoms of left atrial hypertension 5 years before her catheterization, suggesting that she was in stage II (see Fig. 31–3) of mitral stenosis at that time. At the time of presentation to us, she had evidence of advanced right heart failure and pulmonary hypertension. This woman has "two stenoses," and both are severe: the mitral orifice area is less than one tenth normal at 0.3 cm^2, and the pulmonary arteriolar (vascular) resistance is approximately 18 times normal at 1838 dynes-sec-cm^{-5}! She is in late stage IV of mitral stenosis, as diagrammed in Figure 31–3.

MITRAL REGURGITATION

Mitral incompetence, failure of the valve to prevent regurgitation of blood from the left ventricle to the left atrium during ventricular systole, may be caused by functional or anatomic inadequacy of any one of the components of the mitral valve apparatus, which consists of two valve leaflets, two papillary muscles with their chordae tendineae, and the valve ring or annulus.

Mitral regurgitation may occur when there is destruction or deformation of the valve leaflets as a result of rheumatic fever or bacterial endocarditis. Mitral regurgitation begins during "isometric" ventricular contraction and continues throughout systole, thus giving rise to a holosystolic murmur. A fibromyxomatous process in the mitral valve leaflets and chordae tendineae may give rise to the "floppy valve syndrome." There may or may not be other evidence of Marfan's syndrome in these patients. The papillary muscles are usually normal, but there is a marked redundancy of the valve leaflets and chordae with resulting prolapse into the left atrium during systole and accompanying regurgitation.

The papillary muscles are particularly vulnerable to ischemia from coronary artery disease as well as to damage from viral myocarditis. The posterior papillary muscle derives its blood supply from the right coronary and left circumflex arteries. Ischemic dysfunction of this muscle may occur in association with either an inferior or posterolateral myocardial infarction. Less frequently, ischemic involvement of the anterior papillary muscle in an anterior or anterolateral infarction produces mitral regurgitation. Papillary-chordal integrity is maintained to a point when the left ventricle dilates. The common occurrence of a mitral regurgitant murmur in patients with large left ventricles, however, may reflect a simple anatomic loss of this integrity, an involvement of the papillary muscle with the same disease that causes the left ventricle to dilate, or an abnormality of contraction of the mitral annulus.

Mitral regurgitation from whatever cause implies a *double outlet to the left ventricle:* during systole, blood exits through both aortic and mitral valves. Total left ventricular output rises, that going into the aorta may fall, and that regurgitating through the mitral valve depends largely on the size of the regurgitant orifice, left atrial compliance, the systolic mean pressure difference between left ventricle and left atrium, and the duration of systole. Although hypertension aggravates and lowering of blood pressure lessens mitral regurgitation, the most important factor is probably the size of the regurgitant orifice.

In patients with mitral regurgitation, cardiac catheterization is important to provide a complete hemodynamic and angiographic assessment of the severity of the valvular lesion.

Hemodynamic Assessment[3–8]

First, it is important to assess the hemodynamic consequences of the mitral regurgitation by measuring cardiac output and right and left heart pressures.

Interpretation of V Waves in the Pulmonary Capillary Wedge Tracing. With *acute* mitral regurgitation (e.g., ruptured chordae tendineae), giant V waves will be seen in the left atrial or pulmonary artery pressure tracing (Fig. 31–4). In this regard, our Fellows and Residents frequently ask, "How large must a V wave be in order to be diagnostic of severe mitral regurgitation?" In my experience, V waves up to twice the mean left atrial pressure can be seen in the absence of any mitral regurgitation. The patient with left ventricular failure from any cause may have a distended, noncompliant left atrium and the *normal V wave* (which is due to left atrial filling from the pulmonary veins during left ventricular systole) will be prominent in this circumstance.[7] When pulmonary blood flow is increased, the normal V wave increases in prominence correspondingly: this is particularly striking in **acute ventricular septal defect** complicating myocardial infarction, in which enormous V waves (≥50 mmHg) can be seen in the absence of any mitral regurgitation.

V waves *greater than twice the mean* left atrial (or pulmonary capillary wedge) pressure are suggestive of severe mitral regurgitation, and when the height of *the V wave is three times the mean pulmonary capillary wedge* or left atrial pressure, a diagnosis of severe mitral regurgitation is virtually certain (Fig. 31–4). I hasten to point out, however, that the absence of a prominent V wave by no means rules out severe mitral regurgitation. Slowly developing chronic mitral regurgitation commonly leads to marked left atrial enlargement, and the dilated left atrium can accept an enormous regurgitant volume per beat *without any increase in mean pressure or height of the V wave.*[9] Also, the level of afterload, as determined by systemic vascular resistance, may greatly affect the height of the regurgitant or V wave in patients with mitral regurgitation.[4] As seen in Figure 31–5, a patient with severe mitral regurgitation had a V wave of 48 mmHg at a time when LV systolic pressure was approximately 140 mmHg. With sodium nitroprusside (right hand panel, Fig. 31–5), the LV systolic pressure came down to 120 mmHg and the V wave was essentially abolished.[10,11] Although this patient's regurgitant fraction was reduced with sodium nitroprusside (from 80% to 64%), it still remained in the range of severe mitral regurgitation (see subsequent text).

Exercise Hemodynamics. Another important hemodynamic parameter in the assessment of mitral regurgitation is the forward cardiac output. Low cardiac output is common in advanced mitral regurgitation and may account for much of the clinical picture. If resting cardiac output is near normal, and if the patient's primary symptoms are related to exertion (i.e., easy fatigability and dyspnea on exertion), dynamic exercise during cardiac catheterization may be revealing. If the symptoms are cardiac in origin, the patient usually fails to increase cardiac output appropriately with exercise; i.e., the increase in cardiac output will be ≤80% predicted (see formula for prediction of cardiac output increase with exercise in Chapter 17). In addition, pulmonary capillary wedge or left atrial mean pressure will rise with exercise, commonly reaching levels ≥35

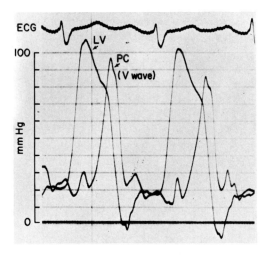

Fig. 31–4. Left ventricular (LV) and pulmonary capillary wedge (PC) pressure tracings taken in a patient with ruptured chordae tendineae and acute mitral insufficiency. The giant V wave results from regurgitation of blood into a relatively small and noncompliant left atrium. Electrocardiogram (ECG) illustrates the timing of the PC V wave, whose peak follows ventricular repolarization, as manifested by the T wave of the ECG.

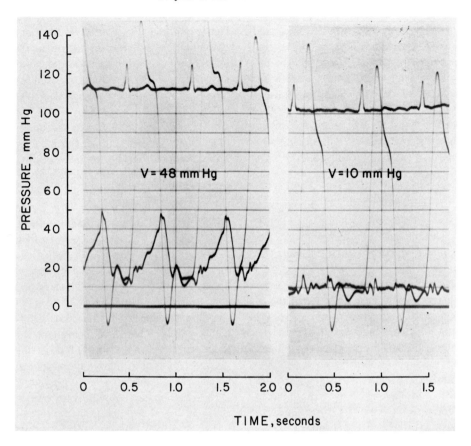

Fig. 31–5. Left ventricular and pulmonary capillary wedge pressures before (left) and during (right) an infusion of sodium nitroprusside in a patient with severe mitral regurgitation and atrial fibrillation. This illustrates the sensitivity of the V wave height to LV afterload in patients with mitral regurgitation. See text for discussion. (From Harshaw CW et al: Reduced systemic vascular resistance as therapy for severe mitral regurgitation of valvular origin. Ann Intern Med 83:312, 1975.)

mmHg by 4 to 5 minutes of supine bicycle exercise, even if the control value was nearly normal. A case demonstrating this point is illustrated in Figure 17–6, Chapter 17.

Angiographic Assessment

The second objective of cardiac catheterization in patients with mitral regurgitation is the angiographic assessment of the severity of the regurgitation by left ventriculography. The assessment may be qualitative, by noting the degree of opacification of the left atrium due to regurgitation back through the incompetent valve, using a scale of 1 + (mild), 2 + (moderate), 3 + (moderately severe), and 4 + (severe) regurgitation. These grades are essentially subjective, but certain criteria can be used to enhance consistency of their usage. Regurgitation that is 1 + essentially clears with each beat and never opacifies the entire left atrium. When regurgitation is 2 + (moderate), it does not clear with one beat and generally does opacify the entire left atrium (albeit faintly) after several beats; however, opacification of the left atrium does not equal that of the left ventricle. In 3 + regurgitation (moderately severe), the left atrium is completely opacified and achieves equal opacification with the left ventricle. In 4 + regurgitation (severe), opacification of the entire left atrium occurs within one beat, the opacification becomes progressively more dense with each beat, and contrast can be seen refluxing into the pulmonary veins during left ventricular systole.

Regurgitant Fraction. The angiographic assessment of severity of mitral regurgitation may also be made more quantitative by calculation of the *regurgitant fraction*. This entails measurement of total left ventricular stroke volume (TSV) from the left ventriculogram and the amount that goes forward by way of the aorta to the body (the forward stroke volume, FSV) by Fick or indicator-dilution technique. The TSV is calculated as the difference between end-diastolic and end-systolic left ventricular volumes (EDV − ESV = TSV), as described in Chapter 19. Regurgitant stroke volume (RSV, regurgitant volume/beat) is then given as RSV = TSV − FSV. Regurgitant fraction (RF) is then calculated as RF = RSV/TSV.

The accuracy of these calculations depends on many factors. Because FSV is calculated by dividing cardiac output by heart rate at the time of the Fick (or other) cardiac output determination, it is an average stroke volume. The particular beat chosen from the left ventriculogram for volume determination must therefore be an ''average'' or representative beat; alternatively, volumes from multiple beats must be calculated and averaged. Thus, in patients with atrial fibrillation or extrasystoles during ventriculography, the regurgitant stroke volume and regurgitant fraction may be highly inaccurate, and we do not calculate them in such patients. It should also be obvious that the accuracy of the regurgitant fraction depends on a similar physiologic state prevailing between the cardiac output and angiographic phases of the catheterization procedure. An increase in arterial blood pressure may substantially increase the mitral regurgitation and decrease forward output. Therefore, if blood pressure or other hemodynamic variables change significantly between the time of cardiac output determination and left ventriculography, it is pointless to calculate regurgitant fraction. Finally, regurgitant fraction quantifies, at best, the *total* amount of regurgitation. Thus, if a patient has both mitral and aortic regurgitation, the regurgitant fraction gives an assessment of the regurgitation due to *both* lesions combined.

A study from the University of Texas at Dallas analyzed the interrelationship of qualitative and quantitative angiographic grading in 230 patients with either aortic or mitral regurgitation.[12] These authors showed a stepwise correlation between actual regurgitant volume (L/min/M^2) and 1+ to 4+ regurgitation graded visually, using the definitions given in this chapter. For the 147 patients with mitral regurgitation, 1+ regurgitation was associated with a mean regurgitant flow of 0.61 L/min/M^2, 2+ regurgitation with 1.14 L/min/M^2, 3+ regurgitation with 2.14 L/min/M^2, and 4+ regurgitation with 4.60 L/min/M^2 and the regurgitant fractions showed similar correlation (L. David Hillis, M.D., personal communication). There was considerable scatter in the data, however, so that much overlap of actual flow values existed.

Within the context of these caveats and qualifications, we regard the regurgitant fraction as a useful parameter in the quantitative assessment of mitral regurgitation. In general, RF <20% is mild, 20% to 40% is moderate, 40% to 60% is moderately severe, and >60% is severe mitral regurgitation.

The third objective of cardiac catheterization in patients with mitral regurgitation is the assessment of left ventricular function by measuring the left ventricular diastolic pressure and more importantly by measuring the left ventricular ejection fraction and end-systolic volume. As others have emphasized, the nearer the preoperative ejection fraction is to normal, the greater is the degree of postoperative restoration to full activity. Specific parameters of left ventricular function are discussed in Chapters 19 and 20.

Catheterization Protocol

1. Right heart catheterization for evaluation of right atrial pressure (to detect possible tricuspid valve disease or right ventricular failure), pulmonary artery pressure (degree of pulmonary hypertension), and wedge pressure (V wave height). In severe, acute mitral regurgitation, a V wave may actually be seen in the pulmonary artery as a second or late systolic hump in the pressure wave form.[8]

2. Left heart catheterization for measurement of LVEDP and assessment of gradients (if any) across mitral or aortic valves. A characteristic of severe mitral regurgitation is that the LVEDP is usually much lower than the LA or PCW mean pressure. In contrast, in LV failure due to cardiomyopathy or coronary artery disease, LVEDP is usually close to or equals the PCW mean pressure, while in aortic regurgitation or LV aneurysm, LVEDP is usually much higher than PCW mean pressure.

3. Cardiac output by Fick or indicator-dilution technique. This measures the fraction of blood going out by way of the aorta to the body, and by itself yields no information about regurgitant flow. The response of forward cardiac output to dynamic exercise may provide useful information, however, because patients with severe mitral regurgitation are generally incapable of increasing forward output commensurate with the needs of the body, as estimated by the increased oxygen consumption (see Chapter 17).

4. Cineangiography of the left ventricle is the definitive method for evaluating mitral regurgitation. By this method, it is possible to measure the total left ventricular volumes and regurgitant fraction, as discussed previously.

5. Pharmacologic intervention. An infusion of sodium nitroprusside (Fig. 31–5) often has a dramatic and salutary effect on the hemodynamic abnormalities in mitral regurgitation and may have both therapeutic and diagnostic value. Although TSV may not change, RSV decreases and FSV increases, leading to increased cardiac output.

Case 4

G.A. was a 59-year-old woman with no history of rheumatic fever in childhood. She was healthy and active until 6 months before admission, when she noticed both dyspnea and lower chest discomfort on mild exertion but no other symptoms of heart failure. There was no past history of bacterial endocarditis.

On physical examination, she had normal body habitus. Blood pressure was 130/70 mmHg; pulse, 80 beats/min and regular. The jugular veins were not distended, the carotid pulsations were normal, and the lungs were clear. The apical impulse was diffuse; S_1 was diminished. There was a grade 3 apical pansystolic murmur transmitted to the axilla. No opening snap, S_3, or diastolic murmurs were heard. There were no aortic murmurs.

The ECG showed normal sinus rhythm, complete right bundle branch block, and left axis deviation.

Chest roentgenogram showed enlargement of the left ventricle and left atrium. No valvular calcification was seen.

Cardiac catheterization, left ventricular angiography, and coronary angiography were performed with the following findings:

Body surface area, m²	1.95
O₂ consumption, ml/min	200
A-V O₂ difference, ml/L	52
Cardiac output, L/min	
Total left ventricular output	
(angiographic)	10.4
Forward flow (Fick)	3.9
Regurgitant flow	6.5
Heart rate/min	67
Stroke volume, ml/beat	
End-diastolic LV volume, ml	
(angiography)	197
End-systolic LV volume, ml	
(angiography)	42
Total LV stroke volume, ml	
(angiography)	155
Forward stroke volume, ml	
(Fick)	58
Regurgitant stroke volume,	
ml	97
Ejection fraction (155 ÷ 197)	0.79
Regurgitant fraction	
(97 ÷ 155)	0.63
Pressures, mmHg:	
Brachial artery	140/84, $\overline{105}$
Left ventricle	140/14
Systolic mean	112
Systolic ejection period,	
sec/beat	0.28
Pulmonary capillary wedge,	
mean	12
V wave	24
Pulmonary artery	30/14, $\overline{19}$

Right ventricle	30/6
Right atrium, mean	4
Pulmonary vascular resistance	143
Systemic vascular resistance, dynes-sec-cm^{-5}	2071

Left ventricular cineangiography showed an excellent and uniform contraction of the left ventricle and a large regurgitant jet into the left atrium, which was completely filled within one beat. The mitral valve did not prolapse into the left atrium.

Coronary arteriograms with selective injections into both left and right coronary arteries revealed normal vasculature, no irregularities or narrowings, and normal run-off.

Interpretation. Mitral regurgitation was identified and quantified. There were no other valvular lesions. Although the left ventricular end diastolic pressure and volume were above normal, the left ventricle contracted uniformly and vigorously as judged by cineangiography. The ejection fraction of 0.79 and the end-systolic volume were normal. The slight elevation of pulmonary vascular resistance was mainly related to the low pulmonary blood flow (forward cardiac output) of 3.9 L/min (cardiac index = 2.0 L/min/M^2).

Systemic vascular resistance was increased substantially, perhaps representing excessive vasoconstriction in response to the decreased forward cardiac output. The increased systemic vascular resistance presented an augmented afterload to the left ventricle, thereby worsening this patient's mitral regurgitation. Reduced systemic vascular resistance, induced by vasodilator therapy with hydralazine, prazosin, or a converting enzyme inhibitor, would probably improve this patient's cardiac output and symptoms of dyspnea on exertion.

AORTIC STENOSIS

Aortic stenosis may be valvular, subvalvular, or supravalvular. Valvular aortic stenosis is most often of the acquired calcific type, which develops on the substrate of a congenitally deformed (e.g., bicuspid) aortic valve. Valvular aortic stenosis may also be present from birth (congenital aortic stenosis) or may develop as a consequence of rheumatic fever. Subaortic stenosis is of various types. Supravalvular stenosis is rare. All produce a significant systolic pressure difference between the left ventricle and the aorta. In subaortic stenosis, the gradient is between the main portion of the left ventricle and its outflow tract, although in "tunnel" subaortic stenosis there may be no discrete subvalvular chamber. In supravalvular stenosis, the gradient is between the proximal and distal aorta just beyond the aortic valve. To facilitate surgical intervention, it is important to identify the site and nature of the obstruction in each instance. This is determined by both hemodynamics and angiography. In addition, left ventricular function and the presence or absence of aortic and mitral regurgitation should be evaluated. The left ventricle becomes progressively hypertrophied in aortic stenosis. The cardiac output is well maintained until the left ventricle dilates and fails; it then becomes progressively reduced. The following discussion will focus on valvular aortic stenosis in the adult.

The cardinal indications for cardiac catheterization in anticipation of surgery for all three types of aortic stenosis are left ventricular failure, angina pectoris, or syncope. Coronary angiography should be performed in essentially all adults being studied for evaluation of hemodynamically significant aortic stenosis.

Hemodynamic Assessment

In the hemodynamic assessment of valvular aortic stenosis, primary importance should be placed on obtaining simultaneous measurement of pressure and flow across the aortic valve. As discussed in Chapter 11, this permits calculation of the aortic orifice or valve area (AVA). In the typical adult with symptomatic aortic stenosis, AVA is reduced to ≤0.7 cm^2. Occasionally a valve of 0.8 to 0.9 cm^2 results in a symptomatic presentation, especially when there is concomitant coronary artery disease or hypertension, or when the absolute value of cardiac output is high (e.g., a large

Table 31–1. *Correlation Between Clinical Severity of Acquired Aortic Stenosis in Adults and Aortic Valve Area*

Aortic Valve Area	Clinical Severity
AVA ≥1.0 cm²	Mild: symptoms rare in absence of other heart disease (coronary disease, other valve lesions)
1.0 cm² > AVA >0.7 cm²	Moderate: symptoms with unusual stress, such as vigorous exercise, rapid atrial fibrillation, influenza
0.7 cm² > AVA >0.5 cm²	Moderately severe: symptoms with ordinary activities of daily living
AVA ≤0.5 cm²	Severe: symptoms at rest or minimal exertion, biventricular failure

patient, anemia, fever, or thyrotoxicosis). When AVA is ≤0.5 cm², severe aortic stenosis is present and cardiac reserve is minimal or absent.

For the typical adult patient with acquired aortic stenosis, correlation between clinical severity and aortic valve area calculated by the Gorlin equation (see Chapter 11) is summarized in Table 31–1. If other cardiac disease is present (e.g., coronary disease, other valve disease, cardiomyopathy), the correlations listed in Table 31–1 will not be applicable.

Most patients with aortic stenosis, particularly those with the clinical presentation of

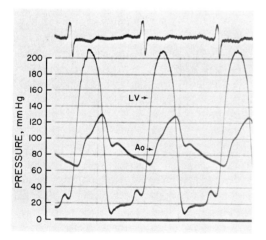

Fig. 31–6. Left ventricular (LV) and aortic (Ao) pressure tracings in an elderly man with severe calcific aortic stenosis. The large A wave in the LV tracing is consistent with decreased compliance of the massively hypertrophied ventricle. The LV pressure was measured with a micromanometer catheter, and aortic pressure was measured with a fluid-filled catheter system attached via tubing to a P23Db transducer. This accounts in part for the delay in onset of Ao upstroke relative to LV pressure rise.

angina and/or syncope, have a normal cardiac output/index, normal right heart and PCW mean pressures, and normal LV ejection fraction. The LVEDP is usually increased, reflecting a stiff LV chamber, and there is a prominent A wave in PCW, LA, and LV pressure tracings (Fig. 31–6). In more advanced cases, LV ejection fraction and cardiac output are depressed, and right heart and PCW mean pressures are elevated. Severe pulmonary hypertension with right heart failure, ascites, and edema may come to dominate the picture. In these patients, the low output state may lead to a reduction in the intensity of the characteristic systolic murmur, obscuring the diagnosis.

Carabello's Sign. An interesting hemodynamic finding, described by Carabello, and coworkers,[13] is a rise in arterial blood pressure during left heart catheter pull-back in patients with severe aortic stenosis (Fig. 31–7). Pressure tracings from 42 patients with aortic stenosis who underwent continuous arterial pressure recording during left heart catheter pull-back (withdrawal from LV to central aorta of a catheter that had been placed in the LV by retrograde technique) were examined. Increases in peripheral arterial pressure of ≥5 mmHg were noted during withdrawal of the retrograde catheter from left ventricle to central aorta in 15 of the 42 patients. Fifteen of 20 patients (75%) with AVA ≤0.6 cm² demonstrated this phenomenon, but none of 22 patients with AVA ≥0.7 cm² showed such an increase. It was concluded that a rise in peak arterial pressure during LV catheter withdrawal is an ancillary hemodynamic finding of

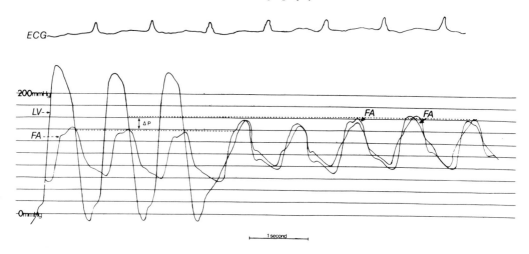

Fig. 31–7. Left ventricular (LV) and femoral artery (FA) pressure tracings in a patient with severe aortic stenosis (aortic valve area, 0.4 cm²). During pullback of the retrograde catheter from LV to ascending aorta, the peak systolic femoral artery pressure can be seen to increase (ΔP) by approximately 20 mmHg. This sign is seen only in patients with aortic valve areas <0.6 cm². The mechanism of this phenomenon is believed to be partial obstruction of an already narrowed aortic orifice by the retrograde catheter and relief of this obstruction with catheter withdrawal. (From Carabello BA et al: Changes in arterial pressure during left heart pull-back in patients with aortic stenosis. Am J Cardiol 44:424, 1979.)

critical aortic stenosis (Fig. 31–7). Although the mechanism of this phenomenon is uncertain, partial obstruction of an already narrowed aortic orifice by the retrograde catheter and relief of this obstruction with catheter withdrawal may be operative.

Angiographic Assessment

In patients with aortic stenosis, left ventriculography can yield important information, and we believe that it should generally be part of the catheterization procedure. It must be emphasized, however, that patients with LV failure and high PCW pressures due to aortic stenosis may not tolerate the radiographic contrast load of left ventriculography. Adequate preventriculography preparation (e.g., IV furosemide, morphine, or oxygen) and use of non-ionic or low-osmolality contrast agents, as outlined in Chapter 14, is mandatory in such patients, and ventriculography should not be done in such patients without careful consideration of risk vs benefit. The value to be obtained from left ventriculography includes assessment of the mitral valve (is there significant mitral regurgitation?), detection of

regional wall motion abnormalities or LV aneurysm indicative of major coronary disease, and overall assessment of LV function. In addition, wall thickness and LV mass may be measured from the ventriculogram.

Aortography is generally not required in the patient with aortic stenosis, unless the gradient is small and the aortic pulse pressure is wide. Selective coronary arteriography should be done in most patients with acquired calcific aortic stenosis, especially if chest pain is present.

Catheterization Protocol

1. Right heart catheterization for measurement of right heart pressures and cardiac output.

2. Left heart catheterization for measurement of pressure gradient across aortic valve, LVEDP, and assessment of presence or absence of a transmitral gradient (concomitant mitral stenosis). Retrograde crossing of a tight aortic valve may be difficult. From the *brachial approach*, I have been successful in crossing a tight aortic valve, most often using a Sones catheter. The Cordis polyurethane

Sones catheter has high torque control and tapers to a 5.5 French tip, which can often be negotiated across a stenotic aortic valve without the aid of a guide wire. When a guide wire is required, a 0.35-inch diameter straight wire passes easily through the Sones catheter and can help in crossing the aortic valve.

With a *femoral approach,* the use of a pigtail catheter together with a straight guide wire protruded a short distance beyond the catheter tip is my standard first approach to retrograde catheterization of the left ventricle in the patient with aortic stenosis: this method is illustrated in Chapter 5, Figure 5–5. On occasion, a right or left Judkins coronary catheter used together with a straight guide wire is successful in crossing a tight aortic valve in a patient with aortic stenosis. We recently had one patient in whom all these approaches failed, but a left L-2 Amplatz catheter with straight guide wire was successfully introduced in retrograde catheterization of the left ventricle in a patient with calcific aortic stenosis and a very eccentric aortic valve orifice.

An improved catheter design for crossing stenosed aortic valves has been developed by Feldman and co-workers[14] at the University of Chicago. Using this catheter (Cook Inc., Feldman A catheter), the authors found that the median time to cross the aortic valve retrograde was 30 to 40 seconds in a group of 17 patients with a mean aortic valve area of 0.75 cm^2.

If these approaches are not successful (or are not desirable in a particular patient), a transseptal approach may be used. In some laboratories, the transseptal approach is the primary technique for patients with aortic stenosis.

3. Angiography following the guidelines just discussed.

Left ventriculography demonstrates the stenotic orifice of the valve during systole as outlined by a jet of contrast material ejected into the aorta. The valve cusps may appear irregular, their mobility may be reduced, and the number of cusps may be frequently identified. In congenital aortic stenosis, the valve often forms a funnel during systole. The ascending

aorta is dilated (poststenotic dilatation), but the subvalvular area is widely patent. A subaortic membrane, with a small central orifice, or a subvalvular muscular ring may be seen. The characteristic changes of idiopathic hypertrophic subaortic stenosis may be observed. In supravalvular stenosis, the narrowing of the proximal aorta can be seen.

Aortography also can be helpful in evaluation of the patient with aortic stenosis. In "pure" aortic stenosis (no concomitant aortic regurgitation), aortography often demonstrates a negative jet of radiolucent blood exiting focally from the left ventricle. In congenital aortic stenosis, there may be upward doming of the aortic valve leaflets which together with the central negative jet gives the so-called Prussian helmet sign (Fig. 31–8). In the patient with aortic stenosis when some aortic regurgitation is also present, aortography permits a rough quantitation of the severity of the regurgitation. If new catheter techniques (e.g., balloon valvuloplasty) are under consideration, determination of the extent of associated

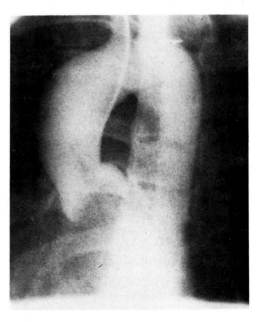

Fig. 31–8. Aortogram in a young man with congenital aortic stenosis; 45-degree LAO cine projection. Catheter positioned clear of the aortic valve. Systolic frame shows doming of the valve cusps with negative jet of blood (the Prussian helmet sign). Note also the poststenotic dilatation of the ascending aorta.

aortic regurgitation may become important in clinical decision making. Hemodynamic assessment can often detect the presence of mixed significant aortic stenosis and regurgitation, as illustrated by the patient whose pressure tracings are shown in Figure 31–9. This 78-year-old man had the unusual combination of hemodynamically significant aortic stenosis (70 mmHg gradient) *and* significant aortic regurgitation (3+, regurgitant fraction 48%).

Case 5

Aortic Stenosis Without Appreciable Cardiomegaly. L.C. was a 48-year-old married woman with a history of rheumatic fever in childhood. Six months before admission, she noted increasing exertional dyspnea and decreased effort tolerance. She had had dizziness, but no syncope or angina.

Physical examination was normal except for the heart. There was a somewhat forceful apex impulse in the midclavicular line in the fifth interspace. Rhythm was regular. S_1 and S_2 were normal. The only murmur was a grade 2 ejection type systolic murmur, maximal along the left sternal border transmitted to apex and into the carotids. No thrill was detected. The carotid pulsations exhibited a slow upstroke but were of normal amplitude.

The ECG revealed left ventricular hypertrophy and strain.

Chest radiographs showed a heart of normal overall size. There was a little rounding in the region of the left ventricle. The other cardiac chambers appeared normal, as did the lungs. At fluoroscopy there was calcification in the region of the aortic valve.

The findings at cardiac catheterization were as follows:

Body surface area, m^2	1.87
O$_2$ consumption, ml/min	225
A-V O$_2$ difference, ml/L	40
Cardiac output, L/min	5.6
Heart rate/min	70
Pressures, mmHg:	
Brachial artery	100/66
Systolic mean	84
Left ventricle	176/16
Systolic mean	140
Diastolic mean	10
Systolic ejection period, sec/beat	0.35
Pulmonary capillary wedge, mean	10
Pulmonary artery	25/11, $\overline{15}$
Right ventricle	25/5
Right atrium, mean	5
Pulmonary vascular resistance, dynes-sec-cm^{-5}	72
Calculated aortic valve area, cm^2	0.7
Ejection fraction	0.69

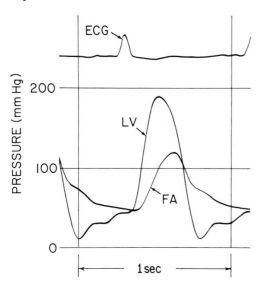

Fig. 31–9. Left ventricular (LV) and femoral artery (FA) pressure tracings in a 78-year-old man with increasing dyspnea on exertion and one episode of pulmonary edema. In this case, femoral artery and central aortic pressures were nearly superimposable. There is a 70 mmHg peak-to-peak systolic gradient, but there is also unusually rapid aortic diastolic runoff with equilibration (diastasis) of end-diastolic LV and FA pressures. This latter finding suggested significant aortic regurgitation, which was confirmed by aortography.

Cineangiography showed a vigorously contracting normal-sized left ventricle and a calcified aortic valve with three cusps. The cusps were almost immobile. A jet was seen passing through the valve which almost immediately became obscured by the radiopacity of the aorta. There was a rather discrete poststenotic dilation of the ascending aorta just above the aortic valve.

Interpretation. The moderately severe calcific aortic stenosis in this woman was probably rheumatic in origin. The left ventricle contracted well, as indicated by an ejection fraction of 0.69 and a normal cardiac output. The elevated LV end-diastolic pressure at rest was compatible with a decreased chamber distensibility from hypertrophy.

Case 6

Aortic Stenosis With Appreciable Cardiomegaly. A.H., a 77-year-old man, was well until 3 years before admission, when exertional dyspnea, orthopnea, fatigue, and peripheral edema appeared. Despite therapy, these symptoms increased progressively to the point of invalidism. He had mild angina, and had had two syncopal episodes.

On physical examination, the blood pressure was 110/80 mmHg; the pulse, 78 beats/min, and regular; respirations, 24 per minute. The carotids were of small volume with slow upstroke. Neck veins were moderately distended. There were basilar rales to the angles of the scapulae over both lungs. The PMI was in the sixth interspace 2 cm within the anterior axillary line, diffuse and forceful. There was no parasternal heave. A grade 2/6 aortic systolic ejection murmur was heard all along the left sternal border and over both carotid arteries. The liver was two fingerbreadths below the costal margin. There was slight pitting edema of both lower legs. The ECG showed left ventricular hypertrophy and strain pattern.

Chest roentgenogram showed enlargement of the left ventricle, calcification in the region of the aortic valve, moderate redistribution of vascular markings to the upper lobes of the lungs, and a small amount of pleural fluid on the right.

Cardiac catheterization yielded the following results:

Body surface area, m^2	1.76
O$_2$ consumption, ml/min	218
A-V O$_2$ difference, ml/L	81
Cardiac output, L/min	2.7

Heart rate/min	90
Pressures, mmHg	
Brachial artery	135/78
Systolic mean	100
Left ventricle	184/35
Systolic mean	140
Diastolic mean	28
Systolic ejection period, sec/beat	0.27
Pulmonary capillary wedge, mean	29
Pulmonary artery	75/40, $\overline{52}$
Right ventricle	75/12
Right atrium, mean	10
Pulmonary vascular resistance, dynes-sec-cm^{-5}	683
Calculated aortic valve area, cm^2	0.4
Ejection fraction	0.30

Left ventriculography was performed only after pretreatment with intravenous furosemide, and showed a large dilated left ventricle with uniformly poor contractions in systole. There was no mitral or aortic regurgitation. The aortic valve had two cusps that appeared ragged and were heavily calcified. There was considerable dilation of the ascending aorta. Left ventriculography was tolerated well, and coronary angiography (two injections of the left coronary artery and one injection of the right coronary artery) revealed the absence of significant coronary artery obstruction.

Interpretation. There was severe calcific aortic stenosis as indicated by a calculated valve area of 0.4 cm^2. Severe left ventricular failure was present, as indicated by left ventricular dilatation, high left ventricular mean and end-diastolic pressures, uniformly poor contraction by cineangiography, an ejection fraction of only 0.30, and a very low cardiac output. The aortic obstruction was severe, and the left ventricle was so decompensated that it generated a peak systolic pressure of only 184 mmHg (instead of 250 to 300 mmHg, as would be expected with a normal cardiac output), and the transaortic mean pressure difference was only 40 mmHg.

The pulmonary capillary wedge pressure of

29 mmHg explained the rales heard at both lung bases as well as the patient's shortness of breath. The pulmonary hypertension was due in part to the elevated left ventricular diastolic pressure (passive rise), and in part to reactive pulmonary hypertension as revealed by the finding of a pulmonary vascular resistance of 683 dynes-sec-cm^{-5}, more than five times normal.

The pressure load on the right ventricle resulted in its decompensation, as indicated by a mild elevation of the right ventricular diastolic and right atrial pressures. The clinical counterpart was slight distension of neck veins, enlarged liver, and edema.

AORTIC REGURGITATION

The dynamic effects of aortic regurgitation are caused by regurgitation of blood from aorta to left ventricle in diastole. The magnitude of the regurgitation depends on the size of the regurgitant orifice, the pressure difference between aorta and left ventricle in diastole, and the duration of diastole. The size of the regurgitant aperture may be as large as 1.0 cm^2, but regurgitation is generally severe when it is more than 0.5 cm^2. The total left ventricular stroke volume increases and equals that which supplies the body (forward flow), plus that which is regurgitated. The amount of blood regurgitated may be as much as 60% or more of the systolic discharge and usually occurs mainly in early diastole.

Hemodynamic Assessment

The large stroke volume entering the aorta with systole produces an elevated systolic pressure, whereas the regurgitation produces a lowered aortic diastolic pressure (Fig. 31–10). Left ventricular workload increases progressively with the magnitude of regurgitation. This is due not only to the raised stroke volume and to the rise of systolic pressure, but also to the high intramyocardial tension that must be developed by the dilated left ventricle to produce a given pressure (LaPlace's law). Dilatation and hypertrophy of the left ventricle

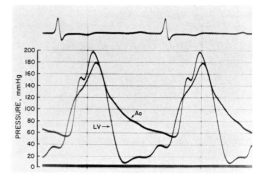

Fig. 31–10.   Left ventricular (LV) and aortic (Ao) pressure tracings in a patient with severe aortic insufficiency secondary to rheumatic heart disease. In this condition, the aortic and left ventricular pressures may equalize in late diastole, a phenomenon occasionally termed "diastasis."

are invariable consequences of aortic regurgitation. The heart may become the largest encountered in cardiac pathology—the so-called cor bovinum. Up to a point, the forward output is well maintained. The addition of blood regurgitated to the normal inflow from the left atrium increases the diastolic volume of the left ventricle, leading to a more forceful contraction (Starling's law). With time the fraction of end-diastolic volume ejected per beat (ejection fraction) becomes diminished, reflecting impaired myocardial function. Furthermore, the left ventricle may operate with an excessive end-systolic volume—another index of left ventricular dysfunction.

Premature Mitral Valve Closure. The reflux of blood into the left ventricle in diastole encounters that streaming through the mitral valve from the left atrium. The mitral valve may close prematurely because the regurgitating blood may raise the left ventricular diastolic pressure to exceed that in the left atrium. This is particularly common in acute aortic regurgitation, in which the sudden onset of severe regurgitation into a normal-sized left ventricle leads to striking elevations in LV diastolic pressure (Fig. 31–11). In the case illustrated in Figure 31–11, LVEDP approaches 50 mmHg, and LV diastolic pressure exceeds left atrial (or wedge) pressure for nearly half of diastole. This reversal of pressures is as-

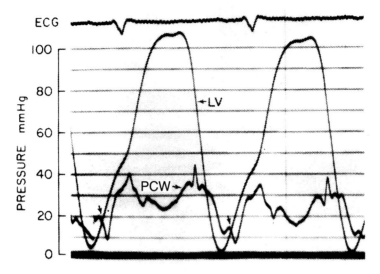

Fig. 31–11. Left ventricular (LV) and pulmonary capillary wedge (PCW) pressures in a patient with acute aortic regurgitation due to infective endocarditis. Note the unusual wave form of the LV pressure with its striking late diastolic rise, loss of clear A wave, and high elevation of LVEDP (approximately 45 to 50 mmHg). LV diastolic pressure rises in late diastole to exceed left atrial and pulmonary wedge pressures (arrow), forcing premature closure of the mitral valve. (From Mann T et al: Assessing the hemodynamic severity of acute aortic regurgitation due to infective endocarditis. N Engl J Med 293:108, 1975.)

sociated with premature mitral valve closure, which may be seen on the echocardiogram.

Another example of premature closure of the mitral valve in association with severe aortic regurgitation is shown in Figure 31–12.

These tracings were recorded during cardiac catheterization of a 71-year-old man who had previously had aortic valve replacement for aortic stenosis. After doing extremely well for more than 5 years, he suddenly developed

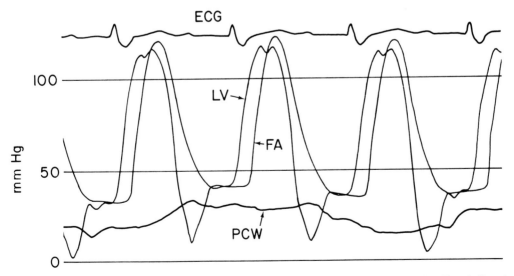

Fig. 31–12. Severe aortic regurgitation developing in a 71-year-old man with a prosthetic aortic valve. There is diastasis between left ventricle (LV) and aorta. Also, LV diastolic pressure exceeds pulmonary capillary wedge (PCW) pressure early in diastole. Femoral artery = FA. See text for details.

marked shortness of breath and a new murmur of aortic regurgitation. Pressure recordings show that left ventricular diastolic pressure exceeds left atrial (pulmonary capillary wedge pressure) by the end of the first third of the diastolic filling period. Also, complete diastasis of aortic and left ventricular pressures occurs by mid-diastole, at which point aortic regurgitation ceases because there is no longer any gradient driving the regurgitant flow. As expected, this patient's diastolic murmur was blowing in quality, decrescendo, and ended by mid-diastole.

Acute vs Chronic Aortic Regurgitation. The typical hemodynamic findings in acute vs chronic aortic regurgitation have been reported by Mann et al,[15] and are presented in Table 31–2. As can be seen, widened pulse pressure is characteristic only of chronic aortic regurgitation, reflecting both the enormous stroke volume associated with this condition, and the tachycardia commonly seen in patients with acute aortic regurgitation. This may give rise to a situation where there exists a high *end*-diastolic pressure in the noncompliant left ventricle in the presence of little if any elevation of the mean pressure in the left atrium. With

time and with the severity of the leak, the *mean* diastolic pressure of the ventricle rises, and when this happens, left atrial and pulmonary capillary wedge pressure rise.

Another hemodynamic finding in aortic regurgitation is the amplification of peak systolic pressure in peripheral arteries (especially the femoral and popliteal), so that peak systolic femoral artery pressure may exceed central aortic pressure by 20 to 50 mmHg. This is essentially an exaggeration of a normal phenomenon (see Chapter 9), but emphasizes the importance of central aortic pressure measurement in aortic regurgitation.

Angiographic Assessment

Aortic cineangiography yields a graphic demonstration of the severity and dynamics of the regurgitation. Qualitative assessment is subjective, as for mitral regurgitation. We use a scale of 1 + to 4 +, employing the following definitions to aid discrimination of these four degrees of regurgitation. In 1 + regurgitation (mild), a small amount of contrast material enters the left ventricle in diastole; it is essentially cleared with each beat and never fills the

Table 31–2. *Comparison of Hemodynamic and Angiographic Findings in Acute and Chronic Aortic Regurgitation*

	Acute AR	Chronic AR	P Value
Age (years)	33 ± 14	40 ± 15	NS
Regurgitant fraction	0.6 ± 0.1	0.7 ± 0.1	NS
LVEDP (mmHg)	41 ± 12	36 ± 13	NS
Ejection fraction	0.6 ± 0.1	0.6 ± 0.1	NS
Heart rate (beats/min)	108 ± 15	71 ± 14	<0.01
LV volumes (ml/m²)			
EDV	146 ± 28	264 ± 64	<0.01
ESV	57 ± 23	101 ± 42	<0.02
TSV	89 ± 22	163 ± 57	<0.01
Aortic pressure (mmHg):			
Systolic	110 ± 14	155 ± 26	<0.01
Diastolic	56 ± 11	50 ± 6	NS
Mean	78 ± 12	90 ± 8	<0.02
Pulse pressure (mmHg)	55 ± 7	105 ± 22	<0.01
Systemic Vascular Resistance			
(dynes-sec-cm⁻⁵)	1326 ± 372	1341 ± 461	NS

Mean $\pm$ SD; EDV, ESV and TSV are LV end-diastolic, end-systolic and total stroke volumes; AR, aortic regurgitation; LVEDP, left ventricular end-diastolic pressure. (Modified from Mann JT et al: Assessing the hemodynamic severity of acute aortic regurgitation due to infective endocarditis. N Engl J Med 293:108, 1975.)

ventricular chamber. More contrast material enters with each diastole in 2+ (moderate) regurgitation, and faint opacification of the entire chamber occurs. With moderately severe (3+) regurgitation, the LV chamber is well opacified, and equal in density with the ascending aorta. Severe (4+) aortic regurgitation is characterized by complete, dense opacification of the LV chamber on the first beat, and there is the appearance that the left ventricle is more densely opacified than the ascending aorta.

Quantitative assessment of aortic regurgitation involves calculation of the regurgitant fraction (RF), as described in Chapter 19. The same scale of interpretation holds as for mitral regurgitation with RF <20% corresponding to mild regurgitation; 20% to 40%, moderate; 40% to 60%, moderately severe; and >60%, severe aortic regurgitation.

Part of the angiographic assessment of aortic regurgitation involves assessment of the aortic valve leaflets (mobility, calcification, number of cusps), the ascending aorta (extent and type of dilatation), and possible associated abnormalities (e.g., coronary lesions, sinus of Valsalva aneurysm, dissecting aneurysm of the aorta, and ventricular septal defect). All these aspects are best evaluated in the LAO view.

Catheterization Protocol

1. Right heart catheterization for measurement of right heart pressures and cardiac output.

2. Left heart catheterization for measurement of central aortic pulse pressure, LVEDP, detection of transvalvular gradients (if any), of diastasis between LV and aorta, if this is present (Fig. 31–12), and of relative height of LVEDP compared to PCW or LA mean pressure.

3. Angiography, including left ventriculography, aortography, and possibly coronary angiography (if indicated clinically).

4. If resting hemodynamics are normal, consider stress intervention, such as dynamic exercise.

TRICUSPID REGURGITATION

Tricuspid regurgitation can be functional or organic. Functional tricuspid regurgitation is thought to be due to right ventricular dilatation and failure as a result of excessive right ventricular afterload. Most commonly, this is caused by pulmonary hypertension from mitral stenosis, left ventricular failure, cor pulmonale, or pulmonary embolism.

''Organic'' tricuspid regurgitation implies disease of the tricuspid valve or its supporting apparatus, and is most commonly seen with rheumatic heart disease, bacterial endocarditis, or right ventricular infarction.

Hemodynamic Assessment

In tricuspid regurgitation, either organic or functional, the primary hemodynamic finding is a large systolic wave in the right atrial pressure tracing. Tracings of jugular venous pulsations have distinguished A, C, and V waves in the normal subject; in the patient with moderate tricuspid regurgitation there is a fourth pulsation, the S wave. This systolic wave pre-

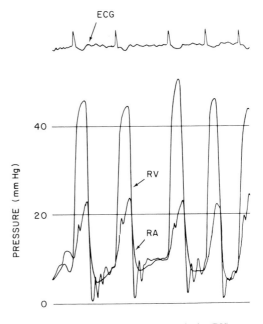

Fig. 31–13. Right atrial (RA) and ventricular (RV) pressures in a 75-year-old woman with rheumatic heart disease. There is severe organic tricuspid regurgitation with RA waveform resembling RV pressure.

cedes and blends with the normal ventricular filling (V) wave, and in severe tricuspid regurgitation, the S and V waves form a single regurgitant systolic wave (Fig. 31–13). As can be seen in Figure 31–13, the right atrial pressure tracing in severe tricuspid regurgitation resembles the right ventricular pressure tracing. In the most extreme cases, the pressure tracings are virtually superimposable, which is to be expected because the right atrium and ventricle are physiologically a common chamber in such cases.

The hemodynamic distinction between organic and functional tricuspid regurgitation is difficult. Generally, if the patient with severe tricuspid regurgitation has a right ventricular systolic pressure greater than 60 mmHg, the tricuspid regurgitation is functional, whereas if the right ventricular systolic pressure is ≤40 mmHg, there is a substantial organic component. This distinction is of practical importance in terms of surgical correction because functional tricuspid regurgitation will improve substantially solely with correction of the right ventricular hypertension (e.g., following corrective surgery for mitral stenosis), whereas the patient with major organic tricuspid regurgitation may not survive cardiac surgery unless the operation includes tricuspid valve replacement or tricuspid annuloplasty.

Angiographic Assessment

The angiographic demonstration of tricuspid regurgitation is generally accomplished by right ventricular cineangiography in the RAO projection, as discussed in Chapter 14. Some artificial tricuspid regurgitation is seen because of the presence of the catheter across the tricuspid valve, but this is usually minor. It is important to choose a catheter type, position, and injection rate that will avoid extrasystoles because a run of ventricular tachycardia makes it impossible to evaluate the degree of tricuspid regurgitation; these considerations are discussed in Chapter 14. We like the Grollman, pigtail or Eppendorf catheters situated in mid-RV or RV outflow tract, with injection rates of 12 to 18 ml/sec depending on RV size and

irritability. A scale of 1+ to 4+ is used to grade the severity of tricuspid regurgitation, using criteria of definition similar to those described for mitral regurgitation. In some circumstances, a right atrial cineangiogram in RAO projection can be used for assessment of tricuspid regurgitation; in this instance, a negative jet (unopacified blood) from RV to RA shows the regurgitation. A catheter technique for assessing tricuspid regurgitation using a specially shaped no. 7 NIH catheter has been described with excellent results in a series of 60 patients.[16]

Cardiac catheterization protocol depends upon the associated conditions.

TRICUSPID STENOSIS

Previously, this rare condition was seen only in patients with rheumatic heart disease and mitral stenosis. Today, however, stenosis of a prosthetic tricuspid valve (placed originally as treatment for tricuspid regurgitation) accounts for the majority of the cases seen in most major medical centers. The clinical diagnosis may be difficult, especially if the patient is in atrial fibrillation. Diagnosis is aided by the characteristic finding of an increased jugular venous pressure with blunting or absence of the Y descent. One patient seen by the author had severe stenosis of her native mitral, aortic, and tricuspid valves. This was a 43-year-old woman with a history of repeated bouts of rheumatic fever in childhood, whose major complaint was fatigue and "blackouts."

Hemodynamic Assessment

The sine qua non of tricuspid stenosis is a pandiastolic gradient across the tricuspid valve. The gradient is usually small (4 to 8 mmHg) and may be missed unless a careful assessment is made. Two catheters (or a single catheter with double lumen) and simultaneous measurement of RA and RV pressures should be used if there is any doubt about the presence of this condition. A careful RV to RA pullback using a standard catheter, however, will serve to confirm or eliminate this diagnosis with reliability in most cases. The tricuspid valve area is calculated using the formula given in Chapter 11. Tricuspid stenosis is usually of clinical and hemodynamic significance when the tricuspid valve area is <1.3 cm².

Angiographic Assessment

The valve is usually calcified and shows decreased mobility. There may be associated right atrial dilatation and some tricuspid regurgitation.

Cardiac catheterization protocol depends on associated lesions.

PULMONIC STENOSIS AND REGURGITATION

Pulmonic stenosis is essentially a congenital condition. Pulmonic regurgitation is usually functional and a consequence of severe pulmonary hypertension. When the pulmonary artery pressure exceeds 100 mmHg systolic, there is usually some pulmonic regurgitation. This may lead to widening of the pulmonary artery pulse pressure and an increase in RVEDP. Angiographic assessment of pulmonic regurgitation is difficult because the angiographic catheter lying across the pulmonic valve may cause artifactual regurgitation. Cineangiography in RAO or LAO projection with contrast injection at 20 to 25 ml/sec into the main pulmonary artery will demonstrate the pulmonic valve and allow some assessment of regurgitation.

Cardiac catheterization protocol depends on associated conditions.

RELATIVE STENOSIS OF PROSTHETIC VALVES

An unusual case of *relative* tricuspid stenosis, mitral stenosis, and aortic stenosis in a 60-year-old man is shown in Figure 31–14 and illustrates an important point concerning function of prosthetic cardiac valves. This man had mitral valve replacement with a Harken disc valve in 1969 for rheumatic mitral regurgitation. He then did well until 1980, when he presented with left and right heart failure and was found at cardiac catheterization to have severe aortic and tricuspid regurgitation, but normal function of the mitral prosthetic valve. Aortic valve replacement (Starr-Edwards prosthesis) and tricuspid valve replacement (porcine prosthesis) led to improvement, but over the following years he required large amounts of diuretic therapy to remain free of edema and pulmonary congestion. Echocardiographic assessment of his prosthetic valves demonstrated apparently normal function, and left ventricular contraction was vigorous.

Because of persistent left and right heart failure, cardiac catheterization was undertaken in 1985. The porcine tricuspid valve was crossed antegrade with a Swan-Ganz catheter, and the Starr-Edwards aortic prosthesis was crossed retrograde with a Sones catheter to obtain the pressure measurements shown in Figure 31–14. As can be seen, significant pressure gradients were present across tricuspid, mitral, and aortic prostheses. A surprising finding, however, was an elevated cardiac output, measured by both Fick and thermodilution methods. Oxygen consumption index was 148 ml/min/M² and arteriovenous oxygen difference was 29 ml O₂/L giving a Fick cardiac index of 5 L/min/M² and a cardiac output of 10 L/min. Using the Gorlin formula (Chapter 11), calculated aortic valve area was 1.3 cm², mitral valve was 1.6 cm², and tricuspid valve area was 2.4 cm²: these values were all consistent with the known effective orifice areas of the particular prosthetic valves implanted, and did not signify prosthetic valve dysfunction or stenosis. Thus, a *high cardiac output state* caused substantial pressure gradients to occur across the patient's three prosthetic valves, resulting in the clinical picture of biventricular failure. Thyroid function tests were normal and a search for other causes of high output state (e.g., arteriovenous fistula, Paget's disease) was unrevealing. This patient responded nicely to thiamine supplementation, beta blockade, and diuretic therapy with spironolactone and furosemide: evidence of high output state receded and a vigorous diuresis ensued.

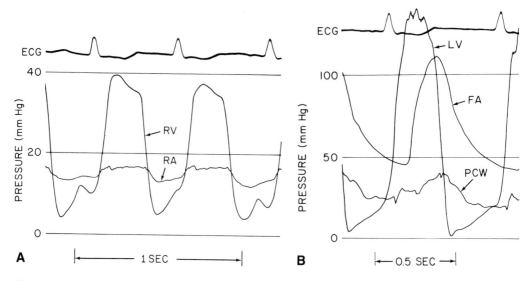

Fig. 31–14.   Pressure tracings in a 60-year-old man with high cardiac output and significant pressure gradients across normally functioning tricuspid, mitral, and aortic valve prostheses. (A) From the right ventricle (RV) and right atrium (RA). (B) From the left ventricle (LV), femoral artery (FA), and pulmonary capillary wedge position (PCW).

Catheter Passage Across Prosthetic Valves

As illustrated in the case just described, it has become routine to cross prosthetic valves with catheters in an attempt to assess their function or the function of other valves. Published reports have documented the safety of this procedure in a large number of patients[17,18] with a variety of prosthetic valves. Based on my own experience and anecdotal experience reported to me by many others, I offer the following guidelines.

First, porcine valves may be crossed retrograde or antegrade safely with a variety of catheters. For retrograde crossing of a *porcine prosthetic valve* in the aortic position, a pigtail catheter is generally my first approach. The pigtail catheter tip is rested on top of the valve's leaflets as they protrude into the aorta high above the sewing ring and is gently advanced until it prolapses into the left ventricular chamber. Antegrade crossing of a *porcine tricuspid prosthesis* is accomplished easily using a balloon-flotation catheter, as described in the preceding section. Retrograde crossing of a *ball valve* (e.g., Starr-Edwards) prosthesis in the aortic position may be accomplished easily using a 7F or 8F Sones catheter with or without guide wire assistance. The pigtail catheter also may be advanced into the left ventricle over a guide wire across a ball valve prosthesis, but the wire should be reinserted for catheter withdrawal, to avoid hooking the pigtail on the metal cage. Although some operators have crossed *low profile disc-valve prostheses* (e.g., Bjork-Shiley valve) retrograde without complications, instances where catheter entrapment occurred with retrograde crossing of such valves have been reported.[19] Also, Dr. Viking Bjork has specifically stated that the Bjork-Shiley valve must not be crossed retrograde, based on his own large experience. When restudy has been required in his patients, a transseptal approach has been used. Accordingly, it is our practice never to attempt to cross a Bjork-Shiley valve or any low profile disc valve prosthesis retrograde.

REFERENCES

1. Lewis BM et al: Clinical and physiological correlations in patients with mitral stenosis. Am Heart J 43:2, 1952.
2. Erny RE et al: Hemodynamic results and follow-up of patients with iatrogenic atrial septal defects following balloon mitral valvuloplasty. J Am Coll Cardiol 13:70A, 1989.

3. Braunwald E: Mitral regurgitation. Physiologic, clinical and surgical considerations. N Engl J Med 281:425, 1969.

4. Braunwald E, Welch GH Jr, Morrow AG: The effects of acutely increased systemic resistance on the left atrial pressure pulse: A method for the clinical detection of mitral insufficiency. J Clin Invest 37:35, 1958.

5. Brody W, Criley JM: Intermittent severe mitral regurgitation. Hemodynamic studies in a patient with recurrent acute left-sided heart failure. N Engl J Med 183:673, 1970.

6. Baxley WA, Kennedy JW, Feild B, Dodge HT: Hemodynamics in ruptured chordae tendineae and chronic rheumatic mitral regurgitation. Circulation 48:1288, 1973.

7. Pichard AD et al: Large V waves in the pulmonary wedge pressure tracing in the absence of mitral regurgitation. Am J Cardiol 50:1044, 1982.

8. Grose R, Strain J, Cohen MV: Pulmonary arterial V waves in mitral regurgitation: Clinical and experimental observations. Circulation 69:214, 1984.

9. Fuchs RM, Heuser RP, Yin FCP, Brinker JA: Limitations of pulmonary wedge V waves in diagnosing mitral regurgitation. Am J Cardiol 49:849, 1982.

10. Harshaw CW, Munro AB, McLaurin LP, Grossman W: Reduced systemic vascular resistance as therapy for severe mitral regurgitation of valvular origin. Ann Intern Med 83:312, 1975.

11. Grossman W et al: Lowered aortic impedance as therapy for severe mitral regurgitation. JAMA 230:1011, 1974.

12. Croft CH et al: Limitations of qualitative angiographic grading in aortic or mitral regurgitation. Am J Cardiol 53:1593, 1984.

13. Carabello BA, Barry WH, Grossman W: Changes in arterial pressure during left heart pullback in patients with aortic stenosis: a sign of severe aortic stenosis. Am J Cardiol 44:424, 1979.

14. Feldman T, Carroll JD, Chin YC: An improved catheter design for crossing stenosed aortic valves. Cath Cardiovasc Diagn 16:279, 1989.

15. Mann T, McLaurin LP, Grossman W, Craige E: Assessing the hemodynamic severity of acute aortic regurgitation due to infective endocarditis. N Engl J Med 293:108, 1975.

16. Lingamneni R et al: Tricuspid regurgitation: clinical and angiographic assessment. Cath Cardiovasc Diag 5:7, 1979.

17. Kosinski EJ, Cohn PF, Grossman W, Cohn LH: Severe stenosis occurring in antibiotic sterilised homograft valves. Br Heart J 40:194, 1978.

18. Rigaud M et al: Retrograde catheterization of left ventricle through mechanical aortic prostheses. Eur Heart J 8:689, 1987.

19. Kober G, Hilgermann R: Catheter entrapment in a Bjork-Shiley prosthesis in aortic position. Cathet Cardiovasc Diagn 13:262, 1987.

32

Profiles in Coronary Artery Disease

RICHARD C. PASTERNAK and GREGG J. REIS

Coronary angiography, left ventriculography, and hemodynamic measurements are integral to the evaluation of many patients with suspected or known coronary artery disease. In addition to the diagnostic value of these studies, they are useful for prognostic purposes and for planning therapeutic interventions such as coronary artery bypass surgery. Coronary angiography is also performed in association with newer forms of therapy, such as percutaneous transluminal coronary angioplasty (PTCA) and thrombolysis, thus expanding cardiac catheterization beyond its role as a diagnostic procedure into the realm of therapeutics. The evaluation of ventricular function by angiography and the measurement of hemodynamics allow assessment of possible mechanical compromise caused by coronary artery disease. Additionally, the effect of pharmacologic or mechanical therapies can be determined accurately, and therapeutic strategies may be adjusted based on the results of these studies.

Coronary angiography itself remains the most definitive way to make the diagnosis of coronary artery disease. Although often the diagnosis of coronary artery disease can be made from the history or by noninvasive techniques, angiography may be necessary for diagnostic purposes in patients with recurrent chest pain and atypical features of coronary disease. Important prognostic information can be obtained by defining the coronary anatomy.

Although the most simple prognostic system is based on the number of coronary vessels diseased, more complex systems have been proposed. However, none is so widely used as the "one-, two-, or three vessel disease" categorization. A more accurate determination of prognosis may be made by combining information about ventricular function and various other clinical factors with coronary pathoanatomy. Definition of the coronary anatomy is an absolute necessity before coronary artery bypass surgery, and it is an integral part of percutaneous transluminal coronary interventions. Additionally, in selected patients, the diagnosis of coronary artery spasm can be made by provocative testing with ergonovine.

Left ventriculography is useful for defining prognosis in patients with coronary artery disease. For prediction of survival, analysis of left ventricular function, as determined from a left ventricular cineangiogram, is probably more useful than the definition of the number of diseased coronary vessels.[1] The determination of baseline left ventricular function also affects the choice of therapeutic approaches, both mechanical and pharmacologic. Ventriculography is useful for the detection of complications of coronary artery disease such as mitral regurgitation or ventricular aneurysm. Finally, left ventriculography may be important in defining the relationship between coronary pathoanatomy and electrocardiographic evidence of myocardial infarction. For example, a total coronary artery occlusion may occur in the absence of any myocardial damage, leaving a patient with normal left ventricular function (and a normal electrocardiogram) as long as the portion of heart muscle initially supplied by the occluded artery is adequately supplied by collaterals. Conversely, only minimal narrowing of a coronary artery may be present following an acute myocardial infarction if recanalization of a coronary artery thrombus or relaxation of prolonged coronary spasm has occurred. In such patients, extensive myocardial dysfunction may be demonstrated by left ventriculography, and the electrocardiogram may show Q waves indicative of transmural infarction, in spite of the absence of a critical coronary artery stenosis.

Hemodynamic measurements may aid in the evaluation of abnormalities caused by coronary artery disease. Assessment of the presence and degree of systolic and diastolic dysfunction may be important in devising a medical program that involves choosing from a wide variety of drugs with different pharmacologic actions. As has already been discussed in detail (Chapter 18), pacing may be combined with hemodynamic studies, lactate measurements, thallium scintigraphy, and even contrast echocardiography in the evaluation of certain patients with coronary disease. Such studies are particularly useful when noninvasive testing has failed to lead to clear diagnostic conclusions or the effect of a particular therapy needs to be assessed relatively rapidly.

To illustrate these points, several cases across the spectrum of coronary artery disease will be described. The cases are representative profiles of patients referred to the Cardiac Catheterization Laboratory for evaluation or management. Before the discussion of cases, a brief review of catheterization procedures for patients with ischemic heart disease is presented.

CATHETERIZATION PROTOCOL

For patients with suspected or known coronary artery disease, the catheterization pro-

cedure itself is generally standardized regardless of the exact indications for the study. In many laboratories, combined right and left heart procedures are performed on most patients. Right heart catheterization is undertaken both to assess the hemodynamics and to provide access to the central circulation for diagnostic and therapeutic pharmacologic maneuvers. We generally perform right-sided catheterization using a balloon-tipped, flow-guided catheter inserted by way of a brachial vein or through a sheath in the femoral vein. If the measurements of right heart hemodynamics and saturations are deemed unnecessary, access to the central circulation should still be provided through a well-secured, large-bore venous cannula. Left-heart catheterization is performed by either the brachial or femoral techniques as outlined in previous chapters. Patients undergoing complete cardiac catheterization usually have the study undertaken in the following sequence:

1. The right heart catheter is inserted and right atrial, right ventricular, and pulmonary arterial pressures are measured. Superior vena cava and pulmonary arterial saturations are determined. The balloon of the flow-directed catheter is then inflated, and pulmonary capillary wedge pressure is measured. The mean wedge pressure is recorded, as well as the height of the A wave and V wave, and the balloon is then deflated.

2. Left heart catheterization is then performed, and measurements of central aortic, left ventricular systolic, and end diastolic pressures are made.

3. Cardiac output is determined by either the Fick method (during measurement or estimation of oxygen consumption) or the thermodilution technique (see Chapter 8).

4. Contrast left ventriculography is undertaken with careful attention to segmental wall motion, inclusion of the entire ventricular silhouette for calculation of ejection fraction, and attention to the left atrium for detection of the presence of mitral regurgitation (see Chapter 14).

5. Selective cineangiography of the coronary arteries is then undertaken. Angiograms

are filmed in multiple projections. When stenoses are noted, views providing a minimum of vessel overlap are performed to optimally outline lesions (see Chapter 13).

6. Further interventions such as atrial pacing or ergonovine testing are performed in some patients, following the routine diagnostic procedures.

Although the above procedures are usually followed in sequence for routine diagnostic cases, modification of this sequence or the procedures is appropriate in certain circumstances, particularly when the patient is critically ill. In the latter instance, the procedure is often tailored to allow obtaining the most *important* information first. For example, in a patient with refractory unstable angina in whom left main coronary artery stenosis is suspected, angiography of the left coronary artery system may be performed before left ventriculography or right coronary artery cineangiography. In occasional patients, left ventriculography is omitted, such as when severe renal disease exists (meriting a minimum use of contrast agent) or when severe ventricular dysfunction is present and the risk of further hemodynamic compromise is greater than the need to obtain angiographic information. In the latter case, information from a two-dimensional echocardiogram or radionuclide ventriculogram can often be substituted for left ventricular cineangiography.

CASE STUDIES

Atypical Chest Pain—Normal Coronary Arteries

Registry data from the Society of Cardiac Angiography indicate that the frequency of finding normal coronary arteries at cardiac catheterization is about 20% with an additional 7% of patients having minimal disease.[2] These rates, however, vary considerably in different laboratories. This variability undoubtedly reflects differing referral practices, and the extent to which noninvasive testing is utilized prior to cardiac catheterization. While assessment of the relative risk/benefit ratio is always

necessary when one considers the use of an invasive test, there are situations when cardiac catheterization is appropriate for patients with atypical symptoms and a low risk of coronary artery disease, even after careful noninvasive screening.

Patients with recurrent chest pain not typical for classic angina pectoris may occasionally present a difficult problem even for the most experienced clinician. Studies of patients found to have normal coronary arteries at cardiac catheterization, many of whom have atypical chest pain, have failed to provide a unifying pathophysiologic explanation for this problematic syndrome.[3] Individual causes or relationships that have been identified include: mitral valve prolapse, costochondritis, esophageal spasm, epicardial coronary artery spasm, abnormally reduced coronary vasodilator reserve, cardiomyopathy (of various types), and occult atherosclerotic coronary disease (i.e., undetectable by conventional angiography). An extremely good prognosis has been noted in patients with either classic angina or atypical chest pain who are found to have angiographically normal or near normal coronary arteries.[3] Thus, the performance of coronary angiography to place such a patient in this favorable prognostic group may become necessary for either clinical or professional (such as for airline pilots) reasons. The following case demonstrates some of these issues and findings in one such patient.

Case 1. A 42-year-old woman with a family history of coronary artery disease has had chest pain for 3 years. She had experienced similar pain 30 years earlier, but was then symptom-free until the pain recurred intermittently over the course of the last 3 years. Her pain occurred both at rest and with exertion, and at times it was relieved by nitroglycerin. She has never experienced syncope and does not complain of dyspnea on exertion, but has noted that palpitations occur during periods when the chest pain is more frequent. On three separate occasions she has been hospitalized following prolonged episodes of chest pain. On each admission a myocardial infarction was ruled out. Physical examination was entirely normal with the exception of an early systolic click. Resting ECG shows T wave inversions in the inferior leads. Exercise stress testing reveals fluctuating T wave changes with hyperventilation, but no significant ST segment deviation is seen with maximal exercise. A two-dimensional echocardiogram demonstrated moderate prolapse of both the anterior and posterior mitral valve leaflets. A Doppler echocardiogram did not show mitral regurgitation.

At cardiac catheterization, hemodynamic measurements and cardiac output were normal. Left ventriculography revealed normal motion of all walls with a calculated ejection fraction of 0.62. Prolapse of the posterior mitral leaflet was demonstrated on the ventriculogram (Fig. 32–1). No mitral regurgitation was seen. Coronary arteriograms were normal. Ergonovine testing failed to produce chest pain, ECG changes, or angiographic evidence of coronary artery spasm. Impression: Mitral valve prolapse and normal coronary arteries.

Illustrative Points. The appropriate approach to most patients with mitral valve prolapse is one of reassurance and beta blocker therapy to control both the symptoms of palpitations (which may be caused by either su-

praventricular tachyarrhythmias or ventricular arrhythmias) and chest pain.

It is occasionally necessary to undertake cardiac catheterization to rule out coronary artery disease, even in patients with a low probability of that diagnosis. This case demonstrates the potential difficulty faced in managing some patients with chest pain. If the chest pain is in part characteristic of myocardial ischemia, if noninvasive testing is equivocal, and particularly if certain risk factors are present, the physician may be confronted with the potential for recurrent hospital admissions to rule out myocardial infarction. Although cardiac catheterization is probably not appropriate after the first such admission, invasive testing may become necessary before the decision can be made *not* to hospitalize such a patient each time chest pain occurs. In this case, the demonstration of normal coronary arteries allows the clinician to safely and confidently provide the necessary reassurance when confronted with an anxious and uncomfortable patient complaining of chest pain.

The diagnosis of mitral valve prolapse is usually made easily, without left ventriculography. In this case both the physical examination, which demonstrated a systolic click,

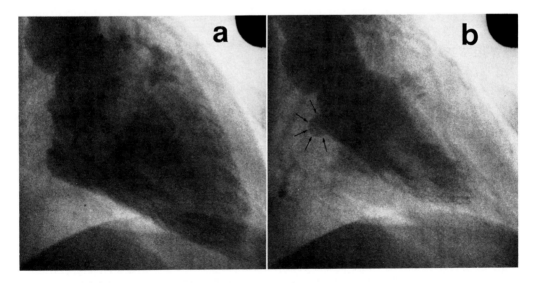

Fig. 32–1. Diastolic (a) and systolic (b) frames of a right anterior oblique left ventriculogram in a 42-year-old woman with chest pain (Case 1). Left ventricular contraction pattern is normal. Note prolapse (leftward bulging) of the posterior leaflet of the mitral valve (arrows, b) during systole.

and the echocardiogram were consistent with mitral valve prolapse. While the echocardiogram is probably the most sensitive diagnostic technique for demonstrating this abnormality, occasionally evidence of mitral valve prolapse may be found only by physical examination or left ventricular cineangiography. Mitral leaflet prolapse, as demonstrated in this case, is most commonly caused by myxomatous degeneration of the mitral valve apparatus. Papillary muscle dysfunction, caused by either myocardial ischemia or infarction, is another frequent cause of mitral valve prolapse.[4] These papillary muscle abnormalities are usually caused by coronary artery disease and most often occur in the context of more widespread evidence of myocardial dysfunction. Abnormal coronary vasodilator reserve (Chap. 13) may be responsible for chest pain in some patients with apparently normal coronary arteries.

Whether or not mitral valve prolapse is present, patients with chest pain and normal coronary arteries have a uniformly good prognosis for both survival and absence of cardiac events. As noted above, no single unifying diagnosis is responsible for pain in most patients with this syndrome. Occasionally, as in the case above, a specific diagnosis can be made which leads to useful therapy.

Variant Angina—Coronary Artery Spasm

The smooth muscle of epicardial coronary arteries is capable of producing a wide range of coronary arterial narrowing, including total occlusion. Coronary artery spasm may occur in the presence or absence of fixed atherosclerotic disease. *Variant angina* occurs when there is transient complete occlusion of a coronary artery causing chest pain and ST-segment elevation in the ECG leads that most closely monitor the area of myocardium that has become ischemic (e.g., inferior ECG leads to right coronary artery spasm or precordial leads for left anterior descending coronary artery spasm). In 1959, Prinzmetal suggested that the association of these ECG changes with reversible ischemic chest pain occurring at rest

was secondary to changes in coronary artery "tonus."[5] Since that time, angiographic demonstration of this phenomenon has been commonly observed, and the terms *Prinzmetal's angina* and *variant angina* have become almost synonymous with coronary artery spasm.

Epicardial coronary artery spasm may occur spontaneously in the course of cardiac catheterization and may be demonstrated by coronary cineangiography. Minor changes in diameter may occur even in normal coronary arteries; such changes are often not apparent subjectively and require specialized techniques for demonstration. Spasm can cause total occlusion of a previously normal or narrowed segment. This phenomenon occurs most frequently in patients with the clinical syndrome of variant angina. An exception to this rule, however, is local spasm occurring at the tip of a coronary catheter. Although such catheter-induced spasm is seen most often at the ostium of the right coronary artery, it may occur at either coronary artery, and with any angiographic catheter. As discussed in Chapter 13, various vasoconstrictor stimuli (e.g., ergonovine maleate) can be used as a diagnostic provocation for coronary artery spasm in patients with suspected variant angina. While normal coronary arteries respond to this pharmacologic stimulus by modest diffuse narrowing, patients with variant angina appear to be particularly sensitive and frequently respond with focal spasm totally occluding the coronary artery. This spasm often occurs at a site of fixed atherosclerotic narrowing which, before spasm, may have been mild, moderate, or severe.

Sudden coronary artery occlusion caused by epicardial coronary artery spasm not only induces chest pain and ECG changes but also is responsible for abnormalities that may be detected by scintigraphic techniques and ventriculography. Thallium scanning during an episode of variant angina shows a perfusion defect in the myocardium supplied by the coronary artery with spasm. Coincident with the onset of ischemia, hemodynamic abnormalities may be detected. Appearing first is evidence of diastolic dysfunction, with an increase in left ventricular end diastolic pressure caused by impaired relaxation of the ischemic segment. During systole, akinesia or even bulging of the ischemic segment may be demonstrated by left ventriculography or echocardiography. If a papillary muscle becomes ischemic as part of this process, transient mitral regurgitation may occur with abnormally tall V waves seen in the pulmonary capillary wedge tracing.

Cardiac catheterization may be unnecessary in some cases of variant angina. This is particularly true when episodes of ischemic pain occur *only* at rest, and the problem responds easily to medical therapy with calcium channel blockers or nitrates. The following case demonstrates a more difficult problem where the diagnosis was obscure and difficulty was encountered with conventional therapy.

Case 2. Intermittently over the past 6 months a 36-year-old woman has had substernal chest pressure that radiates to her left shoulder and back. The discomfort typically occurs with exertion or emotional stress but also has occurred at rest and on occasion has awoken her from sleep. In addition, she has had episodes of epigastric discomfort associated with nausea and dizziness. After a brief syncopal episode she was taken to a local emergency room, where the physical examination and ECG were entirely normal. She was free of symptoms in the emergency room and was sent home, but because of concern about these episodes, an exercise stress test was scheduled. Two weeks later she underwent a graded exercise treadmill test. After 8 minutes of exercise, she experienced precordial substernal chest pressure. Coincident with the onset of this symptom, she developed ST-segment elevation in ECG leads V2 through V4. Exercise was terminated, and she was given one sublingual nitroglycerin. Early during the recovery period a five-beat run of ventricular tachycardia was seen. She was given a second sublingual nitroglycerin, and the pain resolved completely after 6 minutes. When she was pain-free, her electrocardiogram showed T inversions in the same precordial leads that had shown ST-segment elevation minutes earlier.

She was admitted to the hospital to rule out a myocardial infarction. At the time of admission, her physical examination was normal, as was her chest roentgenogram. By the second hospital day, her electrocardiogram was normal as well. Cardiac enzymes were normal. Continuous single-lead bedside monitoring of cardiac rhythm showed no further ventricular ectopy, but fluctuating T wave changes were seen. On the second hospital day, she was placed on diltiazem, 60 mg tid.

Because of her young age and because of electrocardiographic evidence of severe ischemia with exercise, she was referred for cardiac catheterization. Diltiazem was discontinued 36 hours before catheterization. All hemodynamic measurements at rest were within normal limits. Left ventriculography revealed normal left ventricular function with synchronous contraction of all left ventricular walls. Coronary angiography showed a normal right coronary artery (Fig. 32–2a), a normal left circumflex coronary artery, and a minor stenosis of the left anterior descending coronary artery (Fig. 32–2b). She was given 0.05 mg of ergonovine maleate intravenously. Ninety seconds later she noted the onset of both precordial chest discomfort and nausea. The ECG monitor (modified lead V1) showed ST-segment elevation where none had been present previously. Coronary angiography of her right coronary artery now revealed a tapering stenosis (approximately 70%) (Fig. 32–2c). Following injection of contrast medium into the right coronary artery, contrast agent was injected into the left system. This revealed subtotal occlusion of the left anterior descending artery (Fig. 32–2d).

The coronary catheter was passed retrograde into the left ventricle; LVEDP has now risen from 8 to 22 mmHg. Intravenous nitroglycerin (100 μg) was administered immediately after the recognition of provoked coronary artery spasm. Little change was observed in the patient's symptoms, and two minutes later complete heart block developed with a slow ventricular response. The right heart catheter, which had been inserted via a femoral sheath, was immediately withdrawn and a transvenous

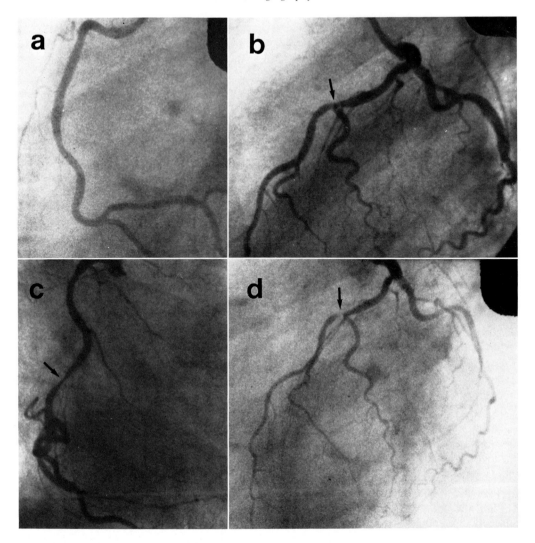

Fig. 32–2. Coronary angiograms in a 36-year-old woman (Case 2) with chest pain and ST segment elevation during exercise. Right (a) and left (b) coronary arteries before ergonovine maleate; note the mild stenosis of the mid-left anterior descending artery (arrow, b) while the patient was asymptomatic. Coronary angiograms after the first dose of ergonovine maleate (0.05 mg) demonstrate spasm with tapering stenosis of the right coronary artery (arrow, c) and a high-grade stenosis of the left anterior descending coronary artery (arrow, d) at the site of the previously noted mild stenosis.

pacemaker was inserted in its place and positioned in the right ventricle with ventricular pacing rapidly achieved. Right and left intracoronary injections of nitroglycerin (200 µg each) were immediately administered. Within 45 seconds the patient began to note abatement of symptoms, and 1 minute later sinus rhythm was restored. A continuous infusion of intravenous nitroglycerin was begun, and after a period of stability, the patient was transferred from the Cardiac Catheterization Laboratory

to the Coronary Care Unit. Over a period of 48 hours a myocardial infarction was ruled out, and the patient was switched to oral isosorbide dinitrate and diltiazem was restarted.

On the third evening after catheterization, the patient's roommate called for a nurse's assistance, having observed the patient collapse suddenly after a brief complaint of dizziness. An electrocardiogram revealed complete heart block with marked ST-segment elevation in the inferior leads. Sublingual nitroglycerin and sublingual nifedipine were immediately administered, and the patient regained consciousness within 3 minutes. The diltiazem dose was increased to 90 mg three times daily; nifedipine was given in gradually increasing doses (finally 30 mg every 6 hours). Additionally, isosorbide dinitrate was given every 4 hours while she was awake with nitropaste applied prior to sleep. On this regimen no further episodes of chest discomfort, nausea, or heart block occurred, and the patient was discharged on the eighth hospital day. At follow-up, intermittently over the next 6 months, the patient reported occasional brief episodes of chest discomfort for which she took sublingual nitroglycerin, but she noted no prolonged episodes and syncope has not recurred.

Illustrative Points. Although Prinzmetal, in his original series, described several patients who, at autopsy, were found to have high grade atherosclerotic narrowing of at least one epicardial coronary artery,[5] it is recognized now that the syndrome of variant angina may occur in patients with any degree of atherosclerotic narrowing, including those totally free (as shown by coronary angiography) of coronary atherosclerosis. This patient demonstrated spasm at the site of a mild atherosclerotic lesion in her left anterior descending coronary artery. She also demonstrated spasm of an angiographically normal right coronary artery.

Many patients with variant angina have spasm at different sites. Only if the spasm occurs at the site of a severe stenosed artery can coronary bypass surgery or coronary angioplasty be expected to be of benefit.[6,7] Such patients usually present with both exercise-induced and rest angina. As was seen in this case, however, even patients with normal or nearly normal coronary arteries may have exercise-induced coronary artery spasm. This case also points out the necessity of obtaining coronary angiograms of the entire coronary system when spasm is demonstrated in one portion because coronary artery spasm may not be limited to a single artery.

Although modest generalized narrowing of the entire coronary arterial system can be seen with ergonovine maleate, particularly at higher doses, severe focal narrowing is the hallmark of variant angina and probably does not occur in the normal population.[8] Even patients with atherosclerotic disease tend not to have focal spasm after ergonovine stimulation unless they also have rest angina. Conversely, the incidence of focal narrowing after ergonovine in patients with rest angina and atherosclerotic fixed narrowing is moderately high.[9] Ergonovine testing should be performed at least 24 hours after discontinuation of nitrates and calcium channel blockers to avoid the possibility of false-negative studies in patients receiving these therapies.

Although most patients with variant angina respond well to the administration of a calcium channel blocker, about 10% of patients with this syndrome require multiple drug therapy. Administration of two different calcium channel blockers in conjunction with intermittent nitrate therapy can control the syndrome in virtually all patients.

Unstable Angina—Atherosclerotic Coronary Disease

Many different terms have been used to describe the syndrome now commonly known as unstable angina. The premonitory syndrome, intermediate syndrome, preinfarction angina, crescendo angina, and coronary insufficiency are among the more commonly used ones. In its broadest definition unstable angina includes patients with new angina, increasingly severe angina, and rest angina. Some investigators, however, use the term *unstable angina* in a more limited way for patients requiring hospital admission because of episodes of rest angina, particularly if such episodes do not respond immediately to medical therapy.

Unstable angina may be present with coronary artery disease of varying severity. Single, double, and triple vessel diseases occur about equally, with left main coronary artery stenosis occurring in about 15% of patients and normal coronary arteries being present in 10%.[10] Although the majority of patients with unstable angina do not go on to develop acute myocardial infarction, an important portion do (10 to 20%).[11] Clinical progression is frequently associated with angiographic progression of coronary artery stenoses to total occlusions.[12] The role of thrombosis superimposed on fixed atherosclerotic plaques is increasingly recognized in both acute myocardial infarction and unstable angina.[13,14] Additionally, plaque hemorrhage and coronary artery spasm are responsible for some cases of unstable angina. Platelet aggregation superimposed on severe coronary stenosis leads to intermittent myocardial ischemia in an animal model of unstable angina[15]; biochemical markers of platelet activation are markedly elevated in patients with unstable coronary syndromes.[16]

As with variant angina, during episodes of unstable angina, evidence of systolic and diastolic dysfunction may appear. Once ischemia occurs, heart rate generally increases, mean arterial pressure rises (unless the quantity of myocardial ischemia is so large that systolic function is severely compromised, in which case blood pressure may fall), and left ventricular end diastolic pressure rises. Mitral and/or tricuspid regurgitation may occur or increase during ischemic episodes. This can be demonstrated by a sudden increase in right-and/or left-sided filling pressures with the presence of a prominent V wave in the pulmonary capillary wedge or right atrial tracings. The height of both the A and the V wave may rise in response to ischemia even when regurgitation across the AV valve is not present. Such a change occurs because ischemia-induced impairment of diastolic relaxation decreases the compliance of the left ventricle so that for the increase in volume occurring with ventricular filling a *greater* increase in pressure is seen than had been present prior to ischemia.

The following two cases are examples of patients with unstable angina. They are chosen to demonstrate both differing pathoanatomy and differing therapeutic options in this syndrome.

Case 3. The patient was a previously asymptomatic 47-year-old sedentary man with moderate hypercholesterolemia and a positive family history for coronary artery disease. He arrived at the emergency room after 2 days of stressful meetings, reporting an episode of substernal chest pressure that was now waning, but that half an hour earlier had been quite severe. Physical examination revealed blood pressure of 155/98 mmHg, heart rate of 94 beats/min., and otherwise normal findings with the exception of a loud fourth heart sound. His electrocardiogram showed T wave inversion in leads V2 through V6, and inverted T waves in leads II, III, and AVF. He was admitted to the Coronary Care Unit.

Twenty-four hours later, his ECG was normal. His cardiac enzymes remained within the normal range, and he was transferred out of the Coronary Care Unit. He was placed on long-acting nitrates and a beta-blocker, and an exercise stress test was scheduled. Twelve hours later, before undergoing exercise testing, he complained of mild-substernal chest pressure. His ECG revealed biphasic T waves in the anterior leads, clearly abnormal and different from his admission electrocardiogram. The chest discomfort and ECG abnormalities reverted promptly after one sublingual nitroglycerin. Because he continued to have symptoms at rest, was reluctant to continue medical therapy indefinitely, and was relatively young, cardiac catheterization was scheduled. He was placed on a calcium channel blocking agent while awaiting catheterization. In the 24 hours before angiography, he suffered two further episodes of chest discomfort, both relieved by sublingual nitroglycerin.

Cardiac catheterization revealed normal hemodynamics and calculated indices. Left ventriculography, which showed normal ventricular function and no mitral regurgitation, was used for calculation of his left ventricular ejection fraction, which was 0.60. Coronary angiography shows an occluded right coronary artery (Fig. 32–3a). The left anterior descending coronary artery had an 85% stenosis proximal to the first septal perforator and to a large diagonal branch (Fig. 32–3b). The left circumflex coronary artery contained no important lesions. The right coronary artery was

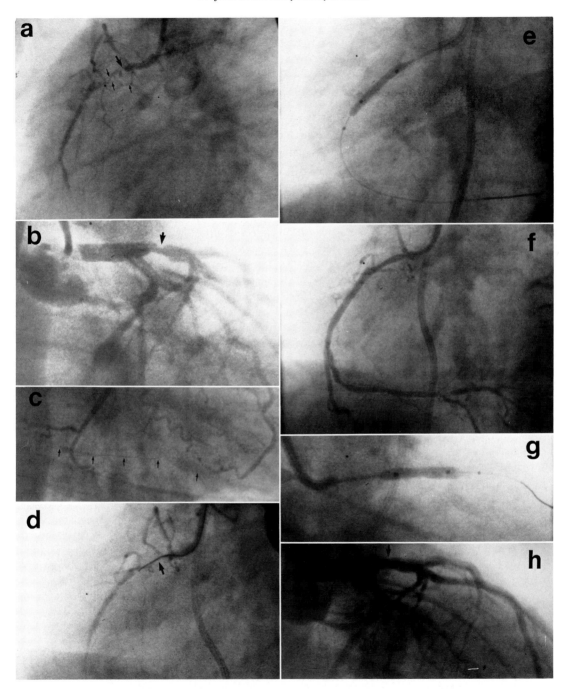

Fig. 32–3. (a) Right coronary angiogram in a 47-year-old man with unstable angina (Case 3) demonstrating a proximal total occlusion (large arrow) with bridging collateral vessels (small arrows) and poor distal runoff. There is a high-grade proximal stenosis of the left anterior descending coronary artery (b, arrow). Faintly visualized collateral vessels from the distal left anterior descending artery to the distal right coronary artery (c, arrows) are seen. A guide wire is used to cross the right coronary artery occlusion (d, arrow); this wire is then used to position the angioplasty balloon at the stenotic site where the balloon is inflated (e). Following angioplasty, the right coronary artery is widely patent (f) and excellent antegrade flow is present. Finally, angioplasty of the proximal left anterior descending stenosis is performed (g) and postangioplasty (h) the stenosis (arrow) is considerably reduced.

dominant, with a posterior descending artery, which had originally received antegrade flow by way of the right coronary artery but now was seen only after contrast injection into the left coronary artery with filling by way of collaterals primarily from the distal portion of the left anterior descending coronary artery (Fig. 32–3c). Thus, the patient had two-vessel coronary artery disease with an occluded right coronary artery and severe stenosis of the left anterior descending coronary artery.

While both lesions could have developed simultaneously, it was far more likely that one was old and the other recent. Severe stenosis of a coronary artery, even coronary artery occlusion, may occur silently if extensive collateralization is present to prevent ischemia of the distal myocardial bed. Once the vessel supplying those collaterals becomes stenosed itself, however, flow through the collaterals is compromised and ischemia may occur over a very wide territory.

Percutaneous transluminal coronary angioplasty (PTCA) may be safely and successfully accomplished in selected cases of total coronary artery occlusion.[17] In this case, PTCA was recommended. The right coronary artery occlusion was traversed with a flexible-tipped steerable guide wire (Fig. 32–3d) over which successful angioplasty was performed in the right coronary artery (Fig. 32–3e and f). Then, the left anterior descending coronary artery stenosis was successfully dilated as well (Fig. 32–3g and h).

Illustrative Points. The presence of multiple risk factors in this relatively young man with typical symptoms of ischemia suggested that the probability of atherosclerotic coronary disease was high. Noninvasive testing was not necessary to make this diagnosis (although in a different setting it might have assisted in risk assessment). Thus, coronary angiography was not necessary for diagnosis, but rather for prognostic and management purposes because his ECG with pain suggested an extensive amount of jeopardized myocardium. Additionally, this busy executive felt strongly opposed to taking medication on a long-term basis, particularly if a relatively safe mechan-

ical alternative was available. In this case, coronary angioplasty could be performed, and was successful. Despite the risk of restenosis at either of the angioplasty sites, the patient willingly chose that risk.

When inferior and anterior ECG changes are seen simultaneously, as in this case, widespread myocardial ischemia must be considered. It has been argued that anatomy as described in the above case is a *true* "left main equivalent."[18] A high-grade stenosis of the left main coronary artery itself may present a precarious clinical situation. The risk with this defect is probably caused by the area of myocardium which becomes ischemic and is thereby threatened by a *single* coronary artery stenosis. Thus, separate left anterior descending coronary artery and left circumflex coronary artery stenoses should not be considered "equivalent" to a left main coronary artery stenosis. When a severe stenosis occurs in one vessel that supplies collaterals to a previously occluded second vessel, however, true left main equivalency may be present (Fig. 32–4). Conversely, as long as the vessel supplying collaterals is not stenosed, extensive collaterals may protect against myocardial ischemia and myocardial infarction. Thus, even in the absence of prior infarction, totally occluded vessels are seen not uncommonly at the time of coronary angiography.

Ischemic ECG changes may persist after symptoms have resolved. It has been suggested that the myocardium remains "stunned" on some occasions after severe ischemia.[19] Persistent ECG changes may reflect metabolic abnormalities that can be present for as long as 7 days.

Case 3 demonstrates the fact that rest angina with relatively severe coronary stenoses may appear as the first manifestation of coronary artery disease. Studies of patients who have had serial catheterizations have demonstrated that coronary occlusion leading to extensive transmural myocardial infarction occurs more frequently in vessels with minimal narrowing at baseline, as opposed to those with severe stenoses.[20] This is presumably because of the development of collateral circulation in pa-

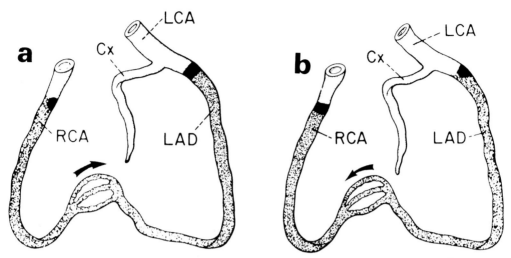

Fig. 32–4. Two examples of possible left main "equivalency." Two-vessel coronary disease with an occluded left anterior descending coronary artery (LAD) and myocardium jeopardized by a right coronary artery (RCA) stenosis (a) or an occluded RCA and myocardium jeopardized by a stenotic LAD (b). LCA = left coronary artery; Cx = circumflex coronary artery. (From Hutter AM Jr: Is there a left main equivalent? Circulation 62:207, 1980.)

tients with long-standing obstruction. The cause of rapid progression of severe stenosis or occlusion presumably involves intraplaque hemorrhage and plaque rupture, with secondary thrombus formation.[21] Although typical exertional angina occurs in many patients with similar coronary pathoanatomy, the first manifestation in some may be unstable angina or acute myocardial infarction. Myocardial ischemia and even infarction may occur silently in as many as a third of all patients with coronary artery disease. Additionally, many patients with angina pectoris have frequent episodes of ischemia (as evidenced by transient ECG changes on ambulatory monitoring) in the absence of perceptible symptoms.[22] Thus, the duration, timing, and severity of symptoms are relatively poor predictors of the *extent* of coronary artery disease present.

Case 4. A 57-year-old insurance salesman noted precordial chest discomfort while jogging. The symptom had been present for 5 months, provoked by progressively less exertion. Over the last 2 weeks chest discomfort had occurred with walking and modest exercise. The patient sought medical attention and an exercise stress test was performed before planned medical therapy. A standard exercise protocol was used, and the patient complained

of moderately severe precordial pressure 4 minutes after beginning exercise. At that point, 3 mm of ST-segment depression was noted in leads V1 through V5, and the patient's systolic blood pressure, which had been 140 mmHg prior to exercise, had fallen to 115 mmHg. Because of the strongly positive stress test with angina, marked ST-segment depression, and a fall in blood pressure, all at a low workload, the patient was referred for cardiac catheterization.

Before angiography, all hemodynamic measurements were normal, including left ventriculography with a calculated ejection fraction of 0.65. Cineangiography of the right coronary artery revealed no focal lesions. In the left coronary artery system a 90% stenosis of the left main coronary artery was present (Fig. 32–5a) with a 70% stenosis of the left anterior descending coronary artery and a total occlusion of the circumflex artery immediately after the origin of its large first marginal branch (Fig. 32–5b). The distal circumflex territory was supplied by collaterals from the right coronary artery. Shortly after the second contrast injection of the left system, the patient began to complain of precordial chest pressure. The ECG monitor lead showed ST-segment depression. Pulmonary capillary wedge pressure

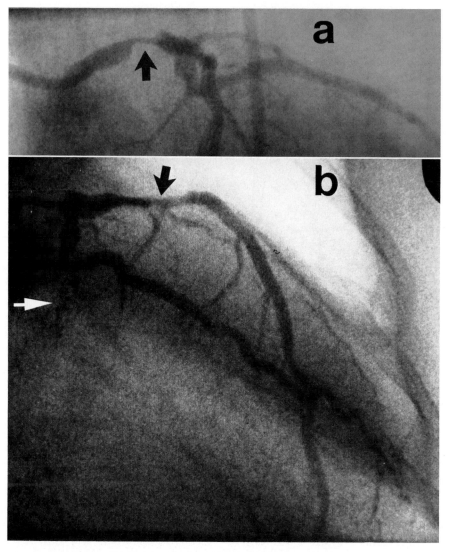

Fig. 32–5. Coronary angiogram in a 57-year-old man with a markedly positive exercise test (Case 4). Selective view of the left main coronary artery (a) showing a severe eccentric stenosis (arrow). Angiogram of the entire left coronary artery system (b) in a right anterior oblique view demonstrating proximal left anterior descending disease (large arrow) and a total occlusion of the circumflex system (small arrow) distal to its first large marginal artery. The distal circumflex artery is only faintly visible in the lower left corner of panel b.

had risen from normal to 18 mmHg. Repeat contrast injection of the left coronary artery system showed no change in the previously visualized stenoses and no focal spasm. The patient was given sublingual nitroglycerin, which briefly diminished his precordial chest pain, but the discomfort returned within 15 minutes. An intravenous nitroglycerin infusion, sublingual nifedipine, and 4 mg of intravenous propranolol (given slowly over 10 minutes) failed to completely relieve the patient's chest discomfort or return his ST-segment depression to baseline.

Thirty minutes after the onset of chest pain, the coronary angiographic catheter was exchanged, over a guide wire, first for a dilator with a larger diameter, and then for a percutaneously introduced intraaortic balloon.

Counterpulsation with the intraaortic balloon pump was rapidly instituted, and within several minutes the patient's precordial chest discomfort was entirely abolished. A 12-lead ECG taken at that time was unchanged from the precatheterization tracing.

The patient remained stable without evidence of myocardial necrosis over a period of 24 hours. On the day after catheterization, coronary artery bypass graft surgery was performed with grafts placed to the left anterior descending artery and both first and second large left circumflex marginal arteries.

Illustrative Points. While a trial of medical therapy is appropriate for most patients with angina pectoris, occasionally it is useful to perform cardiac catheterization early in the course of the disease. A strongly positive exercise stress test, as was present in this case, is considered by many clinicians an indication for early cardiac catheterization. Although the exercise stress test was not necessary for the diagnosis of coronary disease in this case, it was useful for prognostic purposes and did lead to a surgical intervention in precisely the kind of case (left main disease) where surgery has been shown to be of benefit when compared with medical therapy.[23] Percutaneous transluminal coronary angioplasty is not usually recommended for left main coronary artery stenosis. Although the risk of acute occlusion with angioplasty is relatively small (probably less than 10%), the consequences of such an event at the site of a left main stenosis could be catastrophic. In addition, the mortality rate within 3 years of angioplasty of a left main artery not "protected" by a patent bypass graft to the anterior descending or circumflex branches may be as high as 60%,[24] presumably because of restenosis. Results in patients in whom the left main is "protected" are considerably better, with a 3-year mortality rate of 13%.[24]

Intraaortic balloon counterpulsation is of great value in the management of refractory unstable angina. Control of ischemia may often be achieved even when all pharmacologic modalities have been applied maximally and failed. In controlling ischemia with normal

ventricular function, the primary mechanism by which the balloon pump exerts its effect is through the reduction of afterload. By diminishing left ventricular systolic pressure, myocardial oxygen demand is decreased. Although it has been suggested that diastolic augmentation increases coronary flow to the ischemic myocardium, this has not been demonstrated unequivocally in the clinical setting. Percutaneous or surgical insertion of the intraaortic balloon carries significant risks, *including a risk of up to 15%* of limb ischemia requiring vascular surgery.[25] Women, diabetics, and patients with pre-existing peripheral vascular disease are at particularly increased risk. Potential benefits of the procedure must be weighed against risks before proceeding with insertion, and adequacy of peripheral circulation assessed before and after balloon placement. Medically refractory ischemia in the setting of left main coronary stenosis, with surgically operable disease, is an ideal circumstance in which to consider intraaortic balloon pumping.

Multivessel Coronary Disease and Left Ventricular Dysfunction

Necrosis of 40% or more of the left ventricle generally leads to cardiogenic shock, and survival in that situation is rare, although recent evidence suggests that early revascularization with angioplasty or coronary bypass may improve outcome.[27,28] Less extensive myocardial infarction may produce varying degrees of systolic and diastolic dysfunction. The extent of hemodynamic compromise is based on both the area of muscle damaged and its location. For example, extensive damage of the right ventricle may occur with only modest necrosis of the left ventricle. In this circumstance, signs or symptoms of right-sided congestive failure, such as marked peripheral edema, may occur without pulmonary congestion or clinical evidence of low forward cardiac output. In another example, a small infarction involving a papillary muscle and myocardium supporting that papillary muscle may be responsible for intermittent episodes of pulmonary edema due to mitral regurgitation induced by the papillary muscle dysfunction. Thus, assessment of coronary pathoanatomy in conjunction with evaluation of left ventricular function and hemodynamics can be exceedingly important in the management of patients with a wide variety of ischemic syndromes and clinical evidence of ventricular dysfunction. The following case demonstrates that symptoms of congestive heart failure and myocardial ischemia cannot be viewed independently of one another.

Case 5. The patient was a 62-year-old salesman with 10 years of insulin-requiring diabetes mellitus, hyperlipidemia, and a positive family history for premature coronary disease. He had suffered an inferior wall myocardial infarction 15 years ago and a moderately large anterior wall myocardial infarction 6 months ago. Although the latter infarction was not associated with symptoms of heart failure, he developed basilar rales, and diuretic therapy with furosemide was instituted prior to his discharge. At present he reported throat tightness after walking two blocks. The symptom was associated with modest shortness of breath. He had two-pillow orthopnea but no paroxysmal nocturnal dyspnea. His current therapeutic regimen included furosemide, nitroglycerin ointment, and low-dose metoprolol (decreased from higher doses because of his exertional dyspnea, but continued at a low dose because, in its absence, resting tachycardia had been present).

Physical examination revealed a blood pressure of 105/70 mmHg and a regular pulse of 64 beats/min. Jugular venous pressure was approximately 8 cm of water; carotid upstrokes were normal. Lung examination revealed rales at the left base. The cardiac apex was displaced laterally 2 cm. The first heart sound was normal; the second was split paradoxically. A loud fourth heart sound was present and a Grade 1/6 murmur was audible at the apex, with radiation to the base. Peripherally, bilateral trace ankle edema was present and pulses were intact. The electrocardiogram revealed sinus rhythm with left atrial enlargement, left bundle branch block, and inferior and anterior Q waves with diffuse ST and T wave abnormal-

ities. An exercise stress test was performed with thallium imaging. Throat tightness and some precordial discomfort occurred in association with shortness of breath, all beginning within 5 minutes of exercise. Electrocardiographic changes were seen but were uninterpretable because of the pre-existing left bundle branch block. Thallium imaging during stress revealed defects of the inferior—apical, septal, anterior, and posterior—lateral walls. Images obtained 4 hours after exercise showed no change in the anterior and septal defects, but diminution in size of the inferior-apical defect and almost complete disappearance of the posterior-lateral defect. A radionuclide ventriculogram revealed a left ventricular ejection fraction of 0.32.

Because of the patient's activity limitation, with symptoms and evidence by thallium scans of reversible ischemia, despite the presence of congestive heart failure and a depressed ejection fraction, cardiac catheterization is undertaken. That study reveals the following hemodynamics at rest:

Pressures: mmHg

Right atrium, mean	8
Right ventricle	33/9
Pulmonary artery	33/20, $\overline{25}$
Pulmonary capillary wedge, mean	16
Left ventricle	106/25
Aorta	106/60
Cardiac output, L/min	5.2
Cardiac index, L/min/m^2	2.8
Systemic vascular resistance, dynes-sec-cm^{-5}	1108
LV end diastolic volume index, mL/m^2	90
LV end systolic volume index, mL/m^2	53
LV ejection fraction	0.36

Left ventriculography revealed multiple localized wall motion abnormalities with anterior akinesis and inferior-apical hypokinesis (Fig. 32–6a and b). Only trace mitral regurgitation is present. Coronary angiography shows extensive, multivessel disease with a near-total occlusion of the right coronary artery (Fig. 32–6c), a high-grade stenosis of the left anterior descending coronary artery (perhaps representing recanalized thrombus), a stenosis of the proximal left circumflex coronary artery, and severe stenoses of the first and second obtuse marginal branches of that artery (Fig. 32–6d).

Coronary artery bypass surgery was recommended, and the patient accepted this recommendation despite a slight increase in risk related to impaired left ventricular function. The patient underwent four-vessel bypass graft surgery and recovered uneventfully. Two months after surgery, a repeat exercise stress test with thallium was markedly improved, with the patient exercising for 9 minutes before stopping because of exertional dyspnea. No

throat tightness occurred. Thallium scintigraphy demonstrated continued presence of the previously seen persistent defects, but absence of the previously shown reversible posterior-lateral defect.

Illustrative Points. In this case, symptoms of ischemia and congestion occurred nearly simultaneously. This may not always be the case; sometimes symptoms of congestive heart failure may obscure clinical evidence of reversible ischemia. Noninvasive testing may be exceedingly useful in this situation. Exercise-induced ischemia may be apparent from thallium scintigraphy and the effect of ischemia on left ventricular function may be demonstrated by exercise radionuclide ventriculography. When such studies demonstrate the

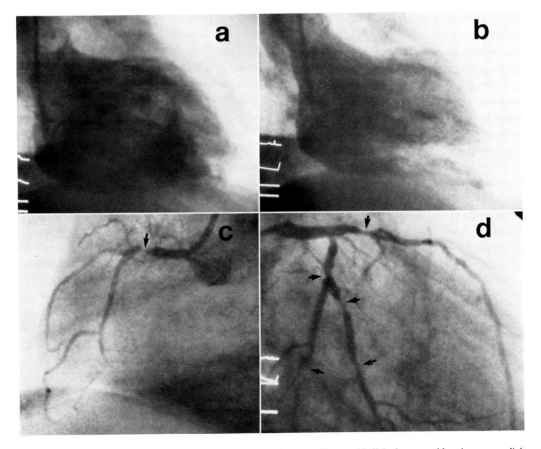

Fig. 32–6. Left ventriculography and coronary angiography in a 62-year-old diabetic man with prior myocardial infarction (Case 5). Diastolic (a) and systolic (b) frames from a left ventriculogram show anterior akinesis and inferior and apical hypokinesis. Coronary angiography reveals a near total occlusion of the proximal right coronary artery (c, arrow), and multiple lesions of the left coronary system (d, arrows).

presence of *both* ventricular dysfunction and active myocardial ischemia, proceeding to invasive examination may be appropriate regardless of the fact that ventricular function is moderately or even severely compromised. The Coronary Artery Surgery Study (CASS) has demonstrated that surgical therapy may be of benefit in asymptomatic patients or those with mild symptoms of ischemia when three-vessel coronary artery disease and left ventricular dysfunction (ejection fraction 0.35 to 0.50) are present.[29] In an earlier era of coronary artery bypass graft surgery, operating on patients with depressed ventricular function was often considered too risky. However, with improved surgical techniques, including better methods for intraoperative myocardial preservation, depressed left ventricular function has a less important impact on operative survival. In fact, it is this group of patients that may benefit most from revascularization, with improved survival and control of angina. In addition, ventricular function may be improved in some patients, particularly during exertion.[30]

Acute Myocardial Infarction— Interventional Therapy

When this textbook was first written, cardiac catheterization was not generally performed on patients during an acute myocardial infarction or early after one. The procedure was avoided both because of a presumed increase in risk and because the diagnostic information obtained from that study was of little use *during* acute myocardial infarction. Advances in our understanding of the pathophysiology of infarction and the availability of newer therapeutic modalities have led to more frequent cardiac catheterization in the early hours of myocardial infarction. It is now generally recognized that coronary artery thrombus is present in the vast majority of patients with acute transmural myocardial infarction.[13] Several large studies have demonstrated improvements in both survival and left ventricular function when thrombolytic agents are ad-

ministered early (less than 6 hours) in the course of myocardial infarction.[31,32] These agents can be given directly into the affected coronary artery but, more importantly, seem to have similar efficacy when given intravenously, which allows more rapid administration and avoids the need for acute cardiac catheterization. The ability to intervene successfully in acute myocardial infarction has led to controversy regarding the role of cardiac catheterization, both immediately and in the days after infarction. Coronary arterial recanalization can be achieved early in the course of acute myocardial infarction by coronary angioplasty in 85% or more of patients.[33] This strategy, however, requires the presence of specialized facilities and personnel, is costly, and is complicated by a significant rate (up to 15%) of early reocclusion. In addition, angioplasty performed immediately after administration of thrombolytic therapy, particularly tissue plasminogen activator (tPA), has been demonstrated to result in a higher rate of major complications than more conservative strategies.[34,35] In 25% or more of cases, however, thrombolytic therapy will fail to open the infarct-related artery. Some investigators have argued that all patients should therefore undergo emergent coronary angiography to identify those with persistent arterial occlusion who may benefit from "salvage" angioplasty. In the absence of clinical signs and/or symptoms of ongoing ischemia (which *are* indications for emergent catheterization), however, the benefits of "salvage" angioplasty have yet to be convincingly demonstrated.

The role of cardiac catheterization in the days and weeks after acute infarction has also been controversial. The Thrombolysis in Myocardial Infarction (TIMI) study[36] demonstrated that patients treated with a "conservative" strategy of thrombolysis, anticoagulation, and beta-blockers had an excellent outcome, with a rate of death or reinfarction of less than 10% in the 6 weeks following infarction. This outcome was not improved by routine performance of cardiac catheterization and angioplasty at 18 to 48 hours following infarction. For this reason, it is recommended that patients treated with thrombolytic therapy for transmural infarction undergo cardiac catheterization only for recurrent symptoms or objective signs (e.g., during exercise testing) of ischemia.

Patients presenting with a non-Q wave infarction have a lower in-hospital but a higher 1 year mortality than patients with Q-wave infarcts.[37] These patients are more likely to have multivessel coronary disease and residual ischemia, and can be considered to be patients with unstable coronary syndromes who may benefit from catheterization. The use of thrombolytic therapy in such patients is under investigation.

The following case was selected to illustrate some of the decision points and findings in the treatment of acute myocardial infarction.

Case 6. The patient was a 38-yr-old plant foreman with a family history of coronary disease and a personal history of heavy cigarette smoking. He noted 2 days of increasingly frequent angina, followed by a prolonged episode of severe substernal chest discomfort. He was taken to a local emergency room, where ST-segment elevation was noted in leads I, AVL, and V1–V6. Intravenous tissue plasminogen activator (tPA) was administered over 3 hours, beginning 2 hours and 45 minutes after the onset of chest pain. Ninety minutes after starting tPA, he had relief of pain, with a decrease in ST segment elevation and an episode of accelerated idioventricular rhythm. Despite continuous infusion of heparin at 1000 units/hr after a 5000 unit bolus, the patient had recurrent chest pain 2 hours after the end of the tPA infusion, accompanied by up to 10 mm of precordial ST-segment elevation. He received an additional 20 mg of tPA, nitrates, and morphine, and was transferred to a hospital with cardiac catheterization facilities.

On arrival, the patient was diaphoretic and pale, and complained of continuing pain. The heart rate was 100 with a blood pressure of 110/80. His chest was clear, the cardiac examination was normal with the exception of a fourth heart sound, and the remainder of his physical examination was within normal limits. The electrocardiogram revealed persistent ST segment elevation.

Four hours after the onset of recurrent pain, the patient entered the Cardiac Catheterization Laboratory. Right heart catheterization revealed a mean right atrial pressure of 13 mmHg and a pulmonary capillary wedge pressure of 25 mmHg. Left ventricular pressure was 115/25 mmHg. Left ventriculography showed akinesis of the anterior, apical, and inferior-apical walls; the overall ejection fraction was 0.37% and there was no mitral regurgitation. The right coronary artery was small and co-dominant. Visualization of the left coronary artery showed minimal atherosclerosis in the large circumflex artery but total occlusion of the midportion of the left anterior descending artery (Fig. 32–7a). No collateral filling of the distal artery was seen. The occlusion was crossed easily with a .014″ guide wire, and angioplasty with 3.0 and 3.5 mm balloons resulted in brisk antegrade flow with a residual stenosis of less than 20% (Fig. 32–7b). After angioplasty, the patient was free of chest pain; electrocardiograms showed a decrease in ST segment elevation with development of Q waves in leads V1 to V4.

The hospital course was complicated by mild pulmonary congestion, treated with diuresis. Afterload reduction with captopril and low-dose beta-blockade was initiated. Anticoagulation was continued with heparin, followed by oral warfarin and aspirin. After a negative submaximal exercise test, the patient was discharged 11 days after infarction.

Illustrative Points. Time is critical in the salvage of ischemic myocardium. Both myocardial oxygen demand and oxygen supply are important in determining the timing of progression from reversible ischemia to necrosis. All studies of intervention in acute myocardial infarction have shown the greatest benefit when therapy is begun within 1 to 2 hours from onset of ischemia.[32] In spite of this, delays in patient presentation, diagnosis, and medication frequently delay treatment beyond this time interval. The maximum length of time after which treatment has no incremental ben-

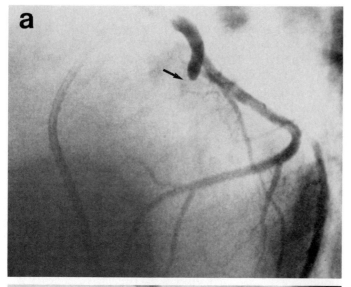

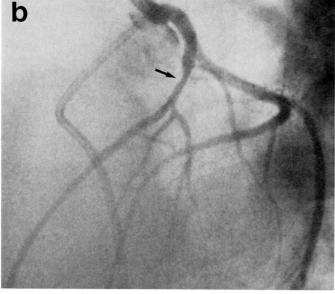

Fig. 32–7. (a) Left coronary angiogram in a 47-year-old man with acute myocardial infarction (Case 6), demonstrating total occlusion of the left anterior descending artery (arrow). (b) After coronary angioplasty, there is a mild residual stenosis (arrow) with brisk antegrade flow.

efit is uncertain, and may depend on the presence of some collateral circulation to the ischemic myocardium; one study[31] has suggested benefit for up to 24 hours. There is evidence that long-term arterial patency decreases the amount of infarct expansion and ventricular dilatation.[38]

Clinical signs of reperfusion include relief of pain, decrease in ST segment abnormalities, and ''reperfusion arrhythmias,'' which may include ventricular ectopy, accelerated idioventricular rhythm, and atrioventricular block.

While complete resolution of pain or ST segment abnormalities is highly predictive of reperfusion,[39] the converse is not true; 50% or more of patients without these signs will also have had reperfusion. The poor predictive value of clinical signs has led to the suggestion that all patients should undergo angiography to identify those with persistently occluded vessels. Until ''salvage'' angioplasty in these patients is clearly demonstrated to be of benefit, this strategy cannot be recommended. This patient had clinical signs of reperfusion but had recurrent ischemia and presumably arterial reocclusion shortly after completion of thrombolytic therapy. Reocclusion rates after successful thrombolytic therapy are reported to be from 10 to 35%; while some are silent, many result in clinical ischemia or reinfarction. Some patients with recurrent ischemia in the first 24 hours after administration of tissue plasminogen activator are given additional doses. To avoid the higher risk of intracranial hemorrhage (which occurs at cumulative doses >100 mg), however, it is often recommended that patients with early reocclusion undergo emergent catheterization, with coronary angioplasty performed if the anatomy is suitable.

Case 7. The patient was a 34-year-old taxi driver with a positive family history of coronary disease and a personal history of heavy cigarette smoking. He developed severe substernal chest pressure, and drove his taxi to the emergency room, where an initial electrocardiogram revealed 3 to 5 mm of ST segment elevation in leads V1 through V5. He was taken to the Cardiac Catheterization Laboratory, where coronary angiography revealed occlusion of the left anterior descending artery in its proximal portion. Intracoronary thrombolytic therapy was administered, with reperfusion of the left anterior descending artery within 30 minutes. Left ventriculography revealed a large area of anterior wall akinesis (Fig. 32–8a and b). Hyperkinesis of the noninfarcted walls was present. The calculated ejection fraction was 0.42. The patient experienced no further signs or symptoms of myocardial ischemia.

Catheterization was repeated 2 weeks later and revealed further improvement of the previously seen left anterior descending artery stenosis. The patient's left ventricular end-diastolic pressure, which was 26 mmHg at the end of the previous procedure, had fallen slightly to 20 mmHg. There was no improvement in his left ventriculogram (Fig. 32–8c and d); in fact, with less vigorous contraction of the noninfarcted segments, his ejection fraction had fallen to 0.33.

Six months later, the patient noted progressively worsening exertional dyspnea. After treatment with digoxin and diuretics, there was a slight improvement in symptoms. A radionuclide ventriculogram obtained at this time revealed marked left ventricular dilatation, a large anterior apical dyskinetic segment, and an ejection fraction of 0.30.

Illustrative Points. Profoundly ischemic heart muscle may demonstrate hypoactive function and metabolic abnormalities as long as 10 days after ischemia is relieved.[19] Thus, left venticulography in the early hours after successful recanalization should not necessarily be expected to show improvement in ventricular function. By 2 weeks, however, the effects of reversible ischemia should no longer be present, and thus the left ventriculogram performed in this patient 14 days after the first procedure provides an accurate picture of myocardial salvage (or lack of salvage). In the months following acute myocardial infarction, remodeling of the ventricle probably occurs.[40] In some cases, actual expansion and thinning of the infarcted area may be present. Bulging of this segment in systole then leads to the characteristic dyskinetic appearance of ventricular aneurysm. The remaining area of ventricle is forced to "take over" for portions of the ventricle that are no longer functional. This increased load on previously normal myocardium may be functionally similar to the volume load introduced with valvular lesions such as aortic and mitral regurgitation. Recent evidence suggests that this "volume load" introduced by the nonfunctioning myocardium frequently produces dilatation of the ventricle not only through infarct expansion but also through expansion of the remaining normal segments.[40] These observations explain, in part, progressive increases in congestive symptoms caused by the rise in left ventricular end-diastolic pressure that may occur with dilatation. Administration of afterload reducing agents such as captopril has been shown to decrease the degree of expansion and reduce left ventricular filling pressures.[41]

Special Situations

Bypass Grafts and New Interventional Technologies. Cardiac catheterization has pro-

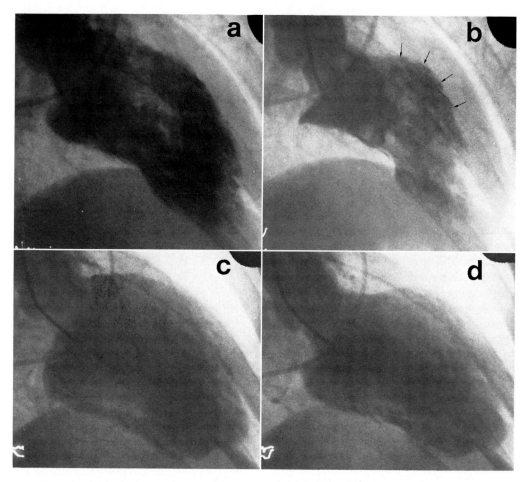

Fig. 32–8. Left ventriculography in Case 7. Diastolic (a) and systolic (b) frames from the left ventriculogram obtained minutes after the successful thrombolysis. Note anterior akinesis (arrows, b) with apical hypokinesis and vigorous contraction of the remaining perimeter. Two weeks later the diastolic volume has increased slightly (c) and anterior wall motion is unimproved (d); contraction of the remaining perimeter is less vigorous than that present on the earlier angiogram.

gressed from a purely diagnostic role to one encompassing many therapeutic techniques. This is particularly relevant for the patient who has previously undergone coronary bypass surgery. Long-term follow-up studies indicate that a high percentage of saphenous vein grafts develop late atherosclerotic narrowing or occlusion.[42] In addition, early graft occlusion, caused by thrombosis and/or fibrointimal proliferation, occurs in up to 20% of patients by 1 year after surgery, despite treatment with anti-platelet agents.[43] Because repeat surgery is associated with increased risk, many of these patients are referred for consideration of coronary angioplasty.

The long-term benefits of angioplasty are limited by the relatively frequent occurrence of restenosis in the dilated segment. Results of angioplasty in patients with multiple prior restenoses are poor; these patients have a 50% or greater restenosis rate.[44] For this reason, alternative interventional technologies are being developed. Intracoronary stents, laser balloon angioplasty, and coronary atherectomy all hold the promise of more reliable initial results and lower restenosis rates. Studies currently in progress will determine if these technologies are indeed superior to standard balloon angioplasty.

Case 8. The patient was a 46-year-old manager with hypercholesterolemia, a strong family history of premature coronary disease, and a personal history of cigarette abuse. He had sustained an anteroseptal myocardial infarction at age 32, and underwent coronary artery bypass surgery with a single saphenous vein graft to the left anterior descending artery. He then did well until age 42, when he sustained a non-Q wave infarction, and was found at cardiac catheterization to have a left dominant system, three-vessel coronary disease, and occlusion of the vein graft. Repeat coronary bypass surgery was performed. A left internal mammary artery graft was placed to the left anterior descending coronary artery; vein grafts were placed to the first and second obtuse marginal branches of the circumflex artery and to the left posterior descending artery. Exertional angina returned, and over 6 weeks symptoms became progressively severe. An exercise stress test with thallium was performed, and after 4 minutes of exercise, the patient developed anginal symptoms accompanied by dyspnea and a fall in systolic blood pressure. Thallium imaging revealed lung uptake with anterior, septal, inferior, and apical defects; there was redistribution at 4 hours in the inferior and apical walls. Because of the strongly positive stress test at a low workload, the patient is referred for cardiac catheterization.

Resting hemodynamics were normal. Left ventriculography showed anterolateral and apical hypokinesis with a calculated ejection fraction of 0.52. The left anterior descending artery was occluded proximally, as were both circumflex marginal branches. There was a 75% stenosis in the left posterior descending artery. The saphenous vein grafts to the second obtuse marginal artery and posterior descending artery were occluded; the graft to the first obtuse marginal artery was patent. The left internal mammary artery graft had a 95% stenosis at the anastomosis with the left anterior descending artery (Fig. 32–9a).

The findings were reviewed with the cardiac surgeon, who was reluctant to perform a third bypass operation. Although coronary angioplasty of the internal mammary artery in this patient was considered a high-risk procedure (because of the amount of jeopardized myocardium and the prior surgery), this procedure was felt to offer the best chance of symptomatic palliation. Angioplasty is performed using a 2.5 mm and then a 3.0 mm balloon, leaving a residual stenosis of only 30% (Fig. 32–9b). Following this, the patient was free of angina; repeat exercise testing to 9 minutes showed no angina, normal blood pressure response, nondiagnostic ST changes, and marked improvement in the ischemia noted previously by thallium imaging.

Illustrative Points. With coronary artery bypass surgery commonly used as a treatment for severe coronary disease, increasing numbers of patients with bypass grafts now present for cardiac catheterization. Studies have shown that 70% or more of saphenous vein grafts will have occlusion or atherosclerotic narrowing within 10 years of bypass surgery.[45] The long-term survival of patients undergoing surgery is adversely affected by graft atherosclerosis, leading to an increase in mortality after 4 to 5 years. The rate of progression of graft atherosclerosis is related to coronary disease risk factors including serum levels of LDL and HDL cholesterol and cigarette smoking.[45] Such lesions are histologically similar to native coronary vessel disease. This is in contrast to the fibrointimal proliferation, which occurs within the first year after bypass surgery or coronary angioplasty, and is a densely cellular process related weakly, if at all, to lipid levels. In addition to graft disease, accelerated atherosclerosis occurs in native coronary arteries after bypass, presumably due to competitive flow.[46] The internal mammary artery graft has vastly superior long-term results with 10-year patency rates of 80 to 90%[47] and correspondingly improved survival in patients receiving this graft. For this reason, internal mammary grafting is now used in the vast majority of bypass operations performed.

Catheterization of the patient with bypass grafts presents special challenges. The most important principle, which cannot be overemphasized, is that the number and location of grafts must be known before catheteriza-

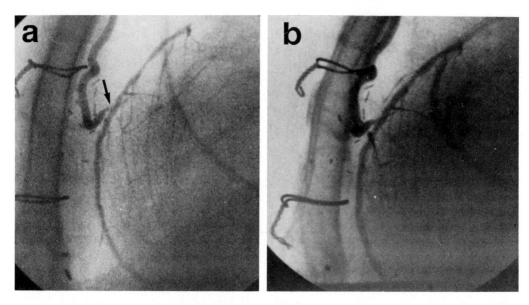

Fig. 32–9. Selective angiography of the left internal mammary artery in a 46-year-old man with angina following coronary bypass surgery (Case 8). There is a severe stenosis at the point of anastomosis with the left anterior descending artery (a, arrow). After angioplasty, the degree of stenosis is significantly reduced (b).

tion. An effort is made to engage the ostia of all saphenous vein grafts, which are usually located on the anterior surface of the ascending aorta and may be marked with radio-opaque rings or surgical clips. All parts of the graft, particularly the ostium and touchdown site, should be well visualized. The internal mammary artery may be engaged selectively from the femoral or brachial approach, although use of the contralateral brachial artery is often difficult. Mammary arteries may be at greater risk for dissection than coronary arteries, and therefore soft-tip catheters specially designed for the mammary artery should be used. Nonionic or dimeric contrast agents are preferred in the subclavian artery to minimize pain and the possibility of central nervous system injury from hyperosmolar contrast agents.

Although angioplasty in patients with previous bypass graft surgery may provide incomplete revascularization, the procedure is sometimes preferable to a high-risk reoperation. This is true in spite of the observation that angioplasty of atherosclerotic saphenous vein grafts carries a risk of distal embolization and has a restenosis rate of about 50% within 6 months.[48] Lesions in the internal mammary artery are usually at the distal anastomosis, and can be dilated successfully, although tortuosity in the proximal artery may make this difficult. In the present case, successful angioplasty resulted in marked symptomatic and objective improvement.

Case 9. The patient was a 34-year-old fireman with a family history of premature coronary disease. He noted the onset of exertional chest pressure accompanied by nausea, weakness, and diaphoresis. Exercise testing was positive for the development of angina and marked ST-segment depression in leads II, III, AVF, and V3–V6 at 9 minutes of a Bruce protocol. Despite treatment with diltiazem, exertional symptoms continued, and the patient was referred for cardiac catheterization.

Resting hemodynamics were normal. Left ventriculography showed normal wall motion, with an ejection fraction of 0.71. Coronary angiography revealed single-vessel coronary disease, with an 80% stenosis in the proximal portion of a very large left anterior descending artery. Coronary angioplasty was performed successfully, with a reduction in stenosis to 20% and no arterial dissection. Discharge medications included diltiazem, isosorbide dinitrate, aspirin, and dipyridamole. Maximal exercise testing 4 days after angioplasty was negative for ischemia.

Three months after angioplasty, anginal symptoms recurred and were rapidly progressive. Repeat exercise testing was dramatically positive (up to 7 mm of ST segment depression) and angiography confirmed the presence of restenosis of the previously dilated segment (Fig. 32–10a). Because of the high risk of recurrent restenosis with conventional angioplasty, percutaneous coronary atherectomy was recommended. A total of 12 cuts (Fig. 32–10b) were performed with the 7 Fr atherectomy catheter, with removal of a substantial amount of white, translucent tissue and reduction in stenosis to less than 10% (Fig. 32–10c). Histopathologic examination of the tissue removed revealed dense sheets of smooth muscle cells, characteristic of restenosis.

The patient was discharged free of angina and returned to work. Repeat exercise testing at 1 week, 3 months, and 6 months after ath-

erectomy was negative for ischemia. Coronary angiography performed 6 months after atherectomy revealed a widely patent artery at the atherectomy site with brisk flow and only a 20 to 30% stenosis.

Illustrative Points. The problem of restenosis remains a significant limitation of coronary angioplasty. Certain risk factors for restenosis have been identified. These include cigarette smoking, diabetes, unstable angina, subtotal or total occlusion of the vessel prior to angioplasty, lesion location in the proximal left anterior descending artery or in a saphenous vein bypass graft, eccentric or highly tortuous lesions, and poor postangioplasty results.[49] Prior restenosis of the segment to be dilated also appears to increase risk of recurrent restenosis, presumably because of the selection of patients with a particularly vigorous smooth muscle cell response.[44]

Despite randomized trials of many agents, including platelet inhibitors (aspirin, dipyridamole, fish oil, ticlopidine), anticoagulants (short-term heparin, warfarin), calcium antag-

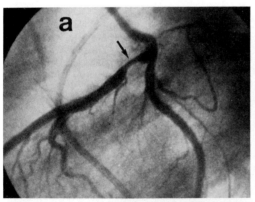

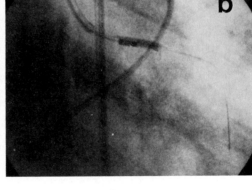

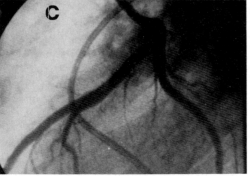

Fig. 32–10. Left coronary angiogram in a 34-year-old man with recurrent angina after coronary angioplasty (Case 9). A severe stenosis is seen in the proximal left anterior descending artery (a, arrow). Several passes are made with the atherectomy device (b, seen in RAO projection) leaving no residual stenosis and a smooth-appearing lumen (c).

onists (nifedipine, diltiazem), and corticosteroids, no treatment has been convincingly demonstrated to reduce the incidence of restenosis. For this reason, an alternative approach has been the use of newer interventional techniques. These include intracoronary stents, coronary atherectomy, and laser balloon angioplasty. Theoretically, a procedure that leaves a smoother, more widely patent lumen will allow better laminar flow across the lesion, producing lower shear force; ideally, this phenomenon will allow more rapid recovery of endothelium and decreased intimal proliferation.[50] Clinical trials of these new techniques are in progress to determine if the theoretical benefits will translate into an actual reduction in rate of restenosis following percutaneous transluminal coronary angioplasty.

REFERENCES

1. Mock MB, et al: Survival of medically treated patients in the coronary artery surgery study (CASS) registry. Circulation 66:562, 1982.
2. Johnson LW, et al: Coronary arteriography 1984–1987: A report of the Registry of the Society for Cardiac Angiography and Interventions. I. Results and complications. Cathet Cardiovasc Diagn 17:5, 1989.
3. Pasternak RC, et al: Chest pain with angiographically insignificant coronary arterial obstruction. Clinical presentation and long-term follow-up. Am J Med 68:813, 1980.
4. Aranda JM, et al: Mitral valve prolapse and coronary artery disease. Clinical hemodynamic and angiographic correlations. Circulation 52:245, 1975.
5. Prinzmetal M, et al: Angina pectoris. I. A variant form of angina pectoris. Am J Med 27:375, 1959.
6. Pasternak RC, et al: Variant angina. Clinical spectrum and results of medical and surgical therapy. J Thorac Cardiovasc Surg 78:614, 1979.
7. Corcos T, et al: Percutaneous transluminal coronary angioplasty for the treatment of variant angina. J Am Coll Cardiol 5:1046–54, 1985.
8. Cipriano PR, et al: The effects of ergonovine maleate on coronary arterial size. Circulation 59:82, 1979.
9. Schroeder JS, et al: Provocation of coronary spasm with ergonovine maleate. Am J Cardiol 40:487, 1977.
10. Alison HW, et al: Coronary anatomy and arteriography in patients with unstable angina pectoris. Am J Cardiol 41:204, 1978.
11. Mulcahy R, et al: Unstable angina: Natural history and determinants of prognosis. Am J Cardiol 48:525, 1981.
12. Neill WA, et al: Acute coronary insufficiency-coronary occlusion after intermittent ischemic attacks. N Engl J Med 302:1157, 1980.
13. DeWood MA, et al: Prevalence of total coronary occlusion during the early hours of transmural myocardial infarction. N Engl J Med 303:898, 1980.
14. Sherman CT, et al: Coronary angioscopy in patients with unstable angina pectoris. N Engl J Med 315:913–9, 1986.
15. Folts JD, Gallagher K, Rowe GG: Blood flow reductions in stenosed canine coronary arteries: vasospasm or platelet aggregation? Circulation 65:248–55, 1982.
16. Fitzgerald DJ, Roy L, Catella F, FitzGerald GA: Platelet activation in unstable coronary disease. N Engl J Med 315:983–9, 1986.
17. Baim DS, Safian RD: Total coronary artery occlusion. Cardiovasc Clin 19:155–67, 1988.
18. Hutter AM: Is there a left main equivalent? Circulation 62:207, 1980.
19. Braunwald E, Kloner RA: The stunned myocardium. Prolonged, postischemic ventricular dysfunction. Circulation 66:1146, 1982.
20. Williams AE, et al: Angiographic morphology in unstable angina pectoris. Am J Cardiol 62:1024, 1988.
21. Fuster V, et al: Insights into the pathogenesis of acute ischemic syndromes. Circulation 77:1213, 1988.
22. Gottlieb SO: Association between silent myocardial ischemia and prognosis: Insensitivity of angina pectoris as a marker of coronary artery disease activity. Am J Cardiol 60:33J, 1987.
23. Chaitman BR, et al: Effect of coronary bypass surgery on survival patterns in subsets of patients with left main coronary artery disease. Am J Cardiol 48:765, 1981.
24. Hartzler GI, et al: Left main coronary angioplasty— A caution. J Am Coll Cardiol 11:61A (abstract), 1988.
25. Alderman JD, et al: Incidence and management of limb ischemia with percutaneous wire guided intraaortic balloon catheters. J Am Coll Cardiol 9:524, 1987.
26. Page DL, et al: Myocardial changes associated with cardiogenic shock. N Engl J Med 285:133, 1971.
27. Lee L, et al: Percutaneous transluminal coronary angioplasty improves survival in acute myocardial infarction complicated by cardiogenic shock. Circulation 78:1345, 1988.
28. Guyton RA, et al: Emergency coronary bypass for cardiogenic shock. Circulation (Suppl V) 76:22, 1987.
29. Passamani E, David KB, Gillespie, MJ, Killip T, and CASS principal investigators and their associates: A randomized trial of coronary artery bypass surgery: survival of patients with a low ejection fraction. N Engl J Med 312:1655, 1985.
30. Kronenberg MW, et al: Left ventricular performance after coronary artery bypass surgery. Ann Intern Med 99:305, 1983.
31. ISIS-2: Randomised trial of intravenous streptokinase, oral aspirin, both, or neither among 17,187 cases of suspected acute myocardial infarction: ISIS-2. Lancet 2:349–360, 1988.
32. Gruppo Italiano per lo Studio Della Streptochinasi Nell'infarto Miocardico (GISSI): Effectiveness of intravenous thrombolytic treatment in acute myocardial infarction. Lancet 1:397, 1986.
33. O'Neill WW: Primary percutaneous coronary angio-

plasty: A protagonist's view. Am J Cardiol 62:15K, 1988.

34. TIMI II: Immediate vs delayed catheterization and angioplasty following thrombolytic therapy for acute myocardial infarction. JAMA 260:2849, 1988.

35. Topol EJ, et al: A randomized trial of immediate versus delayed elective angioplasty after intravenous tissue plasminogen activator in acute myocardial infarction. N Engl J Med 317:581, 1987.

36. TIMI II: Comparison of invasive and conservative strategies after treatment with intravenous tissue plasminogen activator in acute myocardial infarction. N Engl J Med 320:618, 1989.

37. Hutter AM Jr, et al: Nontransmural myocardial infarction: A comparison of hospital and later clinical course of patients with that of matched patients with transmural anterior and transmural inferior myocardial infarction. Am J Cardiol 48:595, 1981.

38. Jeremy RW, et al: Infarct artery perfusion and changes in left ventricular volume in the month after acute myocardial infarction. J Am Coll Cardiol 9:989, 1987.

39. Califf RM, et al: Failure of simple clinical measurements to predict perfusion status after intravenous thrombolysis. Ann Intern Med 108:658, 1988.

40. McKay RG, et al: Left ventricular remodelling following myocardial infarction—A corollary to infarct expansion. Circulation 74:693, 1986.

41. Pfeffer MA, et al: Effect of captopril on progressive ventricular dilatation after anterior myocardial infarction. N Engl J Med 319:80, 1988.

42. Bourassa MG, Campeau L, Lesperance J, Grondin CM: Changes in grafts and coronary arteries after saphenous vein aortocoronary bypass surgery: results at repeat angiography. Circulation 65:90, 1982.

43. Chesebro JH, et al: Effect of dipyridamole and aspirin on late vein-graft patency after coronary bypass operations. N Engl J Med 310:209, 1984.

44. Teirstein PS, et al: Repeat coronary angioplasty: efficacy of a third angioplasty for a second restenosis. J Am Coll Cardiol 13:291, 1989.

45. Campeau L, et al: The relation of risk factors to the development of atherosclerosis in saphenous-vein bypass grafts and the progression of disease in the native circulation. N Engl J Med 311:1329, 1984.

46. Cashin WL, Sanmarco ME, Nessim SA, Blankenhorn DH: Accelerated progression of atherosclerosis in coronary vessels with minimal lesions that are bypassed. N Engl J Med 311:824, 1984.

47. Grondin CM, et al: Comparison of late changes in internal mammary artery and saphenous vein grafts in two consecutive series of patients 10 years after operation. Circulation 70:208, 1984.

48. Cote G, et al: Percutaneous transluminal angioplasty of stenotic coronary artery bypass grafts: 5 years' experience. J Am Coll Cardiol 9:8, 1987.

49. Blackshear JL, O'Callaghan WG, Califf RM: Medical approaches to prevention of restenosis after coronary angioplasty. J Am Coll Cardiol 9:834, 1987.

50. Liu MW, Roubin GS, King SB III: Restenosis after coronary angioplasty: Potential biologic determinants and role of intimal hyperplasia. Circulation 79:1374, 1989.

33

Profiles in Pulmonary Embolism

JOSEPH R. BENOTTI and WILLIAM GROSSMAN

As indicated in Table 33–1, pulmonary embolism usually manifests itself as one or more clinically and hemodynamically distinct syndromes: acute unexplained dyspnea, pulmonary infarction syndrome, cardiogenic shock and cor pulmonale, or chronic pulmonary hypertension with right ventricular failure resulting from persistent or unresolved pulmonary embolism. These syndromes often have somewhat distinct hemodynamic profiles that support the diagnosis and exclude other conditions that would require alternate therapeutic strategies.

DIAGNOSIS

The clinical manifestations of pulmonary embolism are often nonspecific. In previously healthy persons, pulmonary embolism may mimic pneumonia or viral pleurisy;[1] in older patients with underlying cardiopulmonary disease it may present as worsening heart failure or an acute exacerbation of chronic obstructive lung disease.[2] In general, simple laboratory tests are not sufficiently sensitive or specific to be useful in diagnosing pulmonary embolism.[3] At one time, arterial hypoxemia in a patient breathing room air was believed to be sufficiently sensitive to be of value as a screening test for diagnosing pulmonary embolism; however, at least one study has found that approximately 13% of patients with pulmonary embolism have an arterial oxygen tension exceeding 80 mmHg while breathing room air.[4] Normal arterial oxygenation in these patients may be related to a compensatory decline in regional ventilation that complements the reduction in regional perfusion resulting from pulmonary embolism. The end result could be minimal or no ventilation perfusion mismatch and arterial normoxia, which has been reported even in occasional patients with massive pulmonary embolism.[5] Normal arterial blood oxygen saturation is more likely in younger patients without underlying cardiopulmonary disease who sustain a small pulmonary embolus.[6]

Other patients may have fever, hemoptysis, pleurisy, and parenchymal lung infiltrates resulting from a small to moderate size pulmonary embolism—the so-called pulmonary infarction syndrome.[7] Massive pulmonary embolism may present as syncope and shock. Unresolved pulmonary embolism may manifest itself as pulmonary hypertension and right heart failure.[8]

Table 33–1. *Syndromes of Pulmonary Embolism*

I. Acute pulmonary embolism
  A. Unexplained dyspnea
  B. Pulmonary infarction syndrome
  C. Acute cor pulmonale and/or cardiogenic shock
II. Chronic pulmonary embolism
  A. Right ventricular failure from multiple unresolved pulmonary emboli

ECG Findings. Electrocardiographic abnormalities associated with pulmonary embolism are relatively insensitive and nonspecific.[9] Sinus tachycardia, the most common abnormality, is not present with sufficient frequency to be useful for screening and has no specificity. ECG findings that are more suggestive of pulmonary embolism include the $S_1Q_3T_3$ pattern (S wave in lead I, Q wave and inverted T wave in lead III),[10] complete or incomplete right bundle branch block of new onset, and other manifestations of acute right ventricular strain. Unfortunately, these findings are uncommon in pulmonary embolism, and occur primarily in patients with massive embolism.

Femoral Venography. Previous investigations have emphasized the pathophysiologic role of deep venous thrombosis involving the veins above the knee in the genesis of pulmonary embolism. Approximately 90% of patients presenting with pulmonary embolism have evidence of deep venous thrombosis involving the thigh by objective testing using impedance plethysmography or contrast venography.[11] These latter tests are felt by some to be useful as screening procedures for pulmonary embolism. That is, in a patient with a clinical presentation compatible with pulmonary embolism, but with an indeterminate or nondiagnostic ventilation-perfusion lung scan, if concomitant evidence of deep venous thrombosis in the thigh is not demonstrable by objecting testing, the diagnosis of pulmonary embolism is highly unlikely. Conversely, objective evidence of deep venous thrombosis complementing a compatible clinical story enhances the likelihood of pulmonary embolism. The utility of this approach to the diagnosis of pulmonary embolism has been called into serious question, however. Hull et al have demonstrated that approximately 30% of patients with angiographically-proven pulmonary embolism have no evidence of deep venous thrombosis by contrast venography.[12] This finding suggests that in some patients all clots embolized from the thigh veins to the lungs at the same time, or that the pulmonary emboli did not originate in the leg veins, perhaps coming from the pelvic veins, the upper extremity veins, or the right atrium.

Although the importance of deep venous thrombosis of the thigh as the major factor predisposing to pulmonary embolism is incontrovertible, it is often difficult to diagnose deep venous thrombosis or pulmonary embolism by clinical criteria alone.[13,14] Thus, in the individual patient, the diagnosis of pulmonary embolism cannot be reliably substantiated or ruled out by confirming or excluding concomitant deep venous thrombosis. It is important to recognize that approximately 50% of patients with deep venous thrombosis of the thigh established by contrast venography have no suggestive clinical findings (swelling, a palpable chord, tenderness, or erythema).[11,13] Also noteworthy is the observation that approximately 50% of patients with deep venous thrombosis have objective evidence of pulmonary embolism as shown by defects on the perfusion lung scan at the time that the diagnosis of deep venous thrombosis is established.

Lung Scan. The perfusion lung scan is a useful screening procedure for pulmonary embolism. In a patient with a suggestive clinical story, a ***normal*** six-view perfusion lung scan reliably excludes the diagnosis of pulmonary embolism with a certainty approaching 100%.[15,16] In many patients in whom pulmonary embolism is suspected, however, there may be an underlying cardiopulmonary disorder that results in an abnormal perfusion lung scan even in the absence of pulmonary embolism. Such conditions include pneumonia, emphysema, pulmonary blebs, atelectasis, and congestive heart failure.[17] Although careful review of the chest roentgenogram and performance of a simultaneous ventilation lung scan frequently enhances the specificity of the perfusion lung scan in diagnosing pulmonary embolism, many patients with acute cardiopulmonary decompensation compatible with pulmonary embolism have underlying pulmonary parenchymal abnormalities that result in an "indeterminate" ventilation-perfusion lung scan, a study that does little to enhance the clinician's diagnostic certainty in confirming or excluding pulmonary embolism.

In a study of the accuracy of ventilation-perfusion scanning in the diagnosis of pulmonary embolism, the pulmonary angiograms of 55 patients with a clinical presentation consistent with pulmonary embolism were compared with their ventilation-perfusion scans.[15] The scans were assigned to one of four categories: normal, low probability, intermediate probability, and high probability of pulmonary embolism. Three patients had normal scans, and all three had normal pulmonary angiograms. Of 34 patients with "high-probability" ventilation-perfusion lung scans, only 22 (65%) had pulmonary emboli by angiogram; in contrast, of 18 patients with low or intermediate probability scans, 5 (28%) had positive angiograms. Thus, ventilation-perfusion lung scans do not have a high specificity for the diagnosis for pulmonary embolism.[15,16]

SYNDROMES OF PULMONARY EMBOLISM (TABLE 33–1)

Although the clinical and laboratory findings are usually nonspecific, pulmonary embolism frequently presents as one of four hemodynamically and clinically distinct syndromes. These include acute unexplained dyspnea, pulmonary infarction syndrome, acute cardiogenic shock with cor pulmonale, or chronic right ventricular failure with systemic congestion (from multiple unresolved pulmonary emboli).

Acute Unexplained Dyspnea

Acute unexplained dyspnea occurs characteristically in young or middle-aged patients with one or more predispositions to venous thromboembolic disease. Such predispositions include prolonged bed rest as a result of medical or surgical illness, underlying malignancy, use of estrogen-containing preparations (e.g., oral contraceptives), and trauma to the lower extremity. The clinical presentation almost always involves dyspnea and tachypnea of an abrupt onset. After careful clinical evaluation,

however, no obvious underlying cardiopulmonary disorder (e.g., congestive heart failure, pneumonia, atelectasis, pleural effusion, or pneumothorax) is readily identified to account for this presentation.

The pathophysiology of dyspnea resulting from pulmonary embolism has not been clearly established. Nearly 90% of patients with pulmonary embolism and no evidence of prior cardiopulmonary disease, however, have an arterial oxygen tension below 80 mmHg while breathing room air.[4] The mechanism primarily responsible for the development of arterial hypoxia after pulmonary embolism is ventilation/perfusion imbalance with an effective right-to-left shunt within the lungs.

The patient free of chronic cardiopulmonary disease but with acute unexplained dyspnea as the primary manifestation of pulmonary embolism usually demonstrates no reduction in cardiac output, no significant pulmonary hypertension, and no right ventricular failure as a result of the pulmonary embolism. Indeed, the severity of embolic pulmonary artery cross-sectional obstruction is usually less than 50%, the mean pulmonary artery pressure rarely exceeds 20 to 25 mmHg, and the cardiac index is usually elevated (rather than reduced) as a result of the tachycardia resulting from hypoxemia-induced stimulation of the sympathetic nervous system.[18]

Pulmonary Infarction Syndrome

Pathologically, pulmonary infarction represents necrosis of interalveolar septae, with dense alveolar hemorrhage. Fibrosis is prominent in the healing process, and resolution is accompanied by organization and scar formation. Clinically, the pulmonary infarction syndrome is manifested by fever, hemoptysis, pleurisy (with or without an audible pleural friction rub), rales, leukocytosis, and pulmonary infiltrate(s) on chest roentgenogram. Hemoptysis, rales, and the radiologic infiltrate(s) result from intra-alveolar hemorrhage. The pleural effusion is usually blood-tinged to frankly hemorrhagic and exudative in chemical composition. In the patient free of underlying cardiopulmonary disease, when the embolus resolves promptly and alveolar hemorrhage is not associated with necrosis of alveolar septae, healing is usually accompanied by complete resolution with no radiologic or pathologic evidence of scar formation. This is the picture of the so-called incomplete pulmonary infarction. If there is underlying cardiopulmonary disease, it is more likely that healing will be accompanied by scar formation.[19]

The pulmonary infarction syndrome probably results from embolic occlusion of small to moderate-sized pulmonary arteries proximal to the insertion of bronchial-artery-to-pulmonary-artery anastomoses. Sudden occlusion of such a vessel allows unimpeded inflow of blood at high pressure from the bronchial arterial anastomoses into the smaller pulmonary arteries distal to the site of embolic occlusion. Sudden inflow of blood at high pressure probably disrupts the small, thin-walled pulmonary arterial branches and results in alveolar hemorrhage.[7]

Hemodynamic findings in the pulmonary infarction syndrome include tachycardia with little or no pulmonary hypertension. This is not surprising because the emboli to medium-sized vessels causing the pulmonary infarction syndrome usually obstruct less than 50% of the total pulmonary vascular cross-sectional area. Tachycardia and an increased cardiac output result from increased sympathetic outflow, which may be caused by hypoxia and/or pleuritic chest pain. The cardiac output may also be elevated because of increased sympathetic stimulation.

Figure 33–1 illustrates the left lower lobe pulmonary angiogram in a woman who developed pleuritic chest pain, hemoptysis, and a left pleural effusion 8 days following surgery for myocardial revascularization and mitral valve replacement. There are vessel cut-offs and intraluminal filling defects, diagnostic of pulmonary embolism, in several medium-sized branches of the artery to the left lower lobe. Her clinical presentation illustrates the *pulmonary infarction syndrome*.

Cardiogenic Shock and Cor Pulmonale

The *hemodynamic consequences* of pulmonary embolism are determined primarily by

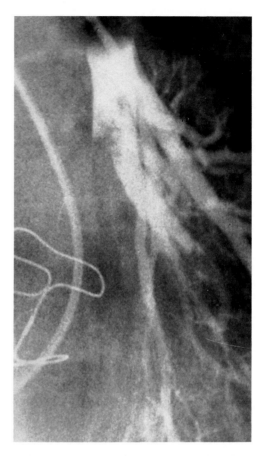

Fig. 33–1. Frame from a pulmonary cineangiogram performed by the technique of balloon occlusion in a woman who developed the pulmonary infarction syndrome following mitral valve replacement and coronary artery bypass surgery. The tip of the catheter is positioned in the most proximal segment of the artery to the left lower lobe, and the balloon has been inflated to a volume of 1.5 cc to occlude arterial inflow. The vessel is opacified selectively by a hand-powered injection of 7 ml of radiographic contrast agent. Multiple vessel cutoffs and intraluminal filling defects diagnostic of pulmonary embolism are visualized.

the size of the pulmonary embolus and whether or not the patient has underlying cardiopulmonary disease. In a patient previously free of cardiopulmonary disease, the hemodynamic impact of pulmonary embolism is related directly to the severity of pulmonary vascular cross-sectional obstruction engendered by the embolus.[6] Significant pulmonary hypertension (mean pulmonary artery pressure exceeding 25 mmHg) does not usually develop in such patients unless emboli obstruct at least 50% of the pulmonary vascular cross-sectional area. When 50 to 75% of the pulmonary arterial tree is obstructed, there is usually mild to moderate pulmonary hypertension (mean pulmonary artery pressure in the range of 25 to 40 mmHg), a normal to reduced pulmonary capillary wedge pressure, a normal or increased cardiac index, mild to moderate elevation in pulmonary vascular resistance (180 to 300 dynes-sec-cm^{-5}), and a normal mean right atrial pressure (<8 mmHg).

With *massive pulmonary embolism* (obstruction of the pulmonary arterial circulation in excess of 75%) and *acute cor pulmonale,* there is sinus tachycardia and the pulmonary artery mean pressure approaches 40 to 45 mmHg. The previously normal right ventricle cannot pump effectively against a pulmonary artery mean pressure elevated acutely to a level exceeding 40 to 45 mmHg. Instead, severe embolic obstruction of this magnitude is usually accompanied by right ventricular dilatation and failure with an increase in mean right atrial pressure to ≥10 mmHg. There is usually a precipitous reduction in stroke output; cardiac output is reduced as well, but to a lesser extent because of compensatory tachycardia. Mean arterial pressure is usually preserved through an adrenergically-mediated reflex increase in systemic vascular resistance. If the patient demonstrates evidence of impaired organ perfusion (confusion or agitation, cool diaphoretic skin, oliguria with elaboration of urine reduced in sodium concentration), the cardiac index is usually below 1.8 to 2 L/min/m^2, the systolic pressure is usually reduced, and the arterial pulse pressure is narrowed.

Figure 33–2 illustrates the pulmonary arteriogram of a patient with acute cor pulmonale. The patient was a 36-year-old man with phlebitis of the right leg, who fainted while having a bowel movement. The right pulmonary artery cineangiogram (Fig. 33–2) demonstrates intraluminal filling defects in the right middle and right upper lobe branches. Two proximal branches originating from the right lower lobe artery are nearly flush-occluded at their origins. Similar thrombi were present throughout the left lung. At the time

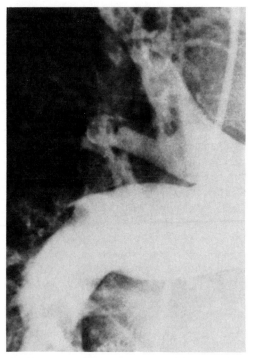

Fig. 33–2. A frame from a right pulmonary artery cineangiogram performed in a 36-year-old man with syncope from massive pulmonary embolism. The tip of an Eppendorf catheter has been positioned 2 to 3 cm proximal to the origin of the artery to the right upper lobe. Intraluminal filling defects diagnostic of pulmonary embolism are visualized in the proximal segments of the right upper and right middle lobe vessels. Although the proximal segment of the right lower lobe artery itself is free of thrombi, several of its proximal branches do not opacify because they are cut off by totally occlusive emboli.

of pulmonary angiography, the patient had markedly elevated right atrial (15 mmHg) and pulmonary artery pressures (65/35 mmHg). The mean pulmonary artery pressure was 45 mmHg. The cardiac index was severely depressed at 1.8 L/min/m^2, but systemic arterial blood pressure was preserved. This case exemplifies massive pulmonary embolism with acute right ventricular failure, a situation in which survival following another pulmonary embolism would be unlikely. Accordingly, he was treated with a thrombolytic agent to promote prompt resolution of the embolic pulmonary artery obstruction.[18,20] Later, an inferior vena cava filter was inserted to prevent subsequent pulmonary embolism.

Cardiogenic shock resulting from massive pulmonary embolism is manifested hemodynamically by tachycardia, a normal to reduced pulmonary capillary wedge pressure ($\leq$12 mmHg), a pulmonary artery mean pressure between 35 and 45 mmHg, an elevated pulmonary vascular resistance (above 500 dynes sec cm^{-5}), an elevated systemic vascular resistance ($>$1600 dynes sec cm^{-5}), right atrial pressure in excess of 10 mmHg, and arterial hypotension, or at least a tendency toward this, with narrowing of the arterial pulse pressure ($<$30 mmHg). Cardiac output is much reduced, and pulmonary arterial blood oxygen saturation is usually $\leq$50%.

The clinical manifestations of cardiogenic shock from pulmonary embolism include severe dyspnea and syncope or light-headedness. There may be chest pain, not necessarily of a pleuritic nature but of a more oppressive retrosternal quality. Objective findings include hypotension, tachycardia, cool and moist skin, central cyanosis, oliguria, mental clouding, jugular venous distention, and a thready arterial pulse. The cardiac examination may be surprisingly unremarkable; however, one should anticipate evidence of pulmonary hypertension. A widely but physiologically split second heart sound (resulting from prolonged right ventricular ejection) with the pulmonic component increased in intensity, a systolic ejection murmur at the base (because of dilatation of the pulmonary trunk) and a left parasternal lift (resulting from pressure overload of the right ventricle with right ventricular dilatation and failure) are commonly present.

The differential diagnosis of cardiogenic shock with an elevated central venous pressure includes cardiac tamponade and right ventricular infarction, in addition to pulmonary embolism. *Cardiac tamponade* is characterized by pulsus paradox and a right atrial pressure over 12 to 16 mmHg with near equalization of the right atrial, right ventricular diastolic, and pulmonary capillary wedge pressures. The pulmonary artery systolic pressure usually exceeds the right ventricular diastolic pressure by no more than 10 mmHg. *Right ventricular infarction* with shock is characterized by a depressed cardiac index ($<$1.8 L/min/m^2), a right atrial mean pressure over 10 mmHg, arterial hypotension, and a mean pulmonary artery and pulmonary artery wedge pressure that usually exceeds right atrial pressure by less than 3 to 5 mmHg. An important hemodynamic differential point is that, with cardiac tamponade or right ventricular infarction, the mean pulmonary artery pressure is usually less than 25 mmHg; however, with massive pulmonary embolism the mean pulmonary artery pressure usually exceeds 35 to 40 mmHg.

Although pulsus paradox is characteristic of cardiac tamponade, occurring in over 90% of patients, it has also been reported in patients with massive pulmonary embolism.[21] A helpful differential point between pulmonary embolism and tamponade is found on the echocardiogram, which almost always demonstrates an anterior and posterior clear space in cardiac tamponade suggestive of a large pericardial effusion. Also, the echocardiogram shows a decrease in the right ventricular end-diastolic dimension during the inspiratory phase of the respiratory cycle in cardiac tamponade because of cardiac compression. These findings are not present in pulmonary embolism, in which the right ventricular chamber is usually dilated.

The findings on bedside hemodynamic monitoring may be somewhat confusing in patients with massive pulmonary embolism, particularly regarding the pulmonary artery phasic pressure as monitored by a flow-directed balloon-tipped catheter. The catheter tip may occasionally engage the soft gelatinous surface of the pulmonary embolus with intermittent damping or loss of the phasic pulmonary artery pressure wave form. Should the catheter intermittently record a very damped pulmonary artery pressure corresponding reasonably well to the previously measured mean pulmonary pressure and catheter manipulation or vigorous flushing restore a more physiologic phasic pulmonary arterial pressure, one should consider intermittent catheter obstruction by in situ thrombus or pulmonary embolus. If the distal thermistor electrode of a thermodilution catheter in the pulmonary artery is intermittently embedded in the thrombus, it will be partially insulated from the injectate bolus delivered to measure cardiac output, and thermodilution cardiac output measurements may be falsely elevated, fluctuating, and inconsistent with other measures of cardiac output (e.g., pulmonary artery blood oxygen saturation).

Unresolved Pulmonary Embolism

Although in an earlier series it was noted that fewer than 1 to 3% of patients fail to demonstrate hemodynamic and angiographic resolution of abnormalities following acute pulmonary embolism,[22] there have been reports of chronic pulmonary hypertension and cor pulmonale resulting from chronic and unresolved pulmonary embolism.[8,23] The clinical manifestations usually suggest pulmonary hypertension. Findings may include dyspnea, orthopnea, cardiomegaly with right ventricular dilatation and failure, distended neck veins, pleural effusions, edema and ascites, and a history compatible with previous thrombophlebitis or pulmonary embolism. The chest roentgenograms usually demonstrate cardiomegaly, dilatation of one or more proximal pulmonary arteries, and pleural effusions. In patients with clinically manifest right ventricular failure, the electrocardiogram almost always demonstrates right ventricular hypertrophy. The perfusion lung scan characteristically reveals segmental, lobar, or whole lung perfusion defects suggesting obstruction in the most proximal segments of at least two or three pulmonary arteries.[24] Although this syndrome is uncommon, it is an important consideration in the evaluation of patients with unexplained

pulmonary hypertension because thromboembolectomy with pulmonary end-arterectomy often can be successful in such cases.[8,23]

Table 33–2 depicts the hemodynamic findings at rest and during supine bicycle exercise in a patient with chronic bilateral pulmonary embolism before and after pulmonary embolectomy. Although the mean pulmonary artery pressure at rest was only minimally elevated, it more than doubled with exercise, and the mean right atrial pressure rose to 15 mmHg. Following pulmonary embolectomy, the patient's dyspnea resolved. The pulmonary artery pressure and pulmonary vascular resistance were reduced at rest and during exercise, compatible with partial relief of the embolic pulmonary vascular obstruction. Figure 33–3 demonstrates the perfusion lung scans and angiograms in this patient before and after embolectomy of a right pulmonary artery thromboembolism. Embolectomy resulted in improved perfusion to the right lung, although segmental defects persisted in the right middle lobe and apex. The postembolectomy pulmonary angiogram demonstrates absence of thrombus in the right main pulmonary artery and improved flow to the right middle, right lower, and left lower lobe arteries.

HEMODYNAMICS OF PULMONARY EMBOLISM IN PATIENTS WITH UNDERLYING CARDIOPULMONARY DISEASE

The hemodynamic impact of pulmonary embolism in patients with underlying cardiopulmonary disease is somewhat different from the effects of pulmonary embolism in patients with

Table 33–2. *Hemodynamic Findings in a Patient with Unresolved Pulmonary Embolism*

		RA	PA	PCW	CO/CI	PVR
Before	Rest	4	38/14 (22)	9	3.7/1.8	281
embolectomy	Exercise	15	101/32 (55)	15	7.2/3.5	444
After	Rest	1	26/8 (16)	8	4.1/2.0	156
embolectomy	Exercise	6	65/20 (40)	21	8.6/4.1	177

RA = mean right atrial pressure (mmHg): PA = pulmonary artery pressure (mmHg), systolic/diastolic (mean); PCW = mean pulmonary artery wedge pressure (mmHg): CO = cardiac output (L/min); CI = cardiac index (L/min/M²); PVR = pulmonary vascular resistance (dynes-sec-cm⁻⁵).

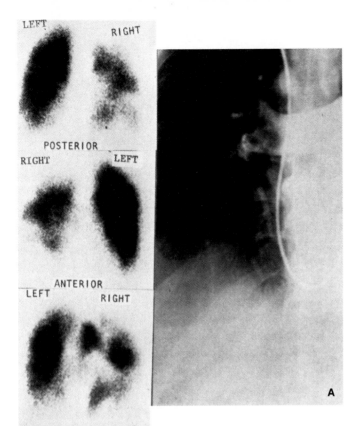

LEFT   RIGHT

POSTERIOR

RIGHT   LEFT

ANTERIOR

LEFT   RIGHT

RIGHT POSTERIOR OBLIQUE

A

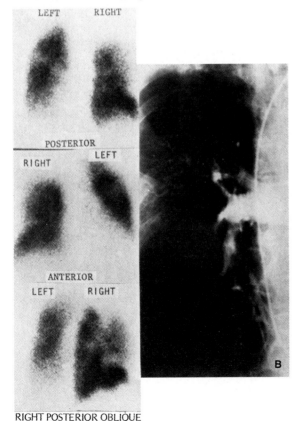

LEFT   RIGHT

POSTERIOR

RIGHT   LEFT

ANTERIOR

LEFT   RIGHT

RIGHT POSTERIOR OBLIQUE

B

Fig. 33–3. A, Pre-embolectomy perfusion scan (left) and right pulmonary artery angiogram (right) in a patient with severe dyspnea on exertion and unresolved pulmonary embolism. The lung scan reveals several segmental and lobar perfusion defects, more prominent in the right lung. The pulmonary angiogram demonstrates virtually absent flow to the right lung. The hemodynamic findings in this patient are depicted in Table 33–2. B, Perfusion lung scan (left) and pulmonary angiogram (right) in the same patient, following pulmonary thrombectomy and endarterectomy. The lung scan demonstrates improved perfusion to the right lung, although segmental defects persist in the right middle lobe and apex. The pulmonary angiogram reveals that the right main pulmonary artery embolus is no longer present and the arteries to the right middle and right lower lobes are better opacified.

normal underlying cardiopulmonary reserve. Patients with underlying cardiopulmonary disease (whether due to chronic left atrial hypertension from coronary, mitral, or aortic valve disease or as a result of pulmonary parenchymal destruction from chronic obstructive lung disease) usually have a reduction in pulmonary vascular cross-sectional area. That is, with any increase in pulmonary blood flow (e.g., with exercise) or with any further reduction in pulmonary cross-sectional area (e.g., due to pulmonary embolism or hypoxia-induced pulmonary vasoconstriction) pulmonary hypertension will develop because pulmonary vascular reserve has been exhausted by the underlying disease process. Such patients may develop severe pulmonary hypertension during exercise, even when the pulmonary artery pressure is normal with the patient at rest. Exercise-induced pulmonary hypertension may also result in some degree of right ventricular hypertrophy in the patient with underlying prior cardiopulmonary disease, so that superimposed acute pulmonary embolism is likely to evoke more severe pulmonary hypertension than pulmonary embolism of similar size in the patient without prior cardiopulmonary disease.

Because of the development of right ventricular hypertrophy as a result of exercise-induced pulmonary hypertension, the patient with underlying cardiopulmonary disease is usually able to develop a mean pulmonary artery pressure well above 40 to 45 mmHg without developing right ventricular dilatation and failure. Thus, a patient with pulmonary embolism demonstrating a mean pulmonary artery pressure exceeding 50 mmHg likely has underlying chronic cardiopulmonary disease that has already resulted in intermittent pulmonary hypertension with consequent right ventricular hypertrophy before the acute event.

REFERENCES

1. Stein PD, Willis PW III, DeMeto DL: History and physical examination in acute pulmonary embolism in patients without prior cardiopulmonary disease. Am J Cardiol 47:218, 1981.
2. Lippman M, Fein A: Pulmonary embolism in the patient with chronic obstructive pulmonary disease. Chest 79:38, 1981.
3. Szucs MM, et al: Diagnostic sensitivity of laboratory findings in acute pulmonary embolism. Ann Intern Med 74:171, 1971.
4. Dantzker DR, Bower JS: Alterations in gas exchange following pulmonary thromboembolism. Chest 81:485, 1982.
5. Jardin F, et al: Hemodynamic factors influencing arterial hypoxemia in massive pulmonary embolism with circulatory failure. Circulation 59:909, 1978.
6. McIntyre KM, Sasahara AA: The hemodynamic response to pulmonary embolism in patients without prior cardiopulmonary disease. Am J Cardiol 28:288, 1971.
7. Dalen JE, et al: Pulmonary embolism: pulmonary hemorrhage and pulmonary infarction. N Engl J Med 296:1431, 1977.
8. Rich S, Levitsky S, Brundage BH: Pulmonary hypertension from chronic pulmonary thromboembolism. Ann Intern Med 108:425, 1988.
9. Stein PD, et al: The electrocardiogram in acute pulmonary embolism. Prog Cardiovasc Dis 17:247, 1975.
10. McGinn S, White PD: Acute cor pulmonale resulting from pulmonary embolism. JAMA 104:1473, 1935.
11. Sasahara AA, Sharma GVRK, Parisi AF: New developments in the detection and prevention of venous thromboembolism. Am J Cardiol 43:1214, 1979.
12. Hull RD, et al: Pulmonary angiography, ventilation lung scanning and venography for clinically suspected pulmonary embolism with abnormal perfusion lung scan. Ann Intern Med 98:891, 1983.
13. Jeffrey PC, Immelman EJ, Benetar SR: Deep-vein thrombosis and pulmonary embolism—an assessment of the accuracy of clinical diagnosis. S Afr Med 57:643, 1980.
14. Moser KM, Lemoine JR: Is embolic risk conditioned by location of deep venous thrombosis? Ann Intern Med 94:438, 1981.
15. Caracci BF, et al: How accurate are ventilation-perfusion scans for pulmonary embolism? Am J Surg 156:477, 1988.
16. McBride K, LaMorte WW, Menzoian JO: Can ventilation-perfusion scans accurately diagnose pulmonary embolism? Arch Surg 121:754, 1986.
17. Newman GE, et al: Scintigraphic perfusion patterns in patients with diffuse lung disease. Radiology 143:227, 1982.
18. A National Cooperative Study: Urokinase pulmonary embolism trial. Circulation 47, April 1973. 47(Suppl. II):1–108, 1973.
19. Hampton AO, Castleman B: Correlation of postmortem chest teleroentgenograms with autopsy findings with special reference to pulmonary embolism and infarction. Am J Roentgenol 43:305, 1940.
20. Goldhaber SZ et al: Randomized controlled trial of recombinant tissue plasminogen activator versus urokinase in the treatment of acute pulmonary embolism. Lancet 2:293, 1988.
21. Cohen SI, et al: Pulsus paradox and Kussmaul's sign in acute pulmonary embolism. Am J Cardiol 32:271, 1973.
22. Dalen JE, Banas JS, Brooks HL, et al: Resolution

rate of acute pulmonary embolism in man. N Engl J Med 280:1194, 1969.

23. Benotti JR, Ockene IS, Alpert JS, Dalen JE: The clinical profile of unresolved pulmonary embolism. Chest 84:669, 1983.

24. Fishman AJ, Moser KM, Fedullo PF: Perfusion lung scans vs. pulmonary angiography in evaluation of suspected primary pulmonary hypertension. Chest 54:678, 1983.

34

Profiles in Dilated (Congestive) and Hypertrophic Cardiomyopathies

WILLIAM GROSSMAN

Cardiomyopathies are primary disorders of heart muscle. Although the term cardiomyopathy is sometimes restricted to refer to cardiac muscle disorders of unknown etiology,[1] most cardiologists include disorders of both unknown and known etiology. For example, the cardiac muscle disorder associated with long-standing ingestion of excessive quantities of ethanol is generally termed alcoholic cardiomyopathy, and that disorder resulting from high-dose doxorubicin therapy for malignancy is called doxorubicin or adriamycin cardiomyopathy.

In general, cardiomyopathies are classified descriptively, as listed in Table 34–1. In this chapter, I shall discuss only the first two types of cardiomyopathy listed in Table 34–1. Restrictive cardiomyopathy is discussed in Chapter 35, along with constrictive pericarditis, with which it is often confused. Obliterative cardiomyopathy is extremely rare in the United States and is beyond the scope of this book.

DILATED (CONGESTIVE) CARDIOMYOPATHY

The clinical syndrome of dilated cardiomyopathy represents a collection of disorders and is also called congestive cardiomyopathy. The term *congestive cardiomyopathy* was in-

troduced initially by Goodwin[2] because the clinical presentation is marked primarily by peripheral and pulmonary edema. Subsequently, Goodwin and associates have preferred the term *dilated cardiomyopathy*, because with current diagnostic techniques (echocardiography, radionuclide ventriculography) it has become possible to diagnose this syndrome before the onset of clinical signs and symptoms of congestion. Also, with effective diuretic and vasodilator management, the congestive component may be eliminated and ventricular filling pressures may be returned to normal. The ventricular chambers remain *dilated*, however, with increased end-systolic and end-diastolic volumes and reduced ventricular ejection fraction.

Cardiac Catheterization Protocol

Study of the patient who is suspected of having dilated cardiomyopathy should include right and left heart catheterization with measurement of pressures, cardiac output, and resistances. As is our routine for right heart catheterization (Chapters 4 and 5), oxygen saturation is measured routinely in blood taken from the superior vena cava and pulmonary artery to detect unsuspected right-to-left shunting. Angiographic studies will need to be tai-

Table 34–1. *Descriptive Classification of Cardiomyopathies*

I. *Dilated (Congestive) Cardiomyopathy:* dilated ventricular chambers with increased end-diastolic and end-systolic volumes and decreased ventricular ejection fraction
  A. Idiopathic
  B. Post-myocarditis
  C. Toxic; 2° to ethanol, doxorubicin, uremia
  D. Peripartum
  E. Chronic overload (e.g., long-standing severe volume overload, untreated hypertension)
  F. Congenital
  G. Miscellaneous (diabetes, autoimmune disease, sarcoid)

II. *Hypertrophic Cardiomyopathy:* hypertrophic ventricular chambers with normal volumes and generally normal contractile function
  A. Asymmetric septal hypertrophy
  B. Apical hypertrophic cardiomyopathy
  C. Diffuse symmetric hypertrophy

III. *Restrictive Cardiomyopathy:* normal ventricular volumes and contractile function, but increased resistance to diastolic filling
  A. Infiltrative type: amyloidosis, hemochromatosis, Fabry's disease
  B. Idiopathic
  C. Diffuse fibrosis (e.g., post-myocarditis, diffuse nontransmural myocardial infarction)

IV. *Obliterative Cardiomyopathy*
  A. Eosinophilic endomyocardial fibroelastosis

lored to the individual case, but left ventriculography and coronary angiography are commonly done as a part of the study in such patients.

Hemodynamic Findings. In the symptomatic patient with dilated cardiomyopathy referred for cardiac catheterization, *left and right ventricular filling pressures* are usually elevated. As mentioned, however, it is possible that the ventricular filling pressures at rest may be normal; this finding is particularly likely in the asymptomatic patient detected early in the course of his disease by noninvasive screening. Also, the patient who has been treated intensively with diuretics (e.g., furosemide and spironolactone) and who is receiving a potent vasodilator (e.g., captopril) may show little or no elevation in resting filling pressures. In general, increases in left and right ventricular filling pressures can be induced easily in such patients by *supine bicycle exercise,* performed as outlined in Chapter 17. With 6 minutes of supine bicycle exercise, pulmonary capillary wedge pressure commonly rises from 10 mmHg to 25 to 40 mmHg, and right atrial pressure increases from 6 mmHg to 15 to 20 mmHg. Supine bicycle exercise provides an acute volume and pressure load on the ventricular myocardium and easily brings out underlying loss of contractile reserve.

Cardiac output is generally reduced in the patient with dilated cardiomyopathy. In the milder cases, the cardiac index may be normal or only slightly reduced and may range from 2.4 to 3.0 L/min/M². In patients with NYHA Class III or IV symptoms from dilated cardiomyopathy, it is common to find the cardiac index depressed more severely. Thus, a cardiac index of 1.6 to 2.3 L/min/M² can be expected in the usual symptomatic patient presenting with dilated cardiomyopathy, and a cardiac index of ≤ 1.5 L/min/M² indicates an advanced depression of myocardial function and a poor prognosis.

The *left ventricular pressure tracing* is typically abnormal in patients with dilated cardiomyopathy. Both the rate of rise and the rate of fall of left ventricular pressure are slow, and this is usually visible to the naked eye (Fig. 34–1). Slowing of the left ventricular pressure upstroke and downstroke gives a *triangular appearance* to the pressure tracing, with the peak systolic pressure representing the apex of the triangle; end-diastolic and minimal (early)-

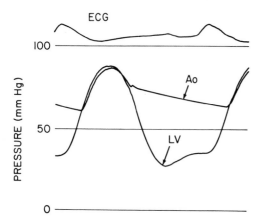

Fig. 34–1. Left ventricular (LV) micromanometer and aortic (Ao) pressure tracings in a 68-year-old woman with advanced dilated cardiomyopathy. Marked slowing of the rates of left ventricular pressure rise and fall give the LV pressure tracing a triangular appearance. Also, the minimal value for left ventricular diastolic pressure is markedly elevated.

diastolic left ventricular pressures define the triangle's base. This deformity accounts for the brief duration of systolic ejection in dilated cardiomyopathy and contrasts with the trapezoidal, almost square-wave appearance of left ventricular pressure in a normal, vigorous heart. A corollary of the triangular wave-form of left ventricular pressure in dilated cardiomyopathy is a normal or low peak systolic pressure.

A second abnormality of the left ventricular pressure tracing in dilated cardiomyopathy is elevation in the value for left ventricular minimal diastolic pressure (Fig. 34–1). Normally, the left ventricular pressure declines briskly after aortic valve closure, reaching a nadir close to 0 mmHg shortly after mitral valve opening. This reflects the normal pattern of rapid myocardial relaxation, acting together with *restoring forces* generated by a vigorous systolic contraction, with end-systolic elastic compression and torsion forces being released during early diastolic filling. In the experimental laboratory under conditions of extremely vigorous contraction (e.g., isoproterenol infusion), or hypovolemia (e.g., hemorrhage), the left ventricular diastolic pressure may actually become negative early in diastole, a phenomenon known as *diastolic*

suction. In dilated cardiomyopathy, diastolic relaxation is generally slow and incomplete,[3] and restoring forces produced by the weakened systolic contraction are minimal. These factors militate against a normal low value for left ventricular minimal diastolic pressure. In addition, end-systolic volume is increased in patients with dilated cardiomyopathy, and this abnormality tends to elevate diastolic volume and pressure above normal.

To appreciate these abnormalities in the left ventricular pressure waveform in dilated cardiomyopathy, one must have pressure tracings of good quality with careful attention to the details discussed in Chapter 9. Micromanometer catheters are not necessary to achieve such high quality tracings, as can be seen in Figure 34–2, where fluid-filled and micromanometer tracings are superimposed.

The left ventricular pressure tracing abnormalities just described can be corrected substantially by acute administration of an inotropic drug.[4-6] Figures 34–2 and 34–3 illustrate the effects of a phosphodiesterase inhibitor (milrinone) and a beta-adrenergic agonist (prenalterol) on the left ventricular pressure contour in patients with dilated cardiomyopathy. As can be seen, early diastolic relaxation is more rapid and more complete after administration of these drugs, as reflected by the steep decline in left ventricular pressure to a value near zero in early diastole.

Patients with dilated cardiomyopathy often have elevations in pulmonary and systemic vascular resistance. It is common to find pulmonary vascular resistance increased to 150 to 300 dynes-sec-cm^{-5}, and patients with values >400 dynes-sec-cm^{-5} are not rare. These increases in pulmonary vascular resistance result in pulmonary hypertension with mean pulmonary artery pressure commonly 30 to 50 mmHg. Systemic vascular resistance is usually ≧1500 dynes-sec-cm^{-5} in untreated patients with advanced dilated cardiomyopathy, probably representing a response to combined elevations in serum levels of angiotensin, vasopressin, and norepinephrine. Because cardiac output is reduced, modest increases in systemic vascular resistance do not result in

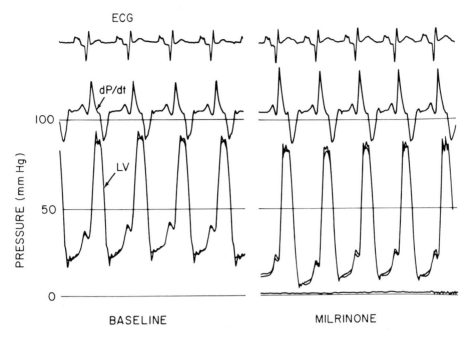

Fig. 34–2. Left ventricular (LV) micromanometer pressure and its first derivative (dP/dt) in a patient with dilated cardiomyopathy before (left) and after (right) intravenous infusion of milrinone. Positive and negative dP/dt have increased without increase in arterial pressure and with a decline in preload, suggesting increased myocardial contractility and relaxation. Left ventricular minimal diastolic pressure is now closer to zero, as is normal. Fluid-filled and micromanometer pressures are displayed simultaneously, indicating the excellent fidelity that can be achieved with fluid-filled systems using the principles described in Chapter 9. (Reproduced with permission from Baim DS, et al: Evaluation of a new bipyridine inotropic agent—milrinone—in patients with severe congestive heart failure. N Engl J Med 309:748, 1983.)

actual elevation of arterial blood pressure, but rather tend to preserve arterial pressure at a normal or only slightly reduced level.

Reduction of systemic and pulmonary vascular resistances to normal by administration of vasodilator agents often results in a striking increase in cardiac output and a simultaneous reduction in left and right ventricular filling pressures. As shown in Figure 34–4, acute administration of sodium nitroprusside[7,8] or captopril[9–11] results in an upward and leftward displacement of the left ventricular filling pressure-stroke volume relationship, since heart rate is affected minimally by these agents in the setting of chronic heart failure.

During cardiac catheterization in patients with dilated cardiomyopathy, it is often wise to test responsiveness to a vasodilator in the laboratory. In my own practice, I do this routinely using the following protocol. After measurement of cardiac output and resting hemodynamics and before angiography, if fill-

ing pressures are elevated significantly (e.g., pulmonary capillary wedge pressure ≥ 16 mmHg) and cardiac output is depressed (e.g., pulmonary artery blood O_2 saturation $\leq 65\%$), I begin an infusion of sodium nitroprusside as long as arterial systolic pressure is > 90 mmHg and has been stable. The starting dose is 15 micrograms/min through a secure, free-flowing intravenous line, and the infusion rate is increased every 3 to 5 minutes to doses of 25, 50, 75, 100, 150, 200, and 300 micrograms/min, if needed, until arterial mean pressure has fallen 10 to 20 mmHg or wedge pressure has fallen by $\geq 50\%$, or pulmonary artery O_2 saturation has increased to $\geq 75\%$. Usually, one of these three end points is achieved at a dose of sodium nitroprusside ≤ 200 micrograms/min; however, I have had occasional patients in whom > 300 micrograms/min were required. If the patient is feeling well during the vasodilator infusion (as is generally the case), I continue the infusion during left ven-

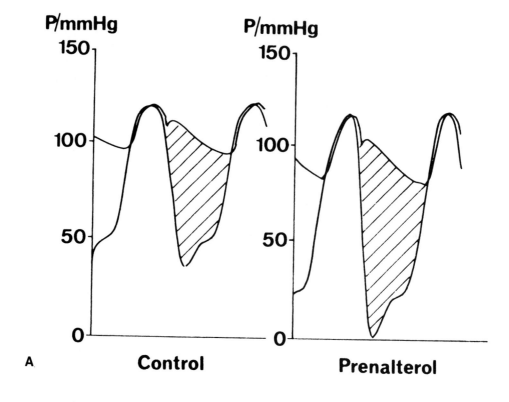

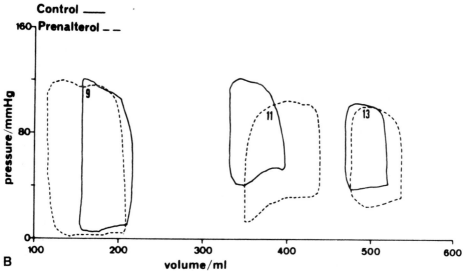

Fig. 34–3. Effects of the beta agonist prenalterol on left ventricular and aortic pressure (A) and left ventricular pressure-volume plots (B) in patients with idiopathic dilated cardiomyopathy. The tracings illustrate the restoration of a normal low value for the left ventricular diastolic pressure nadir, as well as a downward shift in the diastolic pressure volume relationship. (Reproduced with permission from Erbel R, et al: Hemodynamic effects of prenalterol in patients with ischemic heart disease and congestive cardiomyopathy. Circulation 66:361, 1982.)

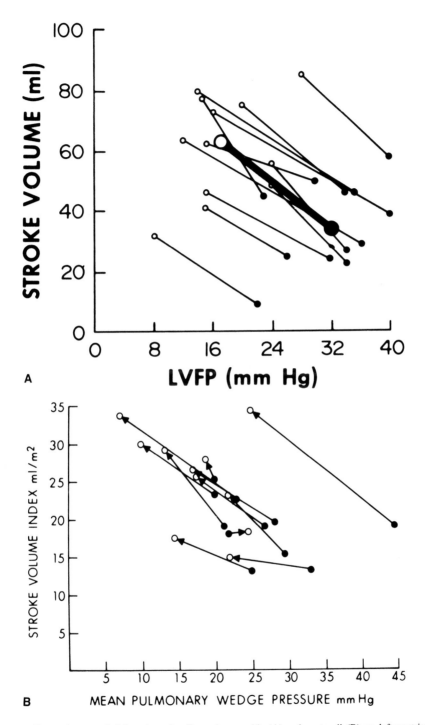

Fig. 34–4. Effects of acute administration of sodium nitroprusside (A) and captopril (B) on left ventricular filling pressure-stoke volume relationships in patients with advanced heart failure. Some of these patients had heart failure on the basis of idiopathic dilated cardiomyopathy, and some had ischemic heart disease. Responses were similar and appeared to be independent of etiology. See text for discussion. (Reproduced with permission from Guiha NH, et al: Treatment of refractory heart failure with infusion of nitroprusside. N Engl J Med 291:587, 1974. (A); and Davis R, et al: Treatment of chronic congestive heart failure with captopril, an oral inhibitor of angiotensin-converting enzyme. N Engl J Med 301:117, 1979 (B).)

triculography and coronary angiography, as a prophylactic measure to protect against pulmonary edema. The dose may have to be reduced if the arterial systolic pressure is ≤ 80 mmHg. A favorable response to sodium nitroprusside in the cardiac catheterization laboratory is not only an aid to the safety of the procedure, but also predicts a favorable response to an oral vasodilator (e.g., captopril) in the patient's long-term management.

Angiographic Studies. Left ventriculography in patients with dilated cardiomyopathy classically reveals extensive hypokinesis. This is usually diffuse in nature, but commonly there are regional wall motion abnormalities that suggest a heterogeneity of the myocardial injury and mimic coronary artery disease. This may represent the consequence of asymmetric injury initially, and in this regard it is of interest that myocarditis may be focal in its inflammatory effects. We have seen several patients in whom biopsy-proven acute myocarditis mimicked regional ischemia and infarction, with left ventriculography showing discrete areas of akinesis or even focal aneurysm formation. These areas of regional dysfunction could also represent the result of coronary emboli from mural thrombus because the occurrence of left ventricular mural thrombus is increased in patients with dilated cardiomyopathy.

Kreulen et al described the angiographic abnormalities associated with dilated cardiomyopathy and pointed out that the dilatation is associated with loss of the normal eccentric shape of the left ventricle.[12] Normally, the ratio of long axis (L) to minor axis (M) is 2:1 for the left ventricular chamber at end-diastole. In dilated cardiomyopathy, L/M approaches 1:1. This change tends to increase meridional wall stress (see Chap. 19) but has an unpredictable effect on longitudinal wall stress, depending on the extent of associated ventricular hypertrophy. In this regard, left ventricular hypertrophy is common in patients with dilated cardiomyopathy.[13] Some authors have reported a substantial beneficial effect of hypertrophy on survival in patients with dilated cardiomyopathy and have suggested that pro-

tection against increasing wall stress might have a protective role for these patients.[13,14]

Endomyocardial Biopsy. Enthusiasm for obtaining endomyocardial biopsy as a part of the diagnostic work-up in patients with suspected dilated cardiomyopathy has been increasing, and at our institution we have shared this enthusiasm. Endomyocardial biopsy is done almost routinely in our laboratory as part of the diagnostic study in patients with advanced heart failure. In over 100 endomyocardial biopsies in nontransplant patients, we found specific heart muscle disorders (inflammatory myocarditis, amyloidosis, hemochromatosis) in approximately 15% of cases. The technique of endomyocardial biopsy and additional specific diseases it can detect is described in detail in Chapter 23. In one study of 100 consecutive endomyocardial biopsies carried out to evaluate heart failure of uncertain etiology,[15] the pathologic information obtained was judged to be clinically useful in 54 patients and not useful in 46 patients. Specific diagnoses that could be made from histologic examination of the biopsy material included inflammatory myocarditis, amyloidosis, sarcoidosis, scleroderma, endomyocardial fibrosis with eosinophilia, doxorubicin cardiomyopathy, radiation-induced cardiomyopathy, and vasculitis.[15]

In summary, a variety of hemodynamic, angiographic, and histologic features can be defined precisely in the course of a single diagnostic cardiac catheterization procedure in patients with suspected dilated cardiomyopathy. Findings from such a study yield valuable information about prognosis[13-17] and help direct appropriate therapy.

HYPERTROPHIC CARDIOMYOPATHY

Cardiac hypertrophy develops to some extent in a wide variety of cardiac diseases. In hypertrophic cardiomyopathy, however, the development of cardiac hypertrophy proceeds without an obvious inciting stimulus or develops out of proportion to the magnitude of the stimulus or stimuli that can be identified.[1,18] While it is commonly regarded as a genetic disorder,[1] many cases appear to be sporadic. Most authors distinguish between obstructive and nonobstructive forms of the disorder, based on the presence or absence of a resting (unprovoked) systolic pressure gradient within the left ventricle,[18] and the presence of a gradient has caused this disorder to be called idiopathic hypertrophic subaortic stenosis (IHSS) or muscular subaortic stenosis (MSS). There remains a great deal of controversy as to whether true "obstruction" occurs in this condition[1,19] because there is some evidence that most of the left ventricular stroke volume has been ejected before development of a significant gradient. There is general agreement, however, that the pressure gradient, when present, has several adverse consequences, including increased systolic wall stress (in cardiac muscle proximal to the site of septal-mitral leaflet contact) and increased myocardial oxygen consumption.

Hypertrophic cardiomyopathy may be diffuse and symmetric, involving all regions of the left ventricle equally, or it may be *asymmetric*. Asymmetric hypertrophic cardiomyopathy commonly involves the high interventricular septum, which is disproportionately hypertrophied so that the ratio of thickness of the diastolic septal wall to thickness of the free (lateral or posterior) left ventricular wall is >1.3. Another form of asymmetric hypertrophic cardiomyopathy, which has been reported from Japan,[20] involves massive apical hypertrophy of the left ventricle. A characteristic electrocardiographic feature is the presence of giant negative T waves in the precordial leads. The apical form of hypertrophic cardiomyopathy has now been recognized to occur in Europe and North America.[21,22]

Hemodynamic Findings. As in the patient with suspected dilated cardiomyopathy, cardiac catheterization in the patient being evaluated for hypertrophic cardiomyopathy should include right and left heart study. Right atrial and right ventricular pressures are usually normal in patients with hypertrophic cardiomyopathy. Rarely, involvement of the right ventricle is said to result in a systolic gradient within the right ventricular chamber, although I have never seen such a case personally. If the hypertrophic process involves the right ventricle, or if the pulmonary capillary wedge pressure is substantially elevated, right ventricular diastolic pressures may be elevated.

Left ventricular end diastolic pressure may be normal in patients with hypertrophic cardiomyopathy but is usually elevated,[18–20] reflecting decreased left ventricular diastolic distensibility. The decreased diastolic distensibility in hypertrophic cardiomyopathy is caused by both increased passive stiffness of the thick-walled left ventricular chamber and decreased rate and extent of myocardial relaxation.[1,23–28] Pulmonary capillary wedge pressure may be elevated, particularly if there is mitral regurgitation, a common finding in patients with hypertrophic cardiomyopathy.[29]

Cardiac output is usually normal or increased in patients with hypertrophic cardiomyopathy, except in the late stages of the disease, when contractility decreases.

The most dramatic hemodynamic features of hypertrophic cardiomyopathy are those related to the systolic intraventricular pressure gradient. As seen in Figure 34–5, the pressure gradient is present between the body and the outflow tract of the left ventricle. A key feature of this systolic gradient and of most of the associated findings is their variability. Most patients with hypertrophic cardiomyopathy do not have a systolic pressure gradient at rest, but may develop one with appropriate provocative maneuvers as listed in Table 34–2.

It should be emphasized that the presence of a systolic gradient at rest or following provocation is a hallmark of only one variety of hypertrophic cardiomyopathy: that form with asymmetric septal hypertrophy. The diffuse hypertrophic variety and the variety associated with massive apical hypertrophy do not exhibit systolic gradients at rest or with provocation.[20]

An interesting aspect of the systolic gradient is an associated deformity that develops in the aortic pressure waveform. This deformity consists of an initial rapid rise in aortic pressure to give a spike early in ejection, followed by a dip in pressure and a secondary rounded or

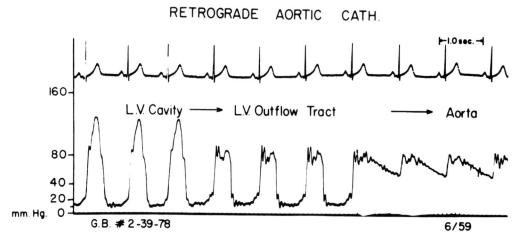

Fig. 34–5. Left ventricular (LV) catheter pullback to the aorta in a patient with hypertrophic cardiomyopathy. There is a significant systolic gradient within the left ventricular cavity, and the LV outflow tract and aortic pressure waveforms exhibit a spike-and-dome contour. (Reproduced with permission from Braunwald E, et al: Idiopathic hypertrophic subaortic stenosis. A description based on an analysis of 65 patients. Circulation 30 (Suppl 4):3, 1964.)

Table 34–2. *Provocative Maneuvers for Development of Systolic Pressure Gradient in Hypertrophic Cardiomyopathy*

1. Valsalva maneuver
2. Amyl nitrite inhalation
3. Postextrasystolic potentiation
4. Isoproterenol
5. Exercise

dome-shaped tidal wave before the dicrotic notch. This spike-and-dome configuration is seen in the central aortic pressure and is transmitted to the carotid pulse and peripheral arterial tracings. It is most evident following an extrasystolic contraction (Fig. 34–6) but is also seen during Valsalva maneuver (Fig. 34–7) and at other times (Fig. 34–8). The mechanism for this spike-and-dome configuration may be related to blending of an initial hyperdynamic ejection velocity leading to the development of a Venturi effect that sucks the anterior mitral leaflet into the outflow tract, thereby impeding mid and late diastolic ejection velocity.

In addition to developing a spike-and-dome pattern, the aortic pulse pressure fails to widen in a postextrasystolic potentiated beat.[18] Normally, a potentiated left ventricular contraction has a larger stroke volume than the preceding sinus beats, and this increased stroke volume

is reflected in an increased aortic pulse pressure. Patients with hypertrophic cardiomyopathy, however, develop a spike-and-dome configuration in which pulse pressure is unchanged or actually reduced following an extrasystolic beat (Fig. 34–6). This sign, which was described by Brockenbrough, Braunwald, and Morrow in 1961,[30] is believed to reflect worsening of obstruction of the left ventricular outflow tract during the potentiated beat, with diminished stroke volume and aortic pulse pressure.

The impaired left ventricular diastolic relaxation seen in hypertrophic cardiomyopathy[23–28] can be dramatic and can affect the contour of the left ventricular diastolic pressure tracing (Fig. 34–9). The patient illustrated in Figure 34–9 was a 55-year-old woman with a family history of hypertrophic cardiomyopathy, who presented with advanced congestive heart failure manifested by paroxysmal nocturnal dyspnea, marked fatigue, and peripheral edema. Echocardiogram showed asymmetric septal hypertrophy. At cardiac catheterization, there was no outflow tract gradient at rest or with provocation. Right atrial mean pressure was increased (11 mmHg), reflecting pulmonary hypertension (60/30, 40 mmHg), which in turn reflected a markedly increased mean pulmonary capillary

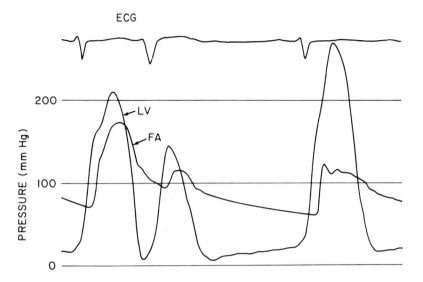

Fig. 34–6. Left ventricular (LV) and femoral artery (FA) pressure tracings in a woman with hypertrophic cardiomyopathy and asymmetric septal hypertrophy, illustrating the increase in gradient and development of a spike-and-dome configuration in the arterial pressure waveform following an extrasystolic beat. Also, arterial pulse pressure clearly narrows in the postextrasystolic beat compared to the control value in the beat before the extrasystole. This narrowing of pulse pressure is known as the Brockenbrough-Braunwald sign.

wedge pressure (32 mmHg). Arteriovenous O_2 difference was wide (71 ml O_2/liter), and cardiac index was depressed (2.0 L/min/M²). Left ventricular ejection fraction was reduced at 41%, a finding sometimes seen in late-stage hypertrophic cardiomyopathy. As seen in Figure 34–9, the left ventricular diastolic pressure did not exhibit its normal rapid decline to a

nadir near zero. Instead, early left ventricular diastolic pressure was increased at approximately 35 mmHg and continued to decline after mitral valve opening until atrial systole produced a diastolic pressure rise coincident with the "a" wave. This striking diastolic relaxation abnormality was largely corrected with nifedipine,[23] as seen in Figure 34–10. The di-

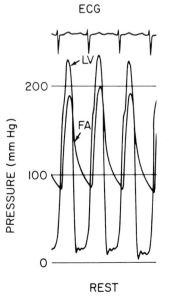

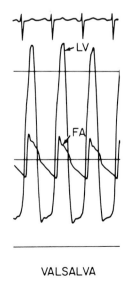

Fig. 34–7. Left ventricular (LV) and femoral artery (FA) pressure tracings in the patient illustrated in Figure 34–6. Valsalva maneuver produces a marked increase in the gradient, as well as a change in the femoral arterial pressure waveform to a spike-and-dome configuration.

REST   VALSALVA

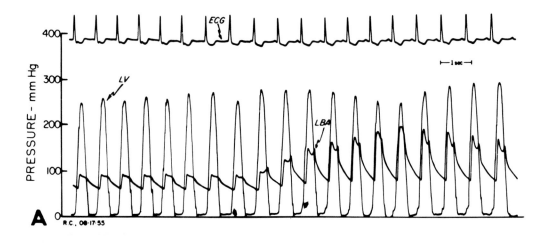

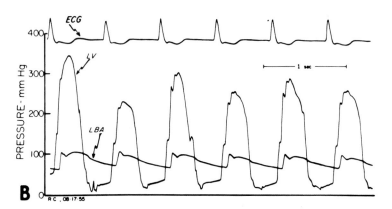

Fig. 34–8. Left ventricular (LV) and left brachial artery (LBA) pressure tracings in a 64-year-old woman with hypertrophic cardiomyopathy. (A) The effect of a spontaneous change from nodal rhythm to sinus rhythm. The short arrows show LV end-diastolic pressure. With restoration of sinus rhythm and a presumed decrease in the obstruction, LV stroke volume increases as reflected in the improved LBA pulse pressure. Also, the loss of atrial kick in patients with a stiff ventricle leads to an acute reduction in cardiac output. (B) Following a premature contraction (not shown) there is LV pulsus alternans. A spike-and-dome pattern is clearly seen in the LBA tracing. (Reproduced with permission from Glancy L, et al: The dynamic nature of left ventricular outflow obstruction in idiopathic hypertrophic subaortic stenosis. Ann Intern Med 75:589, 1971.)

astolic abnormalities of hypertrophic cardiomyopathy are improved by calcium channel blockade,[23,24,31–33] although occasional serious adverse effects have been seen with verapamil.[34]

Diastolic dysfunction is also prominent in **hypertensive hypertrophic cardiomyopathy of the elderly,** a syndrome described by Topol et al.[35] This condition represents a form of hypertrophic cardiomyopathy seen in elderly patients with mild to moderate hypertension who exhibit severe concentric hypertrophy, a small left ventricular cavity, supernormal systolic function characterized by excessive left ventricular emptying, and marked abnormality of diastolic relaxation. In describing this syndrome, Topol and co-workers observed that several of their patients with this condition improved when treatment with digoxin and diuretics was stopped.[35] In contrast, β-adrenergic blocking agents were often effective in relieving dyspnea and chest pain. Left ventriculography in such patients shows a severely hypertrophied ventricular chamber, which demonstrates cavity obliteration at end-systole.

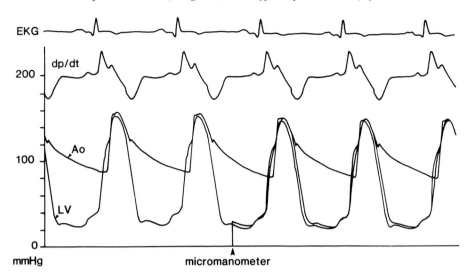

Fig. 34–9. Left ventricular (LV) and aortic (Ao) pressure tracings and rate of LV pressure rise (dP/dt) in a 55-year-old woman with hypertrophic cardiomyopathy. There is no resting pressure gradient. LV diastolic pressure waveform is very abnormal, suggesting marked impairment in myocardial relaxation. Fluid-filled and micromanometer LV tracings are both shown.

Although we will not discuss restrictive cardiomyopathy in this chapter, it is perhaps of value to point out that some unusual forms of infiltrative cardiomyopathy may present with features of both restrictive and hypertrophic cardiomyopathy. Miller et al[36] reported a patient with eosinophilic heart disease who had a left ventricular subaortic gradient of 90 mmHg, a spike-and-dome pattern in the central aortic pressure tracing and a systolic murmur which increased with either amyl nitrate inhalation or Valsalva maneuver. Left and right ventricular end diastolic pressures were elevated at 28 and 16 mmHg, respectively, and left ventricular ejection fraction was markedly increased at 94%. Treatment with prednisone and warfarin resulted in substantial improvement over a 4-month period.[36]

Angiographic Findings. The angiographic findings in hypertrophic cardiomyopathy are rather unique and help to explain some (but not all) of the unusual hemodynamic features just described. In hypertrophic cardiomyopathy with asymmetric septal hypertrophy, left

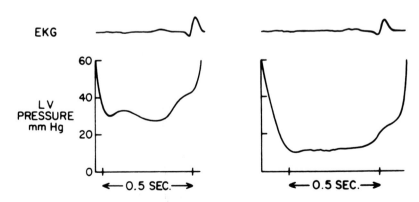

Fig. 34–10. LV diastolic pressure before (left) and after (right) administration of sublingual nifedipine in the patient illustrated in Figure 34–9. There is a lowering of LV diastolic pressure toward normal, as well as a striking improvement in the abnormal relaxation pattern. (Reproduced with permission from Lorell BH, et al: Improved diastolic function and systolic performance in hypertrophic cardiomyopathy after nifedipine. N Engl J Med 303:801, 1980.)

ventriculography shows a thickened intraventricular septum bulging into the left ventricular outflow tract in diastole and systole. In addition to this abnormality, patients with hypertrophic cardiomyopathy in whom a systolic gradient is present within the left ventricular chamber generally show systolic anterior movement (SAM) of the mitral valve's anterior leaflet (Fig. 34–11).

In contrast to hypertrophic cardiomyopathy with asymmetric septal hypertrophy, the patient with asymmetric *apical* hypertrophy does not show systolic anterior motion of the mitral leaflet. In patients with apical hypertrophic cardiomyopathy, the left ventricle shows marked thickening of its anteroapical wall, giving the ventricle a spade-shaped appearance (Fig. 34–12).

Patients with *asymmetric septal hypertrophy* have a distortion of the left ventricle that, in the right anterior oblique view, often resembles a banana, partly because of the large papillary muscles, which appear as filling defects.

In addition to exhibiting abnormal shapes

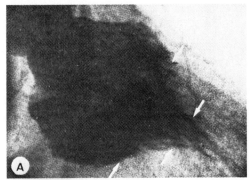
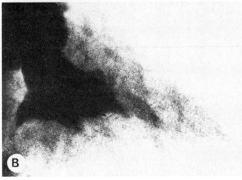

Fig. 34–12. Left ventriculogram at end-diastole (A) and end-systole (B) in a patient with apical hypertrophic cardiomyopathy. There is a spadelike configuration at end-diastole with a marked increase in free wall thickness and an extremely vigorous contraction with almost total cavity obliteration at end-systole. (Reproduced with permission from Yamaguchi H, et al: Hypertrophic non-obstructive cardiomyopathy with giant negative T waves (apical hypertrophy): ventriculographic and echocardiographic features in 30 patients. Am J Cardiol 44:401, 1979.)

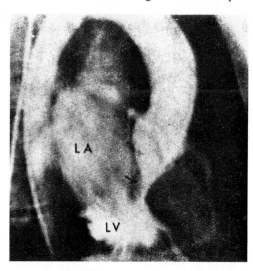

Fig. 34–11. Left ventricular (LV) angiogram in the lateral position in patient with hypertrophic cardiomyopathy with obstruction. The anterior leaflet of the mitral valve moves toward the interventricular septum in systole (arrow), producing marked narrowing of the LV outflow tract. Mitral regurgitation into the left atrium (LA) is present. (Reproduced with permission from Braunwald E, et al: Idiopathic hypertrophic subaortic stenosis. A description based on an analysis of 65 patients. Circulation 30 (Suppl 4):3, 1964.)

(spade, banana) and systolic anterior movement of the mitral valve, patients with hypertrophic cardiomyopathy often exhibit mitral regurgitation on left ventriculography. This is usually mild but may progress to become hemodynamically significant. Coronary angiography may show characteristic abnormalities in hypertrophic cardiomyopathy, with marked systolic compression of septal branches of the left anterior descending artery.[37] In addition, a "sawfish" systolic narrowing of the left anterior descending artery has been reported by Brugada et al[38] and is illustrated in Figure 34–13. The indentations of the left anterior descending artery associated with systolic narrowing of the vessel may represent the effect of contracting hypertrophied

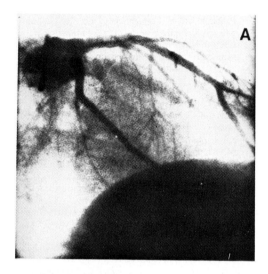

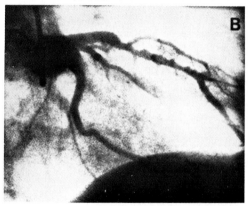

Fig. 34–13. Left coronary angiogram in right anterior oblique projection with caudocranial angulation. Diastolic (A) and systolic (B) frames are shown. A "sawfish" appearance of the left anterior descending artery is seen in association with systolic compression of septal branches in this patient with hypertrophic cardiomyopathy. (Reproduced with permission from Brugada P, et al: "Sawfish" narrowing of the left anterior descending coronary artery: an angiographic sign of hypertrophic cardiomyopathy. Circulation 66:800, 1982.)

and disorganized muscle fiber bundles in the vicinity of the coronary artery.[37]

REFERENCES

1. Goodwin JF: The frontiers of cardiomyopathy. Br Heart J 48:1, 1982.
2. Goodwin JF, Gordon H, Hollman A, Bishop MB: Clinical aspects of cardiomyopathy. Br Med J 1:69, 1961.
3. Grossman W, McLaurin LP, Rolett EL: Alterations in left ventricular relaxation and diastolic compliance in congestive cardiomyopathy. Cardiovasc Res 13:514, 1979.
4. Baim DS, et al: Evaluation of a new bipyridine inotropic agent—milrinone—in patients with severe congestive heart failure. N Engl J Med 309:748, 1983.
5. Monrad ES, et al: Improvement in indices of diastolic performance in patients with congestive heart failure treated with milrinone. Circulation 70:1030, 1984.
6. Erbel R, et al: Hemodynamic effects of prenalterol in patients with ischemic heart disease and congestive cardiomyopathy. Circulation 66:361, 1982.
7. Harshaw CW, Munro AB, McLaurin LP, Grossman W: Reduced systemic vascular resistance as therapy for severe mitral regurgitation of valvular origin. Ann Intern Med 83:312, 1975.
8. Guiha NH, et al: Treatment of refractory heart failure with infusion of nitroprusside. N Engl J Med 291:587, 1974.
9. Davis R, et al: Treatment of chronic congestive heart failure with captopril, an oral inhibitor of angiotensin-converting enzyme. N Engl J Med 301:117, 1979.
10. Dzau VJ, et al: Sustained effectiveness of converting-enzyme inhibition in patients with severe congestive heart failure. N Engl J Med 302:1373, 1980.
11. Ader R, et al: Immediate and sustained hemodynamic and clinical improvement in chronic heart failure by an oral angiotensin-converting enzyme inhibitor. Circulation 61:931, 1980.
12. Kreulen TH, Gorlin R, Herman MV: Ventriculographic patterns and hemodynamics in primary myocardial disease. Circulation 47:299, 1973.
13. Benjamin HJ, Schuster EH, Bulkley BH: Cardiac hypertrophy in idiopathic dilated congestive cardiomyopathy: a clinicopathologic study. Circulation 64:442, 1981.
14. Feild B, et al: Left ventricular function and hypertrophy in cardiomyopathy with depressed ejection fraction. Circulation 47:1022, 1973.
15. Parrillo JE, et al: The results of transvenous endomyocardial biopsy can frequently be used to diagnose myocardial disease in patients with idiopathic heart failure. Circulation 69:93, 1984.
16. Unverferth DV, et al: Factors influencing the one-year mortality of dilated cardiomyopathy. Am J Cardiol 54:147, 1984.
17. Fuster V, et al: The natural history of idiopathic dilated cardiomyopathy. Am J Cardiol 54:525, 1981.
18. Braunwald E, et al: Idiopathic hypertrophic subaortic stenosis. A description based on an analysis of 65 patients. Circulation 30(Suppl 4):3, 1964.
19. Murgo JP, et al: Dynamics of left ventricular ejection in obstructive and nonobstructive hypertrophic cardiomyopathy. J Clin Invest 66:1369, 1980.
20. Yamaguchi H, et al: Hypertrophic nonobstructive cardiomyopathy with giant negative T waves (apical hypertrophy): ventriculographic and echocardiographic features in 30 patients. Am J Cardiol 44:401, 1979.
21. Shapiro LM, McKenna WJ: Distribution of left ventricular hypertrophy in hypertrophic cardiomyopathy: a two-dimensional echocardiographic study. J Am Coll Cardiol 2:437, 1983.
22. Gosselin G, Pasternac A, Lesperance J, Bijak A, Waters DD: Apical hypertrophic cardiomyopathy:

Clinical and angiographic characteristics of the first Canadian series. Can J Cardiol 4:258, 1988.

23. Lorell BH, et al: Improved diastolic function and systolic performance in hypertrophic cardiomyopathy after nifedipine. N Engl J Med 303:801, 1980.

24. Lorell BH, et al: Modification of abnormal left ventricular diastolic properties by nifedipine in patients with hypertrophic cardiomyopathy. Circulation 64:499, 1982.

25. Hanrath P, et al: Effect of verapamil on left ventricular isovolumic relaxation time and regional left ventricular filling in hypertrophic cardiomyopathy. Am J Cardiol 45:1258, 1980.

26. St. John Sutton MG, et al: Echocardiographic assessment of left ventricular filling and septal and posterior wall dynamics in idiopathic hypertrophic subaortic stenosis. Circulation 57:512, 1978.

27. Hanrath P, Mathey DG, Siegert R, Bleifeld W: Left ventricular relaxation and filling pattern in different forms of left ventricular hypertrophy. An echocardiographic study. Am J Cardiol 45:15, 1980.

28. Stewart S, Mason DT, Braunwald E: Impaired rate of left ventricular filling in IHSS and valvular aortic stenosis. Circulation 37:8, 1968.

29. Dinsmore RE, Sanders CA, Harthorne JW: Mitral regurgitation in idiopathic hypertrophic subaortic stenosis. N Engl J Med 275:1225, 1966.

30. Brockenbrough EC, Braunwald E, Morrow AG: A hemodynamic technic for the detection of hypertrophic subaortic stenosis. Circulation 23:189, 1961.

31. Paulus WJ, et al: Comparison of the effects of nitroprusside and nifedipine on diastolic properties in patients with hypertrophic cardiomyopathy: Altered left ventricular loading or improved muscle inactivation? J Am Coll Cardiol 2:879, 1983.

32. Lorell BH: Use of calcium channel blockers in hypertrophic cardiomyopathy. Am J Med 78 (suppl 2B):43, 1985.

33. Bonow RO, et al: Effects of verapamil on left ventricular systolic function and diastolic filling in patients with hypertrophic cardiomyopathy. Circulation 64:787, 1981.

34. Epstein SE, Rosing DR: Verapamil: its potential for causing serious complications in patients with hypertrophic cardiomyopathy. Circulation 64:437, 1981.

35. Topol EJ, Traill FA, Fortuin NJ: Hypertensive hypertrophic cardiomyopathy of the elderly. New Engl J Med 312:277, 1985.

36. Miller W, Walsh RA, McCall D: Eosinophilic heart disease presenting with features suggesting hypertrophic obstructive cardiomyopathy. Cathet Cardiovasc Diagn 13:185, 1987.

37. Pichard AD, et al: Septal perforation compression (narrowing) in idiopathic hypertrophic subaortic stenosis. Am J Cardiol 40:310, 1977.

38. Brugada P, et al: "Sawfish" systolic narrowing of the left anterior descending artery: an angiographic sign of hypertrophic cardiomyopathy. Circulation 66:800, 1982.

35

Profiles in Constrictive Pericarditis, Restrictive Cardiomyopathy, and Cardiac Tamponade

BEVERLY H. LORELL and WILLIAM GROSSMAN

ericarditis from any cause can be followed by three hemodynamic complications: a pericardial effusion under
pressure, resulting in cardiac tamponade; progressive pericardial fibrosis and scarring causing constrictive physiology; a combination of
both. A common feature of each is the presence of diastolic dysfunction caused by external compression of the heart, which prevents
adequate diastolic filling, elevates right and
left heart diastolic pressures, and results ultimately in reduced stroke volume because of
inadequate preload. The diastolic filling pattern during each cardiac cycle and the response
to respiration differ, however, so that distinctive hemodynamic profiles of constrictive
pericarditis, cardiac tamponade, and effusive-
constrictive pericarditis can usually be identified in the cardiac catheterization laboratory.
The hemodynamic and angiographic evaluation must also include consideration of the
presence of restrictive cardiomyopathy, in
which features of impaired diastolic filling
with preserved systolic contractile function
may simulate constrictive pericarditis.[1]

CONSTRICTIVE PERICARDITIS

Clinical Features. Constrictive pericarditis
is a symmetric process in which scarring of

both the parietal and visceral pericardial layers
affects all chambers of the heart. Localized
constriction, which may simulate valvular stenosis, is extremely rare. In the chronic stage,
pericardial calcification may develop, but may
be absent in earlier stages despite severe hemodynamic compromise. Tuberculosis was previously the leading cause of constrictive pericarditis. Today, the most common causes of
subacute or chronic constrictive pericarditis
are recurrent idiopathic or viral pericarditis,
delayed constriction after mediastinal radiation
therapy for malignancy, and pericarditis after
open heart surgery. Less common causes include post-infectious pericarditis, chronic
renal failure, neoplastic pericardial involvement, and connective tissue disorders such as
rheumatoid arthritis and progressive systemic
sclerosis.[2] It is important for cardiologists to
appreciate that high-dose mediastinal irradiation for malignancy may cause severe constrictive pericarditis many years after therapy.[3]
Some patients with acute idiopathic pericarditis with pericardial effusion may go through
a transient phase of mild cardiac constriction,
which spontaneously resolves within 3 months
of the initial illness.[4]

The clinical features of constrictive pericarditis reflect the gradual and often insidious development of systemic and pulmonary venous hypertension. In patients in whom right and left atrial pressures are modestly elevated in the range of 10 to 18 mmHg, symptoms and signs of systemic venous congestion predominate. These include leg edema, postprandial discomfort, hepatic congestion, and ascites. As right and left heart filling pressures become elevated to a level of 18 to 30 mmHg, exertional dyspnea and orthopnea appear, and pleural effusions often develop. The impairment of diastolic filling results initially in an inability to augment stroke volume in response to stress and may cause symptoms of exertional fatigue or hemodynamic instability during dialysis in the uremic patient. As resting cardiac output falls, severe lethargy and cardiac cachexia supervene. The electrocardiogram usually shows reduced voltage and nonspecific ST-T wave abnormalities. Atrial fibrillation is present in about 10% of patients. The chest roentgenogram may show a small, normal, or modestly enlarged silhouette with redistribution of pulmonary blood flow, and the useful marker of pericardial calcification may be present. Advanced tuberculous constrictive pericarditis is associated commonly with dense pericardial calcification, which has been termed "panzerherz" in the German literature, and "concretia cordis" in Latin. Echocardiography can be extremely helpful in suggesting the presence of constrictive pericarditis if a pattern of pericardial thickening, abrupt posterior motion of the interventricular septum in early diastole, and reduced motion of the left ventricular posterior wall is seen. Because of the vague and insidious nature of the symptoms, constrictive pericarditis is often mistaken for primary hepatic disease, intraabdominal malignancy, or nephrotic syndrome.

Constrictive pericarditis should be suspected in any patient with unexplained jugular venous distension, systemic edema, and pleural effusion. Constrictive pericarditis should also be considered in the postoperative heart surgery patient who has unexplained tachycardia, low cardiac output, and venous congestion within the first 2 to 3 months after surgery. Right and left heart cardiac catheterization and angiography should be performed in every patient with this potentially curable disease to: (1) confirm the presence of constrictive physiology and assess its severity before consideration of pericardiectomy; (2) assist in differentiating pericardial disease from restrictive cardiomyopathy; (3) exclude coexisting causes of right atrial hypertension; (4) exclude the rare instances of localized constricting bands, within the atrioventricular groove simulating valvular stenosis, causing external stenosis of the coronary arteries, or producing right ventricular outflow tract obstruction.[5]

Hemodynamic and Angiographic Profile. The symmetric constricting effect of the pericardium usually impairs diastolic filling of all chambers of the heart so that right and left ventricular diastolic pressures are elevated and equal within 5 mmHg or less. Although right and left *ventricular* diastolic pressures are equal in constrictive pericarditis, right and left *atrial* (pulmonary capillary wedge) pressures may differ if coexisting mitral or tricuspid regurgitation is present associated with a large A or V wave in either atrium. For this reason, it is important to record right and left ventricular pressures simultaneously, using equisensitive gains. Care should be taken to calibrate the transducers simultaneously to a column of mercury, and the transducers should be leveled to precisely the same height. Severe pulmonary hypertension is usually absent in constrictive pericarditis unless coexisting heart disease is present, and the pulmonary artery and right ventricular systolic pressures are usually between 35 and 45 mmHg.

The major determinant of the filling pressures is the degree of constriction. Moderate constriction is associated with filling pressures between 12 and 15 mmHg. Hypovolemia, however, may lower these pressures, and it is important to know if the patient has been treated intensively with diuretics and to avoid excessive diuresis immediately before catheterization. In this regard, an entity of "occult" pericardial constriction has been described, in which patients with nondescript chest pain who had normal baseline hemodynamics were shown to develop elevation and equilibration of diastolic pressures suggestive of pericardial constriction after rapid infusion of 1000 ml of normal saline solution.[6] Many of these patients subsequently underwent pericardiectomy, after which their symptoms improved. Caution is in order, however, because the sensitivity and specificity of this volume-challenge test in patients with atypical chest pain is still poorly defined, and there is potential harm with a massive-volume infusion.

The constricting pericardium causes virtually all ventricular filling to occur in early diastole. In severe constrictive pericarditis, in which the heart is encased in a rigid and adherent fibrotic shell, the end-systolic volume is usually less than that defined by the pericardium. Therefore, early diastolic filling is unimpeded and abnormally rapid because of the elevation of venous pressure, but filling halts abruptly in early diastole when total cardiac volume expands to the volume set by the stiff pericardium. The physical finding of a *pericardial knock* is an acoustic marker of the abrupt cessation of early diastolic filling.[7] This pattern of virtually all ventricular filling occurring in early diastole is reflected in the early diastolic dip-and-plateau pattern in the right and left ventricular waveforms. Because right atrial and right ventricular pressures are equilibrated in diastole, the right atrial waveform typically shows a prominent and rapid diastolic Y descent, which indicates that right atrial emptying after tricuspid valve opening is rapid and unimpeded. The Y descent is followed by a steep "A" wave and X descent because the atrium is attempting to eject blood into a right ventricle that is already filled to its capacity. The steep X and Y descent impart to the pressure waveform its characteristic M or W configuration (Fig. 35–1). It is important to avoid an underdamped pressure-transducer system because this causes overshoot in the pressure tracing, which may obscure the presence of the plateau component of the ventricular waveform (Fig. 35–2).

In severe pericardial constriction, negative intrathoracic pressure during inspiration is not communicated to the intrapericardial space and right heart. In contrast to what is seen in normal subjects, systemic venous and right atrial pressures do not fall, and venous flow to the right atrium does not accelerate during inspiration in patients with severe constrictive pericarditis. As illustrated in Figure 35–3, in extreme cases, systemic venous pressure may increase during inspiration (Kussmaul's sign).[8] The lack of phasic augmentation of right heart filling during inspiration accounts for the fact that pulsus paradoxus is minimal or absent in constrictive pericarditis in contrast to cardiac tamponade, in which right heart filling is exaggerated during inspiration at the expense of left heart filling.

Stroke volume is almost always reduced in patients with constrictive pericarditis, but resting cardiac output may be preserved because of tachycardia. Supine dynamic exercise usually causes only a slight rise in cardiac filling pressures, but cardiac output fails to rise appropriately relative to the increase in systemic oxygen consumption. In these patients, enhanced oxygen demand is met almost entirely by increased oxygen extraction and widening of the arteriovenous oxygen difference. In severe cases, resting cardiac index is depressed in association with systemic arterial vasoconstriction and arterial hypotension.

The combination of low stroke volume, low stroke work, and increased ventricular filling pressure indicates failure of cardiac pump function. Pump failure in constrictive pericarditis, however, is usually caused by reduced chamber compliance and diminished myocardial fiber stretch or preload rather than myocardial systolic failure. In the absence of coexisting cardiac disease, left ventricular angiography usually shows that left ventricular volume is moderately to severely reduced. Left ventricular ejection fraction is normal to increased. In the absence of myocardial inflammation or fibrosis, both isovolumic and ejection phase indices of systolic contractile function (e.g., peak dP/dt) are normal.[9] As an important exception, postradiotherapy constriction may be complicated by coexisting radiation-induced myocardial fibrosis with im-

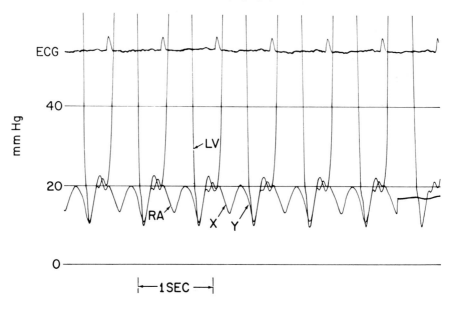

Fig. 35–1. Simultaneous right atrial (RA) and left ventricular (LV) pressure recordings from a patient with constrictive pericarditis, illustrating that both pressures are elevated and equal throughout diastole. Note the prominent Y descent in the right atrial waveform, which indicates that right atrial emptying is rapid and unimpeded in early diastole. The nadir of the Y descent corresponds with the abrupt cessation of early diastolic ventricular filling. The prominent X and Y descents give the right atrial waveform its characteristic M- or W-shaped appearance in constrictive pericarditis.

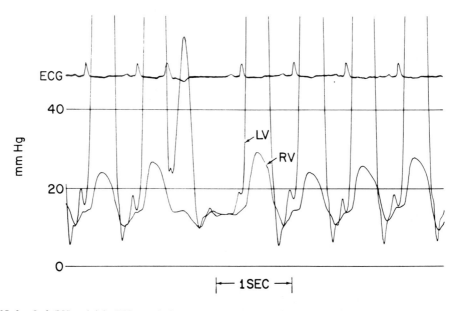

Fig. 35–2. Left (LV) and right (RV) ventricular pressures recorded simultaneously in a patient with surgically confirmed constrictive pericarditis illustrate technical pitfalls in evaluation of pressure tracings. The presence of resting tachycardia partially obscures evaluation of the diastolic waveforms, and underdamping of the left ventricular pressure-transducer system accentuates an undershoot of left ventricular pressure in early diastole and an overshoot during atrial contraction. A long diastole following a premature beat permits the recognition of equilibration of left and right ventricular diastolic pressures and the appreciation of a dip and plateau component of the ventricular waveforms.

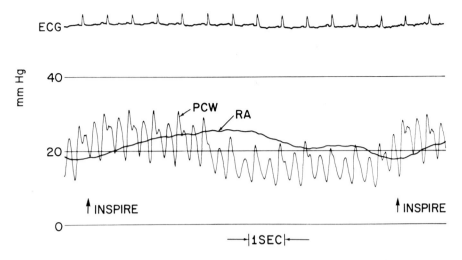

Fig. 35–3. Right atrial (mean, RA) and pulmonary capillary wedge (phasic, PCW) pressure tracings from a patient with constrictive pericarditis. An arrow marks the beginning of the inspiratory phase of each respiratory cycle. Note that mean right atrial pressure increases during inspiration (Kussmaul's sign). The pulmonary capillary wedge pressure is out of phase with right atrial pressure and begins to fall during inspiration as right atrial pressure is rising.

paired systolic contractile function. Superior vena caval angiography can be helpful in selected patients with neoplastic disease to exclude coexisting superior vena caval compression. In patients with constrictive pericarditis, venous angiography may demonstrate dilatation of the superior vena cava, straightening of the right heart border, and pericardial thickening. Coronary angiography should be considered in older patients at increased risk of coronary atherosclerosis before open-heart surgery for extensive pericardiectomy. Coronary angiography is also indicated in all patients with constrictive pericarditis and angina-like chest pain because the pericardial scarring process can rarely cause external pinching or compression of the coronary arteries.[10]

The hemodynamic and angiographic findings may differ somewhat in patients with subacute noncalcific pericarditis of less than one year's duration, in whom the pericardium is characterized by an adherent fluid-fibrin layer in the process of organization rather than a rigid scarred shell. Hancock has compared this relatively *elastic form of constrictive pericarditis* to encircling the heart tightly with rubber bands.[11] In this elastic form of fibroelastic pericardial disease, cardiac compression is present throughout the cardiac cycle, and the pat-

terns of ventricular filling and pressure waveforms are more like those of cardiac tamponade.

RESTRICTIVE CARDIOMYOPATHY

Clinical Features. The differentiation between constrictive pericarditis and restrictive cardiomyopathy is often difficult at the bedside and in the catheterization laboratory. In restrictive cardiomyopathy, the restrictive element resides in the myocardium itself, so that the ventricular walls resist stretch abnormally during cardiac filling. Therefore, the clinical features of patients with restrictive cardiomyopathy caused by idiopathic etiology, metabolic storage diseases, amyloidosis, or hemochromatosis are often similar to those of constrictive pericarditis. In both disorders, ventricular diastolic filling is impaired, ventricular filling pressures are elevated, stroke volume is fixed or reduced, and systolic contractile function is essentially normal.

Hemodynamic and Angiographic Profile. In most cases, careful attention to hemodynamics does permit identification of the patient with restrictive cardiomyopathy. Diastolic pressure in the left ventricle is usually higher than in the right ventricle when both are recorded simultaneously[1,12] (Fig. 35–4). Furthermore, exercise generally increases left ventricular diastolic pressure more than right ventricular diastolic pressure. Pulmonary hypertension is usually more severe in restrictive cardiomyopathy than in constrictive pericarditis, and pulmonary systolic pressures in excess of 50 mmHg are commonly found. In constrictive pericarditis, this degree of pulmonary hypertension is rare, and diastolic plateau pressure usually exceeds one third of the right ventricular systolic pressure.[8] Published data regarding myocardial contractile function are few, but isovolumic and ejection phase indices are often normal.[13,14] In some cases of cardiac amyloidosis, the picture of restrictive cardiomyopathy is absent, and impaired indices of contractile function are present.[12]

In nine patients with restrictive cardiomyopathy and symptoms of either congestive heart failure or chest pain studied at Peter Bent Brigham Hospital, left ventricular ejection fraction was 63 ± 8%, suggestive of normal myocardial contractile function.[15] In these patients, left ventricular end-diastolic pressure

(23 ± 6 mmHg) was substantially higher than right ventricular end-diastolic pressure (16 ± 5 mmHg) and moderate elevation of pulmonary artery systolic pressure was present (49 ± 21 mmHg).

The hemodynamic findings in some patients with restrictive cardiomyopathy, however, are virtually indistinguishable from those of constrictive pericarditis.[13,14,16] Frame-by-frame angiographic analysis of left ventricular filling and the assessment of diastolic filling fractions by radionuclide angiography have been proposed as methods of distinguishing between these two conditions, because early diastolic filling tends to be slower than normal in restrictive cardiomyopathy, but is excessively rapid in constrictive pericarditis.[17,18] The predictive value of this approach, however, has not been established in the individual patient with suspected restrictive myopathy who has a dip-and-plateau ventricular waveform, which itself suggests that early diastolic filling is excessively rapid and abruptly attenuated in mid-diastole. Myocardial biopsy is valuable in documenting the presence of amyloid or other specific causes of restrictive myopathy (myocarditis, hemochromatosis) in some patients in whom cardiac catheterization findings do not differentiate between constrictive pericarditis and restrictive cardiomyopathy.[14,16] It must be kept in mind, however, that amyloidosis and radiation-induced fibrosis may involve both the myocardium and the pericardium.[2,14,16] Furthermore, in many cases, no specific pathologic finding can be identified by biopsy to explain the hemodynamic findings.[15] Thus, in selected patients, exploratory thoracotomy with careful histologic examination of pericardium and myocardium is justified to differentiate the surgically correctable condition of constrictive pericarditis from restrictive cardiomyopathy.

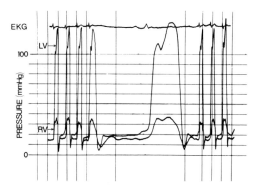

Fig. 35–4. Right and left ventricular (RV and LV) pressure tracings in a 43-year-old woman with idiopathic restrictive cardiomyopathy. A dip and plateau pattern is seen in both ventricles and diastolic pressures are increased. The plateaus, however, are at different absolute levels, approximately 16 mmHg for the RV and 20 mmHg for the LV. In this patient, both RV and LV diastolic pressures increased simultaneously with exercise, and final confirmation of the diagnosis of restrictive cardiomyopathy (versus constrictive pericarditis) was made by thoracotomy. (From Benotti JR, Grossman W, Cohn PF: The clinical profile of restrictive cardiomyopathy. Circulation 61:1206, 1980, by permission of the American Heart Association, Inc.)

OTHER CONDITIONS ASSOCIATED WITH CONSTRICTIVE PHYSIOLOGY

The normal pericardium provides a substantial restraining effect on cardiac dilatation in conditions in which the pericardium has not hypertrophied or stretched to accommodate an increase in cardiac volume. Acute and massive right ventricular infarction with right ventricular dilatation may cause constrictive physiology with elevation and equilibration of right and left ventricular pressures and dip-and-plateau ventricular waveforms.[19] These hemodynamic findings have been shown in animal models of experimental right ventricular infarction to be caused by increased pericardial pressure.[20] Similarly, volume overload caused by subacute tricuspid regurgitation in the presence of an intact pericardium may cause marked elevation and equilibration of ventricular diastolic pressures (Fig. 35–5).

Just as acute volume overload of the right ventricle (as in right ventricular infarction or severe regurgitation) can compress the left ventricle by displacing the elastic shared interventricular septum, overload of the left ventricle can adversely affect right ventricular filling. Bartle and Hermann reported evidence that acute mitral regurgitation in man can present a striking hemodynamic pattern highly suggestive of pericardial constriction.[21] In this instance, significant pulmonary hypertension is an obligatory part of the hemodynamic pattern (Fig. 35–6). This feature allows distinction from the findings in primary right ventricular volume overload (Fig. 35–5), in which pulmonary hypertension will often be absent. Acute massive pulmonary embolism may present with an intermediate picture, whereas pulmonary hypertension causes acute right ventricular failure and dilatation, and this may cause some compression of the left ventricle.

CARDIAC TAMPONADE

Clinical Features. The development of an increase in intrapericardial pressure and the restriction of cardiac filling from a pericardial effusion depend on several factors: (1) the rate

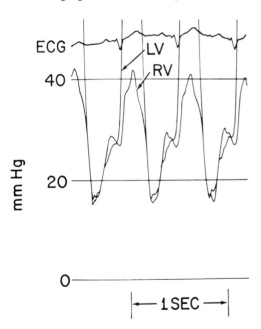

Fig. 35–5. Simultaneous right (RV) and left (LV) ventricular pressure tracings recorded in a patient with several weeks' history of severe tricuspid insufficiency. Note that right and left ventricular end-diastolic pressures are markedly elevated (approximately 28 mmHg) with virtual identity of pressures throughout diastole. Right ventricular systolic pressure is minimally increased, indication that the elevation of right ventricular diastolic pressure is not primarily caused by pulmonary hypertension. These findings suggest a restraining effect of the intact pericardium in the presence of subacute volume overload of the right ventricle.

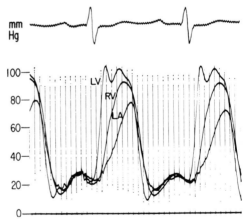

Fig. 35–6. Left and right ventricular (LV, RV) and left atrial (LA) pressure tracings in a 60-year-old man with acute, severe mitral regurgitation. The acute LV and LA volume overloads result in a constrictive physiology, with equalization of LV and RV diastolic pressures because the pericardium has not yet grown sufficiently to accommodate the increased chamber volumes. (Reproduced with permission from Bartle SH, Hermann HJ: Acute mitral regurgitation in man. Hemodynamic evidence and observations indicating an early role for the pericardium. Circulation 36:839, 1967.)

of fluid accumulation; (2) the actual volume of fluid; (3) the distensibility of the pericardium; and (4) the underlying distensibility of the ventricular chambers. The normal unstretched pericardium usually contains less than 50 ml of fluid and can accommodate mild fluctuations in intrapericardial volume with little change in intrapericardial pressure. Using a conventional open-end and fluid-filled catheter system, normal pericardial pressure is zero or negative relative to atmosphere and virtually identical with intrathoracic pressure. Recent studies using special flat balloon catheters suggest the *constraint* pressure exerted by the normal pericardium is nearly equal to right atrial pressure.[22,23] The accurate estimation of normal pericardial pressure in experimental studies is an important controversy; however, this controversy does not detract from the utility of measuring pericardial pressure using fluid-filled catheter systems in patients undergoing pericardiocentesis because interpericardial pressure can be accurately measured by either method once 40 to 50 ml of free fluid is present in the pericardial space.[24] The rapid accumulation of greater than about 150 ml of fluid is associated with a steep rise in intrapericardial pressure. Intracardiac diastolic pressures also rise so that the transmural difference between ventricular diastolic pressure and intrapericardial pressure falls; when equilibration of pericardial and diastolic pressures of either ventricle occurs, transmural distending pressure falls toward zero, and stroke volume falls precipitously.[25] Cardiac output and blood pressure are maintained initially by the compensatory mechanisms of reflex vasoconstriction and tachycardia, but as the impairment of cardiac filling becomes more severe, hypotension and shock ensue.

Cardiac tamponade from acute intrapericardial hemorrhage caused by cardiac trauma may occur when an effusion of less than 200 ml of fluid is sufficient to cause an abrupt rise in intrapericardial pressure to a level above 20 mmHg. Patients exhibit the classic clinical triad described by Beck[26]: (1) elevation of systemic venous pressure; (2) systemic arterial hypotension; (3) a small, quiet heart. Patients

with the acute development of cardiac tamponade are typically agitated and confused and exhibit tachycardia, tachypnea, and profound systemic arterial hypertension. The cardiologist in the catheterization laboratory, however, should recognize that medical patients with chronic pericardial inflammation caused by viral pericarditis, uremia, neoplasm, radiation injury, or collagen vascular disease may slowly accumulate large volumes of fluid, up to 1 to 2 liters, before intrapericardial pressure rises. The clinical picture of slowly developing cardiac tamponade differs from that of acute tamponade caused by cardiac trauma or rupture.[27]

This clinical picture may be further altered in patients with "low-pressure cardiac tamponade" (Fig. 35–7) in whom the development of a pericardial effusion in the setting of severe hypovolemia results in compromised ventricular filling and stroke volume when intrapericardial and right atrial pressures rise and equilibrate at a level of only 5 to 15 mmHg.[28] Low-pressure tamponade is usually associated with severe dehydration and has been reported in neoplastic and tuberculous pericarditis.

In patients with gradual development of cardiac tamponade, the major complaint is usually dyspnea on exertion accompanied by the insidious appearance of systemic problems such as anorexia, edema, and weight loss. In this setting, clinical findings usually include jugular venous distension, moderate tachycardia, pulsus paradoxus, and hepatomegaly, but the classic findings of agitation, severe hypotension, and distant heart sounds ("the small quiet heart") are typically absent.[27]

Depending on the volume of intrapericardial fluid, the cardiac silhouette on the chest roentgenogram may be normal or increased in size. The development of electrical alternation on the electrocardiogram usually reflects pendular, periodic swinging of the heart within the fluid-filled pericardium, but this finding is not specific and may occur in other conditions such as severe heart failure and tension pneumothorax.

In virtually every case of cardiac tamponade, with the possible exception of a moribund

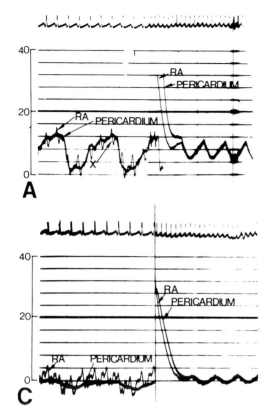

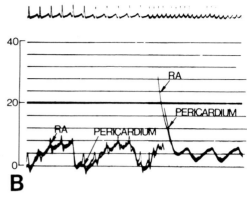

Fig. 35–7. Simultaneous pericardial and right atrial (RA) pressure tracings in a 76-year-old man with "low pressure cardiac tamponade" caused by tuberculous pericardial effusion in the setting of fever and dehydration. The patient had hypotension and pulsus paradoxus, at a mean right atrial pressure of only 8 mmHg (A). Blood pressure improved and pulsus paradoxus disappeared after removal of 200 ml (B) and 600 ml (C) of pericardial fluid. Initially, there is only an X descent in the RA tracing (A). (Reproduced from Antman EM, Cargill V, Grossman W: Low-pressure cardiac tamponade. Ann Intern Med 91:403, 1979.)

patient with an obvious diagnosis (e.g., stab wound of the heart with distended neck veins and marked pulsus paradoxus), an *echocardiogram,* preferably two-dimensional, should be obtained before pericardiocentesis. First, it documents the presence and size of effusion; in this regard, the lack of evidence of an effusion on a good quality echocardiographic study essentially excludes the presence of cardiac tamponade (with the exception of postoperative localized hematoma) and contraindicates needle pericardiocentesis. Second, the probability of success and safety of pericardiocentesis is related to the size of the effusion, because it has been shown that the procedure is likely to be uncomplicated if both anterior and posterior echo-free spaces (greater than 10 mm) are present.[29] Third, the echocardiographic finding of right atrial and right ventricular diastolic collapse occurs early during the development of cardiac tamponade and provides evidence that pericardial pressure is elevated and comprising right ventricular fill-

ing.[30] The hemodynamic implications of right ventricular diastolic collapse are discussed further below.

Combined Cardiac Catheterization and Pericardiocentesis. We recommend a combined procedure of cardiac catheterization and percutaneous catheter pericardiocentesis because: (1) it is the only reliable way to determine the hemodynamic significance of a pericardial effusion; (2) it excludes other important coexisting causes of right atrial hypertension, which may be present in as many as 40% of medical patient with cardiac tamponade;[29] (3) it permits complete drainage of nonloculated pericardial fluid; (4) it allows assessment of adequacy or inadequacy of relieving tamponade physiology; and (5) hemodynamic monitoring and fluoroscopic guidance substantially increase the safety of the procedure. At our center, the use of combined cardiac catheterization and percutaneous catheter pericardiocentesis in 50 consecutive patients with cardiac tamponade relieved tamponade in all patients and no deaths or serious complications.[31] There is rarely justification today for performing blind needle pericardiocentesis at the bedside without hemodynamic monitoring. Percutaneous pericardiocentesis should be attempted only as a temporizing measure in the patient with hemorrhagic traumatic cardiac tamponade and may be difficult or impossible in patients who have a loculated effusion, a localized clot and/or fibrin following cardiac surgery, or absence of an anterior effusion greater than 200 ml in size by echocardiography. Cardiology trainees should probably confine their initial taps to patients with clear-cut echocardiographic evidence of large anterior and posterior effusions.

The combined procedure of cardiac catheterization and percutaneous catheter pericardiocentesis is performed in the cardiac catheterization laboratory with hemodynamic and fluoroscopic monitoring. The pressure transducers for measurement of left heart (pulmonary capillary wedge), right heart, intrapericardial, and arterial pressures are prepared to avoid underdamping and ensure equisensitive pressure measurements (see Chapter 9). The transducer to be used to record intrapericardial pressure should be connected by means of a short length of fluid-filling tubing to the side of a three-way stopcock. The male end of the stopcock is attached to a long (8-inch), thin-walled, 18-gauge hollow pointed needle. In our laboratory, we currently use the 18-gauge hollow needle with a 30-degree bevel supplied in the pericardiocentesis kit of Mansfield Scientific, Inc., Mansfield, Massachusetts. The needle with its stopcock is then attached to a hand-held syringe filled with 1 or 2% lidocaine (Fig. 35–8). The metal needle hub may be attached by sterile connector to the V lead of an electrocardiographic recorder, but equipotential grounding of the apparatus must be ensured to avoid a current leak that could cause ventricular fibrillation.

It is important to measure systemic arterial pressure directly with an intra-arterial catheter or cannula during pericardiocentesis. Right heart catheterization should be carried out with right atrial, ventricular, pulmonary artery and pulmonary capillary wedge pressures measured and recorded. Pulmonary artery and systemic arterial blood samples are then drawn for oxygen content determination, and cardiac output is measured. Before beginning pericardiocentesis, the right heart catheter should be repositioned in the right atrium.

Pericardiocentesis is then performed with the patient's head and thorax propped up with a wedge *so that the patient is sitting at 30-degree or 45-degree elevation,* to promote anterior and inferior pooling of the effusion. *It is critical for the safety of the procedure that the patient be sitting up, at least partially.* We prefer to use the subxiphoid approach, which avoids the major epicardial coronary and internal mammary arteries. The skin is shaved and prepared in aseptic fashion, and both skin and subcutaneous tissues are anesthetized with 1 or 2% lidocaine. The skin is then pierced with a No. 11 blade, about 0.5 cm below and to the left of the xiphoid process, and the subcutaneous tissues are separated with a small mosquito clamp.

The needle, which is connected by means of its three-way stopcock to both the xylocaine-filled syringe and a transducer (Fig. 35–8), is advanced posteriorly until its tip is posterior to the bony rib cage. The hub of the needle is then flattened toward the abdomen, and the needle is advanced cephalad toward the patient's head or either shoulder with approximately a 15-degree posterior tilt. As the needle is slowly advanced, the syringe is aspirated repeatedly (to determine if a fluid-filled space has been entered) and lidocaine is injected frequently to provide adequate anesthesia and to keep the needle clear. The needle is advanced until either the pericardial membrane is felt to give and fluid is freely aspirated, or until an injury current of ST elevation is observed on the lead monitored from the needle. If an injury current is obtained before the fluid can be aspirated, the needle is withdrawn slowly with gentle syringe suction, after first clearing the tip with lidocaine. The needle may then by redirected (preferably with echocardiographic guidance) and advanced once more.

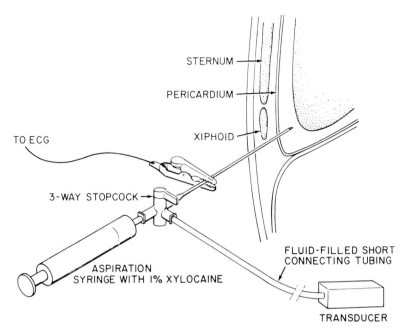

STERNUM

PERICARDIUM

TO ECG   XIPHOID

3-WAY STOPCOCK

FLUID-FILLED SHORT
CONNECTING TUBING

ASPIRATION
SYRINGE WITH 1% XYLOCAINE

TRANSDUCER

Fig. 35–8. Schematic diagram showing the subxiphoid approach to pericardiocentesis. A hollow, thin-walled, 18-gauge needle is connected via a 3-way stopcock to an aspiration syringe filled with 1% or 2% lidocaine and to a short length of fluid-filled tubing to a pressure transducer. A sterile V lead of an electrocardiographic recorder is attached to the metal needle hub. The needle is advanced until pericardial fluid is aspirated or an injury current appears on the V lead monitor recording. Once fluid is aspirated, the stopcock is turned so that needle-tip pressure is displayed against stimultaneously measured right atrial pressure from a right heart catheter. When needle tip position within the pericardial space is thus confirmed, a J-tipped guide wire is passed through the needle into the pericardial space. The needle is then removed, and a catheter with end and side holes is advanced over the guide wire and subsequently connected by means of the 3-way stopcock to both its transducer and its syringe. This permits thorough drainage of the pericardial effusion using a catheter with multiple side holes rather than a sharp needle, and documentation that tamponade physiology is relieved when right atrial pressure falls and intrapericardial pressure is restored to a level at or below zero.

When fluid is freely aspirated, the stopcock is turned into its transducer (Fig. 35–8), and needle tip and right atrial pressures are simultaneously displayed and recorded. If the needle tip is in the pericardial space, and if tamponade is present, intrapericardial and right atrial pressures should be equal and elevated with virtually identical waveforms. If hemorrhagic fluid is aspirated, the pressure waveforms usually enable differentiation of pericardial from right ventricular position of the needle tip. In occasional cases in which it is not immediately obvious from the pressure waveforms whether or not the needle tip is in the pericardial space, a few milliliters of contrast medium can be injected under fluoroscopic observation. If the contrast medium immediately swirls and disappears, the needle is most likely within the right or left ventricle;

sluggish layering of contrast medium inferiorly indicates that the needle is within the pericardial space.

Once the needle tip's position within the pericardial space is confirmed, a floppy-tip 0.038-inch guide wire is passed through the needle into the pericardial space and "wrapped" around the heart as confirmed by fluoroscopy. The needle is removed and a soft tapered large-bore lumen 6 Fr or 7 Fr catheter with end and side holes is advanced over the guide wire, the guide wire is removed, and the catheter hub is connected by means of the three-way stopcock attached to its transducer and to the syringe.

Pressure in the pericardium is now recorded simultaneously with right atrial pressure. As mentioned, if cardiac tamponade is present, right atrial and pericardial pressures will be

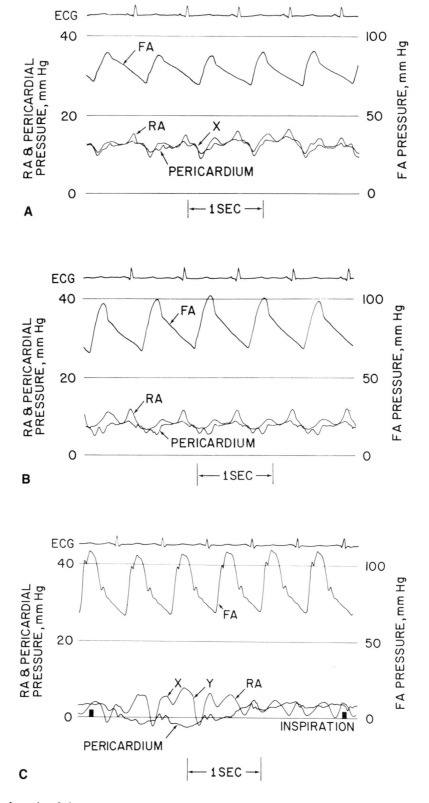

Fig. 35–9. Legend on facing page.

virtually equal, as seen in Figures 35–7 and 35–9. On occasion, the pressures differ by several millimeters of mercury because of un-equal heights of the right atrial and pericardial catheter tips in a patient who is sitting at 30 to 45 degrees of elevation. This gravitational effect may obscure the presence of tamponade physiology. It may be minimized or eliminated by either returning the patient to a supine po-sition (this is safe once the pericardial space has been successfully catheterized) or by checking under fluoroscopy (lateral view) to adjust the catheter tip positions so that both right atrial and pericardial catheter tips are at the same horizontal level, and that the pressure transducers are zeroed at this level.

After pericardial and right atrial pressures (properly zeroed) are recorded, samples of per-icardial fluid are aspirated and sent for chem-ical, bacteriologic, cytologic, and immuno-logic examination. As fluid is then gradually removed, intermittent recording of simulta-neous pericardial and right atrial pressures and systemic arterial pressure is done (Fig. 35–9).

Tamponade physiology is relieved when right atrial and intrapericardial pressures have separated so that (1) intrapericardial pressure has fallen to a mean value of zero and exhibits a negative pressure during inspiration; (2) the right atrial pressure has fallen to a normal level; (3) the right atrial waveform has changed to a normal configuration with reappearance of the diastolic Y descent (Figs. 35–7 and 35–9). Systemic arterial pressure usually rises, and pulsus paradoxus disappears unless res-piratory distress from a coexisting pulmonary process is present. Failure of intrapericardial pressure to fall to a level of 0 to −2 mmHg using a conventional fluid-filled catheter in-dicates that pericardial fluid (free or loculated) under pressure is still present. Failure of right atrial pressure to fall to a normal level below 8 mm Hg indicates that a coexisting cause of right atrial hypertension is present. *Persistent elevation of right atrial pressure with the ap-pearance of a prominent Y descent suggests the presence of effusive-constrictive physiol-ogy.* The jugular veins should also be exam-ined. Continued jugular venous distension after relief of tamponade in patients with sus-pected neoplastic pericarditis mandates exclu-sion of coexisting superior vena caval obstruc-tion. Special attention should be given to right and/or left atrial pressure in patients with car-diac trauma in whom continued pressure ele-vation can be present because of traumatic rup-ture of the atrioventricular valves.

The pericardial pressure-volume curve has a steep slope, so that removal of a small amount of fluid may restore intrapericardial pressure to zero and completely relieve tam-ponade physiology. It is important, however, to realize that a large volume (1 to 2 liters in chronic tamponade) may still be present in the pericardial space. The operator should attempt to remove all fluid that can be aspirated so that reaccumulation of a small volume of fluid will not again cause tamponade. We have found that extremely thorough drainage can be ac-complished reliably by removing the attached

Fig. 35–9. Simultaneous right atrial (RA) and intrapericardial pressure (scale 0 to 40 mmHg) and femoral artery (FA) pressure (scale 0 to 100 mmHg) recorded in a patient with cardiac tamponade. (A) Recordings before pericardiocentesis show the presence of systemic hypotension, and the elevation and equalization of right atrial and intrapericardial pressures. Note that a systolic X descent is present, but the diastolic Y descent is absent, suggesting that right atrial emptying in early diastole is impeded because of cardiac compression by the pericardial effusion. (B) After aspiration of 100 ml of pericardial fluid, right atrial and intrapericardial pressures have fallen and are beginning to separate, and systolic arterial hypertension has improved compared with baseline. (C) After aspiration of a total of 300 ml of pericardial fluid, tamponade physiology is relieved as evidenced by: (1) restoration of intrapericardial pressure to zero; (2) restoration of right atrial pressure to a normal level; (3) reappearance of the diastolic Y descent in the right atrial waveform, indicative of the relief of cardiac compression in early diastole. Note the negative fluctuation in intrapericardial pressure during inspiration, accompanied by an increased steepness in the fall of right atrial pressure during the X and Y descents. Although this degree of fluid aspiration completely relieved tamponade physiology, an additional 1500 ml of fluid was removed from the pericardial space.

syringe from the stopcock and connecting the intrapericardial catheter by way of sterile tubing to a stoppered sterile glass bottle with a vacuum. This should be done only *when a soft catheter is in the pericardial space* as vacuum suction would be very hazardous with sharp needle drainage. The patient may be tilted gently to either side to facilitate complete drainage. Complete drainage is usually present when no more fluid can be aspirated; at this point some patients note the appearance of mild pleuritic chest pain consistent with the apposition of inflamed visceral and parietal pericardial surfaces. Systemic arterial, complete right heart pressures, and cardiac output should be recorded at completion of the procedure to assess the effectiveness of the pericardiocentesis and the presence or absence of any other cardiac abnormality.

The pericardial catheter may be left in place safely for 24 hours and attached securely to a closed drainage system using gravity and not a vacuum for suction. Ordinarily, the catheter should not be left in place for longer than 24 hours because of the hazard of introducing an iatrogenic pericardial infection, and it should be rinsed frequently with 1 to 2 ml of fluid. We no longer routinely inject air or carbon dioxide into the pericardium at the end of the procedure. In general, this procedure is of little value in identifying tumor masses.[29] Presently, two-dimensional echocardiography is a readily available and more accurate method for assessing reaccumulation of an effusion and detecting masses adjacent to the heart. We often find it helpful to obtain an echocardiogram immediately following pericardiocentesis, for future comparison. After pericardiocentesis, most patients should be observed for about 24 hours in an intensive care setting with a flow-directed right heart catheter left in place to monitor for recurrent tamponade, which will be manifest by a progressive increase in right atrial pressure. Patients with underlying left ventricular dysfunction or respiratory distress syndrome should be monitored closely for the development of acute pulmonary edema because of the abrupt increase in pulmonary blood flow after the decompression of cardiac tamponade.[32]

Hemodynamic and Angiographic Profile.

Although cardiac tamponade and constrictive pericarditis are both characterized by elevation of intracardiac pressures, progressive reduction of diastolic filling, and reduction of stroke volume, several important differences between these conditions can be identified in the catheterization laboratory. Unlike pericardial constriction, *cardiac tamponade causes continuous compression of the heart throughout the cardiac cycle,* which prevents rapid emptying of the right atrium into the right ventricle when the tricuspid valve opens. Thus, cardiac tamponade is not characterized by the constrictive pattern of excessively rapid ventricular filling in early diastole. A second important physiologic difference is that in cardiac tamponade, but not in constriction, *negative intrathoracic pressure is transmitted to the fluid-filled intrapericardial space and right atrium during inspiration, associated with an inspiratory increase in right ventricular filling* and stroke volume at the expense of that of the left ventricle. Thus, as will be discussed below, patients with cardiac tamponade differ from patients with constriction in that they show: (1) lack of an early diastolic dip-and-plateau or "square root" pattern in the ventricular waveforms; (2) an attenuated or absent early diastolic Y descent in the right atrial waveform; (3) a fall of right atrial and intrapericardial pressure with inspiration, i.e., absence of Kussmaul's sign; (4) striking pulsus paradoxus caused by inspiratory augmentation of right ventricular filling.

In the normal individual, intrapericardial pressure measured with an open end fluid-filled catheter is zero or actually slightly negative and is identical to fluctuations in intrathoracic pressure.[8] During cardiac tamponade, simultaneous recording of intrapericardial, right, and left heart pressures on equisensitive gain usually shows that intrapericardial, right atrial, and right and left ventricular diastolic pressures are virtually identical and elevated, generally to 15 mmHg or more (Fig. 35–9). In patients with severe hypovolemia, intrapericardial and right atrial pressures may be equal but only modestly elevated. Usually, the pulmonary capillary wedge and left ventricular diastolic pressures are elevated and identical to right atrial and intrapericardial pressure. It is important to appreciate that, in patients with preexisting elevation of left ventricular diastolic pressure, cardiac tamponade can be present when intrapericardial and right heart pressures are elevated and equal, but lower than left ventricular diastolic pressure.[33]

Right ventricular diastolic collapse, a widely used echocardiographic marker of cardiac tamponade, occurs when the critical buckling pressure of the right ventricle is reached. For the normal thin-walled right ventricle, this critical buckling pressure consists of a negative transmural pressure of only 0.05 to 0.1 mmHg![23] This critical relationship between pericardial and right ventricular diastolic pressure can occur when pericardial pressure is lower than left ventricular pressure. This underscores the importance of measuring the intrapericardial pressure in addition to right and left heart filling pressures in the patient with suspected cardiac tamponade. Furthermore, it is important to appreciate that partial right ventricular diastolic collapse, which indicates the development of impaired right heart filling, occurs early in the development of cardiac tamponade and is a poor indicator of both the magnitude of elevation of pericardial pressure and the degree of hemodynamic compromise. In our observations of 50 consecutive patients with echocardiographic findings of pericardial effusion and right heart chamber collapse, there was a wide spectrum of pericardial pressures ranging from 3 to 27 mmHg and over half of the patients had preservation of both a normal systolic blood pressure and cardiac index.[31] Thus, this echocardiographic finding must be evaluated in the context of a careful clinical assessment in making the difficult decision regarding the indications and timing of pericardiocentesis. Pulmonary artery and right ventricular systolic pressures are generally less than 50 mmHg with a narrow pulse pressure reflecting the depressed stroke volume. When tamponade is moderately severe, right ven-

tricular end diastolic pressure equals or exceeds the right ventricular pulse pressure in magnitude. In extremely severe cardiac tamponade, right ventricular systolic pressure may be only minimally higher than right ventricular diastolic pressure.

Because the heart is compressed continuously by fluid under pressure during cardiac tamponade, right ventricular pressure does not fall to near zero in early diastole. Thus, unlike constrictive pericarditis, the right ventricular waveform has an attenuated fall of pressure in early diastole and does not show a dip and plateau. The right atrial waveform is distinctive in that the prominent early diastolic Y descent characteristic of constriction is absent or, indeed, replaced by a positive wave[8] (Fig. 35–9).

Pulsus paradoxus is easily recorded from systemic arterial pressure measurements; in severe cases, peak systolic arterial pressure declines by more than 15 to 20 mmHg during inspiration. The decline in diastolic arterial pressure is less, so that the arterial pulse pressure decreases during inspiration. The predominant mechanism of pulsus paradoxus in cardiac tamponade has been elegantly studied by Shabetai and co-workers,[34] who showed that, when experimental cardiac tamponade was produced in dogs, *pulsus paradoxus depended on the inspiratory expansion of right heart volume at the expense of left heart filling within the heart compressed by fluid.* The role of respiratory preload variation in the genesis of pulsus paradoxus is supported by recent hemodynamic measurements in patients with cardiac tamponade which showed that left ventricular transmural diastolic pressure falls to or below zero during inspiration.[23] Other factors that may contribute to the striking inspiratory fall in left ventricular stroke volume and systemic arterial pressure include inspiratory pooling of pulmonary venous blood, an inspiratory rise in transmural aortic pressure causing an increase in left ventricular afterload, and the fact that the underfilled left ventricle is operating on the steep ascending limb of the Starling curve so that any inspiratory reduction of left heart filling elicits a striking fall in left ventricular stroke volume.[34,35]

These physiologic effects of respiration in cardiac tamponade result in an inspiratory increase of right ventricular stroke volume. As a result, respiratory variation in systolic pulmonary arterial and right ventricular pressures is out of phase by two or three beats with the inspiratory fluctuation in systemic arterial pressure. Pulsus paradoxus may be absent with coexisting atrial septal defect because the inspiratory increase in venous return is distributed between the right and left atria,[36] and in conditions such as aortic regurgitation, in which there is a major contribution to ventricular filling independent of respiration. This is an important consideration when tamponade due to aortic dissection is evaluated. Pulsus paradoxus may also be absent if cardiac compression is caused by localized collections of fluid or thrombus around the heart, as in the postoperative heart patient. In severe tamponade, in which the compensatory mechanisms of sinus tachycardia and an increased systemic resistance are inadequate, systemic hypotension is found.

Aspiration of intrapericardial fluid is accompanied by an initial parallel fall in intrapericardial and right atrial pressures. Further aspiration causes intrapericardial pressure to fall to zero or become negative. Systemic arterial pressure and stroke volume increase, and the magnitude of pulsus paradoxus falls progressively during initial aspirations; these parameters do not change further after pericardial pressure falls below right atrial pressure.

Angiographic studies are rarely indicated if echocardiographic and hemodynamic studies indicate the presence of a pericardial effusion and the physiology of cardiac tamponade. During simple fluoroscopy, as the catheter is advanced to the lateral wall of the right atrium, it is typically not possible to position the catheter tip immediately adjacent to the cardiac silhouette's border, and the catheter tip will appear to pulsate while the cardiac silhouette's border appears immobile. The rapid injection of contrast medium into the superior vena cava will show a separation between the opacified right atrium and the right and outer border of the nonopacified pericardial fluid. The normal convexity of the right heart border is replaced by a straight or, in more severe cases, a concave right atrial border. In traumatic hemopericardium, in which only 100 to 200 ml of fluid may cause cardiac tamponade, the contour of the right atrial border shows characteristic features of tamponade, but the separation of the outer pericardial border from the heart itself may not be evident.

Left ventriculography is usually not useful in evaluation of cardiac tamponade unless there is a suspicion of coexisting left ventricular dysfunction or valvular heart disease. In cardiac tamponade, as in constrictive pericarditis, the fall in stroke volume caused by limitation of diastolic filling is accompanied by a reflex increase in heart rate and contractility from enhanced autonomic tone.[37] Thus, left and right ventricular diastolic volumes are small, but the ejection fraction is high, end-systolic volume is small, and isovolumic contractility indices are normal or supranormal because of enhanced cardiac contractility.[38] When cardiac tamponade is extremely advanced and cardiac output falls, coronary hypoperfusion[39] may reverse these effects followed by the development of profound sinus bradycardia and electromechanical dissociation.

The finding of arterial oxygen desaturation (hypoxemia) in the patient with cardiac tamponade merits comment. Arterial hypoxemia is not a feature of cardiac tamponade. When dyspnea, tachypnea, and hypoxemia are present in a patient after pericardiocentesis, an additional diagnosis should be sought. In patients with cardiac tamponade caused by known or suspected malignancy, the coexisting problem of pulmonary microvascular and lymphangitic carcinomatosis may be present. In such patients, a *pulmonary capillary wedge aspirate* should be obtained for cytologic examination at the time of combined right heart catheterization and pericardiocentesis.[40]

EFFUSIVE-CONSTRICTIVE PERICARDITIS

An intermediate stage in the development of constrictive pericarditis can exist in which a pericardial effusion under pressure is present as well as a constricting visceral pericardium. Hancock called this condition effusive-constrictive pericarditis and emphasized that *its hallmark is the continued elevation of right atrial pressure after pericardial fluid aspiration has restored intrapericardial pressure to zero.*[41] Diagnosis of this common cause of pericardial compression requires simultaneous recording of intrapericardial pressure and cardiac filling pressures during combined pericardiocentesis and cardiac catheterization.[41,42] Initially, intrapericardial, right atrial, right ventricular diastolic, left atrial, and left ventricular diastolic pressures are elevated and equal. Before pericardiocentesis, the hemodynamic features are those of cardiac tamponade. Pulsus paradoxus is usually present, and the right atrial waveform shows a reduced or absent diastolic Y descent, indicating that cardiac compression is present throughout the cardiac cycle, including early diastole. Aspiration of pericardial fluid restores intrapericardial pressure to zero and pulsus paradoxus is relieved. Right atrial pressure remains elevated, however, and the right atrial waveform acquires the configuration of constriction with a prominent Y descent and diminished respiratory fluctuation, as shown in Figure 35–10. Similarly, the right ventricular waveform changes from that of tamponade, in which early diastolic pressure fall is attenuated, to that of constrictive pericarditis with an early diastolic dip-and-plateau configuration. The latter indicates that cardiac compression by the visceral pericardium does not impede ventricular filling until mid-diastole.

Effusive-constrictive pericarditis is usually associated with tuberculosis, mediastinal irradiation, or neoplastic pericardial infiltration.[2,41] It is extremely important to recognize and diagnose accurately during cardiac catheterization. In such patients, the initial pericardiocentesis may improve cardiac output and relieve hypotension. Subsequent long-term relief of cardiac compression, however, requires total visceral and parietal pericardiectomy,[43] rather than repeated pericardiocentesis or a limited subxiphoid pericardial window.

PERCUTANEOUS PERICARDIOSCOPY AND BIOPSY

In patients with chronic large pericardial effusions of unknown cause and in effusions suspected to have an infectious or malignant cause, pericardiocentesis may be performed for fluid analysis to provide a diagnosis. Endrys and coworkers[44] have reported a technique for obtaining pericardial biopsies using an endomyocardial bioptome inserted into the pericardial space by means of a curved 8 Fr Teflon sheath following percutaneous catheter pericardiocentesis. Fluoroscopic guidance of the bioptome to obtain specimens is facilitated by permitting the entry of air into the pericardial space to outline and separate the visceral and parietal layers of the pericardium, after which the air is aspirated. The use of a flexible fiber optic bronchoscope, inserted by means of a subxiphoid incision to allow inspection of the pericardial surface and selective biopsy, has also been reported.[45] These techniques may be useful in yielding diagnostic information in patients with a thickened pericardium and effusion in whom there is a strong suspicion of malignant or tuberculous etiologies. The efficacy and complication rates of these approaches in comparison with surgical exploration and biopsy of the pericardium are not yet known.

OTHER CAUSES OF CARDIAC COMPRESSION

Compression of the heart by masses extrinsic to the pericardium may cause the pathophysiologic abnormalities of cardiac tamponade. Acute compression of the heart by localized cardiac tamponade or an organizing mediastinal hematoma is an increasingly recognized complication in postoperative heart patients, even when the pericardium is left open.[46] In these patients, true fibrotic constrictive pericarditis may gradually develop in association with an organized hematoma.[47]

Wynne and coworkers have reported extrinsic compression of the heart by tumor simulating cardiac tamponade.[48] As shown in Fig-

A. BEFORE PERICARDIOCENTESIS

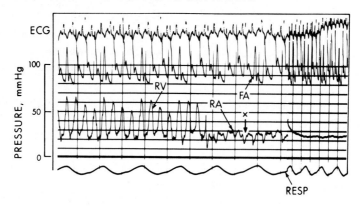

B. AFTER PERICARDIOCENTESIS

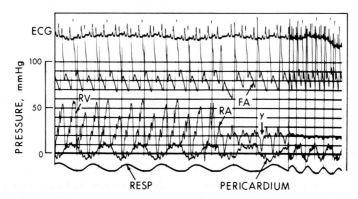

Fig. 35–10. Femoral arterial (FA) and right ventricular (RV) to right atrial (RA) pull-back pressure tracings before (A) and after (B) pericardiocentesis in a patient with effusive-constrictive pericarditis secondary to carcinoma of the lung. After pericardiocentesis and return of pericardial pressure to normal levels (B), there is a loss of the abnormal pulsus paradoxus, but the RV end-diastolic and RA mean pressures remain elevated. Note that a diastolic Y descent is absent in the right atrial waveform before pericardiocentesis (A), and a steep Y descent is the prominent feature of the waveform after pericardiocentesis (B). Time lines are 1 second; a respiratory trace (RESP) is seen with inspiration indicated by a positive (upward) deflection. (From Mann T et al: Effusive-constrictive hemodynamic pattern due to neoplastic involvement of the pericardium. Am J Cardiol 41:781, 1978.)

ure 35–11, a massive posterior sarcoma displaced the heart anteriorly and superiorly, causing increased right and left atrial pressures. Constriction may also be caused by massive neoplastic involvement with tumor encircling the heart (cor en cuirasse). Recent experimental studies by Fowler et al.[25] have added insight into the hemodynamic consequences of regional tamponade with the observation that compression of the right atrium and ventricle has a more pronounced effect on cardiac output and systemic arterial pressure than does left heart compression.

ANOMALIES OF THE PERICARDIUM

Anomalies of the pericardium may cause confusion during cardiac catheterization and angiography unless their characteristic features are recognized. Pericardial cysts, which are filled with clear fluid, are usually located at the right costophrenic angle and come to attention as an unexplained enlargement of the right heart border on the chest roentgenogram. Rarely, they may be associated with atypical chest pain suggestive of angina or pericarditis.

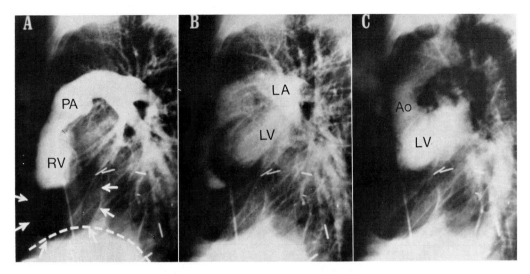

Fig. 35–11. Right ventriculogram (lateral view) in a patient with extrinsic compression of the heart by tumor masquerading as cardiac tamponade. (A) Right ventricular (RV) ejection phase with filling of the pulmonary arteries (PA), and subsequent (B) early and (C) late levo-phase, demonstrating left atrium (LA), left ventricle (LV), and aorta (Ao). Note displacement of both ventricles superiorly and anteriorly by a large radiolucent mass (arrows) interposed between the diaphragm (broken line) and inferior surface of the heart. Metal clips are from the patient's original tumor resection surgery and reflect the location of known persistent tumor mass. (From Wynne J, Markis, JE, and Grossman, W.: Extrinsic compression of the heart by tumor masquerading as cardiac tamponade. Cathet Cardiovasc Diagn 4:81, 1978.)

Contrast angiography is occasionally required to differentiate a cyst from a cardiac aneurysm. Although most patients can be managed conservatively, large pericardial cysts located at the right costophrenic angle can be decompressed in the catheterization laboratory by percutaneous aspiration under fluoroscopic guidance.[49]

Total absence of the pericardium is extremely rare and usually not associated with symptoms. *Absence of the left side of the pericardium* is more common. Patients may come to cardiac catheterization because of chest pain, palpitations, or dyspnea in association with widened splitting of the second heart sound, a systolic murmur at the upper left sternal border, and electrocardiographic abnormalities of right axis deviation and clockwise displacement of the precordial transition zone because of levoposition of the heart. The chest roentgenogram typically shows a leftward position of the heart and a prominent pulmonary artery, and the condition may be confused with other conditions such as pulmonic stenosis or atrial septal defect.[50] Findings at cardiac catheterization are usually normal, and cardiac angiography with diagnostic left pneumothorax to outline the pericardium is indicated rarely today to make the diagnosis if typical clinical and radiologic features are present. In patients with *partial left-sided pericardial defects,* however, angiography can be helpful. Patients frequently complain of chest pain and syncope and are at risk for sudden death related to herniation and strangulation of the heart through the defect. A definitive diagnosis can be made by pulmonary artery angiography with follow-through to the left heart by showing herniation of the left atrium or its appendage beyond the heart border.[51] Partial right-sided pericardial defect can be complicated by severe pleuritic or pericarditis-like chest pain because of inspiratory herniation of the right atrium through the defect.[52] In this condition, right atrial contrast angiography in the left anterior oblique projection may show herniation of the right atrium (and sometimes the right ventricle) through the defect.

REFERENCES

1. Shabetai R, Fowler NO, Fenton JC: Restrictive cardiac disease. Pericarditis and the myocardiopathies. Am Heart J 69:271, 1965.

2. Cameron J, Oesterle SN, Baldwin JC, Hancock EW: The etiologic spectrum of constrictive pericarditis. Am Heart J 113:354, 1987.

3. Applefeld MM, et al: Delayed pericardial disease after radiotherapy. Am J Cardiol 47:210, 1981.

4. Sagrista-Sauleda J, Permanger-Miralda G, Candell-Riera J, Angel J, Soler-Soler J: Transient cardiac constriction: an unrecognized pattern of evolution in effusive acute idiopathic pericarditis. Am J Cardiol 59:961, 1987.

5. Vallance PJT, Gray HH, Oldershaw PJ: Diagnostic features of localized pericardial constriction. Intern J Cardiol 20:416, 1988.

6. Bush CA, Stang JM, Wooley CF, Kilman JW: Occult constrictive pericardial disease: Diagnosis by rapid volume expansion and correction by pericardiectomy. Circulation 56:924, 1977.

7. Tyberg TI, Goodyer AVN, Langou RA: Genesis of pericardial knock in constrictive pericarditis. Am J Cardiol 46:570, 1980.

8. Shabetai R, Fowler NO, Guntheroth WG: The hemodynamics of cardiac tamponade and constrictive pericarditis. Am J Cardiol 26:480, 1970.

9. Gaasch WH, Peterson KL, Shabetai R: Left ventricular function in chronic constrictive pericarditis. Am J Cardiol 34:107, 1974.

10. Goldberg E, Stein J, Berger M, Berdoff RL: Diastolic segmental coronary artery obliteration in constrictive pericarditis. Cathet Cardiovasc Diagn 7:197, 1981.

11. Hancock EW: On the elastic and rigid forms of constrictive pericarditis. Am Heart J 100:917, 1980.

12. Chew C, Ziady GM, Raphael MJ, Oakley GM: The functional defect in amyloid heart disease. The "stiff heart" syndrome. Am J Cardiol 36:438, 1975.

13. Meaney E, et al: Cardiac amyloidosis, constrictive pericarditis and resrictive cardiomyopathy. Am J Cardiol 38:547, 1976.

14. Schoenfeld MH, et al: Restrictive cardiomyopathy versus constrictive pericarditis: Role of endomyocardial biopsy in avoiding unnecessary thoracotomy. Circulation 75:1012, 1987.

15. Benotti JR, Grossman W, Cohn PF: The clinical profile of restrictive cardiomyopathy. Circulation 61:1206, 1980.

16. Kern MJ, Lorell BH, Grossman W: Cardiac amyloidosis masquerading as constrictive pericarditis. Cathet Cardiovasc Diagn 8:629, 1982.

17. Tyberg TI, et al: Left ventricular filling in differentiating restrictive amyloid cardiomyopathy and constrictive pericarditis. Am J Cardiol 47:791, 1981.

18. Aroney CN, et al: Differentiation of restrictive cardiomyopathy from pericardial constriction: Assessment of diastolic function by radionuclide angiography. J Am Coll Cardiol 13:1007, 1989.

19. Lorell BH, et al: Right ventricular infarction. Am J Cardiol 43:465, 1979.

20. Goldstein JA, et al: The role of right ventricular systolic dysfunction and elevated intrapericardial pressure in the genesis of low output in experimental right ventricular infarction. Circulation 65:513, 1982.

21. Bartle SH, Hermann HJ: Acute mitral regurgitation in man. Hemodynamic evidence and observations indicating an early role for the pericardium. Circulation 36:839, 1967.

22. Tyberg JV, et al: The relationship between pericardial pressure and right atrial pressure: An intraoperative study. Circulation 73:428, 1985.

23. Boltwood CM Jr: Ventricular performance related to transmural filling pressure in clinical cardiac tamponade. Circulation 75:941, 1987.

24. Smiseth OA, et al: Assessment of pericardial constraint in dogs. Circulation 71:158, 1985.

25. Fowler NO, Gabel M, Buncher CR: Cardiac tamponade: A comparison of right versus left heart compression. J Am Coll Cardiol 12:187, 1988.

26. Beck CS: Two cardiac compression triads. JAMA 104:714, 1935.

27. Guberman BA, et al: Cardiac tamponade in medical patients. Circulation 64:633, 1981.

28. Antman EM, Cargill V, Grossman W: Low-pressure cardiac tamponade. Ann Intern Med 91:403, 1979.

29. Krikorian JG, Hancock EW: Pericardiocentesis. Am J Med 65:808, 1978.

30. Singh S, et al: Right ventricular and right atrial collapse in patients with cardiac tamponade—a combined echocardiographic and hemodynamic study. Circulation 70:966, 1984.

31. Levine MJ, Lorell BH, Diver DJ, Come PC: Implications of echocardiographically-assisted diagnosis of pericardial tamponade in contemporary medical patients: Detection prior to hemodynamic embarrassment. J Am Coll Cardiol (In press).

32. Vandyke WH, Cure J, Chakko CS, Gheorghiode M: Pulmonary edema after pericardiocentesis for cardiac tamponade. N Engl J Med 309:595 1983.

33. Reddy PS, Curtiss EI, O'Toole JD, Shaver JA: Cardiac tamponade: Hemodynamic observations in man. Circulation 58:265, 1978.

34. Shabetai R, Fowler NO, Fenton JC, Massangkay M: Pulsus paradoxus. J Clin Invest 44:1882, 1965.

35. Friedman HS, Sakurai H, Lejam F: Pulsus paradoxus: A manifestation of a marked reduction in left ventricular end-diastolic volume in cardiac tamponade. J Thorac Cardiovasc Surg 79:74, 1980.

36. Winer HE, Kronzon I: Absence of pulsus paradoxus in patients with cardiac tamponade and atrial septal defects. Am J Cardiol 44:378, 1979.

37. Friedman HS, et al: Effect of autonomic blockade on the hemodynamic findings in acute cardiac tamponade. Am J Physiol 232:H5, 1977.

38. Craig RJ, Whalen RE, Behar VS, McIntosh HD: Pressure and volume changes of the left ventricle in acute pericardial tamponade. Am J Cardiol 22:65, 1968.

39. Jarmakani JM, McHale PA, Greenfield JC, Jr: The effect of cardiac tamponade on coronary hemodynamics in the awake dog. Cardiovasc Res 9:112, 1975.

40. Safian RD, Come SE, Kadin M, Lorell BH: Use of pulmonary capillary wedge aspirates for the antemortem diagnosis of pulmonary microvascular tumor. Cathet Cardiovasc Diagn 17:112, 1989.

41. Hancock EW: Subacute effusive-constrictive pericarditis. Circulation 43:183, 1971.

42. Mann T, Brodie BR, Grossman W, McLaurin LP: Effusive-constrictive hemodynamic pattern due to neoplastic involvement of the pericardium. Am J Cardiol 41:781, 1978.

43. Walsh TJ, Baughman KL, Gardner TJ, Bulkley BH: Constrictive epicarditis as a cause of delayed or absent

response to pericardiectomy. J Thorac Cardiovasc Surg 83:126, 1982.

44. Endrys J, et al: New nonsurgical technique for multiple pericardial biopsies. Cathet Cardiovasc Diagn 15:92, 1988.

45. Kondos GT, Rich S, Levitsky S: Flexible fiberoptic pericardioscopy for the diagnosis of pericardial disease. J Am Coll Cardiol 7:432, 1986.

46. Fyke FE, et al: Detection of intrapericardial hematoma after open heart surgery: The roles of echocardiography and computed tomography. J Am Coll Cardiol 5:1496, 1985.

47. Cimino JJ, Kogan AD: Constrictive pericarditis after cardiac surgery: report of three cases and review of the literature. Am Heart J 118:1292, 1989.

48. Wynne J, Markis JE, Grossman W: Extrinsic compression of the heart by tumor masquerading as cardiac tamponade. Cathet Cardiovasc Diagn 4:81, 1978.

49. Peterson DT, Zatz LM, Popp RL: Pericardial cyst ten years after acute pericarditis. Chest 67:719, 1975.

50. Nasser WK: Congenital absence of the left pericardium. Am J Cardiol 26:466, 1970.

51. Bernal JM, et al: Angiographic demonstration of a partial defect of the pericardium with herniation of the left atrium and ventricle. J Cardiovasc Surg 27:344, 1986.

52. Minocha GK, Falicov RE, Nijensohn E: Partial right-sided congenital pericardial defect with herniation of right atrium and right ventricle. Chest 76:484, 1979.

36

Profiles in Congenital Heart Disease

JAMES E. LOCK, STANTON B. PERRY, and JOHN F. KEANE

Two decades of advances in the diagnosis and management of congenital heart disease have radically altered the population of adults who currently undergo cardiac catheterization. For example, during the period between 1959 and 1964, nearly all adults who underwent cardiac catheterization had relatively simple disease: left-to-right shunts (atrial septal defect, ventricular septal defect, or patent ductus arteriosus) or isolated valvar disease (aortic stenosis, pulmonic stenosis) (Fig. 36–1). In the current era, most of these simpler lesions are diagnosed and corrected in childhood. The surgical management of these lesions is relatively successful (except for aortic stenosis), and these patients now rarely require cardiac management in adult life. In contrast, patients who had complex and highly fatal lesions (transposition of the great arteries, tetralogy of Fallot, single ventricle) are now surviving into adulthood with increasing frequency (Fig. 36–1). Surgical management (even when ''corrective'') has resulted in palliation, however, and these patients require frequent cardiovascular follow-up. Thus, in the half decade from 1979 to 1984, most adults who underwent cardiac catheterization at both the Brigham Hospital and Children's Hospital[1] had either complex heart disease, prior surgery, or both (Fig. 36–2).

This shifting patient population has placed increasing burdens on the catheterizing cardiologist: previously, cardiac catheterization

was designed primarily to establish the diagnosis using pressure tracings, oximetry determinations, angiography, and dye dilution techniques (see Chap. 6). This anatomic diagnostic role of cardiac catheterization in the adult is increasingly accomplished using noninvasive techniques, especially Doppler echocardiography. At present, the more likely indications for catheterization include the search for previously unrecognized associated lesions, assessment of valvar or ventricular function, quantification of abnormalities of the pulmonary vascular bed, electrophysiologic testing, and (most commonly) interventional catheter procedures.

This chapter focuses on the profiles of information one is likely to encounter during cardiac catheterization of the more common congenital cardiac lesions, both preoperatively and postoperatively. These profiles are brief, and include a discussion of the features that may be important in performing transcatheter ''correction'' of the cardiac lesions (see Chap. 30). A much more thorough discussion of the catheterization of congenital heart disease is available elsewhere.[2]

ATRIAL SEPTAL DEFECT

Despite the advances noted above, ASDs are still commonly encountered at cardiac catheterization: physical signs may be relatively subtle in childhood, and symptoms are

654

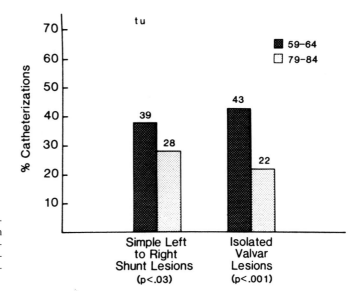

Fig. 36–1. Graph showing frequency with which adult patients with simple forms of congenital heart disease underwent cardiac catheterization 25 years ago and during the recent era.

infrequent until the third decade of a patient's life. Recent advances in transcatheter umbrella closure in ASDs have also renewed catheterization laboratory activity in this condition.

Anatomic Types

Atrial septal defects are broadly categorized into three different types: primum defects (about 30% of all ASDs), secundum defects (about 65%), and sinus venosus defects (about 5%). Ostium primum defects, associated with a counterclockwise superior loop on the elec-

trocardiogram, occur in the most inferior part of the atrial septum. By definition, there is no septal rim between the defect and the atrioventricular valve ring. Ostium primum defects often occur with abnormalities (clefts) of the mitral and tricuspid valves. In such defects, the "atrioventricular" septum (i.e., the part of the heart that separates the right atrium from the left ventricle) is absent, a feature that is best seen echocardiographically; the associated mitral abnormalities frequently result in mitral regurgitation.

Ostium secundum defects are located in the

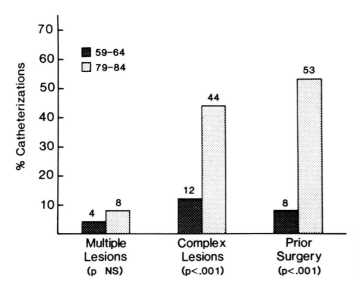

Fig. 36–2. Graph showing that adults with congenital heart disease have increasing frequencies of complex and postoperative diagnoses.

fossa ovalis, below the limbic band, and may represent either failure of closure of the foramen ovale or actual defects within the fossa ovalis. Multiple defects within the fossa ovalis are not rare,[3] and may complicate efforts at transcatheter ASD closure.

Sinus venosus defects are at the most posterior part of the atrial septum with little posterior septal rim. They are usually near the superior vena cava entrance to the heart, and may be associated with a superior P wave axis on electrocardiogram. Anomalous drainage of the right pulmonary veins to the superior vena cava or right atrium is a frequent associated lesion.

Physiology

The size and direction of shunting through an atrial septal defect depend on both the size of the hole and the relative compliances of the two ventricles, factors that decrease right ventricular compliance (e.g., pulmonary stenosis, pulmonary hypertension) induce a smaller left-to-right shunt or a larger right-to-left shunt, while factors that reduce left ventricular compliance (e.g., systemic hypertension, left ventricular infarction) produce a larger left-to-right shunt. In infancy, the right ventricle is normally hypertrophied as a result of intrauterine circulation, and there is little net shunt across an ASD. With increasing age, however, the shunts tend to get larger and larger, resulting in the clinical detection of ASDs in childhood and early adulthood. This tendency for left-to-right shunting to increase throughout life (as arterial blood pressures rise and left ventricular compliance falls) has prompted many authors to advocate a policy of closing all ASDs at the time of diagnosis.[4]

Catheterization Technique

Catheter passage through a secundum ASD from a femoral vein approach is generally straightforward: with the catheter tip in the superior vena cava, withdrawal to the heart with the tip positioned posteroleftward results in the catheter flopping medially across the

limbic band to the fossa ovalis (as is the case for a Brockenbrough maneuver) and from there through the ASD. A primum defect is positioned a bit more inferiorly. Difficulty in crossing a known ASD implies the presence of a sinus venosus defect.

Crossing the atrial septum with a catheter does not demonstrate the presence of an atrial "defect"; a probe patent foramen ovale (where the septum primum and septum secundum overlap each other, but can be separated by a catheter or a marked rise in right atrial pressure) is a normal finding in many children and in 10 to 15% of adults.

Oximetry Data

Atrial defects with left-to-right shunts are characterized by an increase, or step-up, in the oxygen content (or saturation) of blood in the right atrium (Fig. 36–3). Based on the studies of Freed et al. in children,[5] a 10% increase in oxygen saturation between the superior vena cava and the right atrium on a single measurement, or an 8% increase on multiple determinations, indicates an abnormal increase in saturated blood into the right atrium. Studies in adults that have produced similar saturation criteria have generally relied on samples from both the superior and the inferior vena cava. Recognizing the penchant of the inferior vena caval blood to be poorly mixed because of streaming of renal vein blood, multiple IVC samples have proved helpful.

A significant step-up at the right atrial level does not guarantee the presence of an atrial septal defect: patients who have ventricular septal defects or sinus of Valsalva aneurysms into the right ventricle and associated tricuspid regurgitation can have identical oximetric data. Associated abnormalities such as partial anomalous pulmonary venous return to the cava can be difficult to diagnose from oximetry alone, although they are suggested by saturations over 85% in the SVC or IVC.

These oximetry data are used to calculate pulmonary blood flows and shunts. Because oximetry values may vary by 3 to 6% on a random basis, shunts less than 1.5 to 1 cannot

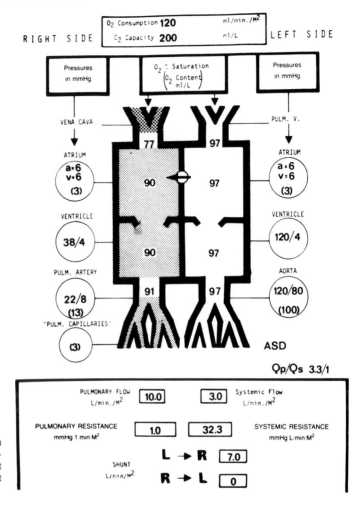

Fig. 36–3. Cardiac catheterization findings in a patient with an atrial septal defect. Note the left-to-right shunt at the atrial level and the flow gradient across the pulmonary valve.

be reliably detected by oximetry. Obviously, the absence of a measured shunt does not exclude an important ASD: with the development of pulmonary vascular disease and progressive right ventricular hypertension, right ventricular compliance may fall, and the left-to-right shunt may become negligible. Further decreases in right ventricular compliance result in cyanosis.

Pressure Data

The hallmark of a moderate or large atrial defect is the equalization of atrial pressures: previous workers have documented that mean atrial pressures are within 1 to 2 mm Hg and a and v wave peaks are within 3 to 4 mm Hg in a good-sized ASD.[6] Obviously, the a and

v waves tend to become similar in both atria with a large defect. We frequently use the pressure gradient across the atrial septum to differentiate a patent foramen ovale from a moderate or large ASD.

Conversely, the absence of a transatrial gradient does not make the diagnosis of an ASD; pericardial tamponade, restrictive physiology, and diseases that raise right atrial pressures all tend to equalize the gradient across the atrial septum.

Angiography

Until recently, angiography was an unimportant part of the catheterization in a patient with an ASD: pressure equalization across the atria, catheter course, and a step-up at the atrial level together make a compelling diagnosis. Most cardiologists have added a left ventriculogram to rule out associated small shunts, as well as the levophase of a pulmonary arteriogram to rule out anomalous pulmonary venous connection. With the advent of an active program to accomplish transcatheter closure of atrial septal defects, we now perform both angiography and balloon sizing of atrial defects to assess the patient's candidacy for transcatheter closure (Fig. 36–4).

Whenever we suspect the presence of an ostium primum ASD in a patient undergoing cardiac catheterization, we always perform a left ventriculogram in a so-called hepatoclavicular view (40 degrees cranial, 40 degrees left anterior oblique). These views outline the presence of associated ventricular defects, which may be present in the most posterior part of the ventricular septum.[7]

Interventional Catheterization

Although patients with sinus venosus defects and ostium primum defects generally have insufficient septal rim to allow transcatheter umbrella closure, about 50 to 60% of patients with secundum ASDs appear to be good candidates.[8,29] In addition to angiography, balloon sizing of the defect with a soft, deformable balloon allows one to assess the stretched

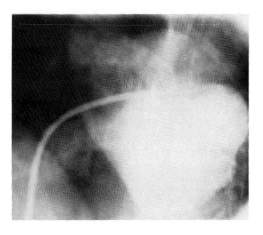

Fig. 36–4. Angiogram across an atrial septal defect in a 40-degree LAO view with cranial angulation. The defect is about 12 mm in diameter.

diameter of the defect. At present, we are closing central defects with stretched diameters of 24 mm or less (Chap. 30).

VENTRICULAR SEPTAL DEFECTS

Ventricular septal defects are an increasingly rare form of heart disease to be subjected to catheterization during adulthood. Loud murmurs permit diagnosis at an early age, large defects produce symptoms early in life and demand early closure, and small defects tend to get smaller with advancing age. Pediatric cardiologists tend to "fish or cut bait" on VSDs by age 2, or certainly by age 5: defects unclosed by that age will probably never require surgical attention.

Nonetheless, patients continue to have congenital, post-traumatic, or postinfarction VSDs that will need diagnostic or interventional cardiac catheterization.

Anatomic Types

Most congenital VSDs are perimembranous: just underneath the aortic valve, they are midway between the anteriormost extent of the ventricular septum (near the pulmonary outflow track) and the posterior septum, between the mitral and tricuspid valve. A-V canal type VSDs are less common, are developmentally related to ostium primum defects, and occur in the posterior septum between the A-V valves. Like ostium primum defects, they tend to be associated with left axis deviation in the ECG frontal plane, and are more commonly seen in patients with Down's syndrome. Subpulmonary VSDs are the most anterior of the membranous VSDs, occur as a deficiency in the conal septum as it lies between the aorta and pulmonary artery. Subpulmonary VSDs (recently referred to as subarterial VSDs) are more commonly diagnosed among Orientals, and are more likely to be associated with aortic valve cusp prolapse and regurgitation.

Muscular VSDs can occur anywhere in the ventricular septum. Most are midmuscular, just below the moderator band in the right ventricle, although defects can occur in the apical septum, the anterior septum, and the posterior septum. Finally, some defects termed "swiss-cheese VSDs" have large openings on the left ventricular side of the septum, but then break up into myriad channels as they pass from left to right.

Once a VSD is thought to be large enough to warrant closure, we continue to recommend cardiac catheterization to exclude additional defects and to assess the pulmonary vascular resistance. Increasing accuracy of noninvasive testing continues to limit the need for catheterization of VSDs to patients in whom closure is needed.

Physiology

Because shunting through a VSD occurs primarily in systole, the size and direction of shunting are determined mostly by the afterload that each ventricle faces: thus, factors that increase left ventricle afterload (hypertension, coarctation) or decrease right ventricular afterload (the fall in pulmonary resistance that occurs normally in early infancy) increase the left-to-right shunt, and factors that decrease left ventricular afterload (vasodilator therapy) or increase right ventricular afterload (the development of pulmonary stenosis or pulmonary vascular disease) decrease the left-to-right shunt or even produce a right-to-left shunt and cyanosis.

In addition, there is a strong natural tendency for VSDs to close with advancing age: most muscular defects close or become small by 5 years of age, and perimembranous defects may close by aneurysm formation or adherence of the septal leaflet of the tricuspid valve to the edges of the defect. Thus, medical management is generally advised initially for any restrictive VSD in an asymptomatic patient.

Catheterization Technique

Until recently, catheter passage through a VSD was avoided for the most part, as it was unnecessary to either make the diagnosis or estimate the size of the shunt. The recent highly successful efforts to close certain VSDs using a transcatheter umbrella approach (Chap. 30) has served to re-emphasize the importance of catheter courses in this defect. For perimembranous defects near the tricuspid valve, the catheter is advanced into the right ventricle and turned posteriorly (counterclockwise) to cross the VSD into the left ventricular outflow track. Midmuscular, apical, and anterior muscular VSDs are difficult to cross from the right ventricle, and are usually crossed with balloon flotation catheters from the left ventricle.

Oximetry Data

As noted previously, a simple right heart pressure/oximetry series with measurements from the wedge position, distal pulmonary arteries, main pulmonary artery, right ventricle and atrium, and the superior vena cava, define the pulmonary artery pressures and estimate the size of the shunt; representative hemodynamics are listed in Figure 36–5.

In cases of elevated pulmonary artery pressure and elevated pulmonary resistance, previous authors have advanced the notion of a "reactive" pulmonary vascular bed: if the resistance falls in response to a vasodilator agent (usually inhaled oxygen), the pulmonary resistance is more likely to fall after corrective surgery. This hypothesis seems to be important in patients who live at high altitude, but has not proved useful in patients with elevated resistance who live at or near sea level.

Pressure Data

Patients with small VSDs have a large pressure drop across the ventricular septum. Equalization of ventricular pressures always occurs with a large VSD, but does not prove the presence of a large defect; small defects with associated pulmonary hypertension may mimic the pressure findings in a large defect. Thus, the size and location of a VSD must be determined by an imaging technique.

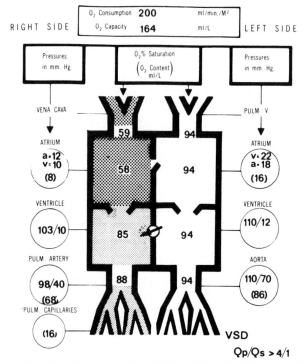

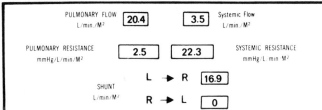

Fig. 36–5. Cardiac catheterization findings in a patient with a large ventricular septal defect. Note the left-to-right shunt at the ventricular level. There is pulmonary hypertension with only slightly elevated pulmonary vascular resistance. Left ventricular filling pressure is increased, reflecting increased flow and perhaps decreased compliance.

Angiography

The angiography of ventricular defects has been revolutionized by the adaptation of the long axial views of Bargeron et al.[10] Because the septum is generally the surface of a cone that points from right back to left front, any x-ray view that is a left anterior view with cranial angulation tends to put the septal surface in its longest (least foreshortened) direction. In general, the midportion of the septum (i.e., the location of perimembranous and midmuscular defects) is best seen with a steep (70 degree) LAO view, the anterior portion of the septum is seen with a straight lateral view (or even an RAO view) and the posterior portion of the septum (the location of atrioventricular canal defects and posterior muscular defects)

is seen with a shallow (40 degree) LAO view. As usual, injection of contrast in the high pressure chamber (the left ventricle) is required; because anatomic definition is needed rather than PVC-free function, we use high-contrast volumes (about 1.5 cc/kg) at rapid rates (less than 1 second injection times) to outline the defect or defects (Fig. 36–6).

Interventional Cardiology

Our recent report of transcatheter closure of selected VSDs using a double umbrella[11] has now been expanded to include over 20 cases at the Children's Hospital in Boston. The results continue to improve. It is likely that transcatheter closure (Chap. 30), using the newest clamshell septal occluding device, will be-

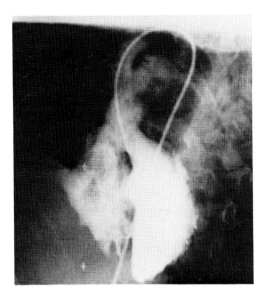

Fig. 36–6. Left ventriculogram in the long axial oblique view, demonstrating multiple VSDs.

come the treatment of choice for muscular defects and for most residual postoperative defects. The role of this technique in the management of postinfarction defects remains an area of active investigation. Considering that the aortic and tricuspid valves are close to the edges of most perimenbranous VSDs, it seems clear that surgery will remain the mainstay of management of these patients at present.

PATENT DUCTUS ARTERIOSUS

Among the more common forms of congenital heart disease, a persistently patent ductus arteriosus (PDA) is usually diagnosed in childhood and corrected at the time of diagnosis. Patency of the ductus is maintained before birth by the production of prostaglandin E. Premature neonates may have an incidence of PDA as high as 40%; medical treatment of these newborns with the arachidonic acid blocker indomethacin eliminates most of these PDAs.

Until recently, the diagnosis of a PDA was made on the basis of physical examination and echocardiography; catheterization was reserved for those patients with unusual findings

or pulmonary hypertension. The development of a safe, reliable method for transcatheter PDA occlusion[12,13] has re-established the importance of catheter techniques in this lesion and brought many more patients with PDA to the catheterization laboratory.

Anatomic Types

PDAs are almost always located off the underside of the aortic arch just distal to the left subclavian, left of the trachea, and proximal to the left mainstem bronchus. Most commonly, they have an hourglass shape with a prominent aortic diverticulum and a narrowing near the pulmonary artery end. Some PDAs are cone-shaped, with a short aortic diverticulum; rarely they are tube-shaped, unrestrictive, and short. An occasional PDA arises from an anomalous left subclavian artery in a patient with a right aortic arch.

Physiology

PDAs are rarely large, except perhaps in patients with Down's syndrome or those who live at high altitudes. A restrictive PDA should produce a measurable step-up in pulmonary arterial saturation, perhaps some pulmonary hypertension, and no change in aortic or right ventricular saturations (Fig. 36–7). The size of the shunt does not appear to change much with the passage of time, although the elderly patient with a PDA is quite likely to tolerate a relatively small shunt poorly. In our experience, patients with small PDAs remain asymptomatic throughout childhood and most of adulthood, but are likely to become symptomatic in their 60s and 70s.

Catheterization Technique

The techniques of a standard right heart catheter study estimate the hemodynamic effects of a PDA. Because, in utero, the ductus arteriosus is merely an extension of the main pulmonary artery, any soft straight catheter usually passes into the PDA from the main pulmonary artery. Because transcatheter clo-

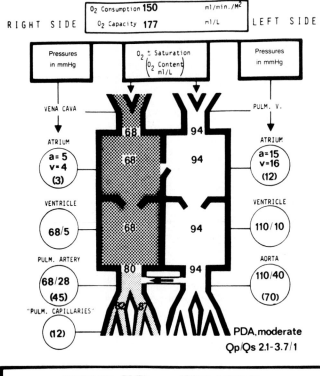

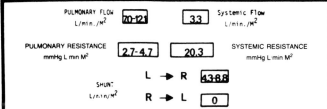

Fig. 36–7. Cardiac catheterization findings in a child with a PDA. There is a left-to-right shunt at the great vessel level, moderate pulmonary hypertension, and disparate saturations in left and right pulmonary arteries.

sure is generally accomplished from the venous side, we use a straight guide wire, advanced from a catheter positioned in the mid MPA, to cross the duct in virtually all cases.

Oximetry Data

Although seemingly straightforward, calculating the shunts in a patient with a PDA is technically difficult. Because aortic blood crosses into the lungs without passing through a mixing chamber, there is considerable streaming in the pulmonary arteries: the cephalad portion of the MPA is often fully saturated, the left pulmonary usually has a higher saturation than the right pulmonary artery, and the "mixed" pulmonary artery saturation cannot be defined accurately. Similarly, in the

presence of a right-to-left shunt, descending aortic blood is bluer than ascending aortic blood. Thus, shunt sizes are estimates at best and do not allow accurate calculation of resistances. If one must determine (in a patient with a hypertensive PDA) whether closing the PDA will result in a fall (or a rise) in pulmonary artery pressure, one must temporarily balloon-occlude the duct and remeasure pressures.

Pressure Data

Most PDAs do not alter right or left heart pressures unless they are large. In the face of any left heart abnormalities (e.g., poor left ventricular function, mitral stenosis) a PDA increases left ventricular systolic and diastolic pressures.

Angiography

Needed to provide an accurate landmark for transcatheter closure, angiographic definition of a PDA is best done in a straight lateral view. A steep LAO may cause the PDA to overlie the underside of the aorta, and make proper definition difficult. The tracheal air column provides an excellent anatomic marker for ductal anatomy, with the narrowest portion of a PDA frequently at the anterior border of the trachea.

Interventional Catheterization

Although a plug and long-wire technique has been used to close PDAs in the catheter laboratory for over 20 years by Porstmann and his colleagues,[14] most workers use a modification of the double umbrella technique of Rashkind[15] (see Chap. 30).

AORTIC STENOSIS

Congenital aortic stenosis, almost always caused by a bicommissural aortic valve, remains a common form of congenital heart disease in both children and adults. The advent of Doppler echocardiography has markedly improved the noninvasive assessment of severity in aortic stenosis, and the need for frequent diagnostic cardiac catheterizations in this lesion has largely disappeared. In general, catheterization is performed just before aortic valvotomy, either surgical or transcatheter. We tend to recommend aortic valvotomy whenever symptoms of cardiac dysfunction appear, or whenever the peak-to-peak valvar gradient (at normal cardiac output) is higher than 50 to 60 mm Hg. Rarely, patients have symptoms or ECG changes out of proportion to their estimated transvalvar gradient, prompting a diagnostic catheterization.

Anatomic Types

Over 75% of children with aortic stenosis have a bicommissural or unicommissural valve, caused by leaflet fusion, and the lesion is present at birth. In these cases, fusion occurs between the right coronary cusp and the noncoronary cusp or, less commonly, between the right and the left coronary cusps. Fusion of the commissure between the left cusp and the noncoronary cusp is essentially unreported. If only one commissure is affected, and the valve is not thickened, there may be little gradient or murmur, with the only finding a fixed aortic ejection click at the apex. Unlike most forms of congenital heart disease, valvar aortic stenosis progresses in severity in one third of cases, making careful follow-up important.[16]

A smaller proportion of patients with aortic stenosis have a lesion below the valve (so-called subaortic stenosis) caused either by a thin fibrous ridge or fibromuscular dysplasia of the left ventricular outflow track. These lesions appear to be progressive in a large proportion of cases, and are known to cause deterioration of the otherwise normal aortic valve, producing aortic regurgitation. Surgery is therefore generally indicated before development of severe stenosis or symptoms, to protect the aortic valve, although the actual value of this treatment approach is uncertain.

Finally, some children have an hourglass deformity above the aortic valve, so-called supravalvar aortic stenosis. Caused at least partly by thickening of the supracoronary ridge, supravalvar aortic stenosis is often seen in association with Williams syndrome and with branch pulmonary artery stenosis.

Physiology

The findings in these patients are similar to those of other patients with aortic obstruction. In addition, patients with supravalvar aortic stenosis usually have unobstructive coronary flow, and hence may develop large coronary vessels and are perhaps less likely to have evidence of ischemia.

Catheterization Technique

Most of what has been written about catheterization in aortic stenosis (Chap. 5) applies to children with congenital aortic stenosis as well. In addition, congenitally narrowed valves tend to have a opening in the posterior part of the valve; once the catheter crosses that valve, it tends to pass posterior to the tensor apparatus of the mitral valve. Because crossing these valves can be difficult, we usually use a side-arm arterial sheath that is one size larger than the catheter; simultaneous pressures are measured from the catheter and the sheath with the catheter in the ascending aorta, to directly measure the amount of pulse delay and pulse amplification. Then, once the catheter is advanced across the valve, a simultaneous measurement of left ventricular and femoral artery pressure allows accurate assessment of the transvalvar gradient and valve area.

Oximetry Data

There are no saturation changes in the left or right heart in these patients. Indeed, the normal variation in right heart oximetry values was established primarily from children with mild valvar aortic and pulmonary stenosis.[5]

Pressure Data

In addition to the simultaneous pressure tracings from the left ventricle and aorta noted previously, a pullback tracing across the aortic valve shouid always be obtained as an internal control. Multihole pigtail catheters are usually used to enter the left ventricle; a pullback tracing with those catheters may not reveal the presence of supravalvar or subvalvar stenosis, making the use of an end-hole catheter necessary.

Angiography

Both aortography and left ventriculography should be obtained in patients with aortic stenosis. Aortography (generally in anteroposterior and lateral views) assesses the degree of aortic regurgitation, annular size, and mobility of the leaflets; and identifies commissural fusion. Ventriculography (left anterior oblique with cranial angulation) helps to estimate ventricular performance, identify subvalvar pathology, and further outline valvar and supravalvar anatomy. Multiple views may be required to best outline the subvalvar region, including a right anterior oblique view with caudal angulation.

Interventional Catheterization

Balloon valvotomy (Chap. 29) has become the treatment of choice for valvar aortic stenosis at our institution.[17] The results are roughly equivalent to those of surgical valvotomy. Although balloon valvotomy may reduce the gradient in many cases of membranous subaortic stenosis, the role of interventional cardiology in that lesion is as yet uncertain.

PULMONIC STENOSIS

Obstructions to the right ventricular outflow track are usually seen in association with other congenital lesions, such as in tetralogy of Fallot, transposition of the great arteries, or single ventricles. Isolated valvar pulmonary stenosis is nonetheless common, although frequently an asymptomatic lesion. Noninvasive assessment of the diagnosis and its severity is now accurate in nearly all circumstances. Catheterization is reserved for patients who require intervention.

Anatomic Types

Valvar pulmonary stenosis accounts for over 80% of isolated obstructions in the right heart. In typical valvar pulmonary stenosis, the annulus is of normal size, the leaflets thin, and the commissures fused, and there is marked poststenotic dilatation. Dysplastic pulmonary valves are different: the annulus is small, the leaflets are markedly thickened (usually thicker than they are long) and do not move during systole, and the leaflets are not fused.

A spectrum of anatomic variants exists between these extremes, although all but the most dysplastic valves can be successfully dilated.

Right ventricular muscle bundles occur as anomalously thickened bundles of muscle within the right ventricular cavity. The pulmonary valve and annulus are generally normal. Unlike other forms of pulmonary stenosis, muscle bundles frequently progress in severity.

The rarest form of pulmonary stenosis is branch pulmonary stenosis, often associated with both supravalvar aortic stenosis and Williams syndrome.

Physiology

Except for anomalous muscle bundles, pulmonary stenosis rarely increases in severity after the first year of life. Severe forms of stenosis in infancy generally worsen right ventricular compliance, increase right atrial pressure, and hence cause a right-to-left shunt across the probe-patent foramen ovale. Thus, severe stenosis commonly presents with cyanosis and rarely with heart failure. Moderate degrees of pulmonary stenosis (e.g., gradients of 40 to 80 mm Hg) rarely present with symptoms. Several studies, however, have documented the fact that patients with moderate pulmonary stenosis have a decreased exercise performance at cardiac catheterization, even in childhood.[18] On the basis of these studies and the extreme safety of balloon dilation in children with pulmonary stenosis, most cardiologists now recommend dilation in any patient with more than mild pulmonary stenosis on an elective basis before age 5 years.

Catheterization Techniques

The foramen ovale is usually open, allowing catheter access to the left heart from a femoral venous approach. Arterial catheters are usually required only for pressure monitoring during balloon dilation. Of note, the opening in the valve of an infant with severe pulmonary stenosis may be extremely small, e.g., less than 1 to 2 mm (Fig. 36–8). Passage of a standard 5 to 6 Fr catheter across such an valve occludes the orifice, stops pulmonary blood flow, and may produce hemodynamic collapse in less than a minute. For this reason, we frequently do not measure pulmonary artery pressure directly in infants with severe pulmonary valve stenosis. Balloon dilation of such valves requires rapid catheter exchanges and fortitude.

Oximetry Data

Most of these patients have no shunts, either right to left or left to right. In severe pulmonary stenosis, however, a right-to-left shunt occurs at the atrial level, producing cyanosis. In these cases, the pressure gradient underestimates the severity of the stenosis (because less than a full cardiac output is crossing the pulmonary valve) and the pulmonary veins are fully saturated (Fig. 36–9).

Rarely, one encounters a patient with both mild pulmonary stenosis and an atrial septal defect. With a large left-to-right shunt at the atrial level, the gradient across the pulmonary valve will be ''falsely'' elevated. Closing the atrial hole reduces the right ventricular pressure.

Pressure Data

In mild pulmonary valve stenosis, the right atrial pressure is normal. As the degree of stenosis increases, the right atrial a wave increases. With severe pulmonary stenosis, right ventricular pressure approaches or exceeds left ventricular pressure, the main pulmonary pressure falls, and the pulse pressure dampens. Marked hypertrophy of the right ventricular wall may cause the RV infundibulum to close during late systole, causing further obstruction.

Angiography

Right ventriculography in a straight lateral view outlines both the valve and subvalvar region (Fig. 36–8). A straight anteroposterior view with cranial angulation demonstrates both the valve and the branch pulmonary ar-

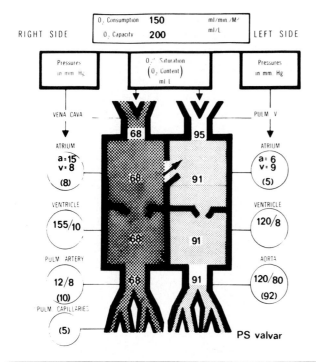

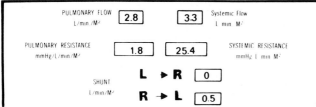

Fig. 36–8. Catheterization findings in a patient with valvar pulmonary stenosis. There is a 143 mm Hg gradient across the valve, and some right-to-left shunting at the atrial level through a patent foramen ovale.

teries; poststenotic dilation of the main pulmonary artery may obscure the origins of the branch pulmonary arteries. Following the contrast until it appears in the left atrium allows one to rule out an associated atrial defect. Further angiography is rarely required.

Interventional Catheterization

As noted in Chapters 29 and 30, balloon dilation, safe and effective at all ages, has become the treatment of choice for this lesion.

COARCTATION OF THE AORTA

Improved noninvasive imaging, including magnetic resonance imaging (MRI), has made precatheterization diagnosis and location of a coarctation virtually certain. Catheterization of

the isolated coarctation is rarely required before surgery. The continued incidence of recurrent coarctation after surgical repair and the common association of coarctation with other forms of congenital heart disease (especially ventricular septal defect, aortic stenosis, subaortic stenosis, and mitral stenosis) make coarctation a common lesion studied at cardiac catheterization.

Anatomic Types

Virtually all forms of coarctation occur at or just distal to the left subclavian artery, at or near the level of the old ductus arteriosus. Coarctations have discrete curtains of tissue indenting the posterior wall of the aorta, although they may be associated with hypoplasia of the transverse aortic arch. Rarely, a coarc-

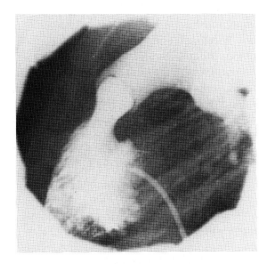

Fig. 36–9. Lateral angiogram in a child with valvar pulmonic stenosis. The valve is thickened and domes during systole, with poststenotic dilation of the main pulmonary artery.

tation may involve a long segment of thoracic or abdominal aorta.

Physiology

The gradient across a coarctation is determined not only by the degree of obstruction, but also by the degree of collateral flow around the obstruction. Most collateral vessels involve the internal mammary arteries or the intercostal arteries (whose enlargement may eventually produce rib notching). Rarely, an obstruction in the transverse aortic arch produces a cerebral steal from the carotids, through the circle of Willis and down the left vertebral artery.

Upper extremity hypertension, the primary sequela of a coarctation, generally resolves after surgical correction. In some children, however, hypertension persists despite adequate anatomic repair. This persistent hypertension is more common when repair occurs late in childhood, prompting the general recommendation to diagnose and correct coarctation before age 3 or 4 years.

Catheterization Technique

Crossing a coarctation is generally straightforward, and not hazardous. Occasionally,

when catheterizing an older patient with coarctation, one may enter an enlarged collateral vessel, thinking it to be the aorta. Complex catheter manipulation in this confined space may prove difficult and even hazardous.

Oximetry Data

Patients with isolated coarctation have no abnormalities in their intracardiac oxygen saturations. Those with associated intracardiac defects (ASD, VSD) have the size of their left-to-right shunt augmented by the coarctation-induced increased afterload.

Pressure Data

Even mild coarctations have a systolic pressure gradient across the coarctation site, although a minimal diastolic gradient is found. As the coarctation severity increases, a gradient is present throughout the cardiac cycle. Finally, the gradient measured by pullback in the catheterization laboratory is frequently smaller than the gradient measured in clinic; while the normal pulse amplification persists in the arms in patients with coarctation, it is frequently absent in the legs, contributing further to the classic examination finding of diminished femoral pulses.

Angiography

A straight lateral aortogram generally provides excellent visualization of the coarctation. If the catheter also opacifies the head and neck vessels, an estimate of collateral flow can be obtained. Such estimates are not precise; if one balloon occludes the coarctation site and measures pressures in the descending aorta, a more precise estimate of collateral adequacy is available.

After surgery has distorted the coarctation site, a lateral aortogram may not define the anatomy well, and various oblique views with cranial or caudal angulation may be needed to define the narrowest site.

Interventional Catheterization

Although balloon dilation frequently reduces the gradient across an unoperated coarctation site, the results are not generally as good as surgical management. Balloon dilation of recurrent coarctation has, however, proven clinically invaluable (Chap. 30).

TETRALOGY OF FALLOT

The most common of cyanotic congenital cardiac conditions, tetralogy of Fallot (the combination of a malalignment VSD, infundibular and valvar pulmonary stenosis, and a resulting overriding aorta and cyanosis) is complex, has a very wide spectrum of abnormalities, and remains a difficult and important surgical challenge. The precise anatomic and physiologic definition provided by cardiac catheterization is invaluable in the management of these patients.

Anatomic Types

All patients with tetralogy of Fallot have, in common, normally related ventricles and great arteries, one or more VSDs, and obstruction to pulmonary blood flow at or below the pulmonary valve. Common additional defects include: (1) branch pulmonary artery stenosis (10% to 20%); (2) pulmonary atresia with PDA-dependent pulmonary blood flow (5 to 10%); (3) additional muscular VSDs (5 to 10%); (4) aortopulmonary collateral arteries supplying blood flow to the lungs (5 to 10%), and coronary arterial anomalies, especially the left anterior descending arising from the right coronary artery (1 to 2%). Each of these variables must be accurately assessed and considered before an attempt at operative repair.

Physiology

The combination of pulmonary obstruction and a VSD produces a right-to-left shunt at the ventricular level. The size of this shunt is unrelated to the size of the VSD (which, in tetralogy of Fallot, is virtually always large and unrestrictive). Rather, the right-to-left shunt and degree of cyanosis are determined primarily by the degree of pulmonary obstruction, and less by the level of systemic vascular resistance. Tetrad spells, or hypercyanotic spells, may be provoked by increased pulmonary obstruction and/or decreased systemic resistance; they are best treated by sedation (which may decrease catecholamine tone and lower the level of muscular pulmonary obstruction), volume, and increasing systemic vascular resistance.

In general, the anatomic obstruction to pulmonary blood flow tends to increase with time, thus increasing the degree of pulmonary obstruction. Thus, aortopulmonary shunts such as the Blalock Taussig shunt (to increase pulmonary blood flow) or complete cardiac correction (relieving the pulmonary stenosis and closing the VSD) are usually required in early childhood.

Catheterization Technique

With a patent foramen ovale as the rule in these patients, one can enter the left heart without difficulty. Similarly, one can generally pass the catheter from the right ventricle both to the aorta and into the pulmonary arteries. Catheter passage into the pulmonary artery, however, often provokes a hypercyanotic spell, and catheter passage from the right ventricle to the aorta often produces transient heart block. Both are to be avoided.

Oximetry Data

Because the VSD in this lesion is just below the aortic valve, there are usually no abnormalities in oxygen saturation at the atrial level or the ventricular level. The right-to-left shunt is documented only in the aorta (Fig. 36–10). Measuring aortic saturation is only moderately important; small changes in the degree of pulmonary arterial obstruction or systemic resistance have major effects on the arterial saturation measured at catheterization. The latter number may have little relationship to the day-

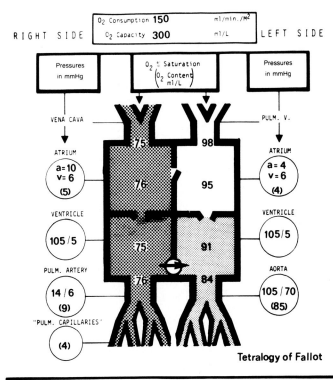

Tetralogy of Fallot

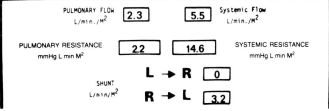

Fig. 36–10. Catheterization findings in a patient with tetralogy of Fallot. There is right-to-left shunting at the atrial and ventricular level, with aortic saturation below left ventricular saturation caused by streaming. Ventricular pressures are equal, and there is a 91 mm Hg peak gradient across the pulmonary outflow track.

to-day arterial saturation (often reflected by the patient's level of blood hemoglobin).

If the cyanosis (and hence the degree of right ventricular obstruction) is severe, a right-to-left shunt may be present at the atrial level, across a patent foramen ovale. These atrial shunts are signs of right ventricular noncompliance, and suggest long-standing right ventricular hypertension.

Pressure Data

Almost by definition, right ventricular pressures equal left ventricular pressures in patients with tetralogy of Fallot. Right and left atrial pressures are usually normal, as are left ventricular and aortic pressures. Pulmonary arterial pressures (when measured) are decreased in cyanotic patients without prior surgery; in the presence of a previous aortopulmonary shunt (e.g., Waterston, Potts), pulmonary arterial pressures may be elevated, even to the level of advanced pulmonary vascular disease.

Angiography

Angiographic definition of anatomic detail is the key to the cardiac catheterization of infants with tetralogy of Fallot. A biplane right ventricular cineangiogram (with cranial angulation of the A-P camera) establishes the diagnosis, defines the anatomy of the pulmonary valve and subpulmonary region, and identifies proximal branch pulmonary arterial obstructions. A left ventriculogram in the so-called long axial oblique view (70-degree LAO with cranial angulation) establishes the presence of multiple VSDs, and may outline the coronary arterial pattern (Fig. 36–11). An aortogram further delineates coronary artery anatomy, and demonstrates the presence or absence of aortopulmonary collateral arteries.

Interventional Catheterization

Interventional procedures are rarely required before surgery in uncomplicated tetralogy of Fallot. In infants with tetralogy of Fallot, pulmonary atresia, and diminutive pulmonary arteries, dilation of hypoplastic pulmonary arteries and coil embolization of aortopulmonary arteries are an essential facet of management. Similarly, interventional procedures are commonly required in patients with postoperative tetralogy of Fallot.

TRANSPOSITION OF THE GREAT ARTERIES

Transposition of great arteries (TGA) remains the most common form of cyanotic congenital heart disease presenting in the first month of life. It was once a uniformly fatal disease, but the outlook for patients with TGA has been dramatically altered by the devel-

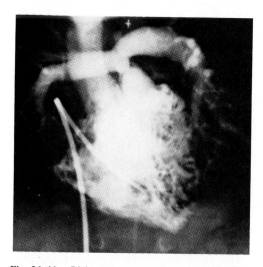

Fig. 36–11. Right ventriculogram in tetralogy of Fallot demonstrates valvar stenosis, small main pulmonary artery, and early filling of the aorta through the ventricular septal defect.

opments of balloon septostomy[19] and PGE1 therapy to raise blood oxygen levels, and by radical surgical correction in infancy to reroute the circulations. Patients with transposition have, in general, the most severe degrees of cyanosis seen in patients with congenital heart disease; the adverse effects of long term cyanosis on the heart, lungs, and brain[20] make early cyanosis relief and repair imperative.

Anatomic Types

Transposition refers to a family of conditions in which the aorta arises from the right ventricle and the pulmonary artery arises from the left ventricle. Most patients have "simple" transposition: an intact ventricular septum and no valvar abnormalities.

A minority of patients have an associated VSD, or pulmonary stenosis, or both. The pulmonary stenosis may be valvar or subvalvar because of a membrane fibromuscular dysplasia. Many other anatomic abnormalities have been associated with the transposition complex, making a complete and precise diagnosis before operative repair important.

Physiology

Unlike the normal circulation (in which blood travels to the lungs and then to the body in a sequential fashion), the circulations in TGA run in parallel: red blood coming back from the lungs returns to the lungs and blue blood coming back to the body returns to the body. Without a defect in the circulation (i.e., ASD, PDA, VSD) to allow red and blue blood to slosh back and forth, the patient would expire in a few minutes. Thus the early goal of therapy is to promote mixing between the circulations by making a hole either in the atrial septum (the Rashkind septostomy) or between the great arteries (the use of prostaglandins to open the ductus arteriosus). These measures may stabilize the patient, but only partially relieve the severe cyanosis associated with TGA. A sequential separation or switching of the circulations, either at the atrial level (the Senning or Mustard procedures) or at the great artery level (the Jatene procedure), is required to restore normal blood oxygenation.

Catheterization Technique

The almost invariable presence of an atrial septal defect in TGA makes the entire heart accessible to a venous catheter. Nonetheless, catheter entry into the pulmonary artery may be difficult; after the catheter enters the left ventricle from the left atrium, it must take a 180-degree turn, over a short distance, to enter the pulmonary artery. The use of a tip deflector wire to bend the catheter at the apex of the left ventricle reliably allows pulmonary arterial cannulation.

Oximetry Data

As noted previously, the well-being of an infant with TGA before repair is determined primarily by the degree of mixing that occurs between the two parallel circuits. Although the mixing can take place at the atrial, ventricular, or great artery level, its net effect is reflected in the levels of aortic and pulmonary arterial saturations. With perfect mixing, the aortic and pulmonary artery saturations are equal (at perhaps 82%). As mixing becomes progressively less adequate, the aortic saturation falls and the pulmonary arterial saturation rises. A difference of more than 10% in these saturations indicates poor mixing (Fig. 36–12) and is generally an indicator to open the atrial septum further with balloon or blade septostomy.

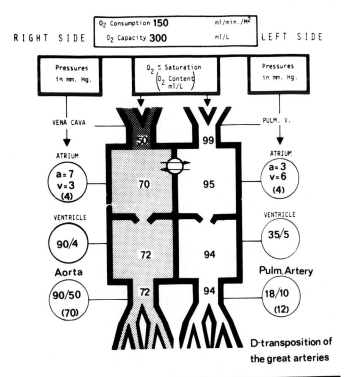

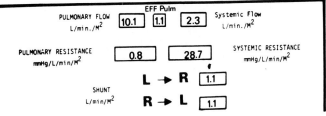

Fig. 36–12. Catheterization findings in an infant with transposition of the great arteries and a small ASD. There is bidirectional shunting at the atrial level, arterial desaturation with poor mixing, and a small systolic pressure gradient across the left ventricular outflow track.

Pressure Data

Because the aorta arises from and is supplied by the right ventricle in TGA, right ventricular pressure is always at or above aortic pressure. In the early neonatal period, persistent patency of the ductus arteriosus causes the pulmonary artery pressure (and hence left ventricular pressure) to be elevated. Over the first few weeks of life, both pulmonary arterial and left ventricular pressures fall, unless there is an associated VSD or pulmonic stenosis. Of note, pulmonary stenosis may be masked if the ductus remains patent, with a pressure gradient developing only when the PDA closes.

In addition, right atrial pressures are elevated, reflecting the elevation in right ventricular pressures. Left atrial pressure varies with the degree of left ventricular pressure elevation, the amount of pulmonary blood flow returning to the left atrium, and the size of the atrial septal defect.

Angiography

Right ventriculography in standard anteroposterior and lateral views establishes the diagnosis, assesses right ventricular function, determines the presence of ventricular septal defects or a patent ductus arteriosus, and assesses tricuspid regurgitation. A left ventriculogram in the long axial oblique view demonstrates the presence and nature of left ventricular outflow tract lesions and demonstrates the location of ventricular septal defects (Fig. 36–13).

With the recent evolution of the neonatal arterial switch operation as the surgical procedure of choice, the precise definition of coronary arterial anatomy in TGA has assumed increased importance. We have recently adopted the laid-back balloon occlusion aortogram[21] as the angiographic procedure to best outline coronary arterial anatomy in TGA (Fig. 36–14). With 45 degrees of caudal angulation, the coronary anatomy is displayed in a transverse section, and in addition, identifies the cusp location of the coronaries as well as their distal courses.

Interventional Catheterization

Even though we now recommend an arterial switch operation electively in the first 10 days of life for most infants with TGA, we continue to perform a balloon atriotomy in the early neonatal period (Chap. 30). Creation of an atrial defect remains the optimum method for

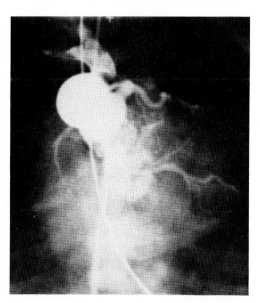

Fig. 36–14. A "laid-back" aortogram produces opacification of the root of the aorta. The circumflex artery arises from the right posterior cusp along with the right coronary artery, and passes posterior to the pulmonary artery before entering the A-V groove. The left anterior descending arises as a separate vessel.

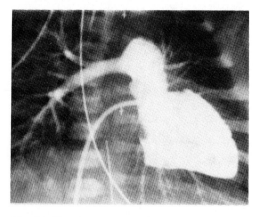

Fig. 36–13. Anteroposterior angiograms in an infant with transposition of the great arteries, demonstrating that the left ventricle supplies a posterior pulmonary artery.

stabilization of these cyanotic infants during several days before a major operative repair.

SINGLE VENTRICLE

The term single ventricle refers to a family of lesions, often complex and with highly variable anatomy, in which there is only one functional ventricular chamber. All of these lesions have the features of a single effective pumping chamber, and may have one or two atrioventricular valves and one or two semilunar valves.

Anatomic Types

The most common form of single ventricle is the highly lethal hypoplastic left heart syndrome (HLHS), usually caused by aortic or mitral atresia. In this syndrome, the left ventricle is diminutive, much too small to sustain life. Although in the past, neonates with HLHS uniformly died when the ductus arteriosus closed, the pioneering efforts of Norwood[22] to create a new aorta surgically and use the right ventricle as a single ventricle has dramatically improved the survival of these children. A less common but similar condition is tricuspid atresia, in which the right heart is hypoplastic, and blood flow to the lungs occurs through a VSD and a small right ventricle, and from there into the lungs. Patients with asplenia and polysplenia (bilateral right-sidedness and left-sidedness respectively) frequently have single ventricles.

Physiology

Previously, all children with single ventricle remained cyanotic and dependent on surgical shunts into their pulmonary arteries to survive. Recently, Fontan demonstrated that atrial pressure alone was enough to maintain a full cardiac output through the lung.[23] This has allowed the separation of the systemic and pulmonary circulations in children with single ventricle, thus eliminating both the volume load on the heart and the deleterious effects of long-standing cyanosis.

Catheterization Technique

The anatomic variability in single ventricles is extremely wide; so are the catheterization techniques for adequate study. Almost all patients with single ventricle have, in common, pulmonary blood flow supplied by an aorto-pulmonary shunt, usually a Blalock-Taussig shunt. Measurement of pulmonary arterial pressure through the shunt is best accomplished by cutting off most of the tip of a pigtail catheter, leaving a 180-degree bend. Placing the catheter into the descending aorta and into the (usually right) subclavian artery and then advancing the soft end of a guide wire out the tip of the pigtail will allow the guide wire to take the acute turn necessary to traverse the Blalock-Taussig shunt. Once the guide wire is securely into the pulmonary artery, the catheter can be advanced over the wire to allow both pressure measurement and angiography.

Oximetry Data

The hallmark of patients with single ventricle is the finding of complete mixing of systemic and pulmonary venous blood at the ventricular level. Because the saturation of pulmonary venous blood is generally near 96%, and because the systemic blood flow is usually normal (producing an arteriovenous oxygen difference of about 17%), the arterial oxygen saturation reflects total pulmonary blood flow: oxygen saturations of 85% or more signify increased pulmonary blood flow, whereas saturations below 75% usually signify decreased pulmonary blood flow. One must, of course, confirm these assumptions at catheterization by direct saturation measurements (Fig. 36–15).

Pressure Measurements

As noted previously, the ultimate palliation for patients with single ventricle is the Fontan procedure, a "repair" that relies on low pulmonary arterial pressures and vascular resistances to allow blood to traverse the lungs without a ventricular pumping chamber. Pulmonary

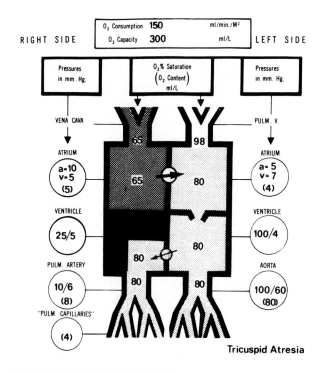

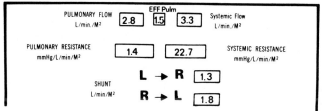

Fig. 36–15. Catheterization findings in a patient with tricuspid atresia, a small ventricular septal defect, and pulmonic stenosis. There is complete mixing of blood in the left atrium with similar saturations in the LA, LV, PA, and aorta. A small interatrial pressure gradient is present.

arterial pressure may be low or elevated because of pulmonary vascular disease from a long-standing large shunt or branch pulmonary arterial stenosis. Again, ventricular pressures are equal to or higher than aortic pressures. Subaortic stenosis is not uncommon in patients with single ventricle, especially those with tricuspid atresia and transposition of the great arteries.

Following repair with a Fontan operation, patients with single ventricle have elevated right atrial pressures, generally between 12 and 18 mm Hg. There should be no gradients between the atrium and the distal pulmonary arteries, and gradients as small as 2 mm Hg may be significant, while gradients of 5 mm Hg or more are high and require reoperation or balloon dilation for correction.

Angiography

Angiographic definition of pulmonary arterial anatomy is vital, and is generally best obtained in straight anteroposterior and lateral views. Ventriculography is used primarily to assess two common late complications of volume-loaded ventricles in patients with cyanosis: global ventricular dysfunction and atrioventricular valve regurgitation.

Finally, additional sources of blood flow to the lungs are badly tolerated in patients about to undergo a Fontan operation. Patients with long-standing cyanosis may develop collateral arteries into the lungs; these arteries must be identified and dealt with before repair using aortography and coil embolization.

Interventional Cardiology

Transcatheter closure of collateral arteries, residual right-to-left shunts, and unnecessary Blalock-Taussig shunts are commonly required in the management of patients with single ventricles, both before and after repair. Balloon dilation of obstructed pulmonary arteries or Fontan anastomoses may also be indicated.

REFERENCES

1. Flanagan MF, Leatherman GF, Carls A, et al: Changing trends of congenital heart disease in adults: A catheterization laboratory perspective. Cathet Cardiovasc Diagn 12:215, 1986.
2. Lock JE, Keane JF, Fellows KE: Diagnostic and Interventional Catheterization in Congenital Heart Disease. Boston, Martinus Nijhoff, 1987.
3. Lewis FJ, Taufic M, Varco RL, Niazi S: The surgical anatomy of atrial septal defects: Experiences with repair under direct vision. Ann Surg 142:401, 1955.
4. Nadas AS, Fyler DC: Pediatric Cardiology. Philadelphia, WB Saunders, 1972.
5. Freed MD, Miettinen OS, Nadas AS: Oximetric detection of intracardiac left-to-right shunts. Br Heart J 42:690, 1979.
6. Levin AR, Spach MS, Boineau JP, et al: Atrial pressure-flow dynamics in atrial septal defects (secundum type). Circulation 37:476, 1968.
7. Elliot LP, Bargeron LM Jr, Bream PR, et al: Axial cineangiography in congenital heart disease. Section II: Specific lesions. Circulation 56:1084, 1977.
8. Lock JE, Rome JJ, Davis R, et al: Transcatheter closure of atrial septal defects: Experimental studies. Circulation 79:1091, 1989.
9. Rome JJ, Keane JF, Perry SB, et al: Double umbrella closure of atrial defects: Initial clinical applications. Circulation, in press, 1990.
10. Bargeron LM Jr, Elliot LP, Soto B, et al: Axial cineangiography in congenital heart disease. Section I: Technical and anatomic considerations. Circulation 56:1075, 1977.
11. Lock JE, Block PC, McKay RG, et al: Transcatheter closure of ventricular septal defects. Circulation 78:361, 1988.
12. Rashkind WJ, Cuaso CC: Transcatheter closure of patent ductus arteriosus. Pediatr Cardiol 1:3, 1979.
13. Wessel DL, Keane JF, Parness I, Lock JE: Outpatient closure of the patent ductus arteriosus. Circulation 77:1068, 1988.
14. Porstmann W, Wierny L, Warnke H, et al: Catheter closure of patent ductus arteriosus, 62 cases treated without thoracotomy. Radiol Clin North Am 9:203, 1971.
15. Rashkind WJ: Transcatheter treatment of congenital heart disease. Circulation 67:711, 1983.
16. Wagner HR, Ellison RC, Keane JF, et al: Clinical course in aortic stenosis. Circulation 56:1-47, 1977.
17. Sholler G, Keane JF, Perry SB, et al: Balloon dilation of congenital aortic stenosis: Results and influence of technical and morphologic features on outcome. Circulation 78:351, 1988.
18. Stone FM, Bessinger FB, Lucas RV, Moller JH: Pre- and postoperative rest and exercise hemodynamics in children with pulmonary stenosis. Circulation 49:1102, 1974.
19. Rashkind WJ, Miller WW: Creation of atrial septal defect without thoracotomy. JAMA 196:991, 1966.
20. Newburger JW, Silbert AR, Buckley LP, Fyler DC: Cognitive function and age at repair of transposition of the great arteries in children. N Engl J Med 310:1495, 1984.
21. Mandell VS, Lock JE, Mayer JE, et al: The "laid-back" aortogram: A new angiographic view for demonstration of coronary arteries in transposition of the great arteries. J Am Coll Cardiol, in press, 1990.
22. Norwood WI, Lang P, Hansen D: Physiologic repair of aortic atresia-hypoplastic left heart syndrome. N Engl J Med 308:23, 1983.
23. Fontan F, Baudet E: Surgical repair of tricuspid atresia. Thorax 26:240, 1971.

Index

Page numbers in *italics* indicate figures; those followed by t indicate tables, by n indicate notes.